Stress, Neuropeptides, and Systemic Disease

Stress, Neuropeptides, and Systemic Disease

Edited by

James A. McCubbin

Department of Behavioral Science
College of Medicine
University of Kentucky
Lexington, Kentucky

Peter G. Kaufmann

Behavioral Medicine Branch
National Institutes of Health
Bethesda, Maryland

Charles B. Nemeroff

Departments of Psychiatry and Pharmacology
Duke University
Durham, North Carolina

Academic Press, Inc.
Harcourt Brace Jovanovich, Publishers
San Diego   New York   Boston   London   Sydney   Tokyo   Toronto

Cover photograph: Triple exposure of a section through the paraventricular nucleus of the hypothalamus in the rat showing the distribution of cells that (1) project to the spinal cord (blue, labeled with the retrogradely transported fluorescent dye, true blue, after injections in the spinal cord), (2) stain immunohistochemically for vasopressin (green, fluorescein fluorescence), or (3) CRF (red, rhodamine fluorescence). Courtesy of Paul E. Sawchenko.

Copyright © 1991 by Academic Press, Inc.
All Rights Reserved.
No part of this publication may be reproduced or transmitted in any form or by any means, electronic or mechanical, including photocopy, recording, or any information storage and retrieval system, without permission in writing from the publisher.

Academic Press, Inc.
San Diego, California 92101

United Kingdom Edition published by
Academic Press Limited
24–28 Oval Road, London NW1 7DX

Library of Congress Cataloging-in-Publication Data

Stress, neuropeptides, and systemic disease / edited by James A.
    McCubbin, Peter G. Kaufmann, Charles B. Nemeroff.
        p.   cm.
    Includes index.
    ISBN   0-12-482490-0   (alk. paper)
    1. Neuropeptides--Physiological effect. 2. Stress (Physiology).
3. Psychoneuroendocrinology.   I. McCubbin, James A. II. Kaufmann,
Peter G. III. Nemeroff, Charles B.
    [DNLM: 1. Neuropeptides--physiology. 2. Stress, Psychological-
-physiopathology.   WL 104 S914]
QP552.N39S74   1991
616.07'1--dc20
DNLM/DLC
for Library of Congress   90-990
                                                            CIP

Printed in the United States of America
91   92   93   94   9 8 7 6 5 4 3 2 1

Contents

v

II
Endocrine Regulation

III
Immune Function

IV
Gastrointestinal Function

V

Cardiovascular Regulation

Contributors

Numbers in parentheses indicate the pages on which the authors' contributions begin.

Shamgar Ben-Eliyahu (261), Department of Psychology, University of California, Los Angeles, California 90024

Donna Benton (221), Geriatric Research, Education and Clinical Center, Sepulveda Veterans Administration Medical Center, Sepulveda, California 91303

Charles J. Billington (327), Neuroendocrine Research Laboratory, Veterans Administration Medical Center, Minneapolis, Minnesota 55417, and Department of Medicine, University of Minnesota, Minneapolis, Minnesota 55455

Garth Bissette (55), Department of Psychiatry, Duke University Medical School, Durham, North Carolina 27710

Marvin R. Brown (73), Autonomic Physiology Laboratory, Department of Medicine, University of California, San Diego, San Diego, California 92103

Thomas F. Burks (303), Department of Pharmacology, College of Medicine, University of Arizona, Tucson, Arizona 85724

Michael F. Callahan (343), Department of Medicine, Wake Forest University Medical Center, Winston-Salem, North Carolina 27103

Daniel B. Carr (409), Departments of Anesthesia and Medicine, Harvard Medical School, Massachusetts General Hospital, Boston, Massachusetts 02114

G. P. Chrousos (287), Developmental Endocrinology Branch, NICHD, Bethesda, Maryland 20892

Belinda J. Cole (119), Department of Neuropsychopharmacology, Schering AG, West Berlin, Federal Republic of Germany

Thomas P. Davis (149), Laboratory of Analytical Chemistry and Mass Spectrometry, Department of Pharmacology, College of Medicine, University of Arizona, Tucson, Arizona 85724

Errol B. De Souza (233), Laboratory of Neurobiology, Neuroscience Branch, National Institute on Drug Abuse, Addiction Research Center, Baltimore, Maryland 21224

P. Murali Doraiswamy (19), Department of Psychiatry, Duke University Medical Center, Department of Psychiatry, Durham, North Carolina 27710

Dwight L. Evans (199), Department of Psychiatry and Medicine, University of North Carolina School of Medicine, Chapel Hill, North Carolina 27599-7160

Laurel A. Fisher (95), Department of Pharmacology, College of Medicine, University of Arizona, Tucson, Arizona 85724

Robert P. Frantz (429), Cardiology Unit, University of Rochester Medical Center, Rochester, New York 14642

Robert P. Gale (261), Department of Medicine, Division of Hematology and Oncology, University of California, Los Angeles, California 90024

P. W. Gold (287), Clinical Neuroendocrinology Branch, National Institute of Mental Health, Bethesda, Maryland 20892

Robert N. Golden (199), Department of Psychiatry, University of North Carolina School of Medicine, Chapel Hill, North Carolina 27599-7160

Thackery S. Gray (37), Department of Anatomy, Loyola University Stritch School of Medicine, Maywood, Illinois 60153

Dimitri E. Grigoriadis (233), Laboratory of Neurobiology, Neuroscience Branch, National Institute on Drug Abuse, Addiction Research Center, Baltimore, Maryland 21224

Kenneth A. Gruber (343), Department of Medicine, Wake Forest University Medical Center, Winston–Salem, North Carolina 27103

George F. Koob (119), Department of Neuropharmacology, Research Institute of Scripps Clinic, La Jolla, California 92037

K. Ranga Rama Krishnan (19), Department of Psychiatry, Duke University Medical Center, Department of Psychiatry, Durham, North Carolina 27710

Allen S. Levine (327), Neuroendocrine Research Laboratory, Veterans Administration Medical Center, Minneapolis, Maryland 55417, and Departments of Food Science and Nutrition, Medicine, Psychiatry, and Surgery, University of Minnesota, Minneapolis/St. Paul, Minnesota 55455

Chang-seng Liang (429), Cardiology Unit, University of Rochester Medical Center, Rochester, New York 14642

John C. Liebeskind (261), Department of Psychology, University of California, Los Angeles, California 90024

Richard McCarty (365), Department of Psychology, University of Virginia, Charlottesville, Virginia 22903

James A. McCubbin (445), Department of Behavioral Science, College of Medicine, University of Kentucky, Lexington, Kentucky 40536-0086

Helen L. Miller (199), Department of Psychiatry, University of North Carolina School of Medicine, Chapel Hill, North Carolina 27599-7160

John E. Morley (221), Geriatric Research, Education and Clinical Center, St. Louis Veterans Administration Medical Center, and Division of Geriatric Medicine, St. Louis University School of Medicine, St. Louis, Missouri 63104

Charles B. Nemeroff (181), Departments of Psychiatry and Pharmacology, Duke University Medical Center, Durham, North Carolina 27710

Diana O. Perkins (199), Department of Psychiatry, University of North Carolina School of Medicine, Chapel Hill, North Carolina 27599-7160

Deborah Reed (19), Department of Psychiatry, Duke University Medical Center, Department of Psychiatry, Durham, North Carolina 27710

James C. Ritchie (19, 181), Department of Psychiatry, Duke University Medical Center, Department of Psychiatry, Durham, North Carolina 27710

Paul E. Sawchenko (3), Laboratory of Neuronal Structure and Function, The Salk Institute for Biological Studies, and The Clayton Foundation for Research-California Division, La Jolla, California 92037

Yehuda Shavit (261), Department of Psychology, The Hebrew University of Jerusalem, Mount Scopus, Jerusalem 91905, Israel

George F. Solomon (221), Geriatric Research, Education and Clinical Center, Sepulveda Veterans Administration Medical Center, Sepulveda, California 91303, and Department of Psychiatry, University of California, Los Angeles, California

Robert A. Stern (199), Department of Psychiatry, University of North Carolina School of Medicine, Chapel Hill, North Carolina 27599-7160

E. M. Sternberg (287), Clinical Neurosciences Branch, National Institute of Mental Health, and Arthritis and Rheumatism Branch, NIAMS, Bethesda, Maryland 20892

Robert E. Stewart (365), Department of Psychology, and Graduate Program in Neuroscience, University of Virginia, Charlottesville, Virginia 22903

Anna N. Taylor (261), Department of Anatomy and Cell Biology, University of California, Los Angeles, California 90024, and West Los Angeles Veterans Administration Center, Brentwood Division, Los Angeles, California

Sanjeev Venkataraman (19), Department of Psychiatry, Duke University Medical Center, Durham, North Carolina 27710

Richard L. Verrier (409), Department of Pharmacology, Georgetown University Medical Center, Washington, D. C. 20007

Elizabeth L. Webster (233), Laboratory of Neurobiology, Neuroscience Branch, National Institute on Drug Abuse, Addiction Research Center, Baltimore, Maryland 21224

Herbert Weiner (261), Department of Psychiatry and Biobehavioral Sciences, University of California, Los Angeles, California 90024

R. L. Wilder (287), Arthritis and Rheumatism Branch, NIAMS, Bethesda, Maryland 20892

Raz Yirmiya (261), Department of Psychology, The Hebrew University of Jerusalem, Mount Scopus, Jerusalem 91905, Israel

Preface

Evolution has provided powerful excitatory and inhibitory mechanisms for rapid physiological adjustment to exceptionally potent environmental stressors. These adaptations have necessitated a higher level of neurochemical processing to more precisely integrate autonomic neuronal outflow and to maintain systemic functioning within normal limits. This modulatory biochemical complex is fueled largely by neuropeptides, a group of newly characterized substances found throughout the central and autonomic nervous systems as well as in various other secretory tissues. Their relatively recent discovery has produced a massive search for the functional significance of these potentially important chemical messengers.

Endogenous peptides act in several distinct ways. These include (1) endocrine properties of systemic release and distant site of action, (2) neurotransmitter functions of classical and corelease exocytosis, and (3) presynaptic autoreceptor neuromodulatory capabilities. The advantages of a peptide-based modulatory system are important from both biosynthetic and receptor-binding aspects. Derivation of several active amino acid sequences from a single parent molecule allows low-cost biosynthetic efficiency. Futhermore, the intricate selectivity of peptidergic receptor subtypes provides a novel mechanism for receptor-based neural integration, operating at a level beyond synaptic connectivity. A disadvantage of this type of system is that a seemingly innocuous peptide abnormality could result in insidious pathophysiological changes, autonomic dysregulation, and subsequent vulnerability to both the acute and chronic harmful effects of stress.

The stressful challenge is a technique that allows dynamic visualization of structural weaknesses. These structural vulnerabilities may eventuate in functional dysregulation and the breakdown of homeostatic processes. Stress appears to extract its toll from a chosen few, and subtle variation in the efficacy of peptide function may determine who copes successfully and who eventually succumbs. Several disease models can be characterized by an inability to maintain homeostasis during stress. These disorders have been viewed as diseases of adaptation, and they encompass various chronic conditions associated with functional dysregulation of the hypothalamic–pituitary–adrenocortical and the sympathetic–adrenomedullary axes. Among these are diverse systemic disorders such as hypertension, heart disease, and immunosuppression. These diseases of adaptation may ultimately encompass other stress-related syndromes including certain affective and anxiety disorders as well as self-regulatory and relapse behaviors involving appetite control, substance abuse, and addiction. Although the relationship between stress and disease has been widely appreciated, the precise psychophysiological mechanisms have never been adequately elucidated. Neuropeptides are now viewed as an integral link between the challenges of our environment and the resilience of our physiological coping.

This book traces the development of this neuropeptide hypothesis from its anatomical substrate to its functional correlates in animal and preclinical human models of stress-induced disease. Histochemical localization of peptide-containing cells and peptidergic receptors provides the anatomical substrate for postulated interactions with central and peripheral autonomic control nuclei. Pharmacological analyses of the functional properties of neuroactive peptides elucidate the potential physiological importance of these substances. Behavioral techniques provide precise characterization of the effects of different types of stress on peptide and target organ function. Specialists in circulatory, endocrine, gastrointestinal, and immunological disorders present evidence of peptidergic influences on normal and abnormal physiology of these various organ systems. Animal models provide preliminary clues about the importance of peptidergic mechanisms in the expression of circulatory, endocrine, gastrointestinal, and immunologic dysregulation in organisms coping with stress. Preclinical studies of humans at risk suggest that subtle individual differences in the efficacy of peptide systems determine stress reactivity and ultimate expression of disease symptoms.

These various research programs have vastly improved our understanding of the role of neuropeptides in brain function. This has led to the realization that minute variations in neuropeptidergic function influence our psychophysiologic efficacy and, in turn, our subsequent vulnerability to the pathogenicity of stress. The results of this conceptual revolution in peptide neurobiology will change the way scientists and physicians view chronic degenerative diseases. A better understanding of basic integrative neuropeptide mechanisms will stimulate development of improved diagnostic procedures and intervention strategies and will undoubtedly provide new tools for the design of novel pharmaceuticals.

The editors gratefully acknowledge the technical assistance of Elizabeth Harlan and Stephen Bruehl in preparation of this book.

James A. McCubbin
Peter G. Kaufmann
Charles B. Nemeroff

I
Basic
Mechanisms

1

A Tale of Three Peptides: Corticotropin-Releasing Factor-, Oxytocin-, and Vasopressin-Containing Pathways Mediating Integrated Hypothalamic Responses to Stress

P. E. Sawchenko

Laboratory of Neuronal Structure and Function
The Salk Institute for Biological Studies, and
The Clayton Foundation for Research—California Division
La Jolla, California 92037

I. Introduction

Virtually any significant challenge, real or perceived, to an organism's well-being results in a neurally mediated release of catecholamines from the adrenal medulla and initiates the neuroendocrine cascade of events that results in the secretion of glucocorticoids from the adrenal cortex. These non-specific events serve to mobilize a well-characterized array of emergency, or stress, responses that involve a number of organ systems and metabolic processes. In addition, though, any given challenge invokes adaptive neuroendocrine and/or autonomic and/or behavioral mechanisms aimed specifically at counteracting the particular imbalance at hand. Thus, the organismic response to stress typically involves common sympatho– and pituitary–adrenal components, but the constellation of ancillary autonomic, endocrine, and behavioral adjustments that is invoked to allow the organism to cope with a particular stressor is unique.

A focus for any consideration of the neural substrates that provide for the integration of stress and other adaptive responses is the hypothalamus. This region harbors magnocellular and parvocellular neurosecretory neurons through which the brain controls secretions of the posterior and anterior lobes of the pituitary, respectively, and cells that influence directly autonomic preganglionic neurons in the brain stem and spinal cord. Three neuropeptides, oxytocin (OT), arginine vasopressin (AVP), and corticotropin-releasing factor (CRF), appear to play privileged roles in integrated hypothalamic function in that they are contained and participate in all three avenues (i.e., via the anterior pituitary, posterior pituitary, and autonomic nervous system) through which the hypothalamus may act to initiate adaptive responses to stress. While each peptide is commonly perceived as being associated with a single cell type and set of functions, it is now clear that their loci of expression and functional associations are more expansive. Recent studies of the localization and regulation of the expression of these peptides have already indicated that the hypothalamic neurons are capable of hitherto unexpected forms of plasticity and regulatory gymnastics.

The present chapter will attempt to highlight recent studies bearing on the organization and control of OT, AVP, and CRF expression and release in hypothalamic neurons, emphasizing the roles of these neuropeptides in both the specific and nonspecific aspects of the response to stress.

II. Effector Neuron Organization

A. Cellular

Retrograde transport studies, buttressed by histochemical staining for OT and AVP peptides and messenger RNAs, have defined clearly the distribution of magnocellular neurosecretory cells that project to the posterior pituitary (e.g., Swanson and Kuypers, 1980; Rhodes et al., 1981; Tanaguchi et al., 1988). These are concentrated in cytoarchitectonically distinct regions of the paraventricular (PVH) and supraoptic (SO) nuclei of the hypothalamus. Their massive input to the posterior lobe is the only established projection of these neurons, though evidence suggesting that at least some of their axons collateralize and interact with as yet ill-defined cells within the hypothalamus has been provided (e.g., Mason et al., 1984).

Unlike the SO, which may be considered to be composed entirely of magnocellular neurosecretory neurons, the PVH contains a prominent and well-differentiated parvocellular division. This includes parvocellular neurosecretory neurons that project to the portal capillary (external) zone of the median eminence for the control of anterior pituitary secretions (Wiegand and Price, 1980), and cells that give rise to long descending projections, which terminate in autonomic-related cell groups in the brainstem and spinal cord (Saper *et al.*, 1979). Among the former is counted a prominent cluster of cells now acknowledged as the principal source for the delivery of CRF to the portal plexus (Swanson *et al.*, 1983; Antoni, 1986). These, along with cells producing other hypophysiotropic principles, such as somatostatin, thyrotropin-releasing hormone, and dopamine, each occupy distinctive aspects of those parts of the parvocellular division in which cells that project to the median eminence are found (see Figure 1).

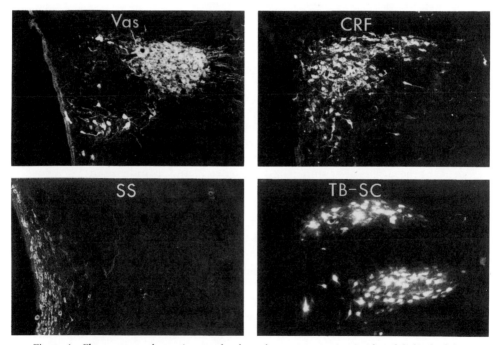

Figure 1 Fluorescence photomicrographs through a representative (midcaudal) level of the PVH to show the mosaic arrangement of anatomically and chemically defined cell types. Vasopressin-immunoreactive (Vas) magnocellular neurosecretory neurons are massed in a laterally situated cluster. Parvocellular neurosecretory neurons, illustrated here by cells stained for corticotropin-releasing factor (CRF) and somatostatin (SS), occupy more medial aspects of the nucleus. Encapsulating the neurosecretory neurons are cells that give rise to long descending projections, represented here by cells retrogradely labeled following injection of the fluorescent tracer true blue in the spinal cord (TB-SC). The three major classes of visceromotor neurons in the PVH are largely separate and topographically organized. The third ventricle is at the left of each micrograph. Reprinted with permission from Cunningham and Sawchenko (1988).

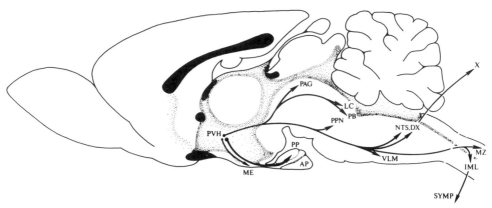

Figure 2 Schematic sagittal view of the rat brain to summarize the major neuroendocrine and descending projections of the PVH in the rat. Abbreviations: AP, anterior pituitary; DX, dorsal motor nucleus of the vagus nerve; IML, (sympathetic) intermediolateral cell column; LC, locus ceruleus; ME, median eminence; MZ, marginal zone; NTS, nucleus of the solitary tract; PAG, periaqueductal gray; PB, parabrachial nucleus; PP, posterior pituitary; PPN, pedunculopontine nucleus; SYMP, sympathetic nervous system; X, vagus nerve. Reprinted with permission from Swanson *et al.* (1986).

Autonomic-related projection neurons in the PVH are clustered in such a manner as to essentially encapsulate neuroendocrine neurons throughout the caudal half of the nucleus. Some of the major projection fields of these cells are summarized in Figure 2, and include inputs to vagal and sympathetic preganglionic neurons, as well as to the principal sensory nucleus of the vagus and several of the "relays" by which visceral sensory information reaches the PVH.

In summary, three major classes of visceromotor neurons are localized in the PVH. These are organized in an intricate mosaic, and occupy topographically distinct regions of the nucleus. Evidence supporting the independence of these output neuron classes has been provided by double-retrograde tracing studies, which have shown that the cells that give rise to autonomic projections are separate from those that project to either the median eminence or the posterior lobe (Swanson and Kuypers, 1980; Swanson *et al.*, 1980).

B. Biochemical

The chemical coding of function is imprecisely superimposed on these distinct groupings of output neurons in the PVH and SO. Certainly OT and AVP are the major secretory products of separate pools of magnocellular neurosecretory neurons. The same is probably true of CRF in its subset of parvocellular neurosecretory neurons, and CRF is almost surely the most abundant secretagogue for corticotropin expressed in these cells. Nonetheless, expression of multiple neuroactive substances within individual neurons is now acknowledged as a widespread phenomenon, and nowhere is this more apparent than in the magnocellular and parvocellular neurosecretory cells under consideration here. Of particular interest here is the fact that CRF has been colocalized within a subset of magnocellular OT neurons (Sawchenko *et al.*, 1984b), and that, under some conditions at least (see below), AVP may be expressed in a majority of parvocellular neurosecretory CRF cells (Kiss *et al.*, 1984; Sawchenko *et al.*, 1984a; Wolfson *et al.*, 1985). Autonomic projection neurons in the PVH do not appear to contain a characterizing "signature" neuroactive agent; instead, small subsets of this population share chemical phenotypes with adjoining neurosecretory cell groups. The predominant markers that have been identified in these neurons thus far are CRF and OT; a smaller contingent of AVP-immunoreactive cells with long descending projections has also been identified (Sawchenko, 1987a; Sawchenko and Swanson, 1982). Thus, the chemical coding of the principal visceromotor projections of the PVH and SO is not fully in register with their anatomical specificity.

C. Regulation and Plasticity

To glean a sense of the significance of the capacity of distinct groups of projection neurons to produce multiple, and partly overlapping, complements of neuroactive peptides, interactions among CRF, OT, and AVP in stimulating corticotropin secretion at the level of the anterior pituitary may be considered. It is now generally acknowledged that CRF neurons in the PVH serve generally to set the stimulatory tone on corticotropes. OT and AVP are also present in hypophyseal portal plasma, and are recognized as secretagogues for corticotropin, with AVP, at least, interacting synergistically with CRF in this context (Plotsky, 1985). Insight into the anatomical arrangement that might allow delivery of the nonapeptides into the portal vasculature was provided when it was shown that diminished corticosteroid feedback, in addition to up-regulating CRF peptide and mRNA levels in parvocellular neurosecretory neurons, also resulted in an apparent induction of AVP expression in a majority of these very cells (Kiss *et al.*, 1984; Sawchenko *et al.*, 1984a) (see Figure 3). This provided a basis for explaining, at least in part, the means by which the CRF–AVP synergy in stimulating corticotropin secretion might be achieved.

Steroid regulation of CRF and AVP expression in parvocellular neurosecretory neurons appears to be mediated by glucocorticoids, and to be quite specific to these peptides, and to this cell type (Sawchenko, 1987b). Other peptides colocalized in CRF neurons but that do not possess corticotropin-releasing activity are ostensibly unaffected by steroid withdrawal.

8 P. E. Sawchenko

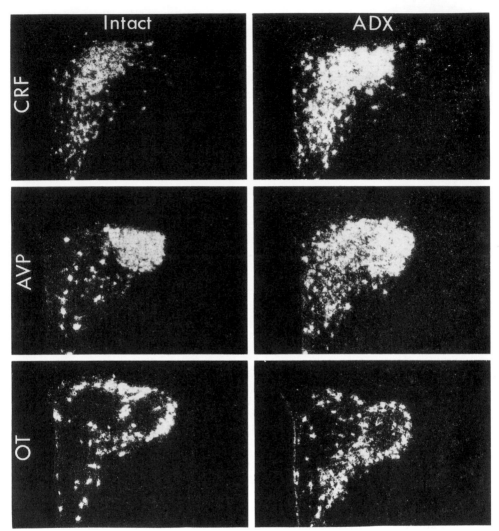

Figure 3 Dark-field micrographs of *in situ* hybridization histochemical material to show the cellular localization of mRNAs encoding CRF, AVP, and OT in the PVH of intact and adrenal-ectomized (ADX) rats. In the intact animal, cells in the more laterally situated magnocellular division that express AVP and OT mRNAs are topographically arranged, and segregated from expressing cells in the parvocellular division. ADX results in an up-regulation of CRF mRNA, and an apparent induction of AVP mRNA, in the parvocellular division of the nucleus, while the distribution and strength of the signals for OT and AVP in the magnocellular division are unchanged.

Neither does adrenalectomy exert pronounced effects on CRF and AVP expression in magnocellular neurosecretory or autonomic-related projections neurons in the PVH (Sawchenko *et al.*, 1984a; Sawchenko, 1987b; Swanson and Simmons, 1989; Young *et al.*, 1986). Here, as in other aspects of the regulation of these peptides that have been studied to date, regulatory influences appear to be exerted differentially, and on the basis of connectivity and functional associations of cell groups, rather than uniformly on all of those that may share any particular biochemical phenotype.

Though steroid modulation of corticotropin secretagogue expression in parvocellular neurosecretory neurons represents one likely means by which the stress response may be modulated, this alone seems clearly insufficient to explain the interactions among CRF, OT, and AVP in this regard. It is unlikely that the contributions from parvocellular neurons can account for the high levels of AVP found in portal plasma (Plotsky and Sawchenko, 1987). Moreover, under no conditions described to date has OT been localized in more than a handful of cells in regions of the PVH that project prominently to the median eminence. Magnocellular neurons are currently the only viable candidate sources for such an influence (Figure 4), and evi-

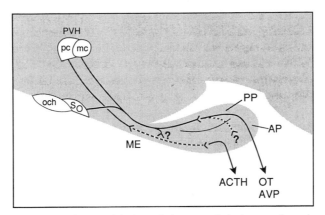

Figure 4 Schematic sagittal view of the hypothalamus and pituitary to show the organization of magnocellular (mc) and parvocellular (pc) neurosecretory components of the PVH, and potential sites at which secretions of magnocellular neurons may interact with the parvocellular system. CRF contained in axonal projections from the parvocellular division of the PVH to the external zone of the median eminence (ME) is transported to the anterior pituitary (AP) via the portal vasculature (dashed line). Projections of magnocellular neurosecretory neurons in the PVH and the supraoptic nucleus (SO) pass through the internal lamina of the median eminence en route to the posterior lobe (PP), where oxytocin (OT) and vasopressin (AVP) are released into the systemic circulation. Magnocellular secretions may gain access to the portal vasculature via exocytotic release at the level of the median eminence, or via vascular links (dashed line) between the posterior and anterior lobes (question marks). The optic chiasm (och) is shown for reference.

dence supporting the notion that axons of magnocellular neurons coursing through the internal lamina of the median eminence can release OT and AVP in proximity to the portal vasculature has been provided. Calcium-dependent, potassium-stimulated release of AVP from isolated median eminence has been demonstrated *in vitro* (Holmes *et al.*, 1986), and exocytotic release of neurosecretory granules has been imaged ultrastructurally from magnocellular axons coursing through the internal lamina (Buma and Nieuwenhuys, 1987). Another avenue permitting nonapeptide–corticotrope interaction, by way of vascular links permitting blood flow from the neural to the anterior lobes, has been suggested (Page, 1986). Magnocellular neurons thus appear capable of releasing secretory products at loci with access to the portal plexus and/or to corticotropes directly (Figure 4). The conditions under which they might do so, and how such release might be integrated with the mechanisms that regulate nonapeptide biosynthesis in the magnocellular nuclei, and secretion from the neurohypophysis, are important and daunting questions that are yet to be explored systematically.

III. Afferent Control

A. Organization of Interoceptive Inputs

Of prime importance in any consideration of substrates that might provide for differential control of functionally and/or chemically defined cell populations in the PVH and SO are the organization and target specificity of neural inputs to the nucleus. The hypothalamic visceral effector neurons under consideration here are under strong visceral sensory control, and pathways carrying this modality will be highlighted here to illustrate organizational principles. Much of what is known of the manner in which pertinent interoceptive information is processed revolves about connections of the nucleus of the solitary tract (NTS), the principal recipient of first-order vagal and glossopharyngeal afferents.

There now exists evidence for a highly differentiated set of pathways linking the NTS to neuroendocrine effector neurons in the PVH and SO (Figure 5). For example, three distinct territories of the NTS, which contain neurons bearing adrenergic, noradrenergic, and multiple peptidergic phenotypes, project to the hypophysiotropic CRF region of the PVH, as do at least two major projection fields of the NTS, the C1 adrenergic cell group and the lateral parabrachial nucleus (Cunningham and Sawchenko, 1988; Cunningham *et al.*, 1990; Saper and Loewy, 1980; Sawchenko *et al.*, 1988a,b). Magnocellular OT neurons also receive a prominent direct NTS projection, but only from peptidergic neurons localized in the caudalmost aspects of the nucleus (Sawchenko *et al.*, 1988a,b) (Figure 6). By contrast,

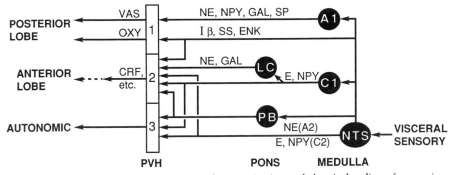

Figure 5 Schematic diagram to represent the organization and chemical coding of some visceral sensory inputs to the PVH. Three major classes of PVH output neurons are numbered, and their principal targets and chemical makeup indicated. The distribution and coding of some major direct and second-order pathways from the NTS to the PVH are also shown. Note the target specificity of each anatomically defined projection, upon which are superimposed complex, and partly overlapping, biochemical specificities. Abbreviations: PB, parabrachial nucleus; LC, locus ceruleus; NE, norepinephrine; E, epinephrine; NPY, neuropeptide Y; GAL, galanin; Iβ, inhibin β; ENK, enkephalin; SP, substance P; SS, somatostatin; VAS, vasopressin; OXY, oxytocin.

magnocellular AVP neurons do not receive a major direct input from the NTS, but are prominently innervated by another target of NTS projections, the A1 noradrenergic cell group of the caudal ventrolateral medulla (Cunningham and Sawchenko, 1988).

Insofar as neurosecretory neurons are concerned, then, ascending visceral sensory inputs appear to be organized on something approaching a point-to-point basis. Autonomic-related projection neurons are not yet known to be discretely targeted by any of these ascending projections but appear to receive minor inputs from several of them. What is clearly needed is an understanding of how specific kinds of interoceptive information are gated through these parallel, yet differentiated, projection systems. What kind(s) of primary afferents end on different groups of NTS projection neurons? How might an extensive set of intra-NTS projections serve to gate afferent traffic through one or more of these output paths to the hypothalamus?

B. Chemical Coding

Chemically defined afferents to the PVH are almost invariably distributed across output neuron classes. Viewed in the light of the more discrete anatomical organization summarized above, such distributions would appear to define potential substrates for invoking in tandem (i.e., integrating) vari-

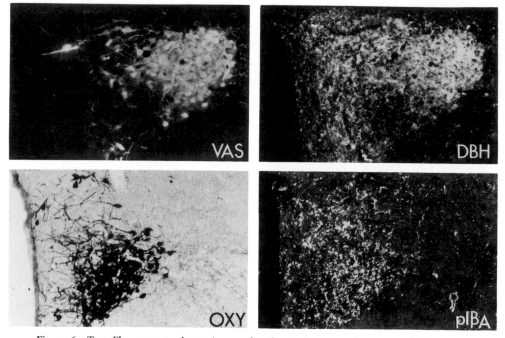

Figure 6 *Top:* Fluorescence photomicrographs of a single section through the PVH stained for both vasopressin (VAS) and dopamine-β-hydroxylase (DBH, a marker for adrenergic and noradrenergic neurons). The DBH-stained terminal field is prominent in the region of vasopressinergic neurons, though the parvocellular division receives an input as well. *Bottom:* Immunoperoxidase preparations of adjacent sections through a slightly more rostral level of the PVH to show the correspondence between an inhibin β (pIβ$_A$) immunoreactive terminal field and oxytocinergic magnocellular neurons. Magnocellular OT and AVP neurons appear differentially innervated by these two chemically specified afferents.

ous combinations of parvocellular neurosecretory, magnocellular neurosecretory and autonomic-related outputs of the nucleus. For example, noradrenergic inputs to the PVH are broadly distributed and touch all major output neuron classes in the PVH (Figure 6). The distribution of projections from each of the three cell groups that contribute to the noradrenergic input are quite distinctive, and appear to innervate preferentially discrete groupings of neurosecretory neurons (Cunningham and Sawchenko, 1988).

Like their hypothalamic targets, each of the principal interoceptive afferents to the PVH neuron expresses multiple neurochemical markers (Figure 5). The patterns of coexpression are varied, ranging from near complete overlap to coexistence within small subsets, and appear generally not to be fully in register with the anatomical organization. For example, neuropeptide Y is contained within the vast majority of brainstem adrenergic neurons that project primarily to the parvocellular division of the PVH, in a subset of A1 noradrenergic neurons that project to the magnocellular division (Sawchenko *et al.*, 1985), and in nonaminergic neurons in the arcuate nucleus of the hypothalamus whose projections to the PVH have not been rigorously defined (Bai *et al.*, 1985). The imprecise superimposition of biochemical phenotypes on a decidedly more discrete anatomical organization would seem to broaden the potential for close regulation of afferent control of the system, though a host of questions remain as to the manner in which coexisting agents in any given neuron may be differentially regulated, and whether any agent expressed in multiple pathways that impinge on the PVH and SO may be subject to common regulatory influences in each.

IV. Integration

Clearly, physiologic conditions exist that may invoke release of OT (e.g., suckling) or AVP (e.g., osmotic challenge) into the systemic circulation in a preferential manner. On the other hand, a stimulus such as hemorrhage increases the electrical activity of magnocellular neurosecretory, parvocellular neurosecretory, and autonomic-related projection neurons in the PVH (Day *et al.*, 1984; Kannan and Yamashita, 1985; Kannan *et al.*, 1987), increases the secretory activity of OT, AVP, and CRF neurons, and increases the concentration of each peptide in hypophyseal portal plasma (Gibbs, 1984; Lang *et al.*, 1983; Plotsky, 1985). The anatomical specificity exhibited by the visceromotor output neurons and their primary visceral afferents would seem to provide a basis for understanding the selectivity of which the system appears capable, but the ability to invoke different groups of output neurons, and even different functions of individual cell groups, remains among the more challenging and intriguing aspects for current studies of hypothalamic function. By way of summary, some of the mechanisms involving AVP-, OT-, and CRF-expressing neurons that may play a role in such integrative mechanisms will be highlighted.

Magnocellular neurosecretory neurons represent at first blush an anatomically simple system that provides for the delivery of OT and AVP to the general circulation in a highly situation-specific manner. There now exists a strong basis to suspect that they are capable of releasing the nonapeptides from preterminal axons in the median eminence, granting them potential access to the portal vasculature where they may interact with CRF in promoting corticotropin secretion. The circumstances under which this might occur, the underlying mechanisms, and the extent to which this may be regulated independently from terminal release in the neural lobe are unknown. Also worthy of consideration is the fact that magnocellular neurosecretory neurons harbor an array of coexisting neuropeptides; the expression of CRF in OT neurons is but one example. These are typically expressed at levels several orders of magnitude lower than OT or AVP, suggesting that they may serve autocrine or paracrine roles at the level of the neural lobe. The observation that CRF can elicit AVP secretion from isolated neurointermediate lobes is consistent with this view (AlZein et al., 1984).

Parvocellular neurosecretory neurons expressing CRF are thought to represent the final common path by which the brain controls the stress response. These cells are capable of expressing additional peptides (e.g., AVP, angiotensin II) that possess corticotropin-releasing activity (Lind et al., 1985), as well as others that do not (e.g., enkephalin, neurotensin). Evidence exists to suggest that AVP expression in parvocellular neurons can occur under normal conditions (Whitnall et al., 1987), though the range of these has yet to be specified. Moreover, the functional significance of the expression of peptides in "CRF neurons" that are ostensibly unrelated to the regulation of the stress response remains to be determined.

Autonomic-related projection neurons of the PVH appear to innervate sympathetic and parasympathetic preganglionic cell groups, as well as the NTS and other relays subserving visceral afferent control of PVH and SO outputs. The neurons that give rise to these projections are biochemically heterogeneous, with CRF, OT, and AVP (among other peptides) expressed in relatively small subsets of projection neurons. This heterogeneity suggests a potential means for encoding target specificity, but the possibility that chemically defined subsets may give rise to topographically distinctive projections has not been examined rigorously. Recent evidence does, however, support the view that cells in the PVH that project to various sympathetically innervated targets exhibit some measure of topographic organization, at least (Strack et al., 1989).

Although the mechanisms that allow for integrated hypothalamic response to a stimulus such as hemorrhage remain to be clearly elaborated, the evidence summarized above has served, if nothing else, to raise possibilities as to the manner in which the generic stress response may be modified and coupled with situation-specific adaptive mechanisms to effectively cope with this kind of challenge. Because of prominence of their involvement in the pertinent output neurons, particularly as regards their interactions in promoting the pituitary–adrenal response to stress, cell types expressing CRF, OT, and AVP will continue to provide a focus for studies of hypothalamic integration. Linear models holding to the traditional "one neuron–one messenger–one function" view are clearly no longer viable.

Acknowledgments

The work from the author's laboratory described here was supported by NIH grants NS-21182 and HL-35137, and was conducted in part by the Clayton Foundation for Research—California Division.

References

AlZein, M., Jeandel, L., Lutz-Bucher, B., and Koch B. (1984). Evidence that CRF stimulates vasopressin secretion from isolated neurointermediate pituitary. *Neuroendocrinol. Lettt.* **6**, 151–155.

Antoni, F. A. (1986). Hypothalamic control of adrenocorticotropin secretion: Advances since the discovery of 41-residue corticotropin-releasing factor. *Endocr. Rev.* **7**, 351–378.

Bai, F. L., Yamano, M., Shiotani, Y., Emson, P. C., Smith, A. D., Powell, J. F., and Tohyama, M. (1985). An arcuato-paraventricular and -dorsomedial hypothalamic neuropeptide Y-containing system which lacks norepinephrine in the rat. *Brain Res.* **331**, 172–175.

Buma, P., and Nieuwenhuys, R. (1987). Ultrastructural demonstration of oxytocin and vasopressin release sites in the neural lobe and median eminence of the rat by tannic acid and immunogold methods. *Neurosci. Lett.* **74**, 151–157.

Cunningham, E. T., Jr., and Sawchenko, P. E. (1988). Anatomical specificity of noradrenergic inputs to the paraventricular and supraoptic nuclei of the rat hypothalamus. *J. Comp. Neurol.* **274**, 60–76.

Cunningham, E. T., Jr., Bohn, M. C., and Sawchenko, P. E. (1990). The organization of adrenergic inputs to the paraventricular and supraoptic nuclei of the rat hypothalamus. *J. Comp. Neurol.* **292**, 651–667.

Day, T. A., Ferguson, A. V., and Renaud, L. P. (1984). Facilitatory influence of noradrenergic afferents on the excitability of rat paraventricular nucleus neurosecretory cells. *J. Physiol. (London)* **355**, 237–249.

Gibbs, D. M. (1984). High concentrations of oxytocin in hypophyseal portal plasma. *Endocrinology (Baltimore)* **114**, 1216–1218.

Holmes, M. C., Antoni, F. A., Aguilera, G., and Catt, K. J. (1986). Magnocellular axons in passage through the median eminence release vasopressin. *Nature (London)* **319**, 326–329.

Kannan, H., and Yamashita, H. (1985). Electrophysiological study of paraventricular nucleus neurons projecting to the dorsomedial medulla and their response to baroreceptor stimulation in rats. *Brain Res.* **279**, 31–40.

Kannan, H., Kasai, M., Osaka, T., and Yamashita, H. (1987). Neurons in the paraventricular nucleus projecting to the median eminence: A study of their afferent connections from peripheral baroreceptors, and from the A1-catecholaminergic area in the ventrolateral medulla. *Brain Res.* **409**, 358–363.

Kiss, J. Z., Mezey, E., and Skirboll, L. (1984). Corticotropin-releasing factor-immunoreactive neurons become vasopressin positive after adrenalectomy. *Proc. Natl. Acad. Sci. U.S.A.* **81**, 1854–1858.

Lang, R. E., Heil, J., Ganten, D., Hermann, K., Unger, T., and Rascher, W. (1983). Oxytocin unlike vasopressin is a stress hormone in the rat. *Neuroendocrinology* **39**, 314–316.

Lind, R. W., Swanson, L. W., and Sawchenko, P. E. (1985). Anatomical evidence that neural circuits related to the subfornical organ contain angiotensin II. *Brain Res. Bull.* **15**, 79–82.

Mason, W. T., Ho, Y. W., and Hatton, G. I. (1984). Axon collaterals of supraoptic neurones: Anatomical and electrophysiological evidence for their existence in the lateral hypothalamus. *Neuroscience* **11**, 169–182.

Page, R. B. (1986). The pituitary portal system. *Curr. Top. Neuroendocrinol.* **7**, 1–47.

Plotsky, P. M. (1985). Hypophyseotropic regulation of adenohypophyseal adrenocorticotropin secretion. *Fed. Proc., Fed. Am. Soc. Exp. Biol.* **44**, 207–213.

Plotsky, P. M., and Sawchenko, P. E. (1987). Hypophysial-portal plasma levels, median eminence content and immunohistochemical staining of corticotropin-releasing factor, arginine vasopressin and oxytocin following pharmacological adrenalectomy. *Endocrinology (Baltimore)* **120**, 1361–1369.

Rhodes, C. H., Morrell, J. I., and Pfaff, D. W. (1981). Immunohistochemical analysis of magnocellular elements in rat hypothalamus: Distribution and numbers of cells containing neurophysin, oxytocin and vasopressin. *J. Comp. Neurol.* **198**, 45–64.

Saper, C. B., and Loewy, A. D. (1980). Efferent connections of the parabrachial nucleus in the rat. *Brain Res.* **197**, 291–317.

Saper, C. B., Loewy, A. D., Swanson, L. W., and Cowan, W. M. (1979). Direct hypothalamo-autonomic connections. *Brain Res.* **117**, 305–312.

Sawchenko, P. E. (1987a). Evidence for differential regulation of CRF- and vasopressin-immunoreactivities in parvocellular neurosecretory and autonomic-related projections of the paraventricular nucleus. *Brain Res.* **437**, 253–263.

Sawchenko, P. E. (1987b). Adrenalectomy-induced enhancement of CRF and vasopressin immunoreactivity in parvocellular neurosecretory neurons: Anatomic, peptide and steroid specificity. *J. Neurosci.* **7**, 1093–1106.

Sawchenko, P. E., and Swanson, L. W. (1982). Immunohistochemical identification of neurons in the paraventricular nucleus of the hypothalamus that project to the medulla or to the spinal cord in the rat. *J. Comp. Neurol.* **205**, 260–272.

Sawchenko, P. E., Swanson, L. W., and Vale, W. W. (1984a). Co-expression of corticotropin-releasing factor and vasopressin immunoreactivity in parvocellular neurosecretory neurons of the adrenalectomized rat. *Proc. Natl. Acad. Sci. U.S.A.* **81**, 1883–1887.

Sawchenko, P. E., Swanson, L. W., and Vale, W. W. (1984b). Corticotropin-releasing factor: Co-expression within distinct subsets of oxytocin-, vasopressin- and neurotensin-immunoreactive neurons in the hypothalamus of the male rat. *J. Neurosci.* **4**, 1118–1129.

Sawchenko, P. E., Swanson, L. W., Grzanna, R., Howe, P. R. C., Bloom, S. R., and Polak, J. M. (1985). Colocalization of neuropeptide Y immunoreactivity in brainstem catecholaminergic neurons that project to the paraventricular and supraoptic nuclei in the rat. *J. Comp. Neurol.* **241**, 138–153.

Sawchenko, P. E., Benoit, R., and Brown, M. R. (1988a). Somatostatin 28-immunoreactive inputs to the paraventricular nucleus: Origin from non-aminergic neurons in the nucleus of the solitary tract. *J. Chem. Neuroanat.* **1**, 81–94.

Sawchenko, P. E., Plotsky, P. M., Cunningham, E. T., Jr., Vaughan, J., Rivier, J., and Vale, W. (1988b). Inhibin -immunoreactivity in a visceral sensory system controlling oxytocin secretion in the rat brain. *Nature (London)* **344**, 315–317.

Strack, A. M., Sawyer, W. B., Hughes, J. H., Platt, K. B., and Loewy, A. D. (1989). A general pattern of CNS innervation of the sympathetic outflow demonstrated by transneuronal pseudorabies viral infection. *Brain Res.* **491**, 156–162.

Swanson, L. W., and Kuypers, H. G. J. M. (1980). The paraventricular nucleus of the hypothalamus: Cytoarchitectonic subdivisions and the organization of projections to the pituitary, dorsal vagal complex and spinal cord as revealed by retrograde fluorescence double labeling methods. *J. Comp. Neurol.* **194**, 555–570.

Swanson, L. W., and Simmons, D. M. (1989). Differential steroid hormone and neural influences on peptide mRNA levels in CRH cells of the paraventricular nucleus: A hybridization histochemical study in the rat. *J. Comp. Neurol.* **285**, 413–435.

Swanson, L. W., Sawchenko, P. E., Wiegand, S. J., and Price, J. L. (1980). Separate neurons in the paraventricular nucleus project to the median eminence and to the medulla or spinal cord. *Brain Res.* **197**, 207–212.

Swanson, L. W., Sawchenko, P. E., Rivier, J., and Vale, W. (1983). Organization of ovine corticotropin-releasing factor immunoreactive cells and fibers in the rat brain: An immunohistochemical study. *Neuroendocrinology* **36**, 165–186.

Swanson, L. W., Sawchenko, P. E., and Lind, R. W. (1986). Regulation of multiple peptides in CRF parvocellular neurosecretory neurons: Implications for the stress response. *Prog. Brain Res.* **68**, 169–190.

Tanaguchi, Y., Yoshida, M., Ishikawa, K., Suzuki, M., and Kurosimi, K. (1988). The distribution of vasopressin- or oxytocin-neurons projecting to the posterior pituitary as revealed by a combination of retrograde transport of horseradish peroxidase and immunohistochemistry. *Arch. Histol. Cytol.* **58**, 83–89.

Whitnall, M. H., Smyth, D., and Gainer, H. (1987). Vasopressin coexists in half of the corticotropin-releasing factor axons in the external zone of the median eminence in normal rats. *Neuroendocrinology* **45**, 420–424.

Wiegand, S. J., and Price, J. L. (1980). The cells of origin of afferent fibers to the median eminence in the rat. *J. Comp. Neurol.* **192**, 1–19.

Wolfson, B., Manning, R. W., Davis, L. G., Arentzen, R., and Baldino, F., Jr. (1985). Colocalization of corticotropin releasing factor and vasopressin mRNA in neurones after adrenalectomy. *Nature (London)* **315**, 59–61.

Young, W. S., III, Mezey, E., and Siegel, R. E. (1986). Quantitative in situ hybridization histochemistry reveals increased levels of corticotropin-releasing factor mRNA after adrenalectomy in rats. *Neurosci. Lett.* **70**, 198–203.

2

Current Concepts in Hypothalamo–Pituitary–Adrenal Axis Regulation

K. Ranga Rama Krishnan   *P. Murali Doraiswamy*

Sanjeev Venkataraman   *Deborah A. Reed*

James C. Richie

Department of Psychiatry
Duke University Medical Center
Durham, North Carolina 27710

I. Basal Regulation of the HPA Axis
   A. Regulation of the Adrenal Cortex
   B. Nonpituitary ACTH Mechanisms
   C. Humoral Factors
   D. Pituitary Corticotroph
II. Physiological Role of CRF and Vasopressin
   A. Role of CRF and Vasopressin in Regulating the ACTH Response to Various Types of Stress
   B. Hemodynamic Stimuli
   C. Insulin Stress
III. Central Regulation of the HPA Axis
   A. Amygdala
   B. Hippocampus
IV. Neural Pathways Mediating HPA Responses to Stimuli
   A. Hemodynamic Changes
   B. Thermal and Noxious Stimuli
   C. Psychological Factors

There is overwhelming evidence suggesting that the hypothalamo–pituitary–adrenal axis (HPA) plays an integral role in the pathophysiology of stress. Recently, there has been a tremendous increase in knowledge about the regulation of the HPA axis. In this chapter, we will discuss the regulation of the HPA axis under basal conditions and the regulation of the system during stress.

I. Basal Regulation of the HPA Axis

For a number of years it has been believed that the limbic system regulates the hypothalamus. The hypothalamus then releases corticotropin-releasing-factor (CRF), which stimulates the pituitary corticotrophs to release adrenocorticotropin (ACTH); which, in turn, releases cortisol from the adrenal cortex. Cortisol exerts a negative feedback on the axis at multiple levels, including the hippocampus, the pituitary and the hypothalamus. Recent evidence, however, suggests that the regulation of this axis is much more complicated than this (see Figure 1 for a schematic representation).

A. Regulation of the Adrenal Cortex

ACTH had been considered the sole agent regulating the release of cortisol from the adrenal cortex; however, new evidence suggests that this view may be incomplete. Krieger and Allen (1975) showed that there were periods when there was a dissociation between plasma ACTH and plasma cortisol concentrations. However, these investigators considered such dissociations to be anomalous episodes. Fehm *et al.* (1984) suggested that there were a number of instances, such as after the noon meal or after the administration of methamphetamine, when cortisol concentrations could rise without a preceding or concomitant change in plasma ACTH concentration. They also showed that in some individuals the early morning rise in cortisol was not always accompanied by a concomitant rise in plasma ACTH concentra-

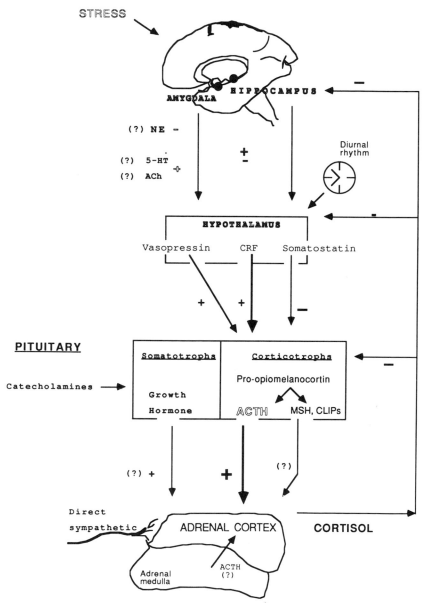

Figure 1   The hypothalamo–pituitary–adrenal axis.

tion. However, the ACTH assay that they used was not very sensitive. This raised the possibility that the increased cortisol secretion that occurred in these patients may have been due to changes in ACTH concentration that were physiologically significant but were below the detection limit of their assay. We (Krishnan *et al.*, 1988a) studied the relationship between plasma ACTH and cortisol concentrations, in normal individuals, during the night and in the early morning period. We found that in about half the instances, there was no significant relationship between the occurrence of cortisol peaks and ACTH peaks. Further, in many instances there was little or no relationship between the magnitude of the cortisol peak and the magnitude of the concomitant ACTH peak. The assay that we used in these studies was extremely sensitive, could detect less than 1 pg/ml of ACTH, and was highly specific (Krishnan *et al.*, 1988a). However, it is possible that even our assay was not sufficiently sensitive to detect small changes in plasma ACTH concentration that could, however, be adequate to cause significant changes in plasma cortisol concentration. In order to answer this question, we next studied the threshold sensitivity of the adrenal cortex to ACTH.

In this study (Krishnan *et al.*, 1988c), we infused low doses, less than 50 ng, of ACTH over a 30-min period in the morning at 9 a.m., after administering 4 mg dexamethasone orally the previous night at 11 p.m. We were able to show significant changes in plasma cortisol concentrations that were not accompanied by changes in plasma ACTH concentration. This further strengthened the distinct possibility that the ACTH–cortisol dissociation, at least in situations where cortisol pulses occurred in the absence of corresponding ACTH pulses, was perhaps a false negative result due to the lack of sensitivity of the assay. However, there were other instances when changes in plasma ACTH occurred without any accompanying change in plasma cortisol concentration. This type of dissociation could not be explained by the ACTH infusion study.

B. Nonpituitary ACTH Mechanisms

At about the same time that these studies suggesting a possible dissociation of ACTH and cortisol appeared in the literature, hitherto unknown extrapituitary ACTH mechanisms capable of regulating the release of cortisol from the adrenal cortex were also described. These putative mechanisms can be categorized into three possibilities. They are (1) direct autonomic innervation of the adrenal cortex, (2) indirect activation of the adrenal cortex by a paracrine mechanism involving the adrenal medulla, and (3) other hormonal peptides that may either directly stimulate the adrenal cortex or modulate the adrenocortical responsiveness to ACTH. These mechanisms are briefly described below. See Krishnan *et al.* (1988a) for additional details and further references.

1. Direct Innervation of the Adrenal Cortex

A sympathetic innervation of the human adrenal cortex has been described by Garcia Alvarez (1979). In addition, there is evidence that neostigmine or physostigmine can release corticosterone in hypophysectomized rats and that adrenocortical sensitivity to ACTH is mediated by cholinergic innervation of the adrenal cortex. These observations have been taken as prima facie evidence for a direct autonomic regulation of the adrenal cortex (Krishnan *et al.*, 1988a).

2. Paracrine Mechanism

In the last few years ACTH has been found in the adrenal medulla, raising the possibility that the ACTH locally released from the adrenal medulla may also play a role in regulating the release of cortisol from the adrenal cortex. Support for this hypothesis has been provided by a case report. Schteingart *et al.* (1972) reported a patient who developed Cushing's syndrome secondary to an adrenal medullary tumor that was a source of ACTH. Additional support comes from the work of Soliman (1982), who showed that the daily rhythm of glucocorticoids persisted in hypophysectomized rats pretreated with ACTH, and that blocking epinephrine synthesis by administration of a phenylethanolamine N-methyltransferase (PNMT) inhibitor abolished the diurnal fluctuation in plasma cortisol. Thus, locally released substances, such as ACTH or epinephrine, may serve as paracrine regulators of the adrenal cortex.

C. Humoral Factors

There are a number of candidates for putative humoral factors regulating the adrenal cortex. These include gamma-3-melanocyte stimulating hormone (gamma-3-MSH), growth hormone, prostaglandins, interferons, and other peptides. Gamma-3-melanocyte stimulating hormone is a cleavage product of the peptide pro-opiomelanocortin (POMC). POMC is the prohormone of ACTH. Gamma-3-MSH has been shown in both *in vitro* and *in vivo* studies to stimulate the release of corticosterone. In general, gamma-3-MSH seems to be cosecreted with ACTH and therefore it may be a factor that primarily increases the sensitivity of the adrenal cortex to ACTH, thus enhancing the effect of ACTH. It probably does not play a role in the absence of ACTH. Growth hormone also potentiates the effects of ACTH on adrenal function in hypophysectomized rats, but it has no direct effect on cortisol secretion. Prostaglandins can increase steroidogenesis, although the physiological significance of prostaglandins in regulating the adrenal cortex is not known. Besides these substances, factors derived from the thyroid and the liver, as well as other factors from the thymus, have also been reported to potentiate ACTH effects on steroidogenesis in isolated or *in vitro* preparations of the adrenal cortex. Other relevant humoral factors may include the lymphokines, derived from the lymphocytes, such as interferons. A possible immune–adrenal interaction has been proposed, but this link remains controversial. For a more detailed review of the regulation of the adrenal cortex, and for the references see Krishnan *et al.* (1988a).

D. Pituitary Corticotroph

The regulation of the pituitary corticotroph is better understood than the regulation of cortisol secretion by the adrenal cortex. A number of factors are known to regulate the pituitary corticotroph. These include corticotropin-releasing-factor, vasopressin, somatostatin, vasoactive intestinal polypeptide, catecholamines (through both alpha-1- and beta-adrenergic mechanisms), angiotensin, and glucocorticoids. A brief discussion of their role follows.

1. Corticotropin-Releasing Factor

The 41 amino acid sequence of CRF in humans and in rats is identical. Structure–activity studies have shown that the carboxy terminal of CRF is critical for its biological activity. The sequence comprising amino acids 15–41 retains the full CRF bioactivity (Vale *et al.*, 1981). The pituitary actions of CRF are primarily on the corticotroph cells. CRF stimulates the synthesis of the precursor POMC and the release of ACTH and other adenohypophyseal products of POMC. CRF binds to high-affinity receptors on cells in the anterior and intermediate lobes of the pituitary gland (reviewed by Owens and Nemeroff, 1988). This step then activates adenylate cyclase to increase the intracellular levels of cyclic AMP and enhance the activity of cyclic-AMP-dependent protein kinases. CRF also increases cytosolic free calcium concentrations. It is believed that the cyclic AMP mechanism is responsible for ACTH secretion and POMC synthesis. CRF is secreted by immunoreactive neurons in the parvocellular subdivision of the paraventricular nucleus (PVN) into the pituitary portal blood. Some of the neurons that synthesize CRF also synthesize vasopressin, while others primarily synthesize CRF (see review by Antoni, 1986). The dynamic characteristics of ACTH response to CRF have been analyzed in great detail (Gold *et al.*, 1986), and it has been found that the ACTH response to CRF pulses depends not only upon the length of the pulse but also on the interval between pulses.

2. Vasopressin

Vasopressin for many years was considered to be the corticotropin-releasing factor. Vasopressin by itself is capable of releasing ACTH from the corticotroph cells. However, this effect is minimal when compared to the effect of CRF on the corticotroph cells. Vasopressin potentiates the effect of CRF on the ACTH cells. It amplifies the effect of CRF on ACTH release two- to threefold, and the slope of the dose-response curve for vasopressin or CRF is usually much more shallow than that of vasopressin in combination with CRF. Vasopressin effects on the corticotroph are mediated by a receptor that appears to be similar to the V_1 or the pressor type of vasopressin receptor, but is different in certain binding characteristics. The exact mechanism by which vasopressin stimulates ACTH and potentiates the ACTH response to CRF is still not known (reviewed by Antoni, 1986).

3. Oxytocin

Oxytocin is also capable of releasing ACTH from corticotroph cells. This effect has mainly been shown in animal studies. In humans, oxytocin is believed to inhibit ACTH secretion. Overall, the role of oxytocin in the regulation of ACTH secretion from the corticotroph cells is unclear (Antoni, 1986).

4. Catecholamines

Catecholamines act directly on the pituitary to increase ACTH secretion through both alpha-1- and beta-adrenergic mechanisms (reviewed by Axelrod and Reisine, 1984). The beta-adrenergic mechanism has been mainly shown in AT20 cells and has not yet been demonstrated in humans. The alpha-1-adrenergic mechanism has not been demonstrated in humans.

5. Angiotensin II

Angiotensin-II has also been identified as an ACTH secretogogue in pituitary cell cultures and *in vivo* studies. However, its physiological role remains unclear (Antoni, 1986).

6. Other Factors

Other factors that may also influence this system include vasoactive intestinal polypeptide (VIP), serotonin, and atrial natriuretic factor (ANF). However, their physiological significance remains uncertain (Antoni, 1986).

II. Physiological Role of CRF and Vasopressin

As noted earlier, CRF and vasopressin, the two peptides that primarily regulate the corticotroph cells, are sometimes colocalized in the same hypothalamic neurons and at other times are not colocalized. Studies that have looked at the concentrations of CRF and vasopressin in portal hypophyseal blood have noted that the secretion of these hormones can be dissociated in various conditions (Antoni, 1986).

The precise interactive role of these two peptides in controlling the diurnal variation of ACTH secretion is not known. However, the role of these peptides has been investigated under various experimental paradigms. One such paradigm, a postadrenalectomy study, sheds some interesting clues regarding this interaction and is mentioned below.

After adrenalectomy (Dallman *et al.*, 1974; Koch and Lutz-Bucher, 1985), in the initial phase there is a marked increase in ACTH release due to a lack of glucocorticoid feedback, which depletes the pituitary store of ACTH and down-regulates the pituitary vasopressin receptors. Hence, pituitary response to CRF and vasopressin is reduced. However, shortly after this initial phase, compensatory changes occur in the pituitary corticotroph resulting in an increase in the concentrations of POMC and in the pituitary content of ACTH. During this period the pituitary response to CRF and vasopressin is enhanced. However, with time there is a marked and long-lasting desensitization (decreased number) of vasopressin and CRF receptors. These studies indicate that glucocorticoids appear to have a permissive type of action in regulating the CRF and vasopressin receptors on the corticotroph and thereby regulating the corticotroph ACTH response to these peptides.

A. Role of CRF and Vasopressin in Regulating the ACTH Response to Various Types of Stress

CRF appears to be the major factor modulating the ACTH response to stress with vasopressin also playing a role. ACTH responses to hemodynamic stimuli and insulin-induced hypoglycemia exemplify this type of regulation (Antoni, 1986).

B. Hemodynamic Stimuli

Hemorrhage increases the secretion of ACTH. Carlson and Gann (1984) studied the ACTH response to hemodynamic stimuli in cats and showed that in animals pretreated with dexamethasone the ACTH response to hemodynamic stress was preserved, indicating that the HPA response to this stimulus is steroid nonsupressible. They then showed that vasopressin anti-serum attenuated the increase in plasma ACTH evoked by hemorrhage. Hypophyseal portal blood collections in the rat have also shown that hemorrhage increases vasopressin concentrations. Thus ACTH responses to hemodynamic stimuli appear, at least in part, to be regulated by vasopressin.

C. Insulin Stress

Insulin-induced hypoglycemia is also a potent stimulus for ACTH secretion. The full ACTH response to this stimulus requires the presence of catecholamines, CRF, and a marked rise in vasopressin. In the rat, the principal mediator of the ACTH response to insulin has been shown to be an increase in vasopressin release (reviewed by Antoni, 1986).

III. Central Regulation of the HPA Axis

The details of the neural pathways and mechanisms subserving the control of the hypothalamo–pituitary–adrenal axis are obscure. In the last few years there has been some progress in defining these pathways and their neurotransmitters. A number of brain structures have been implicated in the regulation of the hypothalamo–pituitary–adrenal axis. These include the amygdala, the hippocampus, septal area, cingulum, orbital, and brainstem regions.

A. Amygdala

Okinaka (1961) stimulated the amygdala in dogs anesthetized with morphine and demonstrated a significant elevation of adrenal 17-hydroxycorticosteroid secretion. Slusher and Hyde (1961) reported a similar phenomenon in cats. They showed that the increase occurred primarily when the medial part of the basal nucleus of the amygdala was stimulated, whereas stimulation of the lateral amygdaloid nucleus generally decreased 17-hydroxycorticosteroid secretion. Mason (1959) showed that electrical stimulation of the amygdala of conscious monkeys led to a marked increase in peripheral plasma 17-hydroxycorticosteroids.

Knigge (1961) and Seggie (1980) failed to find, in rats, a significant effect of bilateral destruction of the amygdala on plasma corticosterone concentrations. However, Knigge and Hays (1963) have also reported that bilateral lesions of the amygdala markedly attenuated the plasma corticosterone response to the stress of ether and intracardiac puncture. These lat-

ter studies and the findings of Allen and Allen (1974) and Ishihara *et al.*
(1964) suggest that the amygdaloid nuclei facilitate the effects of stress on
the pituitary–adreno–cortical secretory activity and that the pathway for
this facilitatory effect may traverse the direct medial amygdaloid projection
to the hypothalamus.

B. Hippocampus

Okinaka (1961) showed that electrical stimulation of the hippocampus led
to a significant but small decrease in adrenal 17-hydroxycorticosterone secretion rate. In humans, electrical stimulation of the hippocampus decreases
peripheral plasma 17 hydroxycorticosteroid concentrations. A sustained inhibitory effect of the hippocampus on pituitary adrenocortical activity was
shown by Kim and Kim (1961), who documented that the responses to
two acute stressors were enhanced by lesions of the hippocampus. Thus the
hippocampus appears to have an inhibitory role in the regulation of the
HPA axis.

The results of studies that addressed the effect of stimulation of the
septum are inconsistent. However, other studies have shown that stimulation of the posterior orbital surface of the cortex has an excitatory effect
on the HPA axis.

IV. Neural Pathways Mediating HPA Responses to Stimuli

Donald Gann and his collaborators (1981) have carried out a number of
elegant studies examining the neural pathways that regulate the HPA axis
response to a variety of stimuli, such as changes in blood volume, body
temperature, and pain.

A. Hemodynamic Changes

Hemodynamic changes can consistently activate the HPA axis (Gann *et al.*,
1981). The receptors responsible for this are located in the right atrium and
in the carotid arteries. The afferent pathways reach the dorsolateral medulla
and the lateral solitary nucleus, which then appear to mediate the response.
These neurons project to the locus ceruleus and also project without synaps-
ing to the hypothalamus. Several studies have shown that electrical stimulation of parts of the locus ceruleus can activate the HPA axis. In addition, a
pathway from the solitary nucleus to the raphe complex may also play a
role in regulating the hypothalamo–pituitary–adrenal axis.

B. Thermal and Noxious Stimuli

The effects of changes in body temperature on the HPA axis are probably mediated by intrinsic circuits within the hypothalamus involving temperature-sensitive neurons in the preoptic area of the hypothalamus and parts of the dorsomedial region of the posterior hypothalamus. However, the pathways for this stimulus have not yet been well delineated.

The ascending pathways for pain run in the lateral spinothalamic tract, with collaterals projecting to the gigantocellular and tegmental fields. Electrical stimulation of these fields in the brainstem leads to ACTH release. The ascending pathway from these fields projects into the ventral tegmental area of the midbrain and into the medial forebrain bundle before terminating in the ventral hypothalamus. The amgydala may also play a role in facilitating this response.

Thus for each of the stimuli mentioned above there appear to be discrete neural pathways that lead to the eventual release of ACTH.

C. Psychological Factors

Gann *et al.* (1981) suggest that psychological factors influence the hypothalamo–pituitary–adrenal axis through the limbic system, possibly by the facilitatory and inhibitory areas in the septum, which project to the ventral hypothalamus through the fornix. In addition, the amygdala, as previously described, may also play a role. Fibers from the amygdala project to the stria terminalis and then into the medial forebrain bundle to reach the medial basal hypothalamus through the supraoptic decussation.

V. Neurotransmitter Mechanisms in the Neural Control of the HPA Axis

A. Catecholamines

1. Norepinephrine

The role of catecholamines in the central regulation of the hypothalamo–pituitary–adrenal axis is controversial. The noradrenergic neuronal system that projects to the basal hypothalamus has been shown to play a role in the regulation of the HPA axis. In a series of studies, Feldman *et al.* (1984) have shown that norepinephrine plays an inhibitory role in regulating this axis. They have also shown that the pathways projecting through the medial forebrain bundle to the hypothalamus may mediate many of the neural stimuli that activate the hypothalamo–pituitary–adrenal axis. Although a few studies have reported a stimulatory effect of norepinephrine, the bulk of the evidence suggests that norepinephrine plays an inhibitory role in controlling CRF–ACTH secretion. The effect of methoxamine on the hypothalamo–pituitary–adrenal axis is believed by some to be mediated through a central alpha-1-adrenergic mechanism. In humans, norepinephrine may exert a stimulatory effect on the basal regulation of the HPA axis, but its effect on stress is somewhat different. The beta-blocker propranolol has no effect on basal plasma cortisol levels, but has been shown to markedly increase the HPA response to insulin stress, suggesting that norepinephrine acting via beta-receptors may play an inhibitory role in the regulation of the HPA axis to stress. These studies suggest that there is a central stimulatory component through an alpha-adrenergic mechanism and an inhibitory component (especially in response to stress) through a beta-adrenergic component.

2. Dopamine

Dopaminergic neurons and terminals are present in the hypothalamic region. Some of these are intrinsic to the hypothalamus while others arise from the mesencephalic dopaminergic nuclei. Dopamine, however, does not seem to play a major role in regulating the HPA axis.

B. Serotonin

Serotonin is believed to primarily play a stimulatory role in regulating the HPA axis. Serotonin has been shown to stimulate CRF secretion from hypothalamic neurons into the portal hypophyseal blood. The serotonergic nerve terminals in the hypothalamus originate from the mesencephalic raphe nuclear cell groups. Serotonin has been shown to play a role in the circadian periodicity of CRF–ACTH secretion, and some studies have suggested that serotonin inhibits ACTH response to stressful stimuli. This, however, remains controversial. In humans, 5-hydroxytryptophan (5-HT) has been shown to release ACTH by some authors, but not by others. Cyproheptadine, a nonselective 5-HT receptor antagonist, and metergoline, a selective 5-HT antagonist, can both reduce plasma cortisol concentrations (Cavagnini *et al.*, 1975). Krieger *et al.* (1975) have used cyproheptadine in the treatment of Cushing's syndrome. The plasma cortisol response to hypoglycemic stress is blocked in humans by cyproheptadine. However, since cyproheptadine has multiple effects, its precise role in inhibiting the HPA response is not known. Fenfluramine has been shown to stimulate the HPA axis in humans, and dose responses for fenfluramine have been established (Lewis and Sherman, 1984) We have shown that 1.5 mg/kg of fenfluramine has a significant stimulatory effect on the hypothalamo–pituitary–adrenal axis (unpublished data) (see Figure 2).

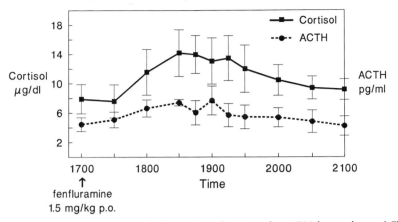

Figure 2 Effects of 1.5 mg/kg po fenfluramine, administered at 1700 h, on plasma ACTH and cortisol (unpublished data).

C. Gamma-Aminobutyric Acid (GABA) and Opioids

GABA is an inhibitory central nervous system (CNS) neurotransmitter, and GABAergic terminals project to the medial hypothalamus. GABA inhibits ACTH release in response to different stimuli. Opioid peptides are known to alter the hypothalamo–pituitary–adrenal axis secretion. In humans, morphine suppresses the early-morning as well as the stress-induced secretion of ACTH. Naloxone blocks this effect, suggesting that morphine and opiates have an inhibitory central effect on the hypothalamo–pituitary–adrenal axis. However, the significance of the opioid peptides and GABA in regulating the HPA axis remains unclear (reviewed by Jones *et al.*, 1984).

VI. Feedback Regulation of the HPA Axis

There are at least three distinct time domains in which negative feedback is exerted by glucocorticoids on the hypothalamo–pituitary–adrenal axis. These time domains have been classified by Keller-Wood and Dallman (1984) as fast, intermediate, and delayed feedback. The feedback effect can occur at several sites. These sites include the corticotroph, hypothalamus, and extrahypothalamic sites, especially the hippocampus. The corticosteroid feedback inhibition that occurs immediately (within minutes) after the administration of cortisol is called fast feedback. The fast feedback has been mainly demonstrated in pathological conditions in humans, such as in Addison's disease, and in animals by showing inhibition of the HPA axis pre-stimulated by stress, or by a direct effect on the corticotroph. This fast feedback is believed to be rate sensitive. In other words, it is dependent upon the rate of rise of the glucocorticoids. In humans this rate-sensitive feedback has not been well demonstrated with regard to its effects on basal secretion of cortisol or on CRF-induced ACTH response. Delayed feedback is a dose-dependent phenomenon, and it occurs a few hours after the increase in cortisol concentration. The feedback regulation at the level of extrahypothalamic sites, such as the hippocampus, has received considerable attention in recent years.

Sapolsky (1988) has shown that the feedback inhibition through the hippocampus is gradually lost with aging, due to destruction of some of the hippocampal neurons. They have speculated that this mechanism may be related to the pathophysiology of dementia in the elderly.

A similar phenomenon may also occur with repeated stress. Sapolsky and McEwen (1988) have demonstrated that with repeated stress there is a gradual destruction of hippocampal neurons and the loss of feedback. They have suggested that this may be an explanation for the nonsuppression in the dexamethasone suppression test (DST) seen in depressed individuals.

The DST is carried out as follows: 1 mg dexamethasone is given at 11:30 p.m., and plasma cortisol is determined the following day at 4:00 p.m. and 11:00 p.m. Normally the plasma cortisol is suppressed below 5 μg/dl, but in many depressed patients the levels are much higher than 5 μg/dl (Carroll *et al.*, 1981).

Recent studies have suggested that nonsuppression on the DST may be correlated with neuroanatomical changes in the brain. The main neuroanatomical index that has been studied so far is the ratio between the size of the lateral ventricles and the brain, the so-called ventricular brain ratio (VBR). We (Rao *et al.*, 1989) have recently studied 82 depressed patients using magnetic resonance imaging (MRI) to assess the VBR and the relationship between the VBR and the DST status. This study was conducted as follows: 82 of the patients admitted to the Affective Disorders Unit at Duke University Medical Center who satisfied the DSM-3 criteria for major depression were studied. The MRIs were performed on the 1.5-tesla GE Signa System. Spin pulse echo sequences were used to generate T1 weighted and T2 weighted images. For both the T1 and T2 weighted images, a series of 5-mm-thick sections, with a 2.5-mm interscan gap, were performed in the axial plane parallel to the orbitomeatal line. VBR was measured using the method of Synek and Rubin (see Rao *et al.*, 1989). The assessment was made on the console, using the CLIPS Program of the GE Signa System. The cursor was used to delineate the regions of interest, and their areas were then calculated with the CLIPS Program. The correlation coefficient for two observers for VBR assessment using this program independent of each other was 0.94. The DST was performed in the standard fashion. Plasma cortisol was measured by an Abbott TDXT analyzer using floracin polarization immunoassay. The interassay and intraassay coefficients of variation were both equal to 8%. The correlation coefficient between the highest postdexamethasone cortisol concentrations and the VBR was 0.34, with a p value of 0.0014. However, the VBR cannot in itself be considered as evidence directly supportive of Sapolsky's hypothesis (Sapolsky and McEwen, 1988). Further work is needed to examine the relationship between highest postdexamethasone cortisol concentrations and the hippocampal volume (which can also be determined by MRI). It is not known whether such changes are reversible, and further studies are under way to determine this. The presence of a strong correlation does not by itself indicate causality, although it does raise the possibility of an interaction between neuroanatomical changes in the brain, stress, and dysregulation of the hypothalamo–pituitary–adrenal axis.

VII. Summary

In this chapter we have presented some current concepts regarding the regulation of the hypothalamo–pituitary–adrenal axis under both basal and stress conditions. The complexity in the dynamics of the regulation of the HPA axis has also been presented, and an attempt has been made to dispel the notion that the regulation of this central nervous system–hypothalamus–pituitary–adrenal gland axis is simple and straightforward. Instead, the multiple interactions of variables at each level, potential alterations over time with aging, and their significance in the pathophysiology of stress have been discussed. These findings have to be borne in mind when designing and interpreting studies of stress in relation to the HPA axis abnormalities.

Acknowledgments

This work was supported in part by a grant from NIMH, MH 40139, NIH supplement to RR-30.

References

Allen, J. P., and Allen, J. F. (1974). Role of the amygdaloid complex in the stress induced release of ACTH in the rat. *Neuroendocrinology* 15, 220.

Antoni, F. A. (1986). Hypothalamic control of adrenocorticotropin secretion: Advances since the discovery of 41-Residue Corticotropin-Releasing-Factor. *Endocr. Rev.*, 7(4), 351–377.

Axelrod, J., and Reisine, T. D. (1984). Stress hormones: Their interaction and regulation. *Science* 224, 452–459.

Carlson, D. E., and Gann, D. S. (1984). Effects of vasopressin antiserum on the response of adrenocorticotropin and cortisol to haemorrhage. *Endocrinology (Baltimore)* 114, 317.

Carroll, B. J., Feinberg, M., and Greden J. F. Tarika, J., Albala, A. A., Haskett, R., James, N. McI., Kronfol, Z., Lohr, N., Steiner, M., de Vigne, J. P., Young, E., (1981). A specific laboratory test for the diagnosis of melancholia. *Arch. Gen. Psychiatry*, 38, 15–22.

Cavagnini, F., Panerai, A. E., Valentini, F., Bulgheroin, P., Peracchi, M., and Pinto, M. (1975). Inhibition of ACTH response in man. *J. Clin. Endocrinol. Metab.* 41, 143–148

Dallman, M. F., De Manincor, D., and Shinsako, J. (1974). Diminishing corticotrop capacity to release ACTH during sustained stimulation: The 24 hrs after bilateral adrenalectomy in the rat. *Endocrinology (Baltimore)* 95, 65.

Fehm, H. L., Holl, R., Klein, E., and Voigt, K. H. (1984). Evidence for ACTH unrelated mechanisms in the regulation of cortisol secretion in man. *Klin. Wochenschr.* 62, 19–24.

Feldman, S., Melamed, E., Conforti, N., and Weidenfeld, J. (1984). Inhibition in cortico-trophin and corticosterone secretion following photic stimulation in rats with 6-hydroxydopamine injection into the medial forebrain bundle. *J. Neurosci. Res.* 12, 87–92.

Gann, D. S., Dallman, M. F., and Engeland, W. C. (1981). Reflex control and modulation of ACTH and Corticosteroids. *In* Endocrine Physiology III, McCann, SM (Ed) Univ. Park Press, Baltimore.

Ganong, W. F., Bernhard, W. F., and McMurrey, J. D. (1977). Neurotransmitters in the control of ACTH secretion: Catecholamines. *Ann. N.Y. Acad. Sci.* 297, 509–517

Garcia-Alvarez. (1979). *Anatomica (Zaragoza)* 19, 267.

Gold, P. W., Loriaux, D. X., Roy, A., Kling, M. A., Calabrese, J. R., Kellner, C. H., Nieman, L. K., Post, R. M., Pickar, D. Gallucci, W. Avgerinos, P. Paul, S. Oldfield, E. H., Cutler, G. B. Chrousos, G. P. (1986). Responses to CRF in the hypercortisolism of depression and in patients with Cushing's disease. *N. Engl. J. Med.* 314, 1329.

Ishihara, I., Komori, Y., and Maruyama, T. (1964). Amygdala and adrenocortical response. *Annu. Rep. Environ. Med. Nagoya Univ.* 12, 9–17.

Jones, M. T., Gillham, B., Altaher, A. R. H., Nicholson, S. A., Campbell, E. A., Watts, S. M., and Thody, A. (1984). Clinical and experimental studies on the role of GABA in the regulation of ACTH secretion: A review. *Psychoneuroendocrinology* 9(2), 107–123.

Keller-Wood, M. E., and Dallman, M. (1984). Corticosteroid inhibition of ACTH secretion. *Endocr. Rev.* 5, 1.

Kim, C., and Kim, C. U. (1961). Effect of partial hippocampal resection on stress mechanism in rats. *Am. J. Physiol.* 201, 337–340.

Knigge, K. M. (1961). Adrenocortical response to stress in rats with lesions in hippocampus and amygdala. *Proc. Soc. Exp. Biol. Med.* 108, 18–21.

Knigge, K. M., and Hays, M. (1963). Evidence of inhibitive role of hippocampus in neural regulation of ACTH release. *Proc. Soc. Exp. Biol. Med.* 114, 67–69.

Koch, B., and Lutz-Bucher, B. (1985). Specific receptors for vasopressin in the pituitary gland: Evidence for down regulation and desensitization to adrenocorticotropin releasing factors. *Endocrinology (Baltimore)* 116, 671.

Krieger, D. T., and Allen, W. (1975). Relationship of bioassayable and immunoassayable plasma ACTH and cortisol concentration in normal subjects and in patients with Cushing's syndrome. *J. Clin. Endocrinol. Metab.* 10, 675–687.

Krieger, D. T., Amorosa, L., and Linick, F. (1975). Cyproheptadine induced remission of Cushings disease. *N. Engl J. Med.* **293**, 893–896.

Krishnan, K. R., Manepalli, A., Ritchie, J. C., Venkatraman, S., France, R., Nemeroff, C. B., and Carroll, B. J. (1988a). What is the relationship between plasma ACTH & plasma cortisol in normal humans and depressed patients. *In* "The Hypothalamic-Pituitary-Adrenal Axis: Physiology, Pathophysiology and Psychiatric Implications" (A. F. Schatzberg and C. B. Nemeroff, eds.), pp. 115–131. Raven Press, New York.

Krishnan, K. R., Goli, V., Ellinwood, E. H., France, R. D., Blazer, D. G., and Nemeroff, C. B. (1988b). Leukoencephalopathy in patients with major depression. *Biol. Psychiatry* **23**, 519–522.

Krishnan, K. R., Ritchie, J. C., Manepalli, A. N., Nemeroff, C. B., Carroll, B. J. (1988c). Adrenocortical sensitivity to ACTH in humans. *Biol. Psychiatry* **24**, 105–108.

Lewis, D. A., and Sherman, B. M. (1984). Serotonergic stimulation of adrenocorticotropin secretion in man. *J. Clin. Endocrinol. Metab.* **58**, 458–462.

Mason, J. W. (1959). Plasma 17 hydroxycorticosteroid levels during electrical stimulation of the amygdala in conscious monkeys. *Am. J. Physiol.* **196**, 44–48.

Okinaka, S. (1961). Die regulation der hypophysennebennierenfunktion durch das limbic system and den mitt elhirnanteil der formatio retrarlaris. *Acta Neuroveg.* **23**, 15–20.

Owens, M., and Nemeroff, C. B. (1988). The neurobiology of Corticotropin-Releasing Factor: Implications for affective disorders. *In* "The Hypothalamic-Pituitary-Adrenal Axis: Physiology, Pathophy-siology and Psychiatric Implications A. F. (Schatzberg, and C. B. Nemeroff, eds.), pp. 1–36. Raven Press, New York.

Plotsky, P. M., Bruhn, T. O., and Vale, W. W. (1985). Hypophysiotropic regulation of ACTH secretion in response to insulin-induced hypoglycemia. *Endocrinology (Baltimore)* **116**, 633.

Rao, V., Krishnan, K. R., Goli, V., Blazer, D. G., Ellinwood, E. H., and Nemeroff, C. B. (1989). Neuroanatomical changes and HPA axis abnormalities. *Biol. Psychiatry* **26**:729–732.

Sapolsky, R. M., and McEwen, B. S. (1988). Why dexamethasone resistance? Two possible neundendocrine mechanisms. *In* "The Hypothalamic-Pituitary-Adrenal Axis: Physiology, Pathophysiology and Psychiatric Implications" A. F. (Schatzberg, and C. B. Nemeroff, eds.), pp. 155–169. Raven Press, New York.

Schteingart, D. E., Conn, J. W., Orth, D. N., Harrison, T. S., Fox, J. E., Bookstein, J. J. (1972). Secretion of ACTH and β-MSH by an adrenal paraganglioma. *J. Clin. Endocrinol. Metab.* **34**, 676.

Seggie, J. (1980). Amygdala lesions and 24 hour variation in plasma corticosterone, growth hormone and prolactin levels. *Can. J. Physiol. Pharmacol.* **58**, 249–253.

Sharp, B., and Sowers, J. R. (1983). Adrenocortical response to Corticotropin is inhibited by gamma-MSH antisera in normotensive and spontaneously hypertensive rats. *Biochem. Biophys. Res. Commun.* **110**, 357.

Slusher, M. A., and Hyde, J. E. (1961). Effect of limbic stimulation on release of corticosteroids into adrenal venous effluent of the cat. *Endocrinology (Baltimore)* **69**, 1080–1084.

Soliman, K. F. A. (1982). Peripheral regulation of the glucocorticoids diurnal rhythm. *In* "Towards Chrono Pharmacology" (R. Takaboshi *et al.*, eds.), p. 235. Pergamon, London.

Vale, W., Spiess, J., Rivier, C., and Rivier, J. (1981). Characterization of a 41-residue ovine hypothalamic peptide that stimulates secretion of ACTH and β-endorphin. *Science* **213**, 1394.

3

Amygdala: Role in Autonomic and Neuroendocrine Responses to Stress

Thackery S. Gray

Department of Anatomy
Loyola University Stritch School of Medicine
Maywood, Illinois 60153

I. Introduction

The purpose of this chapter is to review the various neurobiological studies that provide evidence for a role of the amygdala in autonomic and neuroendocrine responses to stress. Prevailing scientific literature indicates that the amygdala is involved in many behavioral functions including defensive, reproductive, and ingestive behaviors as well as other adaptive behaviors that serve to promote the survival of the organism. However, this chapter is not intended to be comprehensive and will concentrate on reviewing literature that establishes relationships between the amygdala, neurotransmitters, and anatomical circuitry that are important in the mediation of stress and related pathologies. Experimental and clinical experiments available in the literature and data published by the author will be discussed. Several more complete reviews on the amygdala have been recently published (LeDoux, 1987; Price *et al.*, 1987; Sarter and Markowitsch, 1985).

II. Anatomical and Functional Studies

The amygdala is an anatomically defined region within the temporal lobes of mammals including humans. The amygdala is an important component of the limbic system and as such is considered a pivotal region for mediating the perception and the expression of fear and anxiety. Anatomically the limbic system is composed primarily of diencephalic and telencephalic structures that provide an interface between the neocortex and regions within the brainstem and spinal cord that control somatomotor, visceromotor, and neuroendocrine systems. Figure 1 schematically presents the anatomic relationships between the amygdala, forebrain, limbic system, and brainstem–spinal cord. The amygdala is special among limbic structures in that it has direct anatomic connections with neocortex, hypothalamic neuroendocrine cells, and preganglionic autonomic regions of the brainstem. Thus, based on anatomic evidence the amygdala may contribute the final common pathways for limbic-system-mediated somatomotor and visceromotor adjustment to environmental changes. It should be noted that amygdaloid projections to brainstem autonomic regions (i.e., areas related to preganglionic autonomic neurons) originate mainly from one part of the amygdala, the central nucleus. Most studies on autonomic and neuroendocrine functions of the amygdala have focused on the central amygdaloid nucleus.

A wealth of data from behavioral and physiological studies indicate that the amygdala is important for the mediation of normal responses to fear-evoking or anxiety-producing stimuli. Electrical stimulation of the amygdala in conscious human subjects elicits fully integrated experiences of fear and anxiety (Chapman *et al.*, 1954; Gloor, 1986). Compared to other stimulation sites within the brain, the perceptions of fear following amygdaloid stimulation are strikingly realistic and are usually associated with spe-

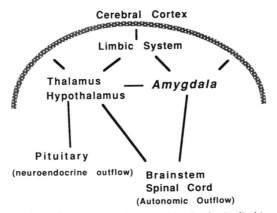

Figure 1   Anatomic relationships between the amygdala, forebrain, limbic system, and brainstem–spinal cord.

cific stimuli or events encountered in the past. Accompanying stimulation-induced fear are autonomic changes including increases in heart rate and blood pressure, pupillary dilatation, and pallor, as well as appropriate facial expressions. Similar responses have been observed following stimulation of the amygdala in conscious animals. Electrical stimulation of the amygdala in awake animals causes increases in heart rate, blood pressure, and respiratory responses that occur during fearful and anxious behavior. This constellation of somato- and visceromotor changes is often characterized as the "defense response" (Kaada, 1972; Hilton and Zbrozyna, 1963; Stock *et al.*, 1981; Galeno and Brody, 1983; Iwata *et al.*, 1987; Harper *et al.*, 1984). It is important that amygdaloid stimulation occur in a conscious animal, because increases in cardiovascular parameters are attenuated or are not observed when animals are anesthetized or asleep (Harper *et al.*, 1984; Galeno and Brody, 1983).

Fear or anxiety that is associated with real or perceived threat constitutes psychological stress. This "stress" or so-called defense response is composed of a set of relatively well-defined biological changes as described above. These changes help to promote the readiness and execution of behaviors that will ultimately increase the probability of survival of the organism. Thus, these alterations in the cardiovascular, respiratory, and other visceral systems are adaptive in nature and have a strong learned component to them. Destruction of the amygdala markedly affects various measures of fear/anxiety and blunts learned visceral/somatomotor responses to fear-provoking stimuli. It has been known since the classical work of Kluver and Bucy (1939) that amygdaloid lesions markedly reduce emotional responsiveness. More localized amygdaloid lesion studies indicate that a specific part of the amygdala, the central nucleus, is important for mediation of autonomic changes associated with stress. Bilateral ablation of the central amygdaloid nucleus attenuates learned heart-rate responses in rabbits (Kapp *et al.*, 1985). Cryogenic treatment of the central amygdaloid nucleus blocked learned blood pressure and respiratory response in the cat (Zhang *et al.* 1986). In rats, lesions of the central amygdala impede increases in heart rate and blood pressure that occur to a tone associated with shock (Iwata *et al.*, 1986). The increases in heart rate and blood pressure to the shock alone were unaffected by amygdaloid lesions. Destruction of the central amygdala in rats also reduced stimulus-induced exaggerated increases in cardiovascular responses (Folkow *et al.*, 1982; Galeno *et al.*, 1982). Lesions of the central amygdala also reduced defecation associated with a tone that signals shock (Vanderwolf *et al.*, 1986). The amygdala probably does not function in normal homeostatic functions as it is not active during sleep or anesthetic states. In addition, the amygdala is not necessary for mediation of cardiovascular response to physical stressors. Rather, the amygdala probably functions to alter basal autonomic activity during responses to threatening or anxiety-provoking stimuli. Finally, a high density of benzodiazepine receptors has been localized within the amygdala, suggesting it is an important site for anxiolytic drug actions (Niehoff and Kuhar, 1983). The benzodiazepine receptors are localized within the basolateral amygdaloid nucleus, an important intraamygdaloid input to the central amygdaloid nucleus.

III. Amygdala and Peptides

A majority of the peptides that have been localized with neurons of the brain are found within either neuronal cells bodies or terminals of the amygdala. Table I summarizes the neuropeptides and their localization within cell bodies and/or terminals within the rat central nucleus of the amygdala (cf. Price *et al.*, 1987; Gray, 1989).

The main output neurons of the amygdala are corticotropin-releasing factor, neurotensin, somatostatin, galanin, and substance P (Gray, 1989; Gray and Magnuson, 1987a,b; Milner and Pickel, 1986; Moga and Gray, 1985; Moga *et al.*, 1989; Veening *et al.*, 1984). Table II summarizes the organization of peptide efferent and afferent pathways. Amygdaloid peptide-containing cells project mainly to the brainstem, although hypothalamic projections have been also reported (Sakanaka *et al.*, 1981). Most, if not all, peptidergic cell types innervate the bed nucleus of the stria terminalis (cf. Gray, 1989). Enkephalin neurons participate in a reciprocal pathway between the central nucleus of the amygdala and lateral part of the bed nucleus of the stria terminalis (Uhl *et al.*, 1978; Palkovits *et al.*, 1981). The presently identified brainstem targets are the midbrain central

Table I

Amygdala Peptide-Containing Cell Bodies and Terminals

Cell bodies and terminals	Mainly terminals
Corticotropin-releasing factor	Angiotensin II
Dynorphin	Atriopeptin
Enkephalin	Bombesin
Galanin	Cholecystokinin
Neurotensin	Calcitonin gene-related peptide
Somatostatin	Neuropeptide Y
Substance P	Pro-opiomelanocortins
	Thyrotropin-releasing factor
	Vasoactive intestinal polypeptide

grey, the parabrachial nuclei, and the dorsal vagal complex. A somatostatin input to the A8 catecholamine group has been identified (Deutch *et al.*, 1988).

Peptidergic axonal inputs to the amygdala are numerous and arise from many different regions. Unlike the peptidergic outputs of the amygdala, some peptidergic terminal inputs show clear single source specificity. For example, calcitonin gene-related peptide terminals arise exclusively from cells within the parabrachial nucleus (Schwaber *et al.*, 1988; Yamano *et al.*, 1988), and cholecystokinin terminals come from cells within the region of the substantia nigra (Hökfelt *et al.*, 1980). Many peptide inputs originate from multiple regions. Neurotensin and enkephalin terminals are provided by cells within the parabrachial nucleus and nucleus of the solitary tract (Block *et al.*, 1989; Zardetto-Smith and Gray, 1986).

There is some evidence of coexistence of peptides or monamines within cell bodies and/or terminals of the amygdala. Enkephalin and gamma-aminobutyric acid (GABA) coexist within the cells of the amygdala (Oertel *et al.*, 1983). Cholecystokinin and dopamine terminals of the amygdala originate in part from the same neurons within the substantia nigra (Hökfelt *et al.*, 1980). Substance P and calcitonin gene-related peptide coexist within parabrachial cells and probably axons that project to the amygdala (Yamano *et al.*, 1988). Other monoaminergic inputs include serotonin

Table II
Amygdaloid Peptide Neuronal Outputs and Inputs

Outputs	Inputs
Bed nucleus of the stria terminalis	Hypothalamus
A8 Dopaminergic cell group	Dynorphin (lateral hypothalmus)
Midbrain central gray	Pro-opiomelanocortin (arcuate
	nucleus)
Parabrachial region	Substantia nigra/ventral tegmental area
Nucleus of the solitary tract	Cholecystokinin
Medullary reticular formation	Dynorphin
Corticotropin-releasing factor	Midbrain central grey/raphé nuclei
Neurotensin	Vasoactive intestinal polypeptide
Somatostatin	Parabrachial nucleus
Galanin	Enkephalin
Substance P	Calcitonin gene-related peptide
	Neurotensin
	Substance P
	Nucleus of the solitary tract
	Neuropeptide Y
	Enkephalin
	Neurotensin

from the raphe nuclei (Fallon, 1981), noradrenaline from locus coeruleus (Fallon, 1981), and noradrenaline/adrenaline from the dorsal and ventrolateral medulla (Fallon, 1981; Zardetto-Smith and Gray, 1988). It is likely that many of these monoaminergic inputs also contain neuropeptides. For example, vasoactive intestinal polypeptide arises from cells of the dorsal raphe region (Marley *et al.*, 1981).

From these data it is apparent that the function of neuropeptides within the pathways of the amygdala is quite complicated. The output neurons appear to project in a more generalized fashion in that multiple targets tend to receive the same peptidergic inputs. The differential effects of these peptides on their target regions could form the substrates for differential activation of components of the defense response. One possibility is that different target regions of the amygdala mediate different components of responses to aversive stimuli. Experimental lesions of the midbrain central gray will abolish freezing responses to a tone that signals electric shock in rats (Liebman *et al.*, 1970; LeDoux *et al.*, 1988). However, ablation of the central gray will not affect the cardiovascular response to the tone (LeDoux *et al.*, 1988). Destruction of cells within the lateral hypothalamus will affect the cardiovascular response to the tone, but not the freezing response. This suggests that the stress or defense response may be differentially organized by target regions of amygdaloid neurons. However, it should be noted that integrated defense responses have been elicited by stimulation of amygdaloid pathways from the amygdala through the hypothalamus and into the central gray (Hilton and Zbrozyna, 1963). The neurochemical inputs to the amygdala and their possible function are even more complicated than the outputs. However, modulation of the amygdaloid functions by other brain regions can be to some degree coded according to peptide type, its source, and whether it coexists with another putative neurotransmitter. For example, as noted above, calcitonin gene-related peptide arises only from cells within the parabrachial region. Injections of calcitonin gene-related peptide within the amygdala results in increases in heart rate, blood pressure, and plasma catecholamines (Nguyen *et al.*, 1986; Brown and Gray, 1988). This suggests that the parabrachial nucleus calcitonin gene-related peptide pathway to the amygdala acts to promote the amygdala-mediated autonomic components of the stress response. Thyrotropin-releasing factor injections into the amygdala also increase heart rate, blood pressure, and plasma catecholamine levels, but bombesin, somatostatin, and angiotensin II only increase blood pressure (Brown and Gray, 1988). The source of these latter peptidergic terminals is unknown; however, it is likely that they are of hypothalamic and/or brainstem origin.

Neuropeptides have also been localized within neurons of the human amygdala. The peptides identified within human amygdala include neurotensin, substance P, cholecystokinin, neuropeptide Y, vasoactive intestinal polypeptide, met-enkephalin, and somatostatin (Roberts *et al.*, 1983; Michel *et al.*, 1986; Zech *et al.*, 1986). Zech *et al.* (1986) examined the amygdala of controls, schizophrenics, and patients that had suffered from Huntington's chorea. There were no striking differences in peptide immunoreactivity between normal and schizophrenic brain specimens, although vasoactive intestinal polypeptide immunoreactivity was slightly increased in the central amygdaloid nucleus of schizophrenic patients. In the Huntington's chorea brain specimens the amygdala exhibited significant atrophy and reduced peptide immunoreactivity.

IV. Amygdala and Catecholamines

A relationship between stress and the release of central and peripheral catecholamines is well established in that there is considerable evidence that noradrenergic, adrenergic, and dopaminergic brain cells are involved in responses to stress (Dunn and Kramarcy, 1984; Tilders and Berkenbosch, 1986). Indeed, stimulation of the locus ceruleus produces a cardiovascular response similar to amygdaloid stimulation (Stock *et al.*, 1981). Cells that produce catecholamines are distributed throughout the brainstem in designated groups (for recent map, see Hökfelt *et al.*, 1984). Generally, dopamine is found within the midbrain (A8–10 cell groups), noradrenaline within the pons (A4–6 cell groups) and to a lesser extent within the medulla (A1, A2 cell groups), and adrenaline within the medulla (C1, C2 cell groups). Recent data in our laboratory indicate that the amygdala innervates relatively specific subsets of brainstem catecholaminergic cells (Wallace *et al.*, 1989). Amygdaloid neurons heavily innervate a continuum of dopaminergic cells that extend from lateral substantia nigra (A9) into the retrorubral field (A8). In the pons, amygdaloid terminals were found on noradrenergic cells within rostral portions of the locus ceruleus (A6). Adrenergic cells within the nucleus of the solitary tract and ventrolateral medulla also were associated with amygdaloid terminals. Noradrenergic cells within the caudal part of the nucleus of the solitary tract were also innervated by the amygdala. Areas that did not receive many amygdaloid terminals included dopaminergic cells of the ventral tegmental area (A10) and more medial parts of the substantia nigra, the main body of the locus ceruleus, the subceruleus, and the Kolliker–Fuse nucleus. Amygdaloid terminals were not observed contacting cells of the A5 catecholamine group and the noradrenergic cells of the caudal ventrolateral medulla.

Thus, the amygdala can selectively affect the activity of specific dopaminergic cells of the midbrain, the rostral locus ceruleus, and noradrenergic/

adrenergic cells of the medulla. The functions of these pathways are not clear, but we can speculate based on the postulated function of these catecholaminergic cell groups. The dopaminergic cells of the midbrain contribute fibers to the mesostriatal pathway and the mesolimbocortical pathway (Deutch *et al.*, 1988; cf. Hökfelt *et al.*, 1984). Both the mesostriatal and mesolimbocortical systems have postulated roles during stress. The mesolimbocortical pathway projects back to the amygdala and is thought to be important in the maintenance of gastric mucosal integrity in the presence of stressors (Ray *et al.*, 1988). The protective effect of dopamine may be related to amygdaloid neuronal processing of reward-related behaviors (Nakano *et al.*, 1987). There is also an important interaction in terms of stress-induced gastric pathology and thyrotropin-releasing hormone (TRH), neurotensin, and dopamine within the amygdala (Henke *et al.*, 1988). The amygdala may also be affecting other regions of the limbic system through its projections to the midbrain dopaminergic cell groups. Various types of stressors elevate dopamine levels within the prefrontal cortex, presumably through activation of the mesolimbocortical dopaminergic system (Deutch *et al.*, 1989; Dunn and Kramarcy, 1984). The amygdala could be partially responsible for cortical release of dopamine. In addition, the mesostriatal pathway is involved in the central control of thermoregulation by its action upon heat dissipation mechanisms (Lee *et al.*, 1985). Perhaps this could be related to temperature changes observed during stress.

As stated above, the rostral part of the locus ceruleus noradrenergic cell group was also innervated by the amygdala. Intermittent electrical stimulation of the amygdala over a period of 3–4 hr in cats will repeatedly produce the defense response and will also reduce overall levels of cerebral noradrenaline (Reis and Gunne, 1965). It is the rostral part of the locus ceruleus that projects back upon the amygdala, hypothalamus, and limbic system (Loughlin *et al.*, 1986). Stimulation of the amygdala causes an increase in plasma noradrenaline (Brown and Gray, 1988). Given these findings, it is not surprising that there is a close temporal relationship between the release of noradrenaline within the amygdala and plasma increases of noradrenaline (Dietl, 1985). This pathway could function to further facilitate or inhibit limbic system activity. For example, injection of α_2-adrenergic receptor agonists into the central amygdala of rats prevents air stress from increasing renal nerve activity (Koepke *et al.*, 1987). This treatment did not inhibit increases of blood pressure that are normally observed in response to noise stress. Injections of beta-adrenoreceptor antagonists into the amygdala did not affect renal nerve activity or blood pressure increases. In contrast, administration of beta-adrenoreceptor antagonists into the amygdala does block learned cardiovascular responses to aversive stimuli in rabbits (Kapp *et al.*, 1985). Perhaps cardiovascular and sympathetic modulation may be organized separately depending on differential receptor activation of peptidergic neurons within the amygdala. The exact mechanisms by which this could occur are unclear. However, disruption of the noradrenergic input to the amygdala alters neurotensin immunoreactivity with the cell bodies of the amygdaloid central nucleus (Kawakami et al., 1984). This could occur through differential receptor activation of amygdaloid peptide-producing neurons.

Adrenergic C2 and noradrenergic A2 cell groups of the nucleus of the solitary tract (NTS) were frequently contacted by amygdaloid axons (Wallace et al., 1989). Stimulation of the central nucleus of the amygdala attenuates the baroreceptor reflex (Stock et al., 1981), and adrenaline and noradrenaline administration within the NTS decreases the activity of neurons that activate the baroreceptor reflex (Felman and Moises, 1987; Saavedra et al., 1983). Via this mechanism amygdaloid neurons could effect local release of adrenaline and/or noradrenaline within the NTS, which would have an inhibitory action on the baroreceptive modulating neurons. This postulated baroreceptor reflex inhibition could account for amygdaloid stimulation-induced hypertensive responses.

V. Amygdala and Neuroendocrine Responses

Stimulation of the amygdala in a variety of animal species alters corticosterone and/or other neuroendocrine-related hormones (Kaada, 1972; Hayward, 1972). Plasma corticosterone or ACTH levels are altered following electrical stimulation of the amygdala in awake rats and cats (Dunn and Whitener, 1986; Matheson et al., 1971; Redgate and Fahringer, 1973). Increases and decreases in corticosterone responses have been observed, although corticomedial amygdaloid stimulation increases corticosterone levels in alert animals (Matheson et al., 1971; Redgate and Fahringer, 1973). Amygdala ablations inhibit adrenocortical responses to stress-inducing somatosensory and olfactory stimuli (Feldman and Conforti, 1981). Lesions of the amygdala also reduce compensatory hypersecretion of ACTH seen after adrenalectomy (Allen and Allen, 1974). More current lesion studies of the amygdala have identified the importance of the central amygdaloid nucleus in the mediation of ACTH release. Central amygdaloid nucleus destruction significantly attenuated ACTH responses to immobilization stress (Beaulieu et al., 1987), although baseline secretion of ACTH is unaffected. Ablations of the central nucleus increased the serotonergic activity within the hypothalamus and the amygdala (Beaulieu et al., 1987). This finding is of interest because studies have emphasized the importance of the serotonergic system in the delayed negative feedback actions of glucocorticoid feedback to the ACTH-stimulating parts of the hypothalamus (cf. Beaulieu *et al.*, 1987). Possibly the removal of the central nucleus and the subsequent effect upon the serotonergic neurons could account for the attenuated ACTH hypersecretion observed after adrenalectomy (Allen and Allen, 1974).

The anatomical pathways by which the amygdala can affect hypothalamic neuroendocrine output have not been identified with certainty. There are at least three routes by which the amygdala can communicate with hypothalamic cells that affect pituitary function. One route is a direct projection to the medial and lateral parvocellular parts of the paraventricular hypothalamic nucleus (PVN) (Gray *et al.*, 1989; Magnuson and Gray 1988). Amygdaloid axons appear to directly contact CRF-, vasopressin-, and oxytocin-containing cells. However, this pathway is relatively sparse compared to an indirect projection to the bed nucleus of the stria terminalis, which in turn projects massively into the PVN and with terminals contacting both magnocellular and parvocellular neurons (Swanson, 1987; Magnuson and Gray, 1989). A last group of pathways by which the amygdala can affect neuroendocrine output is through its projections to the brainstem, which in turn project back upon the hypothalamus (Van Der Kooy *et al.*, 1984).

VI. Summary and Conclusions

Over 10 years ago Gloor (1978) proposed a model for how the amygdala functions in relationship to the limbic system and related brain regions. Figure 2 schematically illustrates an extended version of this model. Cortical and thalamic inputs to the amygdala probably convey input on the sensory properties of a stimulus. The significance (i.e., threatening or nonthreatening) of the stimulus may be coded via interactions through associated neural circuitry (e.g., cortex, thalamus, and hippocampus) and/or within amygdala itself. The amygdala activates appropriate regions of the hypothalamus, other limbic regions, and the brainstem. The mechanisms through which this occurs most likely involve activation of multiple peptidergic and monoaminergic systems as well as other neurotransmitter systems.

Feedback from the brainstem probably reflects summation of visceral sensory input and descending forebrain influences. This input could function to reduce or increase amygdaloid activity. For example, input to the amygdala could augment or attenuate the emotional perception of the threatening circumstances, depending on the function of the particular neural circuitry and the anxiety or arousal state of the animal. It is likely that altered visceral functions are detected by people at conscious and uncon-

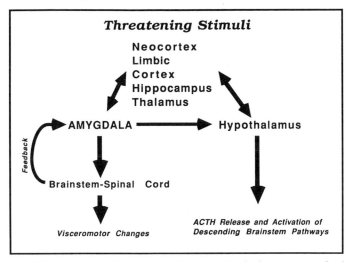

Figure 2   Model of amygdala functions in relation to the limbic system and related brain regions.

scious levels. Consciously, visceral changes are perceived (e.g., "twisted feelings in the gut") and permit us to define the seriousness of the threat or stressor that confronts us. Within the central nervous system the visceral feedback contributes to the formation of an "emotional or affective" significance to the threatening stimulus (i.e., learning). In addition, reflexes occur in an attempt to maintain autonomic homeostasis. For example, the baroreceptor reflex serves to maintain heart rate and blood pressure at a relatively steady state. Amygdaloid activity normally overrides this reflex, but as amygdaloid activity is reduced, the baroreceptor reflex may serve to further return amygdaloid as well as brainstem activity to normal basal levels.

Thus, the amygdala is important for learned visceral, somatic, and neuroendocrine responses to environmental stressors. It is not surprising that the studies have demonstrated the amygdala's importance in the expression of a variety of animal models of "stress-related" pathologies. Chronic stimulation of the amygdala produces gastric ulcers (cf. Henke, 1988). Bilateral ablations of the central amygdala reduce the incidence and severity of immobilization stress-induced ulcers in rats (Henke, 1988). The amygdala has been implicated in the development and/or expression of hypertension in the the spontaneously hypertensive rat (Folkow *et al.*, 1982; Galeno *et al.*, 1982). Lesions of the amygdala slow the development of hypertension in spontaneously hypertensive rats (Folkow *et al.*, 1982; Galeno *et al.*, 1982). Amygdaloid removal also attenuates the exaggerated hemodynamic response to stress that is typically observed in adult hypertensive rats (Folkow *et al.*, 1982). A subregion of the amygdala called the central nucleus is particularly important in this regard. However, it is apparent that the amygdala is only one important interactive region and must be studied in the context of its neural connections with the hypothalamus and brainstem. Additional studies are needed to focus on the interactions of peptides and neural circuitry with the more established neurotransmitter candidates such as the catecholamines, serotonin, GABA, and acetylcholine.

Acknowledgments

The author thanks Debra J. Magnuson for her helpful criticism and excellent technical assistance. The author's work described in this chapter was supported by NIH grant NS 20041 and a grant from the Office of Naval Research, ONR 4414809.

References

Allen, J. P., and Allen, C. F. (1974). Role of amygdaloid complexes in the stress-induced release of ACTH in the rat. *Neuroendocrinology* 15, 220–230.

Beaulieu, S., Di Paolo, T., and Barden, N. (1986). Control of ACTH secretion by the central nucleus of the amygdala: Implication of the serotonergic system and its relevance to the glucocorticoid delayed feedback mechanism. *Neuroendocrinology* 44, 247–254.

Beaulieu, S., Di Paolo, T., Cote, J., and Barden, N. (1987). Participation of the central amygdaloid nucleus in the response of adrenocorticotropin (ACTH) secretion to immobilization stress: Opposing roles of the noradrenergic and dopaminergic systems. *Neuroendocrinology* 45, 37–46.

Beaulieu, S., Peletier, G., Vaudry, H., and Barden, N. (1989). Influence of the central nucleus of the amygdala on the content of corticotropin-releasing factor in the median eminence. *Neuroendocrinology* 49, 255–261.

Block, C. H., Hoffman, G., and Kapp, B. S. (1989). Peptide containing pathways from the parabrachial complex to the central nucleus of the amygdala. *Peptides (N.Y.)* 10, 465–471.

Brown, M. R., and Gray, T. S. (1988). Peptide injections into the amygdala of conscious rats: Effects on blood pressure, heart rate and plasma catecholamines. *Regul. Pept.* 21, 95–10.

Chapman, W. P., Schroeder, H. R., Geyer, G., Brazier, M. A. B., Fager, C., Poppen, J. L., Solomon, H. C., and Yakovlev, P. I. (1954). Physiological evidence concerning importance of the amygdaloid nuclear region in the integration of circulatory function in man. *Science* 120, 949–950.

Deutch, A. Y., Bean, A. J., and Roth, R. H. (1988). Regulation of A8 dopamine neurons by somatostatin. *Eur. J. Pharmacol.* 147, 317–320.

Deutch, A. Y., Goldstein, M., Baldino, F. B., Jr., and Roth, R. H. (1988). Telencephalic projections of the A8 dopamine cell group. *In* "The Mesocorticolimbic Dopamine System" (P. W. Kalivas and C. B. Nemeroff, eds), pp. 27–50. *Ann. N. Y. Acad. Sci.,* New York.

Dietl, H. (1985). Temporal relationship between noradrenaline release in the central amygdala and plasma noradrenaline secretion in rats and tree shrews. *Neurosci. Lett.* **55**, 41–46.

Dunn, A. J., and Kramarcy, M. R. (1984). Neurochemical responses during stress: Relationships between the hypothalamic-pituitary-adrenal and catecholamine systems. *In* "Handbook of Psychopharmacology" (L. I. Iversen, S. D. Iversen, and S. H. Snyder, eds.), Vol. 18, pp. 455–515. Plenum, New York.

Dunn, J. D., and Whitener, J. (1986). Plasma corticosterone responses to electrical stimulation of the amygdaloid complex: Cytoarchitectural specificity. *Neuroendocrinology* **42**, 211–217.

Fallon, J. H. (1981). Histochemical characterization of dopaminergic, noradrenergic and serotonergic projections to the amygdala. *In* "The Amygdaloid Complex" (Y. Ben-Ari, ed.), pp. 175–184. Elsevier North-Holland, Amsterdam.

Feldman, S., and Conforti, N. (1981). Amygdalectomy inhibits adrenocorticotropin responses to somatosensory and olfactory stimulation. *Neuroendocrinology* **5**, 1323–1329.

Felman, P. D., and Moises, H. C. (1987). Adrenergic responses of baroreceptor cells in the nucleus tractus solitarii of the rat: A microiontophoretic study. *Brain Res.* **420**, 351–361.

Folkow, B., Hallback-Norlander, M., Martner, J., and Nordborg, C. (1982). Influence of amygdala lesions on cardiovascular responses to alerting stimuli, on behaviour and on blood pressure development in spontaneously hypertensive rats. *Acta Physiol. Scand.* **116**, 133–139.

Galeno, T. M., and Brody, M. J. (1983). Hemodynamic responses to amygdaloid stimulation in spontaneously hypertensive rats. *Am. J. Physiol.* **245**, R281-R286.

Galeno, T. M., Van Hoesen, B. W., Maixner, W., Johnson, A. K., and Brody, M. J. (1982). Contribution of the amygdala to the development of spontaneous hypertension. *Brain Res.* **246**, 1–6.

Gloor, P. (1978). Inputs and outputs of the amygdala: What the amygdala is trying to tell the rest of the brain. *In* "Limbic Mechanisms. The Continuing Evolution of the Limbic System Concept," (K. E. Livingston and O. Hornykiewicz, eds.) pp. 189–209. Plenum, New York.

Gloor, P. (1986). Role of the human limbic system in perception, memory, and affect: Lessons from temporal lobe epilepsy. *In* "The Limbic System: Functional Organization and Clinical Disorders (B. K. Doan and K. E. Livingston, eds.), pp. 159–169. Raven Press, New York.

Gray, T. S. (1989). Autonomic neuropeptide connections of the amygdala. *In* Neuropeptides and Stress: (Y. Tache, J. E. Morley, and M. R. Brown, eds.), pp. 92–106. Springer-Verlag, New York.

Gray, T. S., and Magnuson, D. J. (1987a). Galanin-immunoreactive neurons in amygdala and hypothalamus innervate the midbrain central gray in rat. *Neurosc. Lett.* **83**, 163–166.

Gray, T. S., and Magnuson, D. J. (1987b). Neuropeptide neuronal efferents from the bed nucleus of the stria terminalis and central amygdaloid nucleus to the dorsal vagal complex in the rat. *J. Comp. Neurol.* **262**, 365–374.

Gray, T. S., Carney, M. E., and Magnuson, D. J. (1989). Direct projections from the central amygdaloid nucleus to the hypothalamic paraventricular nucleus: Possible role in stress-induced ACTH release. *Neuroendocrinology* **50**, 433–446.

Harper, R. M., Frysinger, R. C., Trelease, R. B., and Marks, J. D. (1984). State dependent alteration of respiratory cycle timing by stimulation of the central nucleus of amygdala. *Brain Res.* **306**, 1–8.

Hayward, J. N. (1972). The amygdaloid nuclear complex and mechanisms of release of vasopressin from the neurohypophysis. *In* "The Neurobiology of the Amygdala" (B. E. Eleuthériou, ed.), pp. 685–740. Plenum, New York.

Henke, P. G. (1988). Recent studies of the central nucleus of the amygdala and stress ulcers. *Neurosci. Biobehav. Rev.* **12**, 143–150.

Henke, P. G., Sullivan, R. M., and Ray, A. (1988). Interactions of thyrotropin-releasing hormone (TRH) with neurotensin and dopamine in the central nucleus of the amygdala during stress ulcer formation in rats. *Neuroscience Lett.* **91**, 95–100.

Hilton, S. B., and Zbrozyna, A. W. (1963), Amygdaloid region for defense reaction and its efferents pathway to the brain stem. *J. Physiol. (London)* **165**, 106–184.

Hökfelt, T., Skirboll, L., Rehfeld, J. F., Goldstein, M., Markey, K., and Dann, O. (1980). A subpopulation of mesencephalic dopamine neurons projecting to limbic areas contains a cholecystokinin-like peptide: Evidence from immunohistochemistry combined with retrograde tracing. *Neuroscience* **5**, 2093–2124.

Hökfelt, T., Martensson, R., Bjorklund, A., Kleinau, S., and Goldstein, M., (1984). Distributional maps of tyrosine hydroxylase-immunoreactive neurons in the rat brain. *In* "Handbook of Chemical Neuroanatomy" (A. Bjorklund and T. Hökfelt, eds.), Vol.2, Part I, pp. 277–379. Am. Elsevier, New York.

Iwata, J., LeDoux, J., Meeley, M. P., Arneric, S., and Reis, D. J. (1986). Intrinsic neurons in the amygdaloid field projected to by the medial geniculate body mediate emotional responses conditioned to acoustic stimuli. *Brain Res.* **383**, 195–214.

Iwata, J., Chida, K., and LeDoux, J. E. (1987). Cardiovascular responses elicited by stimulation of neurons in the central nucleus of amygdala in awake, but not anesthetized rats, resemble conditioned emotional responses. *Brain Res.* **418**, 183–188.

Kaada, B. R. (1972). Stimulation and regional ablation of the amygdaloid complex with reference to functional representations. *In* "The Neurobiology of the Amygdala" (B. E. Eleforiou, ed.), pp. 205–281. Plenum, New York.

Kapp, B. S., Pascoe, J. P., and Bixler, M. A. (1985). The amygdala: A neuroanatomical systems approach to its contribution to aversive conditioning. *In* "The Neuropsychology of Memory" (N. Butters and L. Squire, eds.), pp. 473–488. Guilford Press, New York.

Kawakami, F., Fukui, K., Okamura H., Morimoto N., Yanaihara, N., Nakajima, T., and Ibata, Y. (1984). Influence of ascending noradrenergic fibers on the neurotensin-like immunoreactive perikarya and evidence of direct projection of ascending neurotensin-like immunoreactive fibers in the rat. *Neurosci. Lett.* **51**, 231–234.

Kluver, H., and Bucy, P. C. (1939). Preliminary analysis of functions of the temporal lobe in monkeys. *Arch. Neurol. Psychiatry* **42**, 979–1000.

Koepke, J. P., Jones, S., and DiBona, G. F. (1987). α_2-Adrenoreceptors in amygdala control renal sympathetic nerve activity and renal function in conscious spontaneously hypertensive rat. *Brain Res.* **404**, 80–88.

LeDoux, J. E. (1987). Emotion. *In* "Handbook of Physiology" (F. Plum, ed), Sect. 5 Chapter 10, pp. 419–459. Waverly press, Baltimore, Maryland.

LeDoux, J. E., Iwata, J., Cicchetti, P., and Reis, D. J. (1988). Different projections of the central amygdaloid nucleus mediate autonomic and behavioral correlates of conditioned fear. *J. Neurosci.* **8**, 2517–2529.

Lee, T. F., Mora, F., and Myers, R. D. (1985). Dopamine and thermoregulation: An evaluation with special reference to dopaminergic pathways. *Neurosci. Biobehav. Rev.* **9**, 589–598.

Liebman, J., Mayer, D. J., and Liebsekin, J. C. (1970). Mesencephalic central grey lesions and few-motivated behavior in rats. *Brain Res.* **23**, 353–370.

Loughlin, S. E., Foote, S. L., and Grzanna, R. (1986). Efferent projections of nucleus locus coeruleus: Morphologcial subpopulations have different efferent targets. *Neuroscience* **18**, 307–319.

Magnuson, D. J., and Gray, T. S. (1988). Amygdala directly innervates parvocellular paraventricular hypothalamic CRF, vasopressin and oxytocin containing cells. *Soc. Neurosci. Abstr.* **14**, 1288.

Magnuson, D. J., and Gray, T. S. (1989). Bed nucleus of the stria terminalis directly innervates parvocellular paraventricular hypothalamic CRF, vasopressin and oxytocin containing cells. *Soc. Neurosci. Abstr.* **15**:135.

Marley, P. D., Emson, P. C., Hunt, S. P., and Fahrenkrug, J. (1981). A long ascending projection in the rat brain containing vasoactive intestinal polypeptide. *Neurosci. Lett.* **27**, 261–266.

Matheson, B. K., Branch, B. J., and Taylor, A. N. (1971). Effects of amygdaloid stimulation on pituitary-adrenal activity in conscious cats. *Brain Res.* **32**, 151–167.

Michel, J.-P., Sakanoto, N., Kopp, N., and Pearson, J. (1986). Neurotensin immunoreactive structures in the human infant striatum, septum, amygdala and cerebral cortex. *Brain Res.* **397**, 93–102.

Milner, T. A., and Pickel, V. M. (1986). Ultratructural localization and afferent sources of substance P in the rat parabrachial region. *Neuroscience* **17**, 687–707.

Moga, M. M., and Gray, T. S. (1985). Evidence for corticotropin releasing factor, neurotensin and somatostatin within the neural pathway from the central nucleus of the amygdala to the parabrachial nucleus. *J. Comp. Neurol* **241**, 272–284.

Moga, M. M., Saper, C. B., and Gray, T. S. (1989). The bed nucleus of the stria terminalis: Cytoarchitecture, immunohistochemistry and projections to the parabrachial nucleus in the rat. *J. Comp. Neurol.* **283**, 315–332.

Nakano, Y., Lenard, L., Oomura, Y., Nishino, H., Aou, S., and Yamamoto, T. (1987). Functional involvement of catecholamines in reward-related neuronal activity of the monkey amygdala. *J. Neurophysiol.* **57**, 72–91.

Nguyen, K. Q., Sills, M. A., and Jacobowitz, D. M. (1986). Cardiovascular effects produced by microinjections of calcitonin gene-related peptide in the rat central amygdaloid nucleus. *Peptides (N.Y.)* **7**, 337–339.

Niehoff, D. L., and Kuhar, M. J. (1983). Benzodiazephine receptors: Localization in rat amygdala. *J. Neurosci.* **3**, 2091–2097.

Oertel, W. H., Riethmuller, G., Mugniani, E., Schemechel, E. E., Weindl, A., Gramsch, C., and Herz, A. (1983). Opioid peptide-like immunoreactivity localized in GABA-ergic neurons of the rat neostriatum and central amygdaloid nucleus. *Life Sci.* **33**, 73–76.

Palkovits, M., Epelbaum, J., and Gros, C. (1981). Met-enkephalin concentrations in individual brain nuclei of the ansa lenticularis and stria terminalis transected rats. *Brain Res.* **303**, 337–357.

Price, J. L., Russchen, F. T., and Amaral, D. G. (1987). The limbic region. II. The amygdaloid complex. *In* "Handbook of Chemical Neuroanatomy" (P. C. Emson, ed.), Vol. 5, Part I, pp. 279–388. Raven Press, New York.

Ray, A., Henke, P. G., and Sullivan, R. M. (1988). Central dopamine systems and gastric stress pathology in rats. *Physiol. Behav.* **42**, 359–364.

Redgate, E. S., and Fahringer, E. E. (1973). A comparison of the pituitary-adrenal activity elicited by electrical stimulation of preoptic, amygdaloid and hypothalamic sites in the rat brain. *Neuroendocrinology* **12**, 334–343.

Reis, D. J., and Gunne, L.-M. (1965). Brain catecholamines: Relation to the defense reaction evoked by brain stimulation in the cat. *Science* **156**, 1768–1770.

Roberts, G. W., Crow, T. J., Bloom, S. R., and Polak, J. M. (1983). Distribution of peptides in human amygdala. *Histochem. J.* **15**, Suppl. 3, 11.

Saavedra, J. M., Fernandez-Pardal, J., Torda, T., Reis, D., and Ross, C. (1983). Dissociation between rat hypothalamic and brainstem PNMT after stress and between hypothalamic catecholamines and PNMT after midbrain hemitransections. *In* "Stress: The Role of

Catecholamines and Other Neurotransmitters" (E. Usdin, E. Kvetnansky, and J. Axelrod, eds.), Vol. 1, pp. 137–146. Gordon & Breach, New York.

Sakanaka, M., Shiosaka, S., Takatsuki, K., Inagaki, S., Takagi, H., Senba, E., Kawai, Y., Matsuzaki, T., and Tohyama, M. (1981). Experimental immunohistochemical studies on the amygdalofugal peptidergic (substance P and somatostatin) fibers in the stria terminalis of the rat. *Brain Res.* **221**, 231–242.

Sarter, M., and Markowitsch, H. J. (1985). Involvement of the amygdala in learning and memory: A critical review with emphasis on anatomical relations. *Behav. Neurosci.* **99**, 342–380.

Schwaber, J. S., Sternini, C., Brecha, N. C., Rogers, W. T., and Card, J. P. (1988). Neurons containing calcitonin gene-related peptide in the parabrachial nucleus project to the central nucleus of the amygdala. *J. Comp. Neurol.* **270**, 416–426.

Shiosaka, S., Sakanaka, M., Inagaki, S., Senba, E., Hara, Y., Takatsuki, K., Takagi, H., Kawai, Y., and Tohyama, M. (1983). Putative neurotransmitters in the amygdaloid complex with special reference to peptidergic pathways. *In* "Chemical Neuroanatomy" (P. C. Emson, ed.), pp. 359–388. Raven Press, New York.

Stock, G., Rupprecht, U., Stumpf, H., and Schlor, K. H. (1981). Cardiovascular changes during arousal elicited by stimulation of amygdala, hypothalamus and locus coeruleus. *J. Auton. Nerv. Syst.* **3**, 503–510.

Svenson, T. H. (1987). Peripheral, autonomic regulation of locus coeruleus noradrenergic neurons in brain: Putative implications for psychiatry and psychopharmacology. *Psychopharmacology* **92**, 1–7.

Swanson, L. W. (1987). The hypothalamus. *In* "Handbook of Chemical Neuroanatomy" (A. Bjorklund, T. Hökfelt, and L. W. Swanson, eds), Part I, pp. 1–124. Elsevier/North-Holland Biomedical Press, Amsterdam.

Tilders, F. J. H., and Berkenbosch, F. (1986). CRF and catecholamines; their place in central and peripheral regulation of the stress response. *Acta Endocrinol. (Copenhagen)* **276**, 63–75.

Uhl, G. R., Kuhar, M. G., and Snyder, S. H. (1978). Enkephalin-containing pathway: Amygdaloid efferents in stria terminalis. *Brain Res.* **149**, 223–228.

Van Der Kooy, D., Koda, L. Y., McGinty, J. R., Gerfen, C. R., and Bloom, F. E. (1984). The organization of projections from the cortex, amygdala, and hypothalamus to the nucleus of the solitary tract in rat. *J. Comp. Neurol.* **224**, 1–24.

Vanderwolf, C. H., Kelly, M. E., Kraemer, P., and Streather, A. (1986). Are emotion and motivation localized in the limbic system and nucleus accumbens? *Behav. Brain Res.* **27**, 45–58.

Veening, J. G., Swanson, L. W., and Sawchenko, P. E. (1984). The organization of projections from the central nucleus of the amygdala to brainstem sites involved in central autonomic regulation: A combined retrograde transport-immunohistochemical study. *Brain Res.* **303**, 337–357.

Wallace, D. M., Magnuson, D. J., and Gray, T. S. (1989). The amygdalo-brainstem pathway: Selective innervation of dopaminergic, noradrenergic and adrenergic cells in the rat. *Neurosci. Lett.* **97**, 252–258.

Yamano, M., Hillyard, C. J., Girgis, S., MacIntyre, I., Emson, P. C., and Tohyama, M. (1988). Presence of a substance P-like immunoreactive neurone system from the parabrachial area to the central amygdaloid nucleus of the rat with reference to coexistence with calcitonin gene-related peptide. *Brain Res.* **451**, 179–188.

Zardetto-Smith, A. M., and Gray, T. S. (1986). Peptidergic projections from the nucleus tractus solitarius to the central nucleus of the amygdala in the rat. *Anat. Rec.* **214**, 150A.

Zardetto-Smith, A. M., and Gray, T. S. (1988). Catecholaminergic cells of the ventrolateral medulla and nucleus of the solitary tract innervate the central nucleus of the amygdala in the rat. *Soc. Neurosci. Abstr.* **14**, 1318.

Zech, M., Roberts, G. W., Bogerts, B., Crow, T. J., and Polak, J. M. (1986). Neuropeptides in the amygdala of controls, schizophrenics and patients suffering from Huntington's chorea: An immunohistochemical study. *Acta Neuropathol.* **71**, 259–266.

Zhang, J.-X., Harper, R. M., and Ni, H. (1986). Cryogenic blockade of the central nucleus of the amygdala attenuates aversively conditioned blood pressure and respiratory responses. *Brain Res.* **386**, 136–145.

Zolovick, A. J. (1972). Effects of lesions and electrical stimulation of the amygdala on hypothalamic-hypophyseal regulation. *In* "The Neurobiology of the Amygdala" (B. E. Eleftheriou, ed.), pp. 643–684. Plenum, New York.

4

Neuropeptides Involved in Stress and Their Distribution in the Mammalian Central Nervous System

Garth Bissette
Department of Psychiatry
Duke University Medical School
Durham, North Carolina 27710

Text

References

In the last decade, our understanding of the various physiological alterations that occur after exposure to stressful stimuli has significantly increased. The plethora of data generated in this period has broadened the scope of central nervous system (CNS) transmitter systems that appear to be involved in the stress response. The first neuropeptides found in the brain were thought to be primarily involved in endocrine regulation but are now known to act as neurotransmitters as well as hormones. As endocrine changes have long been associated with stressful stimuli, the involvement of CNS neuropeptides in many of the physiological and behavioral responses to stress are not surprising. A neuropeptide with consistently altered concentrations in discrete brain regions in response to a variety of stressors can be considered to play a role in the stress response. The most obvious candidates elicit some relevant physiological or behavioral response that allows survival or that facilitates a return to the relatively unstressed state. A neuropeptide that is consistently altered in regional concentration by a variety of qualitatively different stressors may be considered to participate in the stress response even though the exact physiological relevance of its alteration presently remains obscure. However, it is important to remember that not every neuropeptide that exhibits concentration changes after administration of a stressful stimulus can be assumed to play a physiological role in the stress response. The ability of certain stressors to activate non-stress-specific systems that mediate other aspects of homeostasis must also be appreciated. Thus exposure to cold stress will activate thermoregulatory mechanisms that would not necessarily be involved in the stress response to hemorrhage or electric shock. Similarly, a stress that produces pain will encompass pain-specific neuronal mechanisms during the response. This review will focus on direct alteration of CNS neuropeptide systems in response to various stressors and will not include the voluminous literature on pituitary or peripheral hormone alterations, although these may well be regulated or initiated by CNS neuropeptide release in response to stress.

The hypothalamic–pituitary–adrenal (HPA) axis has been the focus of many investigations on the physiological manifestation of the stress response since Selye's (1936) seminal description of adrenal hypertrophy and lymphatic atrophy in response to chronic stress. With the discovery of corticotropin-releasing factor (CRF) by Vale and co-workers (1981), the hypothalamic component of this axis became available for investigation. It has long been recognized that blood levels of adrenocorticotrophic hormone (ACTH) and corticosterone are increased by exposure to stress, but the ability of vasopressin to also release ACTH complicated the natural assumption that the HPA axis was responding to CRF alterations due to stress. Several surveys of hypothalamic and extrahypothalamic brain regions containing CRF have now been conducted in laboratory animals following exposure to acute or chronic stressors. The CRF that is released from the median eminence of the hypothalamus into the pituitary portal system is synthesized by neurons with cell bodies residing in the paraventricular nucleus (PVN) of the hypothalamus (Swanson et al., 1983; Bloom et al., 1982; Bugnon et al., 1982; Roth et al., 1983; Olschowka et al., 1982; Joseph and Knigge, 1983; Merchenthaler et al., 1983). Lesions of the PVN reduce median eminence CRF by 90% with a resulting 80% reduction in ACTH release after ether stress (Bruhn et al., 1984). Paraventricular nucleus neurons (Sawchenko et al., 1984a; Roth et al., 1987; Piekut and Joseph, 1986; Whitnall and Gainer, 1988) as well as axons (Whitnall et al., 1987) and vesicles of the median eminence (Whitnall et al., 1985) that coexpress CRF and vasopressin have been described.

Several studies have examined the release of CRF from the median eminence after exposure to stress. Plotsky and Vale (1984) measured CRF in hypophyseal portal plasma and reported a twofold increase in CRF 30 min after removal of 15% of the blood volume of urethane-anesthetized rats. Haas and George (1988) found that a single 5-min exposure to restraint would raise the CRF concentration of the median eminence after 24 h, but saw no other change in CRF at earlier time points, although plasma ACTH increased within 15 min of the stress. Median eminence CRF was decreased 24 h after colchicine-induced blockade of axonal transport, while colchicine administration and anisomycin inhibition of protein synthesis during restraint also resulted in decreased CRF content in the median eminence 24 h later. In contrast, our group (Chappell et al., 1986) found median eminence CRF to be significantly decreased (> 55%) after either a single, acute 3-h restraint at 4°C or a 2-week regimen of daily exposure to one of several varied stressors, which included cold swim, tail pinch, cold restraint, and ether stress.

Ixart *et al.* (1987) used push–pull cannulae implanted in the median eminence to assess the effects of ether stress on CRF release. A 13-fold increase over basal levels of CRF release was observed within 15 min of a single 2-min ether exposure. Suemaru *et al.* (1985) found that ether/laparotomy stress raised whole-hypothalamus CRF concentrations at 2.5 min with a decrease after 5 min that rebounded to prestress levels by 30 min. Cold-restraint stress reduced hypothalamic CRF at 15 min with an increase after 180 min. Medulla oblongata CRF content was decreased at 60 min by ether/laparotomy stress and at 180 min by restraint stress. Moldow *et al.* (1987) also reported decreased CRF content in whole hypothalamus 15 and 30 min after restraint stress followed by an increase at 60 min that is abolished by cyclohexamide inhibition of protein synthesis. Berkenbosch *et al.*, (1989) recently demonstrated that in laboratory animals with colchicine-induced blockade of axonal transport, both CRF and arginine vasopressin (AVP) are decreased in the median eminence after insulin-induced hypoglycemic stress. These investigators assessed CRF and AVP by both radioimmunoassay and quantitative immunocytochemistry with excellent agreement ($r = 0.99$) between these two complimentary methods. Hashimoto *et al.* (1988) observed a 40% decrease in median eminence CRF 5 min after a 1-min ether exposure. A similar CRF decrease after ether stress was observed in either naïve or chronically restrained rats. Murakami *et al.* (1989) also observed a transient increase in median eminence CRF at 2.5 min after stress induced by either ether exposure or angiotension II injection. From 5 to 20 min after the stressor, CRF content of the median eminence steadily declined. No change in CRF content was observed in midbrain, cortex, or the paraventricular nucleus at these time points.

Thus, the concatenation of these results is that the application of an acute or chronic stress induces immediate release of CRF from the median eminence with a resulting measurable decrease that is immediately masked by synthesis and subsequent transport of CRF from the paraventricular nucleus (PVN) in the first minute or two. This replenishment is eventually outstripped by continued release of CRF, resulting in decreased median eminence concentrations of CRF over the course of several hours until synthesis again is able to overcome release. This interpretation is also supported by data from Hauger *et al.* (1988) demonstrating pituitary CRF receptor down-regulation after 18 and 48 h of restraint but no change at 2.5 h. Silverman *et al.* (1989) confirmed the presence of CRF terminals impinging upon CRF-containing PVN neurons, which supports CRF as a potential modulator of its own release.

Table I

CRF Concentration of Various Rat Brain Nuclei or Regions

Brain nucleus or region	CRF concentration (pg/mg protein ± SEM)[a]
Hypothalamus	
Median eminence/arcuate nucleus	5054 ± 674
Paraventricular nucleus	498 ± 44
Periventricular nucleus	316 ± 15
Medial preoptic nucleus	142 ± 11
Lateral preoptic nucleus	86 ± 6
Anterior hypothalamic nucleus	93 ± 7
Ventromedial nucleus	97 ± 15
Dorsomedial nucleus	114 ± 7
Limbic system	
Olfactory tubercles	94 ± 7
Nucleus tractus diagonalis	64 ± 4
Lateral septal nucleus	68 ± 7
Medial septal nucleus	86 ± 9
Nucleus accumbens	94 ± 12
Bed nucleus of the stria terminalis	136 ± 14
Dorsal hippocampus	31 ± 2
Ventral hippocampus	34 ± 2
Lateral habenula	72 ± 8
Substantia innominata	98 ± 5
Cortical amygdaloid nucleus	148 ± 21
Basal amygdaloid nucleus	85 ± 3
Central amygdaloid nucleus	192 ± 17
Medial amygdaloid nucleus	110 ± 10
Lateral amygdaloid nucleus	77 ± 5
Cerebral cortex	
Medial prefrontal cortex	22 ± 1
Pyriform cortex	28 ± 2
Cingulate cortex	Not detectable
Entorhinal cortex	27 ± 3
Midbrain	
Ventral tegmental area	134 ± 11
Zona reticularis of the substantia nigra	94 ± 7
Zona compacta of the substantia nigra	190 ± 13
Pars lateralis of the substantia nigra	129 ± 7
Periaqueductal gray	144 ± 18
Pons	
Medial raphe nucleus	241 ± 18
Dorsal raphe nucleus	236 ± 28
Locus ceruleus	148 ± 9
Medulla	
Dorsal vagal complex	193 ± 15

[a]Values represent means ±SEM of micropunch dissected regions from 10 individual animals. See Chappell et al. (1986) for details.

   While the paraventricular nucleus projection to the median eminence remains the major source of brain CRF, other, extrahypothalamic CRF-staining cells have been visualized in the nucleus of the solitary tract, the locus ceruleus, ventral tegmental area, central nucleus of the amygdala, the bed nucleus of the stria terminalis, septum, diagonal band/preoptic area, and as scattered cortical interneurons (Swanson *et al.*, 1983; Petrusz *et al.*, 1985; Merchenthaler, 1984; Sakanaka *et al.*, 1987). Receptors for CRF have also been mapped and have a generally similar distribution (DeSouza, 1986). Our group (Chappell *et al.*, 1986) has measured CRF concentration in 36 brain regions during a micropunch survey (see Table I). Several of these regions exhibited alterations in CRF concentration after exposure to a single acute stress or 2 weeks of daily exposure to novel stressors (see Table II). There is obviously an anatomically heterogeneous response in regional CRF concentrations after acute and chronic stress, as seen in the significant increases in CRF concentration in the locus ceruleus (116%) after both acute and chronic stress paradigms. Chronic stress significantly increased the anterior hypothalamic (80%) and the periventricular nucleus (39%) concentrations of CRF. Chronic stress decreased the CRF content of the paraventricular nucleus (30%), but this did not reach statistical significance. Decreases in CRF in the central nucleus of the amygdala (15%) and

Table II

Acute and Chronic Stress Alterations in CRF Concentration That Correspond to CRF Neuronal Pathways

Brain region	CRF concentration (pg/mg protein)		
	Control	Acute stress[a]	Chronic stress[a]
Median eminence	5054 ± 674	2425 ± 528*	2783 ± 572*
Paraventricular nucleus	498 ± 44	478 ± 81	361 ± 45
Periventricular nucleus	316 ± 15	326 ± 16	440 ± 41*
Anterior hypothalamic nucleus	93 ± 7	132 ± 20	116 ± 11*
Medial preoptic	142 ± 11	97 ± 5*	119 ± 10
Lateral septum	68 ± 7	52 ± 5	53 ± 3
Medial septum	86 ± 9	118 ± 10	112 ± 17
Bed nucleus of the stria terminalis	136 ± 14	244 ± 52	283 ± 45
Basal nucleus of the amygdala	85 ± 3	100 ± 6	103 ± 10
Central nucleus of the amygdala	192 ± 17	166 ± 17	166 ± 19
Locus ceruleus	148 ± 9	306 ± 50*	321 ± 36*
Dorsal vagal complex	193 ± 15	150 ± 19	128 ± 11*

[a]Asterisk indicates a statistically significant difference from controls of $p \leq 0.05$. See Chappell *et al.* (1986) for details.

increases in the bed nucleus of the stria terminalis (85%) were also indicated but again did not reach statistical significance. The medial preoptic and dorsal vagal content of CRF was decreased by both stressors but only reached statistical significance for acute and chronic stress, respectively. Several other lines of research have also suggested a clear distinction between CRF systems of the hypothalamus and extrahypothalamic CRF.

Our present knowledge of CRF pathways allows only speculation as to which of these extrahypothalamic CRF changes are relevant to the stress response, but progress is being rapidly achieved. Of the regions known to change CRF concentration after stress, perhaps the most intriguing is the increase in CRF in the locus ceruleus. Valentino and Foote (1988) have elegantly demonstrated that CRF applied to locus ceruleus neurons increases their firing rate. Immunocytochemistry has demonstrated CRF terminals adjacent to noradrenergic locus ceruleus neurons (Foote and Cha, 1988), and this region is known to exhibit increased noradrenergic turnover (Thierry *et al.*, 1968; Cassens *et al.*, 1980) and increased neuronal firing rates (Cedarbaum and Aghajanian, 1978; Elam *et al.*, 1984) in response to stress or arousal. Alonso *et al.* (1986) demonstrated that noradrenergic input from the locus ceruleus stimulates synthesis and release of CRF from PVN neurons as well. Sawchenko and Swanson (1982) have previously identified a noradrenergic pathway from the locus ceruleus to the PVN, and Mermet and Ganon (1988) have demonstrated that ether stress stimulates the release of norepinephrine in the PVN. Hornby and Piekut (1989) have shown CRF neurons of various hypothalamic and limbic regions to be intimately associated with nerve fibers that stain for the noradrenergic marker, dopamine β-hydroxylase. Our group has recently shown (Owens *et al.*, 1989) that acute systemic administration of triazolobenzodiazepines has effects on locus ceruleus and PVN concentrations of CRF that are opposite the changes seen after acute or chronic stress.

Within the PVN, CRF neurons that contain multiple peptides have been described, including neurotensin, enkephalin, cholecystokinin, galanin, and vasoactive intestinal peptide (Ceccatelli *et al.*, 1989) in one study and oxytocin, vasopressin, and neurotensin (Sawchenko *et al.*, 1984b) in another. CRF is colocalized with neurotensin in the bed nucleus of the stria terminalis and the central nucleus of the amygdala (Shimada *et al.*, 1989). CRF has also been shown to be colocalized with dynorphin 1–8 in the hypothalamus (Roth *et al.*, 1983) and with substance P in lateral dorsal tegmental neurons (Crawley *et al.*, 1985). Several CRF pathways in addition to the PVN projection to the median eminence have now been characterized. Lind and Swanson (1984) reported a CRF projection from neurons of the lateral parabrachial nucleus after injection of horseradish peroxidase (HRP) into the median preoptic nucleus. Moga and Gray (1985) identified a pathway containing CRF, neurotensin, and somatostatin that originated in the central nucleus of the amygdala and projected to the parabrachial nucleus. Sakanaka *et al.* (1986) used cobalt-enhanced immunohistochemistry and retrograde transport of horseradish peroxidase to demonstrate topographic projections of CRF neurons in the central, basolateral, and medial amygdaloid nuclei. CRF in the central amygdala projected to the dorsal and ventral parabrachial nuclei through fiber tracts contained in the lateral hypothalamus and mesencephalic reticular formation. CRF projections to the ventromedial hypothalamus, which contains the PVN, arose from cell bodies in the corticomedial nucleus of the amygdala and the subiculum of the hippocampus. This same method was later used to demonstrate CRF pathways from the paraventricular region and the anterior hypothalamus to the lateral septum (Sakanaka *et al.*, 1988). Beaulieu *et al.* (1989) found that lesions of the central amygdaloid nucleus would deplete CRF from the external median eminence and hypothesized a projection from CRF cell bodies in the amygdala to the paraventricular nucleus of the hypothalamus. Gray and Magnusson (1987) demonstrated a pathway between CRF neurons in the central amygdala and bed nucleus of the stria terminalis to the dorsal vagal complex of the rat metencephalon. These pathways resonate remarkably with the alterations in CRF content observed by our group (Chappell *et al.*, 1986) after acute and chronic stress (see Table II).

Several other lines of evidence support a specific role for CRF in stress-induced behaviors. Alpha-helical CRF is a synthetic antagonist of CRF (Rivier *et al.*, 1984) that has been shown to inhibit footshock-induced fighting in rats (Tazi *et al.*, 1987). Kalin *et al.* (1988) used intraventricular alpha-helical CRF to block footshock-induced freezing behavior in rats. CRF did not exhibit any analgesic effect; thus the effect seems to be mediated through other behavioral mechanisms. Lightman and Young (1989) have recently demonstrated that lactating female rats are able to block the increase in hypothalamic CRF and oxytocin mRNA that is seen in nonlactating females after a hypertonic saline stress. Several studies have now shown increased cerebrospinal fluid concentrations of CRF in psychiatric patients with major depression (Nemeroff *et al.*, 1984; Banki *et al.*, 1987; Arato *et al.*, 1989). Patients with this disease often present with HPA dysfunction, and CRF hypersecretion may underly some of these changes. A decrease in CRF receptor number in frontal cortex of suicide victims supports this hypothesis (Nemeroff *et al.*, 1988). Thus CRF concentrations, receptors, and messenger RNA levels are altered in discrete brain regions by a variety of stressors, and these CRF alterations are anatomically positioned in brain regions known to subserve physiological and behavioral responses seen during response to stress.

Thyrotropin-releasing hormone (TRH) is another CNS neuropeptide with an extrahypothalamic distribution that seems to be involved in the stress response. Several groups have now reported alteration in TRH concentrations of various brain regions in response to such diverse stresses as hypothermia, electroconvulsive shock, restraint, and hemorrhage. Bissette (1987) reported increased TRH content in 5 of 11 mouse brain regions, including the hypothalamus and preoptic region, after 5 days of daily 3-h exposure to 4°C. More recently, Okuda et al. (1988a) described a paradigm where rats were restrained and then exposed to cold or maintained at room temperature for up to 4–5 h. TRH content in the hypothalamus and midbrain was decreased at 120 min after exposure to cold. TRH concentration changes were also seen in some cortical regions as well as the medulla oblongata after cold exposure, but these regions were not consistently changed in the same direction when compared to the controls at different time points. In contrast to Okuda et al. (1988a), Lin et al. (1989) reported increased TRH content in the rat hypothalamus after either cold stress or injection of a pyrogen. Rats were restrained and subjected to either 8, 22, or 30°C ambient temperature until body temperature stabilized or for 120 min after injection of pyrogen. Both exposure to 8°C and pyrogen injection increased metabolism and cutaneous vasoconstriction in addition to doubling hypothalamic TRH concentration. The conflicting results of these two reports are further complicated by an earlier finding of Koivusalo and Leppaluoto (1979) showing hypothalamic TRH concentration increases of greater than 40% within 10 s of immobilization in rats and increases within 10 min of room transfer, but finding no change in hypothalamic TRH concentration after 45 min of acute 4°C cold exposure. In addition, these researchers reported hypothalamic circadian rhythms in rats with daytime hypothalamic TRH peaks but with an opposite rhythm for brainstem TRH. TRH has been hypothesized to play a role in thermoregulation since the discovery of its ability to reverse the sedation and hypothermia of several CNS depressants including ethanol and pentobarbital. TRH-containing neuronal cell bodies are found in the PVN, the periventricular nucleus, the preoptic hypothalamus, the septum, and several brainstem nuclei (Hökfelt et al., 1975, 1989). Known TRH neuronal pathways include PVN and periventricular TRH perikarya with projections to the median eminence (Ishikawa et al., 1988) and projections from TRH neurons of the lateral preoptic nucleus and bed nucleus of the stria terminalis to the septum (Ishikawa et al., 1986). Siaud et al. (1987) have shown decreased TRH concentration in the nucleus of the solitary tract after lesions of the hypothalamic paraventricular nucleus. TRH is colocalized in dorsal raphe neurons containing substance P and 5-hydroxytryptamine (5-HT) (Johansson et al., 1981). TRH is currently hypothesized to play a role in maintainence of thermoneutrality and is particularly implicated in the CNS response to cold exposure. Thus, central administration of TRH causes hyperthermia in many species (Boschi and Rips, 1981), and intraventricular administration of TRH antiserum induces hypothermia (Prasad *et al.*, 1980). TRH content of ventricular cerebrospinal fluid (CSF) is increased and TRH is released from the median eminence after exposure of rats to 4°C cold (Arancibia *et al.*, 1983). Iontophoresis of TRH onto warm-and-cold-sensitive neurons of the preoptic hypothalamus increases the firing rate of cold-sensitive neurons and decreases the firing rate of warm-sensitive neurons (Hori *et al.*, 1988).

However, brain TRH concentration is also changed by stressors that do not present a thermoregulatory challenge. In an elegant study, Takayama *et al.* (1986) investigated the effects of 0.5, 1, and 3 h of immobilization stress on TRH, substance P, and methionine enkephalin concentration and receptor contents of the frontal cortex, septum, striatum, amygdala with pyriform cortex, hypothalamus, thalamus and midbrain, hippocampus, pons, and medulla oblongata. Three hours of immobilization stress significantly reduced TRH concentration in the frontal cortex, amygdala with pyriform cortex, pons, and medulla oblongata, while septum and spinal-cord content of TRH was significantly reduced at 0.5 h. Hypothalamic TRH declined over time with immobilization stress but did not reach statistical significance. After 1 h of immobilization, receptors for TRH were reduced in number in the septum and hypothalamus, and at 0.5 h in the amygdala and pyriform cortex.

Hemorrhage stress has also been shown to alter TRH concentrations in brain. Ono *et al.* (1989) described changes in TRH concentration and TRH receptor content in frontal cortex, striatum, septum, hypothalamus, hippocampus, midbrain, and hindbrain after hemorrhage stress. Rats were chronically cannulated via the femoral artery and blood volume equal to 3.5% of body weight was removed over 30 min before decapitation and dissection. Compared to cannulated but nonhemorrhaged controls, TRH was significantly decreased in frontal cortex, septum, hippocampus, and hindbrain of hemorrhage stressed rats. TRH receptors were significantly decreased in number in the septum and hindbrain. Okuda *et al.* (1988b) also used hemorrhage stress to investigate TRH concentration changes in ventricular fluid drawn from conscious, freely moving rats by push–pull cannulae. The concentration of TRH in CSF from the fourth ventricle increased 30% in rats that had 30% of their total blood volume withdrawn over 2 min from indwelling femoral artery catheters. Concomitant administration of TRH antisera through the fourth ventricle push–pull cannula prevented the hemorrhage-induced hypotension that was normally seen after blood withdrawal. Mizobe and Okuda (1988) reported that, in contrast to the findings of Ono *et al.* (1989), reversible and irreversible hemorrhage increased TRH in several brain regions. In this paradigm, 4 ml of blood was initially withdrawn from indwelling femoral artery catheter and further 1-ml bleeds were performed at 5, 15, 30, and 60 min, resulting in 50% of total blood volume being withdrawn. Animals that survived this severe shock for 24 h consistently (>99%) had plasma lactate levels lower than 3.8 mEq/l after the stress. When TRH brain region concentrations were compared in animals that had been sacrificed after the 60-min bleed, those animals with plasma lactate below 3.8 mEq/l and that would almost certainly have recovered had significantly higher TRH concentrations in the frontal cortex, striatum, cerebellum, midbrain, and medulla oblongata, but not in the hypothalamus or hippocampus. Perhaps the differences in amount of hemorrhage, time point chosen, and antisera specificity between these two studies are responsible for the contradictory findings. Like CRF, TRH has been shown to be altered in concentration after a variety of stressors, and these changes are often seen in brain regions thought to mediate relevant physiological responses to the stressor presented. TRH has also been shown to be elevated in the CSF of patients with major depression, a psychiatric disorder often associated with stress (Banki et al., 1988).

Several other neuropeptides have been shown to be altered by stressful stimuli. Some of these reports involve colocalized transmitters within brain regions thought to be involved in the stress response, although many of the findings are limited to presentation of a single type of stressor. Neurotensin and cholecystokinin (CCK) are found within dopamine neurons of the ventral tegmental area (VTA) (Hökfelt et al., 1984; Kalivas and Miller, 1984; Seroogy et al., 1988) while caudate nucleus substance P neurons are regulated by nigrostriatal dopamine neurons (Bannon, 1988). Footshock has been shown to activate VTA neurons specifically (Thierry et al., 1976; Deutch et al., 1985), as the adjacent substantia nigra does not respond in a similar fashion. Substance P has been reported to be decreased in the VTA after footshock (Lisoprawski et al., 1981), and antisera to substance P injected into the VTA prevents the increase in dopamine metabolites in the nucleus accumbens and striatum after footshock (Bannon et al., 1983). Siegel et al. (1987) demonstrated that footshock stress could reduce the concentration of substance P and CCK in the ventromedial and dorsomedial hypothalamus as well as the anterior lateral hypothalamic area. In the arcuate nucleus of the hypothalamus, footshock increased the concentration of CCK within 60 min while substance P was unchanged. This group has also reported concentration changes in these peptides in extrahypothalamic regions after footshock (Siegel et al., 1984). These include CCK concentration increases in the lateral and medial septum and frontal cortex. Substance P depletions in the olfactory tubercles and increased substance P concentrations in the medial, but not lateral, septum were also observed. Deutch et al. (1987) showed that neurotensin concentrations in the VTA were increased by mild footshock with no change in somatostatin or CRF. No stress associated alterations of these peptides were observed in the substantia nigra, retrorubral field, prefrontal cortex, nucleus accumbens, or striatum.

However, neurotransmitter colocalization does not necessarily assume parallel changes in concentration after stress. Neuropeptide Y is known to be colocalized with norepinephrine in certain brainstem nuclei. Cold stress that increases noradrenergic turnover in brainstem does not alter neuropeptide Y concentration (Schon *et al.*, 1986). Somatostatin is colocalized with substance P in the bed nucleus of the stria terminalis and central amygdaloid nucleus (Shimada *et al.*, 1989), but these two peptides respond differently to hemorrhage shock. Feuerstein *et al.* (1984) removed 8 ml of blood from 300-g rats and reported the concentration of substance P to be significantly decreased 2 h later in the paraventricular nucleus and the nucleus tractus solitarius. Somatostatin was decreased in the nucleus ambiguus, the nucleus tractus solitarius, the paraventricular nucleus, and the supraoptic nucleus 2 h after bleeding. Using push–pull cannulae techniques, Arancibia *et al.* (1984) have reported somatostatin to be released from rat median eminence after hypertonic K^+ infusion or 3 min of tail pinch. Alterations in brain somatostatin have also been reported after both exercise stress and immobilization. Terry and Crawley (1980) examined the somatostatin concentration of 12 micropunch dissected brain regions from rats forced to swim in 37°C water for 30 min. The somatostatin concentrations of both the caudate nucleus and the median eminence were decreased in the exercised rats compared to controls, with no change in several other hypothalamic, limbic, and mesencephalic regions. Negro-Vilar and Saavedra (1980) also reported decreased somatostatin and vasopressin concentrations in the median eminence of both normotensive Wistar–Kyoto rats and spontaneously hypertensive rats after 4 h of immobilization. However, these two rat strains showed very different extrahypothalamic somatostatin responses. The hypertensive, immobilized rats exhibited significantly increased somatostatin concentration in the organum vasculosum of the laminae terminalis, the subfornical organ, the stria medullaris, and the dorsal and ventral bed nuclei of the stria terminalis. Hypertensive rats also had significantly increased concentrations of vasopressin in the periventricular nucleus, the superchiasmatic nucleus, the arcuate nucleus, and the paraventricular and dorsomedial hypothalamic nuclei. Vasopressin concentrations in rat cervical and lumbosacral spinal cord were recently reported to be changed after hand restraint for 1 min, with no change in hypothalamus or the pons–medulla (Miaskowski *et al.*, 1988). Oxytocin concentrations of thoracic and lumbosacral spinal cord were significantly increased by 1 min of restraint with significant decreases in the hypothalamus and pons–medulla. Burbach *et al.* (1984) have reported that 2% sodium chloride in drinking water increases vasopressin concentrations in plasma over ninefold, increases vasopressin–neurophysin mRNA content fivefold in the supraoptic nucleus, and doubles the concentration of this mRNA in the paraventricular nucleus. This represents an example of a physiological response in order to maintain sodium balance that involves a substance also reported to be released in response to noxious stress. As the tools of molecular biology become more available and can be used in concert with radioimmunoassay of concentration and assessment of receptor populations, it should be possible to deduce whether the changes in neuropeptide concentration reflect synthesis, release, or degradation of the peptide. At present, such mechanistic distinctions are not possible based upon the available static concentration data.

The current evidence for neuropeptides that participate in CNS mediation of the stress response is strongest for corticotropin-releasing factor and thyrotropin-releasing hormone. In addition to the compelling data that have documented specific regional alterations in the concentration of these peptides induced by a variety of qualitatively different stressors, both of these peptides have been reported to be increased in the CSF of patients with a diagnosis of major depression. Several other neuropeptides (neurotensin, somatostatin, vasopressin, and substance P) are also implicated as playing some role in response to certain stressful stimuli. This response is often either paradigm-specific or the reported alterations have not yet been confirmed in other laboratories. In several cases, outright conflicting results have been reported. If past history is any guide, it is quite possible that there remain some as yet undiscovered neurochemical substances that are also integrally involved in the stress response. As our laboratory techniques and knowledge about stress and the physiological responses that mediate it become more refined, rational pharmacotherapy may allow amelioration of some of the more destructive aspects of stress.

Acknowledgments

The author's research is supported by NIMH grants MH-42088, MH-39415, and MH-45975. The author is indebted to Ward Virts for excellent assistance in the preparation of this manuscript.

References

Alonso, G., Szafarczyk, A., Balmfrezol, M., and Assenmacher, I. (1986). Immunocytochemical evidence for stimulatory control by the ventral noradrenergic bundle of parvocellular neurons of the paraventricular nucleus secreting corticotropin-releasing hormone and vasopressin in rats. *Brain Res.* **397**, 297–300.

Arancibia, S., Arancibia, L. T., Assenmacher, I., and Astier, H. (1983). Direct evidence of short-term cold-induced TRH release in the median eminence of unanesthetized rats. *Neuroendocrinology* **37**, 225–228.

Arancibia, S., Epelbaum, J., Boyer, R., and Assenmacher, I. (1984). *In vivo* release of somatostatin from rat median eminence after local K + infusion or delivery of nociceptic stress. *Neurosci. Lett.* **50**, 97–102.

Arato, M., Banki, C. M., Bissette, G., and Nemeroff, C. B. (1989). Elevated CSF CRF in suicide victims. *Biol. Psychiatry* **25**, 355–359.

Banki, C. M., Bissette, G., Arato, M., O'Connor, L., and Nemeroff, C. B. (1987). Cerebrospinal fluid corticotropin-releasing factor-like immunoreactivity in depression and schizophrenia. *Am. J. Psychiatry* **144**, 873–877.

Banki, C. M., Bissette, G., Arato, M., and Nemeroff, C. B. (1988). Elevation of immunoreactive CSF TRH in depressed patients. *Am. J. Psychiatry* **145**, 1525–1531.

Bannon, M. (1988). Dopaminergic modulation of striatal tachykinin biosynthesis. *In* "Pharmacology and Functional Regulation of Dopaminergic Neurons" (P. M. Beart, G. W. Woodruff, and D. M. Jackson eds.), pp. 282–288. Macmillan, London.

Bannon, M. J., Elliot, P. J., Alpert, J. E., Goedert, M., Iversen, S. D., and Iversen, L. L. (1983). Role of endogenous substance P in stress-induced activation of mesocortical dopamine neurons. *Nature (London)* **306**, 791–792.

Beaulieu, S., Pelletier, G., Vaudry, H., and Barden, N. (1989). Influence of the central nucleus of the amygdala on the content of corticotropin-releasing factor in the median eminence. *Neuroendocrinology* **49**, 255–261.

Berkenbosch, F., Goeij, D. C. E., and Tilders, F. J. H. (1989). Hypoglycemia enhances turnover of corticotropin-releasing factor and of vasopressin in the zona externa of the rat median eminence. *Endocrinology (Baltimore)* **125**, 28–34.

Bissette, G. (1987). Cold exposure alters endogenous TRH and neurotensin concentrations in mouse brain regions. *Soc. Neurosci, Abstr.* **13**, 1280.

Bloom, F. E., Battenberg, E. L. F., Rivier, J., and Vale, W. W. (1982). Corticotropin-releasing factor (CRF): Immunoreactive neurons and fibers in rat hypothalamus. *Regul. Pept.* **4**, 43–47.

Boschi, G., and Rips, R. (1981). Effects of thyrotropin releasing hormone injections into different loci of rat brain on core temperature. *Neurosci. Lett.* **23**, 93–98.

Bruhn, T. O., Plotsky, P. M., and Vale, W. W. (1984). Effect of paraventricular lesions on corticotropin-releasing factor (CRF)-like immunoreactivity in the stalk-median eminence: Studies on the adrenocorticotropin response to ether stress and exogenous CRF. *Endocrinology (Baltimore)* **114**, 57–62.

Bugnon, F. E., Fellman, D., Gouget, A., and Cardot, J. (1982). Ontology of the corticoliberin neuroglandular systems in rat brain. *Nature (London)* **298**, 159–160.

Burbach, J. P. H., DeHoop, M. J., Schmale, H., Richter, D., De Kloet, E. R., Ten Haaf, J. A., and DeWied, D. (1984). Differential responses to osmotic stress of vasopressin-neurophysin mRNA in hypothalamic nuclei. *Neuroendocrinology* **39**, 582–584.

Cassens, G., Ruffman, M., Kuruc, A., Orsulak, P. J., and Schildkraut, J. J. (1980). Alteration in brain norepinephrine metabolism induced by environmental stimuli previously paired with inescapable shock. *Science* **209**, 1138–1139.

Ceccatelli, S., Eriksson, M., and Hökfelt, T. (1989). Distribution and coexistence of corticotropin-releasing factor-, neurotensin-, enkephalin-, cholecystokinin-, galanin- and vasoactive intestinal polypeptide/peptide histidine isoleucine-like peptides in the parvocellular part of the paraventricular nucleus. *Neuroendocrinology* **49**, 309–323.

Cedarbaum, J. M., and Aghajanian, G. K. (1978). Activation of locus coeruleus neurons by peripheral stimuli: Modulation by a collateral inhibitory mechanism. *Life Sci.* 23, 1383–1392.

Chappell, P. B., Smith, M. A., Kilts, C. D., Bissette, G., Ritchie, J., Anderson, C., and Nemeroff, C. B. (1986). Alterations in corticotropin-releasing factor-like immunoreactivity in discrete rat brain regions after acute and chronic stress. *J. Neurosci.* 6(10), 2908–2914.

Crawley, J. N., Olschowka, J. A., Diz, D. I., and Jacobowitz, D. M. (1985). Behavioral investigation of the co-existence of substance P, corticotropin releasing factor, and acetylcholinesterase in lateral dorsal tegmental neurons projecting to the medial frontal cortex of the rat. *Peptides (N.Y.)* 6, 891–901.

DeSouza, E. (1986). Corticotropin-releasing factor receptors in the rat central nervous system: Characterization and regional distribution. *J. Neurosci.* 7, 88–92.

Deutch, A. Y., Tam, S. Y., and Roth, R. H. (1985). Footshock and conditioned stress increase 3,4 dihydroxyphenylacetic acid (DOPAC) in the ventral tegmental area but not substantia nigra. *Brain Res.* 333, 143–146.

Deutch, A. Y., Bean, A. L., Bissette, G., Nemeroff, C. B., Robbins, R. J., and Roth, R. H. (1987). Stress-induced alteration in neurotensin, somatostatin and corticotropin-releasing factor in mesotelencephalic dopamine system regions. *Brain Res.* 417, 350–354.

Elam, M., Yao, T., Svensson, T. H., and Thoren, P. (1984). Regulation of locus coeruleus neurons and splanchnic sympathetic nerves. *Brain Res.* 290, 281–287.

Feuerstein, G., Helke, C., and Faden, A. I. (1984). Differential changes in substance P and somatostatin in brain nuclei of rats exposed to hemorrhage shock. *Brain Res.* 300, 305–310.

Foote, S. L., and Cha, C. I. (1988). Distribution of corticotropin-releasing-factor-like immunoreactivity in brainstem of two monkey species (Saimiri sciureus and Macaca fascicularis): And immunohistochemical study. *J. Comp. Neurol.* 276, 239–264.

Gray, T. S., and Magnusson, D. J. (1987). Neuropeptide neuronal efferents from the bed nucleus of the stria terminalis and central amygdaloid nucleus to the dorsal vagal complex in the rat. *J. Comp. Neurol.* 262, 365–374.

Hashimoto, K., Suemaru, S., Takao, T., Sugawara, M., Makino, S., and Ota, Z. (1988). Corticotropin-releasing hormone and pituitary-adrenocortical responses in chronically stressed rats. *Reg. Peptides (N.Y.)* 23, 117–126.

Hass, D. A., and George, S. R. (1988). Single or repeated mild stress increases synthesis and release of hypothalamic corticotropin-releasing factor. *Brain Res.* 461, 230–237.

Hauger, R. L., Millan, M. A., Lorang, M., Harwood, J. P., and Aguilera, G. (1988). Corticotropin-releasing factor receptors and pituitary adrenal responses during immobilization stress. *Endocrinology (Baltimore)* 123, 396–405.

Hökfelt, T., Fuxe, K., Johansson, O., Jeffcoate, S., and White, N. (1975). Distribution of thyrotropin-releasing hormone (TRH) in the central nervous system as revealed with immunohistochemistry. *Eur. J. Pharmacol.* 34, 389–397.

Hökfelt, T., Everitt, B. J., Theodorsson-Norheim, E., and Goldstein, M. (1984). Occurence of neurotensin-like immunoreactivity in sub-populations of hypthalamic, mesencephalic and medullary catecholamine neurons. *J. Comp. Neurol.* 222, 543–559.

Hökfelt, T., Tsaro, Y., Alfhake, B., Cullheim, S., Arvidsson, U., Foster, G. A., Schultzberg, M., Schalling, M., Arborelius, L., Freedman, J., Post, C., and Visser, T. (1989). Distribution of TRH-immunoreactivity with special reference to co-existence with other neuroactive compounds. *Ann. N.Y. Acad. Sci.* 533, 76–105.

Hori, T., Yamasaki, M., Asami, T., Koga, H., and Kiyohara, T. (1988). Responses of anterior hypothalamic-pre-optic thermosensitive neurons to thyrotropin releasing hormone and cyclo(his-pro). *Neuropharmacology* 27, 895–901.

Hornby, P. J., and Piekut, D. T. (1989). Opiocortin and catecholamine input to CRF immuno-reactive neurons in rat forebrain. *Peptides (N.Y.)* 10, 1139–1146.

Ishikawa, K., Taniguchi, Y., Kurosumi, K., and Suzuki, M. (1986). Origin of septal thyrotro-pin-releasing hormone in the rat. *Neuroendocrinology* 44, 54–58.

Ishikawa, K., Taniguchi, Y., Inoue, K., Kurosumi, K., and Suzuki, M. (1988). Immunocyto-chemical delineation of the thyrotropic area: Origin of thyrotropin-releasing hormone in the median eminence. *Neuroendocrinology* 47, 384–388.

Ixart, G., Barbanel, G., Conte-Devolx, B., Grino, M., Oliver, C., and Assenmacher, I. (1987). Evidence for basal and stress-induced release of corticotropin-releasing factor in the push-pull cannulated median eminence of concious free-moving rats. *Neurosci. Lett.* 74, 85–89.

Johansson, O., Hökfelt, T., Pernow, B., Jeffcoate, S. L., White, N., Steinbusch, H. W. M., Verhofstad, A. A. J., Emson, P. C., and Spindel, E. (1981). Immunohistochemical sup-port for three putative transmitters in one neuron: Coexistence of 5-hydroxytryptamine, substance P, abd thyrotropin-releasing hormone-like immunoreactivity in medullary neurons projecting to the spinal cord. *Neuroscience* 6, 1857–1881.

Joseph, S. A., and Knigge, K. M. (1983). Corticotropin-releasing factor: Immunohistochemical localization in rat brain. *Neurosci. Lett.* 35, 135–139.

Kalin, N. H., Sherman, J. E., and Takahashi, L. K. (1988). Antagonism of endogenous CRH systems attenuates stress-induced freezing behavior in rats. *Brain Res.* 457, 130–135.

Kalivas, P. W., and Miller, J. S. (1984). Neurotensin neurons in the ventral tegmental area project to the medial nucleus accumbens. *Brain Res.* 300, 157–160.

Koivusalo, F., and Leppaluoto, J. (1979). Brain TRF immunoreactivity during various physio-logical and stress conditions in the rat. *Neuroendocrinology* 29, 231–236.

Lightman, S. L., and Young, W. S. (1989). Lactation inhibits stress-mediated secretion of corti-costerone and oxytocin and hypothalamic accumulation of corticotropin-releasing fac-tor and enkephalin messenger ribonucleic acids. *Endocrinology (Baltimore)* 124, 2358–2364.

Lin, M. T., Wang, P. S., Chuang, J., Fan, L. J., and Won, S. J. (1989). Cold stress or a pyrogenic substance elevates thyrotropin-releasing hormone levels in the rat hypothalamus and induces thermogenic reactions. *Neuroendocrinology* 50, 177–181.

Lind, R. W., and Swanson, L. W. (1984). Evidence for corticotropin releasing factor and leuen-kephalin in the neural projection from the lateral parabranchial nucleus to the median pre-optic nucleus: A retrograde transport, immunohistochemical double labeling study in the rat. *Brain Res.* 321, 217–224.

Lisoprawski, A., Blanc, G., and Glowinski, J. (1981). Activation by stress of the habenulo-interpenduncular substance P neurons in the rat. *Neurosci. Lett.* 25, 47–51.

Merchenthaler, I. (1984). Corticotropin releasing factor (CRF)-like immunoreactivity in the rat central nervous system. Extrahypothalamic distribution. *Peptides (N.Y.)* 5, 53–69.

Merchenthaler, I., Vigh, S., Petrusz, P., and Schally, A. V. (1983). The paraventriculo-infundib-ular corticotropin releasing factor (CRF)-pathway as revealed by immunocytochemistry in long-term hypophysectomized or adrenalectomized rats. *Regul. Pept.* 5, 295–305.

Mermet, C. C., and Ganon, F. G. (1988). Ether stress stimulates noradrenaline release in the hypothalamic paraventricular nucleus. *Neuroendocrinology* 47, 75–82.

Miaskowski, C., Ong, G. L., Lukic, D., and Haldar, J. (1988). Immobilization stress affects oxytocin and vasopressin levels in hypothalamic and extrahypothalamic sites. *Brain Res.* 458, 137–141.

Mizobe, T., and Okuda, C. (1988). Changes in brain thyrotropin-releasing hormone in revers-ible and irreversible hemorrhage shock in the rat. *Circ. Shock* 26, 245–256.

Moga, M. M., and Gray, T. S. (1985). Evidence for coticotropin-releasing factor, neurotensin and somatostatin in the neural pathway form the central nucleus of the amygdala to the parabrachial nucleus. *J. Comp. Neurol.* **241**, 275–284.

Moldow, R. L., Kastin, A. J., Graf, M., and Fischman, A. J. (1987). Stress mediated changes in hypothalamic corticotropin releasing factor-like immunoreactivity. *Life Sci.* **40**, 413–418.

Murakami, K., Akana, S., Dallman, M. F., and Ganong, W. F. (1989). Correlation between the stress-induced transient increase in corticotropin-releasing hormone content of the median eminence of the hypothalamus and adrenocorticotropic hormone secretion. *Neuroendocrinology* **49**, 233–241.

Negro-Vilar, A., and Saavedra, J. M. (1980). Changes in brain somatostatin and vasopressin levels after stress in spontaneously hypertensive and Wistar-Kyoto rats. *Brain Res. Bull.* **5**, 353–358.

Nemeroff, C. B., Widerlov, E., Bissette, G., Walleus, H., Karlsson, I., Eklund, K., Kilts, C. D., Loosen, P. T., and Vale, W. (1984). Elevated concentrations of CSF corticotropin-releasing factor-like immunoreactivity in depressed patients. *Science* **226**, 1342–1344.

Nemeroff, C. B., Owens, M. J., Bissette, G., Andorn, A. C., and Stanley, M. (1988). Reduced corticotropin-releasing factor (CRF) binding sites in the frontal cortex of suicides. *Arch. Gen. Psychiatry* **45**, 577–579.

Okuda, C., Mizobe, T., and Miyazaki, M. (1988a). Effects of hypothermia on thyrotropin-releasing hormone content in the rat brain. *Pharmacol., Biochem. Behav.* **30**, 941–944.

Okuda, C., Mizobe, T., and Miyazaki, M. (1988b). Involvement of endogenous thyrotropin-releasing hormone in central regulation of the cardiovascular system after bleeding in conscious rats. *Brain Res.* **474**, 399–402.

Olschowka, J. A., O'Donohue, T. L., Mueller, G. P., and Jacobowitz, D. M. (1982). Hypothalamic and extrahypothalamic distribution of CRF-like immunoreactive neurons in the rat brain. *Neuroendocrinology* **35**, 305–311.

Ono, T., Ogawa, N., and Mori, A. (1989). The effects of hemorrhagic shock on thyrotropin releasing hormone and tis receptors in discrete regions of rat brain. *Regul. Pept.* **25**, 215–222.

Owens, M. J., Bissette, G., and Nemeroff, C. B. (1989). Acute effects of alprozolam and adinazolam on the concentrations of corticotropin-releasing factor in the rat brain. *Synapse* **4**, 196–202.

Petrusz, P., Merchenthaler, I., Maderdrut, J. L., and Heitz, P. U. (1985). Central and peripheral distribution of corticotropin-releasing factor. *Fed. Proc., Fed. Am. Soc. Exp. Biol.* **44**, 229–235.

Piekut, D. T., and Joseph, S. A. (1986). Co-existence of CRF and vasopressin immunoreactivity in parvocellular paraventricular neurons of rat hypothalamus. *Peptides (N.Y.)* **7**, 891–898.

Plotsky, P. M., and Vale, W. (1984). Hemorrhage-induced secretion of corticotropin-releasing factor-like immunoreactivity into the rat hypophyseal portal circulation and its inhibition by glucocorticoids. *Endocrinology (Baltimore)* **114**, 164–169.

Prasad, C., Jacobs, J. J., and Wilber, J. F. (1980). Immunological blockade of endogenous thyrotropin-releasing hormone produces hypothermia in rats. *Brain Res.* **193**, 580–583.

Rivier, J., Rivier, C., and Vale, W. (1984). Synthetic competitive antagonists of corticotropin factor: effect upon ACTH secretion in the rat. *Science* **224**, 889–891.

Roth, K. A., Weber, E., and Barchas, J. D. (1982). Immunoreactive corticotropin-releasing factor (CRF) and vasopressin are co-localized in a sub-population of the immunoreactive vasopressin cells in the paraventricular nucleus of the hypothalamus. *Life Sci.* **31**, 1857–1860.

Roth, K. A., Weber, E., Barchas, J. D., Chang, D., and Chang, J. K. (1983). Immunoreactive dynorphin-(1-8) and corticotropin-releasing factor in a subpopulation of hypothalamic neurons. *Science* **219**, 189–191.

Sakanaka, M., Shibasaki, T., and Lederis, K. (1986). Distribution and efferent projections of corticotropin-releasing factor-like immunoreactivity in the rat amygdaloid complex. *Brain Res.* **382**, 213–218.

Sakanaka, M., Shibasaki, T., and Lederis, K. (1987). Corticotropin releasing factor-like immunoreactivity in the rat brain as revealed by a modified cobalt-glucose oxidase-diamino-benzidine method. *J. Comp. Neurol.* **260**, 256–298.

Sakanaka, M., Magari, S., Shibasaki, T., and Lederis, K. (1988). Corticotropin-releasing factor-containing afferents to the lateral septum of the rat brain. *J. Comp. Neurol.* **270**, 404–415.

Sawchenko, P. E., and Swanson, L. W. (1982). The organization of noradrenergic pathways from the brainstem to the paraventricular and supraoptic nuclei in the rat brain. *Brain Res. Rev.* **4**, 285–291.

Sawchenko, P. E., Swanson, L. W., and Vale, W. W. (1984a). Co-expression of corticotropin-releasing factor and vasopressin immunoreactivity in parvocellular neurosecretory neurons of the adrenalectomized rat. *Proc. Natl. Acad. Sci. U.S.A.* **81**, 1883–1887.

Sawchenko, P. E., Swanson, L. W., and Vale, W. W. (1984b). Corticotropin-releasing factor: Co-expression within distinct subsets of oxytocin-, vasopressin- and neurotensin- immunoreactive neurons in the hypothalamus of the male rat. *J. Neurosci.* **4**, 1118–1129.

Schon, F., Allen, J. M., Yeats, J. C., Kent, A., Kelly, J. S., and Bloom, S. R. (1986). The effect of 6-hydroxydopamine, reserpine and cold stress on the neuropeptide Y content of the rat central nervous system. *Neuroscience* **19**, 1247–1250.

Selye, H. (1936) A syndrome produced by diverse noxious agents. *Nature (London)* **138**, 32.

Seroogy, K., Ceccatelli, S., Schalling, M., Hökfelt, T., Frey, P., Walsh, J., Dockray, G., Brown, J., Buchan, A., and Goldstein, M. (1988). A sub-population of dopaminergic neurons in rat ventral mesencephalon contains both neurotensin and cholecystokinin. *Brain Res.* **455**, 88–98.

Shimada, S., Inagaki, S., Kubota, Y., Ogawa, N., Shibasaki, T., and Takagi, H. (1989). Co-existence of peptides (corticotropin releasing factor/neurotensin and substance P/somatostatin) in the bed nucleus of the stria terminalis and central amygdaliod nucleus of the rat. *Neuroscience* **30**, 377–383.

Siaud, P., Arancibia, L. T., Szafarczyk, A., and Alonso, G. (1987). Increase of thyrotropin-releasing hormone immunoreactivity in the nucleus of the solitary tract following bilateral lesions of the paraventricular nuclei. *Neurosci. Lett.* **79**, 47–52.

Siegel, R. A., Duker, E.-M., Fuchs, E., Pahnke, U., and Wüttke, W. (1984). Responsiveness of mesolimbic, mesocortical, septal and hippocampal cholecystokinin and substance P neuronal systems to stress in the male rat. *Neurochem. Int.* **6**, 783–789.

Siegel, R. A., Duker, E. M., Pahnke, U., and Wüttke, W. (1987). Stressed-induced changes in cholecystokinin and substance P concentrations in discrete regions of the hypothalamus. *Neuroendocrinology* **96**, 75–81.

Silverman, A. J., Hou-Yu, A., and Chen, W. P. (1989). Corticotropin-releasing factor synapses within the paraventricular nucleus of the hypothalamus. *Neuroendocrinology* **49**, 291–299.

Suemaru, S., Hashimoto, K., and Ota, Z. (1985). Brain corticotropin-releasing factor (CRF) and catecholamine responses in acutely stressed rats. *Endocrinol. Jpn.* **32**, 709–718.

Swanson, L. W., Sawchenko, P. E., Rivier, J., and Vale, W. W. (1983). Organization of ovine corticotropin-releasing factor immunoreactive cells and fibers in the rat brain: An immunohistochemical study. *Neuroendocrinology* **36**, 165–186.

Takayama, H., Ota, Z., and Ogawa, N. (1986). Effect of immobilization stress on neuropeptides and their receptors in rat central nervous system. *Regul. Pept.* **25**, 239–248.

Tazi, A., Dantzer, R., LeMoal, M., Rivier, J., Vale, W., and Koob, G. F. (1987). Corticotropin-releasing factor antagonist blocks stress-induced fighting in rats. *Regul. Pept.* **18**, 37–42.

Terry, L. C., and Crawley, W. R. (1980). The effects of exercise stress on somatostatin concentrations in discrete brain nuclei. *Brain Res.* **197**, 543–546.

Thierry, A. M., Javoy, F., Glowinski, J., and Kety, S. S. (1968). Effects of stress on the metabolism of norepinephrine, dopamine and serotonin in the central nervous system of the rat. Modification of norepinephrine turnover. *J. Pharmacol. Exp. Ther.* **163**, 163–171.

Thierry, A. M., Tassin, J. P., Blanc, G., and Glowinski, J. (1976). Selective activation of the mesocortical DA system by stress. *Nature (London)* **263**, 242–244.

Vale, W. W., Speiss, J., Rivier, C., and Rivier, J. (1981). Characterization of a 41 residue ovine hypothalamic peptide that stimulates the secretion of corticotropin and β-endorphin. *Science* **213**, 1394–1397.

Valentino, R. J., and Foote, S. L. (1988). Corticotropin-releasing hormone increases tonic but not sensory-evoked activity of noradrenergic locus coeruleus neurons in unanesthetized rats. *J. Neurosci.* **8**, 1016–1025.

Whitnall, M. H., and Gainer, H. (1988). Major pro-vasopressin-expressing and pro-vasopressin-deficient subpopulations of corticotropin-releasing hormone neurons in normal rats. *Neuroendocrinology* **47**, 176–180.

Whitnall, M. H., Mezey, E., and Gainer, H. (1985). Co-localization of corticotropin-releasing factor and vasopressin in median eminence neurosecretory vesicles. *Nature (London)* **317**, 248–250.

Whitnall, M. H., Smyth, D., and Gainer, H. (1987). Vasopressin coexists in half of corticotropin-releasing factor axons present in the external zone of the median eminence in normal rats. *Neuroendocrinology* **45**, 420–424.

5

Neuropeptide-Mediated Regulation of the Neuroendocrine and Autonomic Responses to Stress

Marvin R. Brown

Autonomic Physiology Laboratory
Department of Medicine
University of California, San Diego
San Diego, California 92103

I. Introduction

The central nervous system (CNS) biologic actions of peptides are extensive; however, the physiologic roles that most of these peptides play are uncertain. Some have proven actions as hormones and many have putative roles as neuromodulators or hormones. The only peptides released from the CNS for which physiologic roles have been firmly established are the hypophysiotrophic peptides, corticotropin-releasing factor (CRF), thyrotropin-releasing factor (TRF), somatostatin (SS), luteinizing-hormone releasing factor (LRF), and growth-hormone releasing factor (GRF), and the posterior pituitary hormones oxytocin and vasopressin.

Actions of peptides within the CNS have been demonstrated at cellular, isolated brain fragment, and intact integrated systems levels (Krieger *et al.*, 1983). Relevant to the content of this chapter has been the demonstration by neuroanatomists that many of the peptides present within the CNS are anatomically distributed in brain regions associated with the regulation of the autonomic nervous system (ANS) (Palkovits, 1988). Consistent with this observation, many peptides present within the CNS have been demonstrated to affect ANS activity (Brown, 1989). In this regard, a brain peptide–ANS pharmacology has emerged that may provide the basis for important physiologic regulatory systems and new avenues for pharmacotherapeutic manipulations.

Since peptides inside and outside the brain appear to be intercellular messengers capable of influencing complex systems' functions, it would not be surprising to find that these substances are involved in the normalization of homeostatic disruptions that occur following exposure of animals to stressor events.

This chapter describes studies performed over the last 15 years in my laboratory concerning the CNS actions of CRF, TRF, bombesin, and SS to influence neuroendocrine and ANS function. Clearly, no single peptide is the "stress" peptide. More likely is the possibility that groups of peptide and nonpeptide ligands participate in a dynamic fashion with end-organ chemical or nervous inputs to determine the tone of neuroendocrine and autonomic activities.

II. Corticotropin-Releasing Factor

CRF is a physiologic regulator of pituitary ACTH secretion (Vale *et al.*, 1983). CRF and its receptors are anatomically distributed in brain regions that are involved in the regulation of the ANS (Bloom *et al.*, 1982; Swanson *et al.*, 1983; Palkovits *et al.*, 1985; DeSouza, 1987). For example, CRF-containing cell bodies located within the central nucleus of the amygdala

(CeA) project to the lateral hypothalamus, parabrachial nucleus, and nucleus of the solitary tract (NTS) (Moga and Gray, 1985). This anatomic distribution, in combination with pharmacologic and physiologic studies with CRF, suggests that this peptide may play an important role in the regulation of the ANS.

A. Effects of CRF on the Sympathetic Nervous System and Adrenal Medulla

Intracerebroventricular (icv) administration of CRF to the rat or dog elicits dose-related elevations of plasma epinephrine (Epi) and norepinephrine (NE) concentrations (Brown et al., 1982; Kurosawa et al., 1986). CRF (200 pmol) has been microinjected into 48 different brain sites followed by measurement of plasma concentrations of catecholamines (Brown, 1986). No consistent changes of plasma Epi levels were observed. Numerous sites were identified where CRF microinjection resulted in the elevation of plasma NE levels. The most robust responses occurred in the dorsal hypothalamus, zona incerta, ventromedial hypothalamus, and lateral hypothalamus. However, administration of the same dose of CRF into the third ventricle produced responses similar to those observed in these tissue sites. The site of origin of Epi secretion following icv administration of CRF is the adrenal medulla. The sites of origin of NE release following CRF treatment have been evaluated by assessing the accumulation of tissue dopamine following inhibition of the enzyme dopamine beta-hydroxylase. CRF given icv increased dopamine accumulation in the kidney, but not in any other organs tested (Brown and Fisher, 1985b). The data suggest that CRF elicits an increase in noradrenergic activity in the kidney, while producing a reduction of noradrenergic activity in other sites, such as brown fat and pancreas. Other studies have recently found that icv administration of CRF increases sympathetic activity in brown fat (Arase et al., 1988). The increase of sympathetic activity in brown fat induced by a glucocorticoid antagonist, RU-486, was prevented by icv administration of a CRF receptor antagonist (Hardwick et al., 1989). Whether CRF pathways are involved in physiologic regulation of brown fat metabolism and metabolic efficiency has not been established.

B. Effects of CRF on the Parasympathetic Nervous System

CRF is suspected to act within the CNS to influence the parasympathetic nervous system (PNS) on the basis of the effects of this peptide on heart rate (HR) and gastric acid secretion (Fisher, 1988; Tache et al., 1983). Methyl atropine administration has no effect on CRF-induced tachycardia, suggesting that cardiac vagal tone is largely withdrawn in CRF-treated rats (Fisher,

1988). By virtue of its CNS action to inhibit cardiac vagal activity, CRF reduces the gain and range of baroreflex regulation of HR (Fisher, 1988). That CRF acts within the CNS to influence gastric parasympathetic outflow in the rat is also inferred from the observation that subdiaphragmatic vagotomy prevents the inhibitory effects of icv CRF treatment on gastric acid secretion (Tache et al., 1983).

C. CNS Effects of CRF on Visceral Systems

Table I shows the actions of CRF to influence different visceral organ functions. Some of these will be discussed in detail below.

1. Cardiovascular Effects
CRF injected icv increases mean arterial pressure (MAP) and HR in the dog and rat (Fisher et al., 1982; Brown and Fisher, 1983). In contrast, intravenous (iv) administration of CRF lowers MAP (Lenz et al., 1985). Recent studies in the rat demonstrate that CRF given icv produces an increase in cardiac output (CO) and stroke volume, and a decrease in total peripheral vascular resistance (Brown and Fisher, 1985b; Grosskreutz and Brody, 1988; Overton and Fisher, 1989). These results suggest that the elevation in MAP following icv administration of CRF is largely due to an increase in CO. Consistent with these findings, exercise-induced increase in CO in the rat is prevented by icv administration of a CRF receptor antagonist (Kregel et al., 1988). CRF-induced elevations of MAP and HR are not prevented by hypophysectomy, adrenalectomy, or antero-ventral third ventricle (AV3V) lesions, or by peripheral administration of vasopressin receptor antagonist or the angiotensin-converting enzyme inhibitor captopril (Fisher et al., 1983; Brown and Fisher, 1990). CRF-induced elevations of MAP and HR are prevented by administration of the ganglionic blocker chlorisondamine (Fisher et al., 1983). CRF tachycardia is mediated mainly by cardiac parasympathetic withdrawal, although high levels of circulating catecholamines may contribute to this effect as well.

In summary, CRF acts within the CNS to influence sympathetic and parasympathetic nervous efferents so as to increase venous return and elevate HR, thereby producing an increase in CO. The CRF-induced increase in MAP is secondary to an increase in CO rather than a direct result of an increase in peripheral vascular resistance.

2. Metabolic Effects
CRF given icv produces an increase in plasma glucose concentration that is not prevented by hypophysectomy or adrenalectomy, but is prevented by ganglionic blockade with chlorisondamine or by systemic administration of

SS (Brown *et al.*, 1982). CRF-induced hyperglycemia is accompanied by an elevation of plasma glucagon concentrations and a relative lowering of plasma insulin concentrations. Thus, CRF-induced hyperglycemia is mediated by autonomic nervous-dependent elevations of plasma glucagon levels and suppression of insulin secretion with a resultant increase of hepatic glucose production.

As noted above, CRF may act within the CNS to increase sympathetic outflow to brown fat, resulting in increased oxygen consumption and decreased metabolic efficiency (Hardwick *et al.*, 1989; Brown *et al.*, 1981a). CRF, given icv to normal, genetically obese, or ventral-medial hypothala-

Table I

Mechanism of the Effects of CRF on Visceral Organ Function

Observed changes of visceral function	Neuroendocrine or ANS mechanism
Increase of plasma concentrations of glucose and glucagon	Adrenal Epi release; possible NE release in the pancreas (Brown *et al.*, 1982; Kurosawa *et al.*, 1986; Brown and Fisher, 1985b); possible decrease of parasympathetic influence on the pancreas
Increase of cardiac output	Decreased PNS and increased SNS influence on the heart (Fisher, 1988; Fisher *et al.*, 1982; 1983; Fisher and Brown, 1983)
Increase of HR	Decreased PNS and increased SNS influence on the heart (Fisher, 1988; Fisher *et al.*, 1982, 1983; Fisher and Brown, 1983)
Increase of blood pressure	Decreased PNS and increased SNS influence on the heart (Fisher, 1988; Fisher *et al.*, 1982, 1983; Fisher and Brown, 1983)
Decrease of renal and mesenteric blood flow	Increased SNS outflow (Grosskreutz and Brody, 1988; Overton and Fisher, 1989)
Increase of interscapular brown fat metabolism	Increased SNS outflow (Brown and Fisher, 1985b)
Decrease of gastric acid secretion and motility	Decreased PNS activity (Tache *et al.*, 1983; Druge *et al.*, 1989); increased SNS activity; pituitary beta-endorphin release
Increased duodenal bicarbonate secretion	Increased SNS activity and pituitary beta-endorphin release (Lenz, 1989)
Decreased natural killer cell function	Increased SNS activity (Irwin *et al.*, 1988)
Inhibition of ovulation	Inhibition of LRF and LH secretion (Rivier *et al.*, 1986; Rivier and Vale, 1985)

mus-lesioned rats, prevents weight gain (Arase *et al.*, 1988, 1989; Rohner-Jeanrenaud *et al.*, 1989). Whether CRF plays a physiologic role in this regard remains to be determined.

3. Gastrointestinal Effects

CRF given icv to rats and dogs inhibits basal as well as pentagastrin-, 2-deoxyglucose-, TRF-, and meal-stimulated gastric acid secretion (Tache *et al.*, 1983; Lenz, 1985). Adrenalectomy, cervical cord transection, ganglionic blockade, and opiate and vasopressin antagonists are reported to completely or partially prevent CRF-induced inhibition of gastric acid secretion (Tache *et al.*, 1983; Lenz, 1985). Vagotomy has been reported to prevent CRF-induced inhibition of gastric acid secretion in the rat, but not the dog. A recent study has presented data to support a role of vasopressin and the sympathetic nervous system (SNS) in mediating CRF-induced inhibition of gastric acid secretion (Lenz, 1985). These studies suggest a complex of efferent mechanisms activated by CRF capable of inhibiting gastric acid secretion.

CRF also stimulates duodenal bicarbonate secretion and gastrointestinal motility (Lenz, 1989; Lenz *et al.*, 1988; Tache *et al.*, 1987; Williams *et al.*, 1987). The effects of CRF on bicarbonate secretion are dependent on pituitary beta-endorphin release (Lenz, 1989).

4. Immune Function

Irwin *et al.* (1988) have recently demonstrated that icv administration of CRF produces a suppression of natural killer cell activity in the spleen. This effect of CRF is not prevented by hypophysectomy, but is inhibited by administration of the ganglionic blocking agent, chlorisondamine. These results are consistent with a role of CRF in mediating stress-induced suppression of natural killer cell activity and suggest that this effect results from sympathetic nervous stimulation of the spleen. It is of interest that interleukin-1 (I1-1) acts within the CNS to decrease peripheral immune function (Sundar *et al.*, 1988). We have recently demonstrated that I1-1 acts within the CNS to stimulate an increase of plasma concentrations of catecholamines (Rivier *et al.*, 1989).

5. Reproduction and Growth

CRF given icv elicits an inhibition of pituitary luteinizing hormone (LH) and growth hormone (GH) secretion (Ono *et al.*, 1984; Rivier *et al.*, 1986; Rivier and Vale, 1985). CRF-induced inhibition of LH secretion has been reported to be secondary to the release and action of hypothalamic opioid peptides (Almeida *et al.*, 1988). In an extension of these studies, icv administration of a CRF antagonist has been reported to prevent stress-induced inhibition of LH and GH (Rivier *et al.*, 1986; Rivier and Vale, 1985). These results suggest that stress-induced inhibition of growth and reproductive function is mediated by an action of CRF.

D. Physiologic Role of CRF in Regulating the Autonomic Nervous System

A physiologic role of CRF in the regulation of the ANS is supported by data obtained in experiments utilizing a CRF receptor antagonist (see Table II). The CRF receptor antagonists alpha-helical-CRF$^{9-41}$ or alpha-helical-CRF$^{10-41}$, given icv, prevented CRF-induced elevations of plasma catecholamines, MAP, and HR (Brown *et al.*, 1985b, 1986).

The CRF receptor antagonist alpha-helical-CRF$^{9-41}$ acts within the brain to attenuate adrenal Epi secretion following insulin-induced hypoglycemia, 30% hemorrhage, and exposure to ether vapor (Brown *et al.*, 1985b, 1986). This CRF antagonist given icv does not, however, alter basal MAP or HR in spontaneously hypertensive rats (SHR) (at 6 or 12 weeks of age), and does not influence the cardiovascular responses to administration of sodium nitroprusside, or to electrical stimulation of the CeA or anterior hypothalamus in normotensive rats (Brown *et al.*, 1986, 1988b).

Studies were performed using SHRs in an attempt to identify an animal model in which CRF may participate in a pathophysiologic process. We have found that the SHR exhibits an exaggerated elevation of plasma Epi and glucose concentrations and blunted MAP and HR responses following CNS administration of CRF (Brown *et al.*, 1988b). Efforts have continued to determine if CRF-containing pathways and effector systems are involved in the pathophysiology of these animals. We (M. R. Brown and W. Vale, unpublished data) and others have found decreased concentrations of

Table II
Changes of ANS, Neuroendocrine, or Visceral Organ Function That Are Attenuated by CNS Administration of a CRF Antagonist

Adrenal Epi release induced by ether vapor, insulin-induced hypoglycemia, and 30% hemorrhage (Brown *et al.*, 1985b, 1986).

Restraint-induced decrease of gastric acid secretion and gastrointestinal motility (Druge *et al.*, 1989; Lenz *et al.*, 1988; Williams *et al.*, 1987).

Restraint-induced increase of duodenal bicarbonate secretion (Lenz, 1989).

Inhibition of growth hormone and LH secretion (Rivier *et al.*, 1986; Rivier and Vale, 1985).

Exercise-induced increase of HR, MAP, mesenteric vascular resistance, and iliac blood flow (Kregel *et al.*, 1988).

CRF in some brain regions (Hattori *et al.*, 1986). We also investigated the binding affinity and the number of CRF receptors in SHR and Wistar-Kyoto (WKY) rat brains (Brown *et al.*, 1988b). The results of this study failed to show any difference in receptor number or affinity for CRF among SHR, WKY, and Sprague-Dawley rat brains.

Other putative physiologic CNS actions of CRF are listed in Table II.

III. Thyrotropin-Releasing Factor

Thyrotropin-releasing factor (TRF) was the first of the hypothalamic hypophysiotropic factors to be chemically characterized and to be demonstrated to exert biological actions on the CNS (Vale *et al.*, 1977).

A. Effects of TRF on the Sympathetic Nervous System and Adrenal Medulla

TRF placed into the cerebroventricle or the medial preoptic nucleus of rats elicits an increase of plasma concentrations of Epi and NE (Brown, 1981; Feurstein *et al.*, 1983). Direct measurement of nerve firing rates demonstrates that TRF given icv decreases gastric sympathetic outflow while increasing adrenal sympathetic nerve activity (Somiya and Tonoue, 1984).

B. Effects of TRF on the Parasympathetic Nervous System

TRF acts within the CNS to influence the firing rates of various vagal nerve branches. Thus, CNS administration of TRF increases the firing rates of gastric vagal ramus and superior laryngeal nerve (Somiya and Tonoue, 1984; Tonoue, 1982). In addition, the secretion of gastric and pancreatic juice and the increased colonic activity following CNS administration of TRF are prevented by subdiaphragmatic vagotomy or atropine administration (Kato and Kanno, 1983; Tache *et al.*, 1980b; Smith *et al.*, 1977).

C. Effects of TRF on CRF Release

Studies have been performed to determine if TRF-induced changes in ACTH secretion and sympathoadrenal activity are secondary to stimulation of CRF-containing pathways. In this regard, TRF-induced (given icv) ACTH secretion was prevented by iv administration of CRF antiserum or a CRF receptor antagonist (Brown *et al.*, 1989b). The icv administration of a CRF receptor antagonist has failed to prevent TRF-induced elevation of plasma catecholamine concentrations. Thus, CRF does mediate TRF-induced ACTH secretion, but may not mediate TRF-induced changes of sympathoadrenal activity.

D. Effects of TRF on Physiologic Systems

1. Cardiorespiratory Effects

TRF placed into the CNS produces an increase in respiratory rate in rats and cats (Myers *et al.*, 1977; Hedner *et al.*, 1983; Koivasalo *et al.*, 1979; Diz and Jacobowitz, 1984; Niewoehner *et al.*, 1983). In the rat, the increase of respiratory rate is not dependent on an intact SNS or adrenal medulla (Diz and Jacobowitz, 1984). The medial preoptic nucleus may be a site of action of TRF to increase respiratory rate; however, other sites have not been systematically excluded (Diz and Jacobowitz, 1984).

TRF acts within the CNS to increase HR and MAP (Diz and Jacobowitz, 1984). These effects are prevented by a combination of adrenal demedullation and bretylium administration. TRF is demonstrated to exhibit both CNS and extra-CNS actions to attenuate hypotension induced by endotoxin, hemorrhage, spinal-cord injury, leukotrienes, and anaphylaxis (Holaday and Faden, 1983; Holaday *et al.*, 1981; Faden *et al.*, 1981; Lux *et al.*, 1983a,b), TRF is currently being evaluated for its efficacy in treatment of certain forms of hypotension in humans (Faden, 1984). TRF's effects on hypotension are similar to but dissociable from those of the opiate receptor antagonist, naloxone (Faden, 1984).

2. Metabolic Effects

TRF placed into the lateral ventricles of rats has been reported to produce hyperglycemia or hypoglycemia (Brown, 1981; Amir and Butler, 1988). The hyperglycemia is associated with a rise in glucagon and lowering of insulin concentrations in plasma (Brown, 1981). Adrenalectomy, but not CNS administration of SS-28 or des $AA^{1,2,4,5,12,13}$ [D-Trp^8]-somatostatin, prevents TRF-induced hyperglycemia. Thus, TRF-induced hyperglycemia appears to be mediated by adrenal Epi secretion and subsequent changes in insulin and glucagon secretion leading to enhanced hepatic glucose production. The report of TRF-induced hypoglycemia has not been confirmed by other investigators, but could result from parasympathetic stimulation of insulin secretion (Amir and Butler, 1988).

3. Gastrointestinal and Pancreatic Effects

TRF placed into the CNS elicits an increase of the acidity and volume of gastric secretions and an increase of the volume of pancreatic exocrine secretions (Kato and Kanno, 1983; Tache *et al.*, 1980b). Both of these effects are attenuated by subdiaphragmatic vagotomy or atropine treatment (Kato and Kanno, 1983; Tache *et al.*, 1980b).

E. Physiologic Role of TRF in Regulating the Autonomic Nervous System

A physiologic role of TRF in the regulation of the ANS is supported by the observation that icv administration of a TRF antiserum inhibits the spontaneous electrical discharge of the superior laryngeal nerve (Tonoue *et al.*, 1982). These data are consistent with the above-mentioned finding that TRF acts within the CNS to increase superior laryngeal nerve activity (Somiya and Tonoue, 1984; Tonoue, 1982).

IV. Bombesin and Related Peptides

Bombesin-related peptides range in size from nine to 27 amino acids. Bombesin acts within the mammalian brain to modify ANS activity and visceral organ function. Bombesin-related peptides and their receptors have been identified in brain regions that are involved in the regulation of the ANS and visceral systems (Panula *et al.*, 1982; Moody *et al.*, 1978).

A. Effects of Bombesin on the Adrenal Medulla

Bombesin (57–570 pmol) administered into the lateral or third cerebroventricle, or into the cisternum magnum, produces an increase in the plasma concentration of Epi that is totally prevented by bilateral adrenalectomy (Brown *et al.*, 1979b; Brown and Fisher, 1984). At low doses, bombesin given icv elevates plasma concentration of Epi without affecting plasma NE levels in both the rat and dog (Brown *et al.*, 1979b; Brown and Fisher, 1984). Bombesin-induced elevations of plasma Epi levels are not prevented by icv administration of cholinergic, adrenergic, or dopamine receptor antagonists, or by iv administration of naloxone (M. R. Brown, unpublished observation).

A site of action wherein bombesin increases plasma concentration of Epi has been identified within the brainstem in unanesthetized rats (Brown *et al.*, 1989a). Injection of bombesin (5.7 pmol) into the rostral aspect of the NTS produces a dramatic elevation of plasma concentration of Epi; this effect is not observed when bombesin is injected into neighboring or distant brain sites.

B. Effects of Bombesin on the Sympathetic Nervous System

The icv administration of bombesin stimulates an increase of the plasma concentration of NE that is not prevented by adrenalectomy (Panula *et al.*, 1982; Moody *et al.*, 1978). The site of action of bombesin to increase plasma levels of NE has not been identified; however, it may be the same as the site for this peptide to influence adrenal Epi secretion, that is, the rostral NTS or surrounding area of the brainstem.

C. Effects of Bombesin on the Parasympathetic Nervous System

Bombesin, given icv, decreases the firing rate of the gastric ramus of the vagus while markedly increasing transmission through the superior laryn-geal branch of the vagus in the rat (Somiya and Tonoue, 1984). Icv adminis-tration of bombesin into conscious rats produces profound bradycardia and potent inhibition of gastric emptying (Fisher *et al.*, 1985a; Porreca and Burks, 1983). These actions of bombesin are largely attenuated by methyl atropine treatment and subdiaphragmatic vagotomy, supporting the notion of differential activation or inhibition of various vagal branches.

D. Effects of Bombesin on Cardiorespiratory Function

As noted above, bombesin administered icv has profound effects on cardio-vascular function. Bombesin completely prevents cold-induced tachycardia (Fisher *et al.*, 1985c), while having no effect on cold-induced elevations of MAP. The correlation between bombesin's effect on HR and oxygen con-sumption strongly suggests that CO is also impaired.

Bombesin administered icv to rats housed at room temperature de-creases HR and increases MAP (Fisher *et al.*, 1985a,b). Adrenalectomy pre-vents bombesin-induced increases of MAP, but does not alter the decrease of HR (Fisher *et al.*, 1985b). Thus, the decrease of HR is not a baroreflex-mediated effect resulting from bombesin-induced elevation of MAP. It is assumed, but not proven, that the elevation of MAP following bombesin administration is secondary to adrenomedullary Epi secretion. This conclu-sion is supported by the observation that treatment of animals with the alpha-adrenergic receptor antagonist phentolamine prevents bombesin-in-duced elevations of MAP (Fisher *et al.*, 1985b).

Bombesin-induced bradycardia is partially reversed by methyl atro-pine treatment (Fisher *et al.*, 1985a,b). These results are consistent with the conclusion that bombesin increases parasympathetic–cholinergic outflow to the heart, resulting in slowing of HR (Fisher *et al.*, 1985b). Administration of propranolol does not result in any further slowing of HR in bombesin-treated rats. These results suggest that bombesin functionally inhibits sym-pathetic innervation of the heart, and this effect may contribute to the slow-ing of HR.

In anesthetized rats, icv administration of bombesin increases minute ventilation through elevations of both respiratory rate and tidal volume

(Niewoehner *et al.*, 1983). Likewise, intracisternal injection of bombesin increases minute ventilation and inspiratory drive in anesthetized cats; in this species, both tidal volume and MAP are elevated, but no changes of respiratory or HR are observed (Holtman *et al.*, 1983).

E. Effects of Bombesin on Nutrient Metabolism

Hyperglycemia is observed after administration of bombesin into the lateral ventricle, cisterna magna, ventromedial hypothalamus, or lateral hypothalamic area of the rat, and into the third ventricle or dorsal hypothalamic area of the dog (Brown *et al.*, 1979b; Brown, 1983; Gunion *et al.*, 1984; Iguchi *et al.*, 1984). Bombesin-induced hyperglycemia is associated with an elevation of plasma glucagon levels and an absolute or relative reduction of plasma insulin levels (Brown *et al.*, 1979b). Adrenalectomy prevents the CNS actions of bombesin on circulating levels of glucose, glucagon, and insulin, indicating that these effects are secondary to adrenomedullary Epi secretion (Brown *et al.*, 1977a). Consistent with this notion is the observed inability of bombesin to elicit hyperglycemia when adrenal Epi secretion is inhibited by CNS administration of SS-related peptides (Fisher and Brown, 1980; Brown *et al.*, 1981b). Thus, bombesin-induced hyperglycemia in the rat is most likely mediated by elevated plasma Epi levels, which increase the glucagon/insulin ratio in plasma, thereby enhancing hepatic glucose production.

F. Effects of Bombesin on Autonomic Regulation and Thermoregulation

The first CNS action of bombesin to be characterized was the effect of this peptide to decrease core temperature of cold-exposed rats (Brown *et al.*, 1977b). The CNS effects of bombesin on body temperature vary in parallel with ambient temperature. Thus, bombesin injected icv produces hypothermia in cold-exposed rats, hyperthermia in heat-stressed rats, and no change in body temperature in rats maintained in thermoneutral environments (Tache *et al.*, 1980a).

Bombesin acts within the anterior hypothalamic-preoptic region of the rat brain to decrease body temperature of cold-exposed rats (Pittman *et al.*, 1980; Wunder *et al.*, 1980).

Bombesin-induced decreases of body temperature result from an inhibition of regulatory heat production. Animals placed in a cold environment, below their thermoneutral zone, undergo a dose-dependent decrease of body temperature associated with an impairment of oxygen consumption without evidence of increased heat loss (Brown, 1982). Animals receiving bombesin are not poikilothermic, but they do not have the ability to increase heat production when placed in a cold environment. Effects of bombesin on behavior suggest that a change of thermoregulatory set point may be produced by this peptide (Wunder *et al.*, 1980).

The mechanism by which bombesin inhibits regulatory heat production has been investigated using several types of studies. Bombesin administered icv may inhibit TRF release and/or delivery to the pituitary as thyrotropin release is suppressed in cold-exposed rats (Brown and Vale, 1980). The role of bombesin in influencing brain TRF release and/or its CNS actions on temperature regulation has not been explored in detail. It is of interest, however, that TRF administered icv does reverse bombesin-induced hypothermia (Brown *et al.*, 1977a).

A second possible mechanism by which bombesin influences thermoregulation could be through an action to impair the sympathetic or somatic nervous system responses to cold exposure. Bombesin given icv is a potent stimulus for adrenal Epi secretion, produces modest elevations of plasma NE levels, does not impair shivering, and increases gross motor activity in animals exposed to cold. Although cold-exposed rats receiving bombesin icv exhibit normal elevations of plasma NE levels, this peptide is demonstrated to impair SNS responses to cold exposure. Acute exposure to cold produces an increase in heat production mediated in part through SNS stimulation of interscapular brown fat metabolism. As noted above, bombesin administered icv prevents this cold-induced elevation of SNS innervation to brown fat (Brown *et al.*, 1987). The action of bombesin to impair sympathetic activation of brown fat may be an important factor responsible for the disruption of thermoregulation upon exposure to cold environments.

A third mechanism by which bombesin could impair thermoregulation is by alteration of cardiovascular function resulting in decreased metabolic substrate delivery to cellular site of heat production. The inability to increase heat production may result from diminished CO, since icv administration of bombesin completely abolishes cold-induced tachycardia (Fisher *et al.*, 1985c). If tachycardia is essential for elevating CO, then bombesin administration may compromise blood flow and, hence, nutrient delivery to the sites of cellular heat production. This hypothesis is compatible with the observation that HR and oxygen consumption are tightly coupled in bombesin-treated rats during cold exposure and that CNS administration of SS-related peptides reverses the effects of bombesin on HR, oxygen consumption, and body temperature.

In summary, bombesin acts within the CNS to decrease regulatory heat production and oxygen consumption during cold exposure. This effect is associated with an inhibition of brain TRF release, decreased sympathetic stimulation of interscapular brown fat, and a decrease of HR and CO.

Thus, bombesin acts within the CNS to produce a complement of actions that collectively slow an animal's metabolism. Efforts to evaluate the physiologic significance of endogenous brain bombesin require a useful receptor anatagonist.

V. Somatostatin-Related Peptides

Somatostatins comprise a family of peptides, and their analogs including somatostatin-14 (SS-14), somatostatin-28 (SS-28), and des AA[1,2,3,4,5,12,13] [D-Trp[8]]-somatostatin-14 (ODT8-SS). A unique feature of SS-related peptides compared to all other known peptides is the action of these substances to inhibit the secretions of many anatomically and histologically diverse cell types.

A. Effects of Somatostatin on the Sympathetic Nervous System and Adrenal Medulla

SS-28 and ODT8-SS, but not SS-14, act within the CNS to inhibit basal and stimulate adrenal Epi secretion in the rat and dog (Somiya and Tonoue, 1984; Brown, 1983; Brown and Fisher, 1985a; M. R. Brown and L. A. Fisher, unpublished data, 1984; Brown et al., 1985a). SS-28 and ODT8-SS administered into the lateral cerebroventricle inhibit Epi secretion induced by CRF, bombesin, carbachol, 2-deoxyglucose, insulin-induced hypoglycemia, cold exposure, tail suspension, ether vapor exposure, and ethanol treatment (Somiya and Tonoue, 1984; Brown, 1983; Brown and Fisher, 1985a; M. R. Brown and L. A. Fisher, unpublished data, 1984; Brown et al., 1985a) The rise in plasma NE levels following these treatments is not influenced by CNS administration of either SS-28 or ODT8-SS. Studies in the dog demonstrate that the dorsal hypothalamic area is a site of action of SS-28 and ODT8-SS for inhibiting bombesin-induced adrenal Epi secretion (Brown, 1983). Depletion of brain concentrations of SS-related peptides using cysteamine or CNS administration of an SS-receptor antagonist results in increased adrenal Epi secretion (Brown et al., 1985a). SS-14 given icv is reported to decrease gastric sympathetic and adrenal nerve activity (Somiya and Tonoue, 1984).

B. Effects of Somatostatin on the Parasympathetic Nervous System

ODT8-SS given into the CNS increases gastric acid secretion by increasing vagal outflow to the stomach (Tache et al., 1981). As such, subdiaphragmatic vagotomy prevents ODT8-SS-induced gastric acid secretion. SS-14 acts within the CNS to decrease gastric vagal and superior laryngeal nerve activity (Brown, 1988).

C. Effects of Somatostatin on Vasopressin and Oxytocin Release

The icv administration of SS-28 produces an increase of MAP and a decrease of HR that are secondary to pituitary vasopressin release (Brown, 1988). SS-28 given icv also elevates plasma concentrations of oxytocin (Brown et al., 1988a). Sawchenko has recently described an SS-containing pathway that projects from the NTS to vasopressin- and oxytocin-containing cells in the paraventricular and supraoptic nuclei of the hypothalamus (Sawchenko et al., 1988). Depletion of brain SS using cysteamine attenuates hemorrhage-induced elevation of plasma vasopressin levels (Brown et al., 1988c). SS has been demonstrated to inhibit hypothalamic NE release, providing a possible mechanism by which this peptide may stimulate vasopressin release (Gothert, 1980). Thus, SS-containing neural pathways may be involved in mediating hemorrhage-induced vasopressin secretion.

D. Effects of Somatostatin on Physiologic Systems

1. Cardiovascular Effects

As noted above, icv or paraventricular nucleus injections of SS-28 increase MAP and decrease HR, an effect mediated by the release of vasopressin.

2. Metabolic Effects

The initial rationale to investigate the CNS actions of SS-28 and ODT8-SS on the ANS was based on the observation that these two peptides prevent hyperglycemia induced by a variety of neurally acting stimuli, such as bombesin, carbachol, and 2-deoxyglucose administration and physical and chemical stressors (Brown et al., 1979a). The mechanism by which SS-28 and ODT8-SS prevent hyperglycemia induced by these treatments is through the inhibition of adrenal Epi secretion (Fisher and Brown, 1980; Brown et al., 1981b; Brown, 1983; Brown and Fisher, 1985a; M. R. Brown and L. A. Fisher, unpublished data, 1984).

3. Gastrointestinal Effects

ODT8-SS, but not SS-14, given icv to rats increases gastric acid secretion by a vagal-dependent mechanism (Bueno and Ferre, 1982). This is in contrast to the effects of ODT8-SS or SS-14 to inhibit gastric acid secretion when given systemically. SS-14 placed into the CNS is reported to increase the frequency of the migrating myoelectric complexes of the small intestine (Tache et al., 1981).

E. Physiologic Role of Somatostatin in Regulating the Autonomic Nervous System

It has become evident over the past few years that SS-28 and the SS-14 analog ODT8-SS exhibit similar CNS actions to modify adrenal Epi secretion, gastric acid secretion, and thermoregulation. SS-14, however, is relatively devoid of these actions. Whether these differences are due to differential receptor binding, intrinsic activity, or bioavailability of the SS-related peptides has not been determined. Recent studies using cysteamine to deplete or inactivate endogenous brain somatostatins or using an SS receptor antagonist support the hypothesis that endogenous SS-related peptides may be involved in the physiologic regulation of adrenal Epi and vasopressin secretion (Brown *et al.*, 1985a, 1988c).

References

Almeida, O. F. X., Nikolarakis, K. E., and Herz, A. (1988). Evidence for the involvement of endogenous opioids in the inhibition of luteinizing hormone by corticotropin-releasing factor. *Endocrinology (Baltimore)* **122**, 1034–1041.

Amir, S., and Butler, P. D. (1988). Thyrotropin-releasing hormone blocks neurally-mediated hyperglycemia through central action. *Peptides (N.Y.)* **9**, 31–35.

Arase, K., York, D. A., Shimizu, H., Shargill, N., and Bray, G. A. (1988). Effects of corticotropin-releasing factor on food intake and brown adipose tissue thermogenesis in rats. *Am. J. Physiol.* **255**, E255–E259.

Arase, K., Shargill, N. S., and Bray, G. A. (1989). Effects of intraventricular infusion of corticotropin-releasing factor on VMH-lesioned obese rats. *Am. J. Physiol.* **25**, R751–R756.

Bloom, F. E., Battenberg, E. L. F., Rivier, J., and Vale, W. (1982). Corticotropin releasing factor (CRF): Immunoreactive neurones and fibers in rat hypothalamus. *Regul. Pept.* **4**, 215–219.

Brown, M. R. (1981). Thyrotropin releasing factor: A putative CNS regulator of the autonomic nervous system. *Life Sci.* **28**, 1789–1795.

Brown, M. R. (1982). Bombesin and somatostatin related peptides: Effects on oxygen consumption. *Brain Res.* **242**, 243–246.

Brown, M. R. (1983). Central nervous system sites of action of bombesin and somatostatin to influence plasma epinephrine levels. *Brain Res.* **276**, 253–257.

Brown, M. R. (1986). Corticotropin releasing factor: Central nervous system sites of action. *Brain Res.* **399**, 10–14.

Brown, M. R. (1988). Somatostatin-28 effects on central nervous system regulation of vasopressin secretion and blood pressure. *Neuroendocrinology* **47**, 556–562.

Brown, M. R. (1989). Neuropeptide regulation of the autonomic nervous system. *In* "Neuropeptides and Stress" (T. Tache, J. E. Morley, and M. R. Brown, eds.), pp. 107–120. Springer-Verlag, New York.

Brown, M. R., and Fisher, L. A. (1983). Central nervous system effects of corticotropin releasing factor in the dog. *Brain Res.* **280**, 75–79.

Brown, M. R., and Fisher, L. A. (1984). Brain peptide regulation of adrenal epinephrine secretion. *Am. J. Physiol.* **247**, E41–E46.

Brown, M. R., and Fisher, L. A. (1985a). Central nervous system actions of somatostatin-related peptides. *In* "Somatostatin" (Y. C. Patel and G. S. Tannenbaum, eds.), pp. 217–118. Plenum, New York.

Brown, M. R., and Fisher, L. A. (1985b). Corticotropin-releasing factor: Effects on the autonomic nervous system and visceral systems. *Fed. Proc., Fed. Am. Soc. Exp. Biol.* **44**, 243–248.

Brown, M. R., and Fisher, L. A. (1990). CRF: Regulation of the autonomic nervous system by corticotropin releasing factor. *In* "Corticotropin-Releasing Factor: Basic and Clinical Studies of a Neuropeptide" (E. B. DeSouza and C. B. Nemeroff, eds.), pp. 291–298 CRC Press, Boca Raton, Florida.

Brown, M. R., and Vale, W. (1980). Peptides and thermoregulation. *In* "Thermoregulatory Mechanisms and Their Therapeutic Implications" (B. Cox, P. Lomax, A. S. Milton, and E. Schonbaum, eds.), pp. 186–194. Karger, Basel.

Brown, M. R., Rivier, J., and Vale, W. (1977a). Bombesin affects the central nervous system to produce hyperglycemia in rats. *Life Sci.* **21**, 1729–1734.

Brown, M. R., Rivier, J., and Vale, W. (1977b). Bombesin: Potent effects on thermoregulation in the rat. *Science* **196**, 998–1000.

Brown, M. R., Rivier, J., and Vale, W. (1979a). Somatostatin: Central nervous system actions on glucoregulation. *Endocrinology (Baltimore)* **104**, 1709–1715.

Brown, M. R., Tache, Y., and Fisher, D. (1979b). Central nervous system action of bombesin: Mechanism to induce hyperglycemia. *Endocrinology (Baltimore)* **105**, 660–665.

Brown, M. R., Fisher, L. A., Rivier, J., Spiess, J., Rivier, C., and Vale, W. (1981a). Corticotropin-releasing factor: Effects on the sympathetic nervous system and oxygen consumption. *Life Sci.* **30**, 207–210.

Brown, M. R., Rivier, J., and Vale, W. (1981b). Somatostatin-28: Selective action on the pancreatic beta-cell and brain. *Endocrinology (Baltimore)* **108**, 2391–2393.

Brown, M. R., Fisher, L. A., Spiess, J., Rivier, C., Rivier, J., and Vale, W. (1982). Corticotropin-releasing factor: Actions on the sympathetic nervous system and metabolism. *Endocrinology (Baltimore)* **111**, 928–931.

Brown, M. R., Fisher, L., Mason, R. T., Rivier, J., and Vale, W. (1985a). Neurobiological actions of cysteamine. *Fed. Proc., Fed. Am. Soc. Exp. Biol.* **44**, 2556–2560.

Brown, M. R., Fisher, L. A., Webb, V., Vale, W. W., and Rivier, J. E. (1985b). Corticotropin-releasing factor: A physiologic regulator of adrenal epinephrine secretion. *Brain Res.* **328**, 355–357.

Brown, M. R., Gray, T. S., and Fisher, L. A. (1986). Corticotropin-releasing factor receptor antagonist: Effects on the autonomic nervous system and cardiovascular function. *Regul. Pept.* **16**, 321–329.

Brown, M. R., Allen, R., and Fisher, L. (1987). Bombesin alters the sympathetic nervous system response to cold exposure. *Brain Res.* **400**, 35–39.

Brown, M. R., Crum, R., and Sawchenko, P. (1988a). Somatostatin-28 (SS-28) stimulation of vasopressin (AVP) and oxytocin (OF) secretion. *Endocrinology (Baltimore)* **122**, No. 660.

Brown, M. R., Hauger, R., and Fisher, L. A. (1988b). Autonomic and cardiovascular effects of corticotropin-releasing factor in the spontaneously hypertensive rat. *Brain Res.* **441**, 33–40.

Brown, M. R., Mortrud, M., Crum, R., and Sawchenko, P. (1988c). Role of somatostatin in the regulation of vasopressin secretion. *Brain Res.* **452**, 212–218.

Brown, M. R., Carver, K., and Fisher, L. A. (1989a). Bombesin: Central nervous system actions to affect the autonomic nervous system. *Ann. N.Y. Acad. Sci.* **547**, 174–182.

Brown, M. R., Carver-Moore, K., Gray, T. S., and Rivier, C. (1989b). Thyrotropin releasing factor-induced ACTH secretion is mediated by corticotropin releasing factor. *Endocrinology (Baltimore)* **125**, 2558–2562.

Bueno, L., and Ferre, J. P. (1982). Central regulation of intestinal motility by somatostatin and cholecystokinin octapeptide. *Science* **216**, 1427–1428.

DeSouza, E. B. (1987). Corticotropin-releasing factor receptors in the rat central nervous system: Characterization and regional distribution. *J. Neurosci.* **7**, 88–100.

Diz, D. I., and Jacobowitz, D. M. (1984). Cardiovascular effects produced by injections of thyrotropin-releasing hormone in specific preoptic and hypothalamic nuclei in the rat. *Peptides (N.Y.)* **5**, 801–808.

Druge, G., Raedler, A., Greten, H., and Lenz, H. J. (1989). Pathways mediating CRF-induced inhibition of gastric acid secretion in rats. *Am. J. Physiol.* **256**, G214–G219.

Faden, A. I. (1984). Opiate antagonists and thyrotropin-releasing hormone. I. Potential role in the treatment of shock. *J. Am. Med. Assoc.* **252**, 1177–1180.

Faden, A. I., Jacobs, T. P., and Holaday, J. W. (1981). Thyrotropin-releasing hormone improves neurologic recovery after spinal trauma in cats. *N. Engl. J. Med.* **305**, 1063–1067.

Feuerstein, G., Hassen, A. H., and Faden, A. I. (1983). TRF: Cardiovascular and sympathetic modulation in brain nuclei of the rat. *Peptides (N.Y.)* **4**, 617–620.

Fisher, L. A. (1988). Corticotropin-releasing factor: Central nervous system effects on baroreflex control of heart rate. *Life Sci.* **42**, 2645–2649.

Fisher, L. A., and Brown, M. (1980). Somatostatin analog: Plasma catecholamine suppression mediated by the central nervous system. *Endocrinology (Baltimore)* **107**, 714–718.

Fisher, L. A., and Brown, M. R. (1983). Corticotropin-releasing factor: Central nervous system effects on the sympathetic nervous system and cardiovascular regulation. *Curr. Top. Neuroendocrinol.* **3**, 87–101.

Fisher, L. A., Rivier, J., Rivier, C., Spiess, J., Vale, W., and Brown, M. R. (1982). Corticotropin-releasing factor (CRF): Central effects of mean arterial pressure and heart rate in rats. *Endocrinology (Baltimore)* **110**, 2222–2224.

Fisher, L. A., Jessen, G., and Brown, M. R. (1983). Corticotropin-releasing factor (CRF): Mechanism to elevate mean arterial pressure and heart rate. *Regul. Pept.* **5**, 153–161.

Fisher, L. A., Cave, C. R., and Brown, M. R. (1985a). Bombesin-induced stimulation of cardiac parasympathetic innervation. *Regul. Pept.* **8**, 335–343.

Fisher, L. A., Cave, C. R., and Brown, M. R. (1985b). Central nervous system cardiovascular effects of bombesin in conscious rats. *Am. J. Physiol.* **248**, H425–H431.

Fisher, L. A., Cave, C. R., and Brown, M. R. (1985c). Central nervous system effects of bombesin on the cardiovascular response to cold exposure. *Brain Res.* **341**, 261–268.

Gothert, M. (1980). Somatostatin selectively inhibits noradrenaline release from hypothalamic neurones. *Nature (London)* **288**, 86–88.

Grosskreutz, C. L., and Brody, M. R. (1988). Regional hemodynamic responses to central administration of corticotropin-releasing factor (CRF). *Brain Res.* **442**, 363–367.

Gunion, M. W., Grijalva, C. V., Tache, Y., and Novin, D. (1984). Lateral hypothalamic lesions or transections block bombesin hyperglycemia in rats. *Brain Res.* **299**, 239–246.

Hardwick, A. J., Linton, E. A., and Rothwell, N. J. (1989). Thermogenic effects of the antiglucocorticoid RU-486 in the rat: Involvement of corticotropin-releasing factor and sympathetic activation of brown adipose tissue. *Endocrinology (Baltimore)* **124**, 1684–1688.

Hattori, T., Hashimoto, K., and Ota, A. (1986). Brain corticotropin releasing factor in the spontaneously hypertensive rat. *Hypertension (Dallas)* **8**, 1027–1031.

Hedner, J., Hedner, T., Wessberg, P., Lundberg, D., and Jonason, J. (1983). Effects of TRH and TRH analogues on the central regulation of breathing in the rat. *Acta Physiol. Scand.* **117**, 427–437.

Holaday, J. W., and Faden, A. I. (1983). Thyrotropin releasing hormone: Autonomic effects upon cardiorespiratory function in endotoxic shock. *Regul. Pept.* **7**, 111–125.

Holaday, J. W., D'Amato, R. J., and Faden, A. I. (1981). Thyrotropin-releasing hormone improves cardiovascular function in experimental endotoxic and hemorrhagic shock. *Science* **213**, 216–218.

Holtman, J. R., Jr., Jensen, R. T., Buller, A., Hamoah, P., Taveira De Silva, A. M., and Gillis, R. A. (1983). Central respiratory stimulant effect of bombesin in the cat. *Eur. J. Pharmacol.* **90**, 449–452.

Iguchi, A., Matsunaga, H., Nomura, T., Gotoh, M., and Sakamoto, N. (1984). Glucoregulatory effects of intrahypothalamic injections of bombesin and other peptides. *Endocrinology (Baltimore)* **114**, 2242–2246.

Irwin, M., Hauger, R. L., Brown, M., and Britton, K. T. (1988). CRF activates autonomic nervous system and reduces natural killer cytotoxicity. *Am. J. Physiol.* **255**, R744-R747.

Kato, Y., and Kanno, T. (1983). Thyrotropin-releasing hormone injected intracerebroventricularly in the rat stimulates exocrine pancreatic secretion via the vagus nerve. *Regul. Pept.* **7**, 347–356.

Koivasalo, F., Paakkari, I., Leppaluoto, J., and Karppanen, H. (1979). The effect of centrally administered TRH on blood pressure, heart rate and ventilation in rat. *Acta Physiol. Scand.* **106**, 83–86.

Kregel, K. C., Overton, J. M., Fisher, L. A., Taylor, J. A., Tipton, C. M., and Seals, D. L. (1988). Influence of central CRF^{9-41} injection on the cardiovascular responses to exercise in the rat. *FASEB J.* **2**, A1318, No. 5944.

Krieger, D. T., Brownstein, M. J., and Martin, J. B., ed. (1983). "Brain Peptides." Wiley, New York.

Kurosawa, M., Sato, A., Swenson, R. S., and Takahashi, Y. (1986). Sympathoadrenal medullary functions in response to intracerebroventricularly injected corticotropin-releasing factor in anesthetized rats. *Brain Res.* **367**, 250–257.

Lenz, H. J. (1985). Corticotropin-releasing factor: Mechanisms to inhibit gastric acid secretion in conscious dogs. *J. Clin. Invest.* **75**, 889–895.

Lenz, H. J. (1989). Regulation of duodenal bicarbonate secretion during stress by corticotropin-releasing factor and beta-endorphin. *Proc. Natl. Acad. Sci. U.S.A.* **86**, 1417–1420.

Lenz, H. J., Fisher, L. A., Vale, W. W., and Brown, M. R. (1985). Corticotropin-releasing factor, sauvagine and urotensin-I: Effects on blood flow. *Am. J. Physiol.* **249**, R85-R90.

Lenz, H. J., Raedler, A., Greten, H., Vale, W. W., and Rivier, J. E. (1988). Stress-induced gastrointestinal secretory and motor responses in rats are mediated by endogenous corticotropin-releasing factor. *Gastroenterology* **95**, 1510–1517.

Lux, W. E., Jr., Feuerstein, G., and Faden, A. I. (1983a). Alteration of leukotriene D4 hypotension by thyrotropin releasing hormone. *Nature (London)* **302**, 822–824.

Lux, W. E., Jr., Feuerstein, G., and Faden, A. I. (1983b). Thyrotropin-releasing hormone reverses experimental anaphylactic shock through nonendorphin-related mechanisms. *Eur. J. Pharmacol.* **90**, 301–302.

Moga, M. M., and Gray, T. S. (1985). Evidence for corticotropin-releasing factor, neurotensin, and somatostatin in the neural pathway from the central nucleus of the amygdala to the parabrachial nucleus. *J. Comp. Neurol.* **241**, 275–284.

Moody, T. W., Pert, C. B., Rivier, J., and Brown, M. R. (1978). Bombesin: Specific binding to rat brain membranes. *Proc. Natl. Acad. Sci. U.S.A.* **75**, 5372–5376.

Myers, R. D., Metcalf, G., and Rice, J. C. (1977). Identification by microinjection of TRH-sensitive sites in the cat's brain stem that mediate respiratory, temperature and other autonomic changes. *Brain Res.* **126**, 105–115.

Niewoehner, D. E., Levine, A. S., and Morley, J. E. (1983). Central effects of neuropeptides on ventilation in the rat. *Peptides (N.Y.)* **4**, 277–281.

Ono, N., Lumpkin, M. D., Samson, W. K., McDonald, J. K., and McCann, S. M. (1984). Intrahypothalamic action of corticotropin-releasing factor (CRF) to inhibit growth hormone and LH release in the rat. *Life Sci.* **35**, 1117–1123.

Overton, J. M., and Fisher, L. A. (1989). Differentiated regional hemodynamic responses to peripheral and central administration of corticotropin-releasing factor. *FASEB J.* **3**, A1015, No. 4583.

Palkovits, M. (1988). Distribution of neuropeptides in brain: A review of biochemical and immunohistochemical studies. *In* "Peptide Hormones: Effects and Mechanisms of Action" (A. Negro-Vilar and P. M. Conn, eds.), Vol. 1, pp. 3–67. CRC Press, Boca Raton, Florida.

Palkovits, M., Brownstein, M. J., and Vale, W. (1985). Distribution of corticotropin-releasing factor in rat brain. *Fed. Proc., Fed. Am. Soc. Exp. Biol.* **44**, 215–219.

Panula, P., Yang, H.-Y. T., and Costa, E. (1982). Neuronal location of the bombesin-like immunoreactivity in the central nervous system of the rat. *Regul. Pept.* **4**, 275–283.

Pittman, Q. J., Tache, Y., and Brown, M. R. (1980). Bombesin acts in preoptic area to produce hypothermia in rats. *Life Sci.* **26**, 725–730.

Porreca, F., and Burks, T. F. (1983). Centrally administered bombesin affects gastric emptying and small and large bowel transit in the rat. *Gastroenterology* **85**, 313–317.

Rivier, C., and Vale, W. (1985). Involvement of corticotropin-releasing factor and somatostatin in stress-induced inhibition of growth hormone secretion in the rat. *Endocrinology (Baltimore)* **117**, 2478–2482.

Rivier, C., Rivier, J., and Vale, W. (1986). Stress-induced inhibition of reproductive functions: Role of endogenous corticotropin-releasing factor. *Science* **213**, 607–609.

Rivier, C., Vale, W., and Brown, M. (1989). In the rat, interleukin-1 alpha and beta stimulate ACTH and catecholamine release. *Endocrinology (Baltimore)* **125**, 3096–3102.

Rohner-Jeanrenaud, F., Walker, C.-D., Greco-Perotto, R., and Jeanrenaud, B. (1989). Central corticotropin-releasing factor administration prevents the excessive body weight gain of genetically obese *(fa/fa)* rats. *Endocrinology (Baltimore)* **124**, 733–739.

Sawchenko, P. E., Benoit, R., and Brown, M. R. (1988). Somatostatin 28-immunoreactive inputs to the paraventricular and supraoptic nuclei: Principal origin from non-aminergic neurons in the nucleus of the solitary tract. *J. Chem. Neuroanat.* **1**, 81–94.

Smith, J. R., Lahann, T. R., Chestnut, R. M., Carino, M. A., and Horita, A. (1977). Thyrotropin-releasing hormone: Stimulation of colonic activity following intracerebroventricular administration. *Science* **196**, 660–662.

Somiya, H., and Tonoue, T. (1984). Neuropeptide as central integrators of autonomic nerve activity: Effects of TRH, SRIF, VIP and bombesin on gastric and adrenal nerves. *Regul. Pept.* **9**, 47–52.

Sundar, S. K., Becker, K. J., and Weiss, J. M. (1988). Rapid decrease in peripheral immune responses following intracerebral infusion of interleukin-1 or stimulated endogenous release of Il-1. *Soc. Neurosci.* **14**, No. 513.1, 1281.

Swanson, L. W., Sawchenko, P. E., Rivier, J., and Vale, W. W. (1983). Organization of ovine corticotropin-releasing factor immunoreactive cells and fibers in the rat brain: An immunohistochemical study. *Neuroendocrinology* **36**, 165–186.

Tache, Y., Pittman, Q., and Brown, M. (1980a). Bombesin-induced poikilothermy in rats. *Brain Res.* **188**, 525–530.

Tache, Y., Vale, W., and Brown, M. (1980b). Thyrotropin-releasing hormone-CNS action to stimulate gastric acid secretion. *Nature (London)* **287**, 149–151.

Tache, Y., Rivier, J., Vale, W., and Brown, M. (1981). Is somatostatin or a somatostatin-like peptide involved in central nervous system control of gastric secretion? *Regul. Pept.* **1**, 307–315.

Tache, Y., Goto, Y., Gunion, M. W., Vale, W., Rivier, J., and Brown, M. (1983). Inhibition of gastric acid secretion in rats by intracerebral injection of corticotropin-releasing factor. *Science* **222**, 935–937.

Tache, Y., Maeda-Hagiwara, M., and Turkelson, C. M. (1987). Central nervous system action of corticotropin-releasing factor to inhibit gastric emptying in rats. *Am. J. Physiol.* **253**, G241-G245.

Tonoue, T. (1982). Stimulation by thyrotropin-releasing hormone of vagal outflow to the thyroid gland. *Regul. Pept.* **3**, 29–39.

Tonoue, T., Somiya, H., Matsumoto, H., Ogawa, N., and Leppaluoto, J. (1982). Evidence that endogenous thyrotropin-releasing hormone (TRH) may control vagal efferents to thyroid gland: Neural inhibition by central administration of TRH antiserum. *Regul. Pept.* **4**, 293–298.

Vale, W., Rivier, C., and Brown, M. (1977). Regulatory peptides of the hypothalamus. *Annu. Rev. Physiol.* **39**, 473–527.

Vale, W., Rivier, C., Brown, M. R., Spiess, J., Koob, G., Swanson, L., Bilezikjian, L., Bloom, F., and Rivier, J. (1983). Chemical and biological characterization of corticotropin releasing factor. *Recent Prog. Horm. Res.* **39**, 245–270.

Williams, C. L., Peterson, J. M., Villar, R. G., and Burks, T. F. (1987). Corticotropin-releasing factor directly mediates colonic responses to stress. *Am. J. Physiol.* **253**, G582-G586.

Wunder, B. A., Hawkins, M. F., Avery, D. D., and Swan, H. (1980). The effects of bombesin injected into the anterior and posterior hypothalamus on body temperature and oxygen consumption. *Neuropharmacology* **19**, 1095–1097.

6

Corticotropin-Releasing Factor and Autonomic–Cardiovascular Responses to Stress

Laurel A. Fisher
Department of Pharmacology
College of Medicine
University of Arizona
Tucson, Arizona 85724

I. Introduction

Various physical and psychological stimuli elicit marked effects on the cardiovascular system. In an acute time domain, stress-induced cardiovascular responses are essential for supporting or enabling concomitant behavioral and somatic adaptations. Sustained cardiovascular activation, however, is suspected of engendering deleterious consequences such as hypertension, cardiac rhythm disorders, and stroke. The fundamental mechanisms underlying the transition from homeostatic regulation to the maladaptive state are not understood in great detail and therefore remain under active investigation.

As with stress-induced behavioral, endocrine, and somatic responses, the transduction of external and internal stimuli into acute circulatory changes occurs within the central nervous system (CNS). While important advances have occurred regarding the delineation of the neural circuitry involved in cardiovascular control, our understanding of both tonic and phasic regulatory systems is far from complete. That multiple chemical transmitters act at several central nervous system sites to influence cardiovascular function is evinced by a vast body of data; in all likelihood, the enormous array of neurotransmitters and neuroanatomical loci implicated in cardiovascular control reflects the existence of redundant CNS mechanisms defending against circulatory collapse. Perhaps owing to such redundancy, the predominance of any single transmitter candidate in mediating stress-induced cardiovascular adaptations has not, to date, been demonstrated.

The motivation, nevertheless, to identify neurotransmitters involved in such processes stems from several considerations. First, there is now compelling evidence that information transfer within the brain and spinal cord may be executed not only via synaptic connections but also through various hormonal mechanisms. Thus, in addition to impulse transmission through polysynaptic and monosynaptic circuits, the extracellular fluid may serve as a conduit for communication between distant neurons. In this sense, the composition of interstitial fluid and the distribution of functional (coupled) receptor entities at any given time may be tantamount to hard-wired neural circuits as operational determinants of neurotransmission. Moreover, in most cases of neural dysfunction or disease, chemical imbalances rather than anatomical deficits are hypothesized to be pathogenetic antecedents. As such, a pharmacological approach to the treatment of disease is demanded in terms of both theory and practice. Indeed, manipulation of chemical transmission, whether synaptic or nonsynaptic, through diet and/or drugs, is at present the standard mode of therapy for a variety of neural–visceral ailments.

The rationale to investigate the role of corticotropin-releasing factor (CRF) in mediating stress-induced autonomic and cardiovascular adaptations derives initially from this neuropeptide's established hypophysiotropic function, that is, stimulation of pituitary adrenocorticotropic hormone (ACTH) secretion. Thus, activation of the pituitary–adrenal axis, the hallmark endocrine stress response, is mediated by the release of CRF within the CNS, in this case within the median eminence of the hypothalamus. Importantly, the CNS distribution of immunoreactive CRF and CRF receptors extends beyond the hypophysiotropic zone to include several loci that are implicated in autonomic and cardiovascular regulation. Accordingly, it is tenable to hypothesize that stress-induced CRF release is not restricted to the median eminence and that the coincident expression of endocrine, autonomic, and cardiovascular responses to various stressors may be coordinated and/or integrated by CRF-mediated neurotransmission at multiple CNS sites. As detailed below, this hypothesis is supported by evidence provided from neuroanatomical, neurochemical, and neuropharmacological investigations.

II. CRF Neuronal Systems

A. CRF-Immunoreactive Neurons and Fibers

As alluded to above, cell bodies and fibers containing immunoreactive CRF are distributed both within and outside the hypothalamus (Bloom *et al.*, 1982; Olschowka *et al.*, 1982; Swanson *et al.*, 1983). Indeed, both perikarya and fibers that stain for CRF are located in multiple hypothalamic sites including but not limited to the parvocellular and magnocellular subdivisions of the paraventricular nucleus, the medial and lateral preoptic areas, the lateral hypothalamus, and the periventricular area. Within the hypothalamus, the highest concentration of CRF-containing neurons is located in the medial parvocellular subdivision of the paraventricular nucleus. Many of these cells subserve neural control of pituitary ACTH secretion and thus project to the external layer of the median eminence wherein they terminate on the hypophysial portal vessels. A small population of CRF-immunoreactive parvocellular paraventricular neurons sends axons to the dorsal vagal complex and spinal cord, sites of preganglionic autonomic motor nuclei.

Owing to their close proximity within the paraventricular nucleus, it is conceivable that these differentially projecting populations of CRF-containing cells could be activated simultaneously by a common afferent signal. In this way, endocrine and autonomic outputs could be coordinated by CRF release at disparate sites, and indeed, concomitant activation of the pituitary–adrenal axis and sympathetic nervous outflow is characteristic to various patterned stress responses. This argument is buttressed by the demonstration of an extensive network of CRF-immunoreactive axonal terminals and varicosities within the paraventricular nucleus and recent ultrastructural evidence for such terminals making synaptic contacts with CRF-positive cell bodies (Silverman *et al.*, 1989).

Whether or not such "cross-talk" between CRF-containing paraventricular neurons is extensive is at present unknown, but it is well established that reciprocal projections exist between brainstem autonomic nuclei and paraventricular CRF-containing cells. For example, CRF-positive perikarya within the paraventricular nucleus receive a dense projection from the A2 noradrenergic cells located in the nucleus tractus solitarius (Cunningham and Sawchenko, 1988), the major site of visceral sensory input to the CNS. For the purposes of this discussion, one could speculate that these A2 neurons could transmit information concerning afferent baroreceptor impulse traffic to paraventricular CRF-containing cells, which in turn could modulate the activity of brainstem and spinal autonomic motor neurons mediating cardiac and vascular responses to baroreceptor input.

The parvocellular paraventricular neurons discussed above represent only one component of CRF-containing cells that could influence autonomic and cardiovascular function. Indeed, multiple CNS autonomic areas, such as the nucleus tractus solitarius, dorsal motor vagal nucleus, ventrolateral medullary reticular formation, and intermediolateral nucleus of the spinal cord, contain CRF-positive cell bodies and fibers (Giuliano et al., 1988; Krukoff, 1986; Merchenthaler et al., 1983a,b; Olschowka et al., 1982; Schipper et al., 1983; Skofitsch and Jacobowitz, 1985; Swanson et al., 1983). Of particular relevance to the mediation of stress-induced autonomic and cardiovascular responses is the finding that CRF may be utilized as a neurotransmitter in limbic–autonomic pathways; substantial numbers of CRF-immunoreactive neurons located within the central nucleus of the amygdala and the bed nucleus of the stria terminalis project to the parabrachial nucleus and the dorsal vagal complex (Gray and Magnuson, 1987; Moga and Gray, 1985; Sakanaka et al., 1986). The reciprocal connections between pontine and brainstem autonomic nuclei, limbic structures, and the hypothalamic paraventricular nucleus thus represent viable neuroanatomical substrates for the transduction of stressful and/or emotional stimuli into integrated endocrine and autonomic responses. However, it is not at present known whether impulse transmission through these circuits is ongoing tonically or activated specifically in response to selective stressors. In this regard, the recent demonstration of reduced CRF staining within the median eminence after lesions of the central amygdaloid nucleus is of interest (Beaulieu et al., 1989); that CRF-containing neurons in the amygdala probably do not project directly to the median eminence suggests such potential trophic interactions are mediated through polysynaptic pathways.

In addition to the immunohistochemical evidence described above, immunoreactive CRF is detected in the cerebrospinal fluid (Garrick et al., 1987; Nemeroff et al., 1984; Suda et al., 1983) and in hypothalamic and extrahypothalamic CNS sites (Cote et al., 1983; Fischman and Moldow, 1982; Palkovits et al., 1983, 1985; Skofitsch and Jacobowitz, 1985) by radioimmunoassay. Moreover, blot hybridization analyses and in situ hybridization histochemistry studies demonstrate the existence of CRF messenger RNA in both hypothalamic and extrahypothalamic regions (Beyer et al., 1988; Jingami et al., 1985; Young et al., 1986). Immunohistochemical and radioimmunoassay findings differ with regard to the relative distribution and/or concentrations of immunoreactive CRF, perhaps owing to variable sensitivities and specificities of the different anti-CRF sera employed. Also, chromatographic and radioimmunologic evidence suggests that mammalian

CNS contains multiple CRF-like molecules (Skofitsch and Jacobowitz, 1985). The latter possibility is intriguing in that the nonmammalian peptides sauvagine and urotensin-I share considerable sequence homologies with CRF and produce biological actions in mammals that are similar to those of CRF (Brown *et al.*, 1982c; Lenz *et al.*, 1985).

CRF-containing neurons are subject to dynamic regulation. Concentrations of CRF immunoreactivity in both cerebrospinal fluid (Garrick *et al.*, 1987) and hypothalamus (Moldow and Fischman, 1984; Nicholson *et al.*, 1985) exhibit diurnal changes. Endogenous glucocorticoids exert negative control of CRF neuronal systems, and thus following adrenalectomy, levels of both CRF mRNA (Beyer *et al.*, 1988; Jingami *et al.*, 1985) and immunoreactive CRF (Merchenthaler *et al.*, 1983b; Sawchenko, 1987; Swanson *et al.*, 1983) within the hypothalamic paraventricular nucleus are substantially elevated. Interestingly, enhanced CRF staining after adrenalectomy or hypophysectomy is also evident in the intermediolateral spinal cord (Merchenthaler *et al.*, 1983a) and in extrahypothalamic sites such as the central nucleus of the amygdala and the bed nucleus of the stria terminalis (Merchenthaler *et al.*, 1983b; Sawchenko, 1987); as described above, these latter nuclei contain CRF-positive neurons that project to CNS autonomic areas in the pons and medulla. Most importantly, acute and chronic stressors are demonstrated to alter CRF immunoreactivity in both hypothalamic and extrahypothalamic sites (Chappell *et al.*, 1986; Haas and George, 1988; Moldow *et al.*, 1987; Murakami *et al.*, 1989; Suemaru *et al.*, 1986). Thus, CRF neuronal systems throughout the CNS are sensitive to a variety of stressful stimuli and are positioned to influence both endocrine and autonomic responses to such stimuli.

B. CRF Receptors

Specific, high-affinity CRF receptors are nonuniformly distributed throughout the CNS as determined by autoradiographic and radioligand binding analyses (De Souza, 1987; De Souza *et al.*, 1985). CRF binding sites are, in general, localized in areas containing CRF-immunoreactive fibers. As with other neurotransmitter systems, however, there are several CNS loci in which the relative densities of CRF receptors versus CRF immunoreactivity are disparate. CRF receptors are present in several cortical, limbic, hypothalamic, and spinal sites as well as in brainstem autonomic areas including the parabrachial nucleus, the nucleus of the solitary tract, and medullary reticular nuclei. Moreover, sympathetic ganglia and the adrenal medulla contain CRF receptors, suggesting a potential peripheral site of action of CRF in mediating autonomic regulation (Udelsman *et al.*, 1986).

Although both pituitary (Labrie *et al.*, 1982) and brain (Chen *et al.*,

1986; De Souza, 1987; Wynn et al., 1984) CRF receptors are linked to adenylate cyclase, they appear to be regulated differentially. Thus adrenalectomy (Wynn et al., 1984), exogenous glucocorticoid administration (Hauger et al., 1987), and prolonged immobilization stress (Hauger et al., 1988) are demonstrated to down-regulate pituitary CRF receptors while having no appreciable effect on CRF receptors in selected brain regions. It will be of interest to determine whether different subtypes of CRF receptors exist in light of the previously mentioned possibility of multiple CRF-like molecules in mammalian brain (Skofitsch and Jacobowitz, 1985).

III. CNS Actions of CRF

A. Autonomic Nervous Activity

The coincident activation of the pituitary–adrenal axis and the sympathetic nervous sytem is recognized as a characteristic response of stressful stimuli. Owing to the physiologic role of CRF in mediating stress-induced ACTH secretion and to the neuroanatomical connections discussed above, a pertinent line of inquiry regards the CNS actions of CRF on autonomic nervous function. Indeed, a large body of data demonstrates that CRF acts within the CNS to produce stress-like changes in both sympathetic and parasympathetic nervous activity and adrenomedullary outflow (Brown and Fisher, 1985; Fisher, 1989a).

Administration of CRF into the lateral cerebroventricle (icv), third cerebroventricle, or cisterna magna elevates plasma catecholamine levels in conscious rats (Brown et al., 1982a,b,c; Fisher and Brown , 1984), dogs (Brown and Fisher, 1983; Lenz et al., 1985), and rhesus monkeys (Insel et al., 1984). Consistent with these findings is the demonstration that icv administration of CRF stimulates efferent adrenal and renal nerve activities and increases catecholamine secretion rate into the adrenal vein in anesthetized rats (Kurosawa et al., 1986). The stimulatory effects of CRF on sympathetic nervous and adrenomedullary outflow are dose-related, occur rapidly after injection, and are sustained for periods of up to 3 h.

Intravenous injections of anti-CRF sera do not alter the ability of CRF, administered icv, to elevate plasma levels of epinephrine and norepinephrine (Brown and Fisher, 1985). Thus, CRF acts within the CNS to stimulate sympathetic nervous and sympathoadrenal outflow. A recent study by Brown (1986) indicates that there are multiple CNS sites wherein CRF activates sympathetic nervous activity; elevations of plasma norepinephrine levels are measured after intraparenchymal injections of CRF into several CNS tissue sites in conscious rats. Importantly, these effects are not due to nonspecific actions, as there are several sites wherein CRF injection does not alter plasma norepinephrine concentrations. It is important to note that injection of CRF into any single tissue site, including the central nucleus of the amygdala, does not elicit elevations of plasma norepinephrine levels that are greater than those observed after administration of CRF into the ventricular space (Brown, 1986; Brown and Gray, 1988). This finding suggests that CRF-induced stimulation of sympathetic nervous activity is mediated at a periventricular site(s) of action or alternatively that multiple anatomically distinct sites of action are accessed simultaneously after icv administration of CRF. The latter possibility is likely in that ablation of the periventricular region known as the antero-ventral third ventricle (AV3V) does not modify the elevations of plasma norepinephrine and epinephrine levels evoked by icv CRF administration (Brown and Fisher, 1990).

While it is clear that circulating epinephrine is derived from the adrenal medulla, it is now appreciated that rather discrete and viscerotopic alterations of sympathetic nervous outflow are evoked by different stressors. Accordingly, CRF-induced elevations of plasma norepinephrine levels, although elicited from multiple CNS sites, do not result from a global stimulation of sympathetic nervous activity. Norepinephrine turnover in various peripheral organs is modified differentially after icv administration of CRF (Brown and Fisher, 1985); consistent with measurements of renal nerve activity (Kurosawa et al., 1986), norepinephrine turnover is increased in the kidney. In contrast, CRF-induced reductions of norepinephrine turnover are observed in the pancreas and interscapular brown fat whereas no significant changes are measured in the spleen, duodenum, or heart. It should be borne in mind, however, that the function of all peripheral tissues possessing adrenergic receptors could be influenced by the high circulating catecholamine levels following icv administration of CRF.

At present, there is an unfortunate paucity of methods with which to study the physiological roles of most neuropeptides, including CRF. A growing body of evidence, however, supports the physiological involvement of CRF neuronal systems in mediating stress-induced alterations of sympathoadrenal function. The CRF receptor antagonist α-helical CRF$_{9\text{-}41}$, while not very potent, is fairly effective in inhibiting the CNS actions of CRF on autonomic and cardiovascular function. Thus, it is of particular interest that icv administration of α-helical CRF$_{9\text{-}41}$ blunts the elevations of circulating epinephrine levels provoked by such stressors as ether exposure, insulin-induced hypoglycemia, and 30% hemorrhage (Brown et al., 1985, 1986).

The potential role of CRF in regulating autonomic function has also been studied by attempting to modulate CRF neuronal activity via manipulations of internal glucocorticoid levels. As previously discussed, adrenalectomy produces enhanced CRF staining in both hypothalamic and extrahypothalamic sites (Merchenthaler et al., 1983a,b; Sawchenko, 1987) and conversely, dexamethasone treatment reduces immunoreactive CRF levels in the median eminence (Suda et al., 1984). While parallel effects of such manipulations on CRF mRNA are reported to be restricted to the paraventricular nucleus (Beyer et al., 1988), glucocorticoid receptors are present on CRF-containing neurons in sites outside the hypothalamus including the central nucleus of the amygdala and the bed nucleus of the stria terminalis (Cintra et al., 1987). Thus, it is conceivable that glucocorticoid status could influence the activity of CRF neuronal systems that impact on autonomic function. As such, it is of interest that adrenalectomy and glucocorticoid excess produce reciprocal effects on plasma catecholamine levels (Brown and Fisher, 1986; Szemeredi et al., 1988). Adrenalectomy produces a slight increment in basal levels of plasma norepinephrine and markedly enhances ether stress-induced elevations of plasma norepinephrine levels, both effects being reversible by glucocorticoid replacement. Moreover, dexamethasone and corticosterone produce dose-related attenuations of ether stress-induced elevations of plasma norepinephrine and epinephrine levels (Brown and Fisher, 1986), and chronic cortisol administration lowers basal plasma levels of epinephrine (Szemeredi et al., 1988). It is tempting to speculate that the effects of altered glucocorticoid environments on sympathoadrenal activity are mediated through CRF neuronal systems; however, such hypotheses remain to be proven definitively. Nevertheless, the aggregate data derived from these studies and from experiments utilizing α-helical CRF_{9-41} are certainly compatible with the notion of a physiological role of CRF-containing neurons in regulating autonomic nervous activity.

B. Cardiovascular Function

In that both stressful stimuli and CRF produce similar alterations of autonomic nervous activity, it is reasonable to hypothesize that the CNS actions of CRF on cardiovascular function may likewise be comparable to those of stress. In support of this concept, central administration of CRF is demonstrated to elevate arterial pressure and heart rate in conscious rats (Fisher et al., 1982,1983; Fisher and Brown, 1983,1984; Grosskreutz and Brody, 1988; Saunders and Thornhill, 1986), dogs (Brown and Fisher, 1983; Lenz et al., 1985), and sheep (Scoggins et al., 1984). As shown in Figure 1, CRF-induced pressor and tachycardic responses in conscious rats are dose-related, occur rapidly after injection, and are sustained for at least 1 h. In anesthetized rats, icv administration of CRF is reported to elevate heart rate but not arterial pressure (Kurosawa et al., 1986), whereas slight elevations of arterial pressure are observed in anesthetized rhesus monkeys (Kalin et al., 1983). Although anesthesia modifies the CNS actions of CRF on cardiovascular function, it is important to note that CRF-induced elevations of arterial pressure and heart rate are not merely secondary to the locomotor activation elicited by this peptide (Overton and Fisher, 1989c).

Two lines of evidence support the notion that CRF acts within the CNS to elevate arterial pressure and heart rate. First, intravenous injections of CRF cause dose-related reductions of arterial pressure (Fisher and Brown, 1983; Fisher et al., 1983; Lenz et al., 1985). Second, as shown in Figure 2, icv administration of CRF elevates arterial pressure and heart rate in rats pretreated with intravenous injections of anti-CRF sera. Thus, it is unlikely that CRF leaks from the ventricular space to the peripheral circulation to produce pressor and tachycardic actions; indeed, perhaps owing to delayed leakage, peripheral passive immunization against CRF appears to

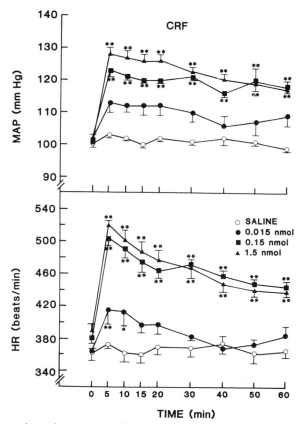

Figure 1 Effects of icv administration of saline or CRF on arterial pressure and heart rate in conscious, unrestrained rats. Each value represents the mean ± SE of six to eight rats.

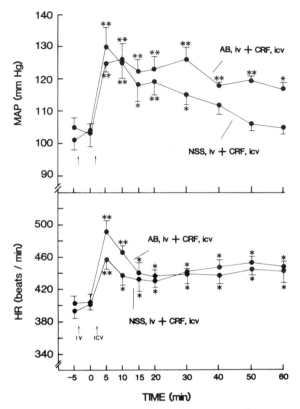

Figure 2 Effects of icv administration of 1.5 nmol CRF on arterial pressure and heart rate in conscious, unrestrained rats pretreated with intravenous (iv) injections of normal sheep serum (NSS) or anti-CRF sera (AB). Each value represents the mean ± SE of six rats.

prolong the elevation of arterial pressure produced by icv administration of CRF. While it is clear that these cardiovascular actions are elicited within the CNS, no particular tissue sites, such as the central nucleus of the amygdala (Brown and Gray, 1988), are identified wherein CRF injection produces greater responses than those observed after icv administration of the peptide. Ablation of the AV3V region does not alter the pressor and tachycardic responses to icv administration of CRF (Brown and Fisher, 1990), ruling out this area as an exclusive site of action of CRF. It is likely that the cardiovascular effects of CRF result from simultaneous activation of multiple CNS sites, similar to the situation described for CRF-induced stimulation of sympathetic outflow.

The cardiovascular actions of CRF are independent from its pituitary effects. Thus, hypophysectomy or dexamethasone treatment does not alter the pressor and tachycardic responses to icv administration of CRF (Fisher *et al.*, 1983). Moreover, although plasma renin activity is elevated after icv administration of CRF, circulating angiotensin II does not mediate the pressor action of CRF as captopril treatment does not modify the expression of CRF-induced cardiovascular changes (Fisher *et al.*, 1983). Likewise, in both rats (Fisher and Brown, 1984; Fisher *et al.*, 1983) and dogs (Brown and Fisher, 1983), pharmacological antagonism of peripheral vasopressin V_1 pressor receptors has no effect on CRF-induced elevations of arterial pressure and heart rate. It is interesting to note that central administration of CRF elevates plasma vasopressin levels in dogs (Brown and Fisher, 1983; Lenz *et al.*, 1985) but not in rats (Fisher and Brown, 1984). Indeed, it is conceivable that, similar to the effects of various stressful stimuli, CRF acts centrally to inhibit vasopressin secretion in rats; potent stimuli for vasopressin secretion, namely, salt loading and water deprivation, are demonstrated to reduce CRF mRNA levels in rat parvocellular paraventricular neurons (Young, 1986).

The CNS actions of CRF on cardiovascular function are dependent on the autonomic nervous system, as prior ganglionic blockade with chlorisondamine prevents CRF-induced elevations of arterial pressure and heart rate in both rats (Fisher and Brown, 1984; Fisher *et al.*, 1982,1983; Grosskreutz and Brody, 1988) and dogs (Brown and Fisher, 1983; Fisher and Brown, 1983). Interestingly, however, pressor and tachycardic responses to CRF are intact in acutely adrenalectomized rats, suggesting that circulating epinephrine does not mediate the cardiovascular actions of CRF (Fisher *et al.*, 1983). Rather, discrete and viscerotopic changes of sympathetic vasomotor outflow follow icv administration of CRF as detected by measurements of regional blood flow (Grosskreutz and Brody, 1988; Overton and Fisher, 1989a,c) in conscious rats; vascular resistance is increased in the renal and mesenteric arteries and decreased in the iliac artery after icv CRF administration. That these effects are mediated within the CNS is supported by the demonstration that intravenous administration of α-helical CRF_{9-41} does not modify their expression (Overton and Fisher, 1989a). Moreover, in both dogs (Lenz *et al.*, 1985) and rats (Overton and Fisher, 1989a), CRF acts peripherally to elevate mesenteric blood flow, an effect opposite to that observed after its icv administration. Importantly, the peripheral actions of CRF on regional blood flow are completely prevented by concomitant intravenous administration of α-helical CRF^{9-41}. Ganglionic blockade inhibits the effects of icv administration of CRF on mesenteric vascular resistance yet increases of iliac blood flow are still evident in this situation (Overton and Fisher, 1989a); most likely, local metabolic mechanisms contribute to the increased iliac blood flow as ganglionic blockade does not prevent CRF-induced locomotor activation.

The pattern of blood flow observed after icv administration of CRF closely resembles that induced by various stressors, namely, shunting of blood from the mesentery to skeletal muscle. Moreover, consistent with stress-induced hemodynamic adaptations, CRF acts within the CNS to elevate cardiac output (Overton *et al.*, 1990b). Thus, CRF-induced pressor responses derive from enhanced cardiac output versus elevated vascular resistance; indeed, total peripheral vascular resistance is reduced after icv administration of CRF (Overton *et al.*, 1990b). The hemodynamic and cardiovascular alterations induced by central administration of CRF are similar to the so-called defense reaction, a patterned response enabling immediate somatomotor and/or behavioral adjustments to real or perceived threats.

The CNS actions of CRF on cardiac baroreflex function are also consistent with those produced by both physical and psychological stressors. Normally, acute elevations of arterial pressure are buffered by baroreceptor reflex-mediated reductions of heart rate. The inverse relationship between arterial pressure and heart rate is, however, not fixed or invariable; CNS processing of baroreceptor information is modulated dynamically, and thus many stressful stimuli elicit simultaneous elevations of arterial pressure and

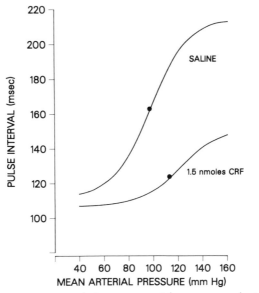

Figure 3 Stimulus-response curves relating mean arterial pressure to pulse interval (reciprocal of heart rate) after icv administration of saline or CRF. Each curve is constructed from the averaged parameter estimates of six conscious, unrestrained rats. Solid dots represent resting levels of arterial pressure and pulse interval.

heart rate (Korner, 1979). That CRF acts within the CNS to increase arterial pressure and heart rate concomitantly suggests, likewise, that this peptide modifies cardiac baroreflex function. Indeed, CRF produces dose-related reductions of reflex gain and range (Fisher, 1988). As shown in Figure 3, icv administration of CRF markedly alters the relationship between arterial pressure and pulse interval (reciprocal of heart rate); the curve relating arterial pressure to pulse interval is shifted downward and to the right. In functional terms, CRF acts within the CNS to elevate heart rate across a wide range of arterial pressure and to blunt the magnitude of reflex bradycardia even at very high levels of arterial pressure. The inhibitory action of CRF on cardiac baroreflex function is mediated by selective suppression of efferent parasympathetic nervous responses to baroreceptor stimulation (Fisher, 1989b). Thus, cardiac vagal tone is withdrawn across all prevailing levels of arterial pressure (Figure 4). CRF-induced elevations of heart rate

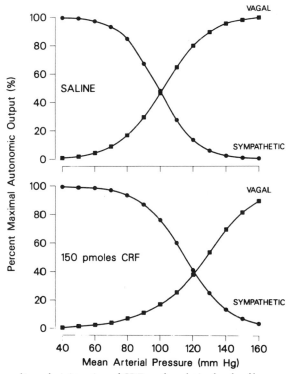

Figure 4   Effects of icv administration of CRF on the relative levels of baroreceptor-dependent cardiac efferent sympathetic and parasympathetic (vagal) tone in conscious, unrestrained rats. Saline and CRF treatment groups consisted of six rats.

are demonstrable after sino-aortic deafferentation, suggesting that vagal inhibition by CRF is not exclusively mediated by suppression of afferent baroreceptor impulse transmission (Overton and Fisher, 1990a). It is possible that CRF acts directly to reduce the activity of cardioinhibitory neurons, as immunoreactive CRF and CRF receptors are distributed within medullary reticular regions in which preganglionic vagal motor neurons are located. In this regard, it is interesting to note that lesions of the paraventricular nucleus blunt baroreceptor denervation-induced elevations of arterial pressure and heart rate (Zhang and Ciriello, 1985).

The CNS actions of CRF on cardiovascular, hemodynamic, and cardiac baroreflex function would enhance cardiovascular capacity in an acute time domain. Chronic autonomic and cardiovascular changes of this nature, however, may be linked to deleterious and maladaptive consequences such as hypertension. Abnormal CNS levels of CRF are measured in the spontaneously hypertensive rat (SHR) model (Hashimoto et al., 1985), and moreover, lesions of the paraventricular nucleus are reported to retard the development of hypertension in this rat strain (Ciriello et al., 1984). Interestingly, icv administration of CRF produces exceedingly attenuated elevations of arterial pressure and heart rate in SHRs versus normotensive rats (Brown et al., 1988). In contrast, CRF-induced elevations of plasma epinephrine levels are markedly enhanced in the SHR (Brown et al., 1988). The mechanisms underlying these altered responses to CRF in the SHR are not yet resolved, although it is unlikely that increased leakage of CRF due to blood–brain barrier deficits accounts for the blunted pressor responses (Fisher and Overton, 1988). It is conceivable that the augmented adrenomedullary epinephrine secretion in the SHR contributes to the attenuated pressor response by an interaction at vasodilatory β_2-adrenergic receptors in selected vascular beds.

Stressful stimuli are suspected of activating endogenous CNS opioid systems. CRF and dynorphin-related peptides coexist within a subpopulation of paraventricular neurons (Roth et al., 1983) suggesting the potential for their simultaneous release and thus perhaps, functional interactions between these peptides. Indeed, CRF and dynorphin-related peptides exhibit reciprocal actions on the release of each other in vitro; CRF stimulates the release of immunoreactive dynorphin from superfused rat hypothalamic slices (Nikolarakis et al., 1986) whereas dynorphin A_{1-17} inhibits the basal release of immunoreactive CRF from perifused rat hypothalami (Yajima et al., 1986). Consistent with the latter observation, in vivo studies in urethane-anesthetized rats demonstrate that icv administration of dynorphin A_{1-13} reduces basal and hypotension-induced secretion of CRF into hypophysial portal blood (Plotsky, 1986). Recent experiments suggest that, in addition to their interactions at the level of release, these peptides may also modulate the CNS actions of each other (Overton and Fisher, 1989b). Thus, a low dose of dynorphin A_{1-17} attenuates CRF-induced elevations of arterial pressure and heart rate (Figure 5). Moreover, similar inhibitory effects of dynorphin A_{1-17} on CRF-induced elevations of plasma catecholamine levels are observed (Overton and Fisher, 1989b). The reciprocal release effects and neuropharmacological interactions between CRF and dynorphin A_{1-17}

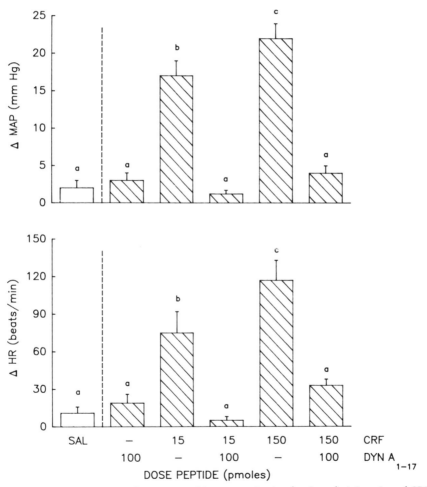

Figure 5 Changes in arterial pressure and heart rate 5 min after icv administration of CRF and dynorphin A_{1-17}, separately and in combination, in conscious, unrestrained rats. Each value represents the mean ± SE of six to eight rats.

suggest that "fine tuning" or feedback regulation of stress-induced autonomic and cardiovascular responses may be achieved by the corelease of multiple neurotransmitters from a single source.

The CRF receptor antagonist, α-helical CRF_{9-41}, has been utilized to examine the physiological role of CRF in mediating cardiovascular regulation. Importantly, the cardiovascular responses to icv administration of CRF are effectively inhibited by coadministration of α-helical CRF_{9-41} (Brown et al., 1986). In anesthetized rats, icv administration of CRF and nitroprusside-induced hypotension produce similar effects on the activity of locus ceruleus neurons, namely, elevations of spontaneous discharge rate and disruption of sensory-evoked phasic firing. The icv administration of α-helical CRF_{9-41} completely blocks the effects of nitroprusside-induced hypotension on locus ceruleus neuronal activity, suggesting that the alterations in neuronal function produced by hemodynamic stress are effected through CRF-mediated neurotransmission (Valentino and Wehby, 1988). Likewise, owing to similar effects of exercise and icv CRF administration on cardiovascular function, one may reasonably speculate that CRF neuronal systems are activated during physical stress. Indeed, icv administration of α-helical CRF_{9-41} significantly attenuates treadmill exercise-induced elevations of arterial pressure, heart rate, mesenteric vascular resistance, and iliac blood flow in rats (Kregel et al., 1990). Importantly, these altered cardiovascular adaptations are detrimental to exercise endurance; rats treated with α-helical CRF_{9-41} have a significantly reduced ability to sustain treadmill running. These findings lend credence to the potential physiological involvement of CRF-containing neurons in mediating exercise-induced cardiovascular responses.

IV. Conclusions

The aggregate neuroanatomical, neurochemical, and neuropharmacological data presented above support the hypothesis that CRF neuronal systems are physiologically involved in mediating autonomic and cardiovascular homeostasis. As depicted in Figure 6, the CNS actions of CRF on endocrine, autonomic nervous, and cardiovascular function are similar to those elicited by stressful stimuli. Thus, the release of CRF within different CNS loci could result in an array of hormonal, neural, and visceral changes that is characteristic of the stress response: pituitary–adrenal activation, enhanced sympathoadrenal outflow, viscerotopic alteration of efferent sympathetic activity, and cardiac vagal withdrawal. That CRF-induced changes in autonomic and cardiovascular function are most potently expressed after icv versus focal intraparenchymal administration suggests multiple CNS sites of action wherein this peptide modifies neurotransmission. Accordingly, it is conceivable that stressful stimuli may simultaneously activate anatomically distinct populations of CRF-containing neurons that project to disparate CNS sites. Alternatively, CRF may act as a brain hormone, circulating via

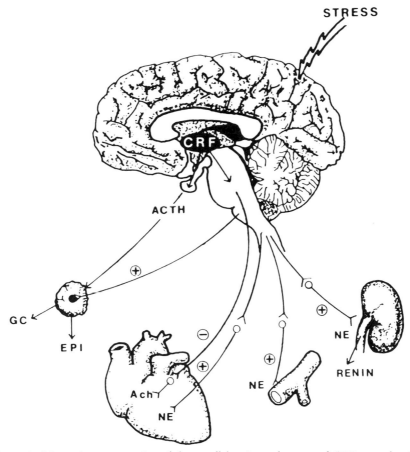

Figure 6 Schematic representation of the parallel actions of stress and CRF on endocrine, autonomic, and cardiovascular function. CRF released within the median eminence is delivered via the portal vessels to the pituitary, where it stimulates the secretion of adrenocorticotropic hormone (ACTH), which in turn evokes glucocorticoid (GC) release from the adrenal cortex. CRF acts at multiple CNS sites to (1) stimulate adrenomedullary epinephrine (EPI) secretion, (2) produce viscerotopic alterations of noradrenergic (NE) sympathetic outflow, and (3) inhibit cardiac vagal (Ach) tone. CRF-induced changes in autonomic nervous outflow result in marked alterations of cardiovascular function.

the interstitial fluid to interact with CRF receptors located throughout the neuraxis.

Consistent with the latter proposal, CRF is cleared rapidly (six times faster than bulk flow) from the ventricular cerebrospinal fluid space, presumably into CNS parenchymal sites because it is not detected in blood following icv administration and it is not degraded readily, as evinced by half-life measurements in blood and cerebrospinal fluid (Oldfield *et al.*, 1985). In fact, there is good evidence that the CNS paravascular interstitial fluid provides an efficient and rapid route for the distribution of even large molecules like horseradish peroxidase from the ventricular cerebrospinal fluid throughout the brain extracellular fluid (Rennels *et al.*, 1985). The notion that neurotransmission within the CNS may not be mediated exclusively by synaptic events is certainly supported by the consistent findings of neuroanatomical mismatches between the relative densities of neuronal terminals containing a particular transmitter and receptors for that transmitter (Herkenham, 1987). Thus, it is conceivable that CRF could interact with CRF receptors located at sites distant from its site of release. If this is the case, then the observed changes in autonomic and cardiovascular function observed after icv CRF administration may be representative of *in vivo* CRF-mediated neurotransmission.

If CRF neuronal systems are physiologically involved in mediating stress-induced autonomic nervous and cardiovascular responses, a valid consideration concerns the role of CRF-containing neurons in the pathogenesis of stress-associated disorders such as cardiovascular disease. The apparent morning-time clustering of fatal heart attacks (Tofler *et al.*, 1987) correlates temporally with the diurnal ACTH surge and hence presumably with CRF release within the CNS. It is thus tempting to speculate that abnormal activity of CRF neuronal systems, perhaps provoked by chronic stress exposure, may be linked to cardiovascular pathologies in humans. At present, whether such speculations are valid remains untested and therefore unknown. It is clear, however, that the animal data collected to date provide a compelling rationale to continue investigations into the role of CRF in mediating stress-induced changes in cardiovascular function.

Acknowledgments

Research from the author's laboratory referred to here is supported by a Presidential Young Investigator Award from the National Science Foundation and an Established Investigatorship from the American Heart Association. The author thanks Rita Wedell for expert assistance with manuscript preparation.

References

Beaulieu, S., Pelletier, G., Vaudry, H., and Barden, N. (1989). Influence of the central nucleus of the amygdala on the content of corticotropin-releasing factor in the median eminence. *Neuroendocrinology* 49, 255–261.

Beyer, H. S., Matta, S. G., and Sharp, B. M. (1988). Regulation of the messenger ribonucleic acid for corticotropin-releasing factor in the paraventricular nucleus and other brain sites of the rat. *Endocrinology (Baltimore)* 123, 2117–2123.

Bloom, F. E., Battenberg, E. L. F., Rivier, J., and Vale, W. (1982). Corticotropin releasing factor (CRF): Immunoreactive neurones and fibers in rat hypothalamus. *Regul. Pept.* 4, 43–48.

Brown, M. (1986). Corticotropin releasing factor: central nervous system sites of action. *Brain Res.* 399, 10–14.

Brown, M. R., and Fisher, L. A. (1983). Central nervous system effects of corticotropin releasing factor in the dog. *Brain Res.* 280, 75–79.

Brown, M. R., and Fisher, L. A. (1985). Corticotropin-releasing factor: Effects on the autonomic nervous system and visceral systems. *Fed. Proc., Fed. Am. Soc. Exp. Biol.* 44, 243–248.

Brown, M. R., and Fisher, L. A. (1986). Glucocorticoid suppression of the sympathetic nervous system and adrenal medulla. *Life Sci.* 39, 1003–1012.

Brown, M. R., and Fisher, L. A. (1990). Regulation of the autonomic nervous system by corticotropin releasing factor. *In* "Corticotropin-Releasing Factor: Basic and Clinical Studies of a Neuropeptide" (E. B. De Souza and C. B. Nemeroff, eds.), pp. 291–298. CRC Press, Boca Raton, Florida.

Brown, M. R., and Gray, T. S. (1988). Peptide injections into the amygdala of conscious rats: Effects on blood pressure, heart rate and plasma catecholamines. *Regul. Pept.* 21, 95–106.

Brown, M. R., Fisher, L. A., Rivier, J., Spiess, J., Rivier, C., and Vale, W. (1982a). Corticotropin-releasing factor: Effects on the sympathetic nervous system and oxygen consumption. *Life Sci.* 30, 207–210.

Brown, M. R., Fisher, L. A., Spiess, J., Rivier, C., Rivier, J., and Vale, W. (1982b). Corticotropin-releasing factor: Actions on the sympathetic nervous system and metabolism. *Endocrinology (Baltimore)* 111, 928–931.

Brown, M. R., Fisher, L. A., Spiess, J., Rivier, J., Rivier, C., and Vale, W. (1982c). Comparison of the biologic actions of corticotropin-releasing factor and sauvagine. *Regul. Pept.* 4, 107–114.

Brown, M. R., Fisher, L. A., Webb, V., Vale, W. W., and Rivier, J. E. (1985). Corticotropin-releasing factor: A physiologic regulator of adrenal epinephrine secretion. *Brain Res.* 328, 355–357.

Brown, M. R., Gray, T. S., and Fisher, L. A. (1986). Corticotropin-releasing factor receptor antagonist: Effects on the autonomic nervous system and cardiovascular function. *Regul. Pept.* 16, 321–329.

Brown, M. R., Hauger, R., and Fisher, L. A. (1988). Autonomic and cardiovascular effects of corticotropin-releasing factor in the spontaneously hypertensive rat. *Brain Res.* 441, 33–40.

Chappell, P. B., Smith, M. A., Kilts, C. D., Bissette, G., Ritchie, J., Anderson, C., and Nemeroff, C. B. (1986). Alterations in corticotropin-releasing factor-like immunoreactivity in discrete rat brain regions after acute and chronic stress. *J. Neurosci.* 6, 2908–2914.

Chen, F. M., Bilezikjian, L. M., Perrin, M. H., Rivier, J., and Vale, W. (1986). Corticotropin releasing factor receptor-mediated stimulation of adenylate cyclase activity in the rat brain. *Brain Res.* **381,** 49–57.

Cintra, A., Fuxe, K., Harfstrand, A., Agnati, L. F., Wikström, A.-C., Okret, S., Vale, W., and Gustafsson, J.-A. (1987). Presence of glucocorticoid receptor immunoreactivity in corticotrophin releasing factor and in growth hormone releasing factor immunoreactive neurons of the rat di- and telencephalon. *Neurosci. Lett.* **77,** 25–30.

Ciriello, J., Kline, R. L., Zhang, T.-X., and Caverson, M. M. (1984). Lesions of the paraventricular nucleus alter the development of spontaneous hypertension in the rat. *Brain Res.* **310,** 355–359.

Cote, J., Lefevre, G., Labrie, F., and Barden, N. (1983). Distribution of corticotropin-releasing factor in ovine brain determined by radioimmunoassay. *Regul. Pept.* **5,** 189–195.

Cunningham, E. T., Jr., and Sawchenko, P. E. (1988). Anatomical specificity of noradrenergic inputs to the paraventricular and supraoptic nuclei of the rat hypothalamus. *J. Comp. Neurol.* **274,** 60–76.

De Souza, E. B. (1987). Corticotropin-releasing factor receptors in the rat central nervous system: characterization and regional distribution. *J. Neurosci.* **7,** 88–100.

De Souza, E. B., Insel, T. R., Perrin, M. H., Rivier, J., Vale, W. W., and Kuhar, M. J. (1985). Corticotropin-releasing factor receptors are widely distributed within the rat central nervous system: an autoradiographic study. *J. Neurosci.* **5,** 3189–3203.

Fischman, A. J., and Moldow, R. L. (1982). Extrahypothalamic distribution of CRF-like immunoreactivity in the rat brain. *Peptides (N.Y.)* **3,** 149–153.

Fisher, L. A. (1988). Corticotropin-releasing factor: central nervous system effects on baroreflex control of heart rate. *Life Sci.* **42,** 2645–2649.

Fisher, L. A. (1989a). Corticotropin-releasing factor: endocrine and autonomic integration of responses to stress. *Trends Pharmacol. Sci.* **10,** 189–193.

Fisher, L. A. (1989b). Central autonomic modulation of cardiac baroreflex by corticotropin-releasing factor. *Am. J. Physiol.* **256,** H949–H955.

Fisher, L. A., and Brown, M. R. (1983). Corticotropin-releasing factor: central nervous system effects on the sympathetic nervous system and cardiovascular regulation. *Curr. Top. Neuroendocrinol.* **3,** 87–101.

Fisher, L. A., and Brown, M. R. (1984). Corticotropin-releasing factor and angiotensin II: Comparison of CNS actions to influence neuroendocrine and cardiovascular function. *Brain Res.* **296,** 41–47.

Fisher, L. A., and Overton, J. M. (1988). Altered cardiovascular response to corticotropin-releasing factor in spontaneously hypertensive rats. *Proc. West. Pharmacol. Soc.* **31,** 317–318.

Fisher, L. A., Rivier, J., Rivier, C., Spiess, J., Vale, W., and Brown, M. R. (1982). Corticotropin-releasing factor (CRF): Central effects on mean arterial pressure and heart rate in rats. *Endocrinology (Baltimore)* **110,** 2222–2224.

Fisher, L. A., Jessen, G., and Brown, M. R. (1983). Corticotropin-releasing factor (CRF): Mechanism to elevate mean arterial pressure and heart rate. *Regul. Pept.* **5,** 153–161.

Garrick, N. A., Hill, J. L., Szele, F. G., Tomai, T. P., Gold, P. W., and Murphy, D. L. (1987). Corticotropin-releasing factor: A marked circadian rhythm in primate cerebrospinal fluid peaks in the evening and is inversely related to the cortisol circadian rhythm. *Endocrinology (Baltimore)* **121,** 1329–1334.

Giuliano, R., Ruggiero, D. A., Milner, T. A., Anwar, M., and Reis, D. J. (1988). Corticotropin-releasing factor: Anatomical substrates of autonomic regulation. *Soc. Neurosci. Abstr.* **14,** 23.

Gray, T. S., and Magnuson, D. J. (1987). Neuropeptide neuronal efferents from the bed nucleus of the stria terminalis and central amygdaloid nucleus to the dorsal vagal complex in the rat. *J. Comp. Neurol.* **262,** 365–374.

Grosskreutz, C. L., and Brody, M. J. (1988). Regional hemodynamic responses to central administration of corticotropin-releasing factor (CRF). *Brain Res.* **442**, 363–367.

Haas, D. A., and George, S. R. (1988). Single or repeated mild stress increases synthesis and release of hypothalamic corticotropin-releasing factor. *Brain Res.* **461**, 230–237.

Hashimoto, K., Hattori, T., Murakami, K., Suemaru, S., Kawada, Y., Kageyama, J., and Ota, Z. (1985). Reduction in brain immunoreactive corticotropin-releasing factor (CRF) in spontaneously hypertensive rats. *Life Sci.* **36**, 643–647.

Hauger, R. L., Millan, M. A., Catt, K. J., and Aguilera, G. (1987). Differential regulation of brain and pituitary corticotropin-releasing factor receptors by corticosterone. *Endocrinology (Baltimore)* **120**, 1527–1533.

Hauger, R. L., Millan, M. A., Lorang, M., Harwood, J. P., and Aguilera, G. (1988). Corticotropin-releasing factor receptors and pituitary adrenal responses during immobilization stress. *Endocrinology (Baltimore)* **123**, 396–405.

Herkenham, M. (1987). Mismatches between neurotransmitter and receptor localizations in brain: Observations and implications. *Neuroscience* **23**, 1–38.

Insel, T. R., Aloi, J. A., Goldstein, D., Wood, J. H., and Jimerson, D. C. (1984). Plasma cortisol and catecholamine responses to intracerebroventricular administration of CRF to rhesus monkeys. *Life Sci.* **34**, 1873–1878.

Jingami, H., Matsukura, S., Numa, S., and Imura, H. (1985). Effects of adrenalectomy and dexamethasone administration on the level of prepro-corticotropin-releasing factor messenger ribonucleic acid (mRNA) in the hypothalamus and adrenocorticotropin/β-lipotropin precursor mRNA in the pituitary in rats. *Endocrinology (Baltimore)* **117**, 1314–1320.

Kalin, N. H., Shelton, S. E., Kraemer, G. W., and McKinney, W. T. (1983). Corticotropin-releasing factor administered intraventricularly to rhesus monkeys. *Peptides (N.Y.)* **4**, 217–220.

Korner, P. I (1979). Central nervous control of autonomic cardiovascular function. *In* "Handbook of Physiology" (R. M. Berne, ed.), Sect. 2, Vol. I, pp. 691–739. Am. Physiol. Soc., Bethesda, Maryland.

Kregel, K. C., Overton, J. M., Seals, D. R., Tipton, C. M., and Fisher, L. A. (1990). Cardiovascular responses to exercise in the rat: role of corticotropin-releasing factor. *J. Appl. Physiol.* **68**, 561–567.

Krukoff, T. L. (1986). Segmental distribution of corticotropin-releasing factor-like and vasoactive intestinal peptide-like immunoreactivities in presumptive sympathetic preganglionic neurons of the cat. *Brain Res.* **382**, 153–157.

Kurosawa, M., Sato, A., Swenson, R. S., and Takahashi, Y. (1986). Sympatho-adrenal medullary functions in response to intracerebroventricularly injected corticotropin-releasing factor in anesthetized rats. *Brain Res.* **367**, 250–257.

Labrie, F., Veilleux, R., Lefevre, G., Coy, D. H., Sueiras-Diaz, J., and Schally, A. V. (1982). Corticotropin-releasing factor stimulates accumulation of adenosine 3′,5′-monophosphate in rat pituitary corticotrophs. *Science* **216**, 1007–1008.

Lenz, H. J., Fisher, L. A., Vale, W. W., and Brown, M. R. (1985). Corticotropin-releasing factor, sauvagine and urotensin-I: Effects on blood flow. *Am. J. Physiol.* **249**, R85–R90.

Merchenthaler, I., Hynes, M. A., Vigh, S., Shally, A. V., and Petrusz, P. (1983a). Immunocytochemical localization of corticotropin releasing factor (CRF) in the rat spinal cord. *Brain Res.* **275**, 373–377.

Merchenthaler, I., Vigh, S., Petrusz, P., and Schally, A. V. (1983b). The paraventriculo-infundibular corticotropin releasing factor (CRF) pathway as revealed by immunocytochemistry in long-term hypophysectomized or adrenalectomized rats. *Regul. Pept.* **5**, 295–305.

Moga, M. M., and Gray, T. S. (1985). Evidence for corticotropin-releasing factor, neurotensin, and somatostatin in the neural pathway from the central nucleus of the amygdala to the parabrachial nucleus. *J. Comp. Neurol.* **241**, 275–284.

Moldow, R. L., and Fischman, A. J. (1984). Circadian rhythm of corticotropin releasing factor-like immunoreactivity in rat hypothalamus. *Peptides (N.Y.)* **5**, 1213–1215.

Moldow, R. L., Kastin, A. J., Graf, M., and Fischman, A. J. (1987). Stress mediated changes in hypothalamic corticotropin releasing factor-like immunoreactivity. *Life Sci.* **40**, 413–418.

Murakami, K., Akana, S., Dallman, M. F., and Ganong, W. F. (1989). Correlation between the stress-induced transient increase in corticotropin-releasing hormone content of the median eminence of the hypothalamus and adrenocorticotropic hormone secretion. *Neuroendocrinology* **49**, 233–241.

Nemeroff, C. B., Widerlov, E., Bissette, G., Walleus, H., Karlsson, I., Eklund, K., Kilts, C. D., Loosen, P. T., and Vale, W. (1984). Elevated concentrations of CSF corticotropin-releasing factor-like immunoreactivity in depressed patients. *Science* **226**, 1342–1344.

Nicholson, S., Lin, J.-H., Mahmoud, S., Campbell, E., Gillham, B., and Jones, M. (1985). Diurnal variations in responsiveness of the hypothalamo-pituitary-adrenocortical axis of the rat. *Neuroendocrinology* **40**, 217–224.

Nikolarakis, K. E., Almeida, O. F. X., and Herz, A. (1986). Stimulation of hypothalamic β-endorphin and dynorphin release by corticotropin-releasing factor (in vitro). *Brain Res.* **399**, 152–155.

Oldfield, E. H., Schulte, H. M., Chrousos, G. P., Rock, J. P., Kornblith, P. L., O'Neill, D. L., Poplack, D. G., Gold, P. W., Cutler, G. B., Jr., and Loriaux, L. (1985). Active clearance of corticotropin-releasing factor from the cerebrospinal fluid. *Neuroendocrinology* **40**, 84–87.

Olschowka, J. A., O'Donohue, T. L., Mueller, G. P., and Jacobowitz, D. M. (1982). The distribution of corticotropin releasing factor-like immunoreactive neurons in rat brain. *Peptides (N.Y.)* **3**, 995–1015.

Overton, J. M., and Fisher, L. A. (1989a). Differentiated regional hemodynamic responses to peripheral and central administration of corticotropin-releasing factor. *FASEB J.* **3**, A1015.

Overton, J. M., and Fisher, L. A. (1989b). Modulation of central nervous system actions of corticotropin-releasing factor by dynorphin-related peptides. *Brain Res.* **488**, 233–240.

Overton, J. M., and Fisher, L. A. (1989c). Central nervous system actions of corticotropin-releasing factor on cardiovascular function in the absence of locomotor activity. *Regul. Pept.* **25**, 315–324.

Overton, J. M., Davis-Gorman, G., and Fisher, L. A. (1990a). Central nervous system cardiovascular actions of CRF in sinoaortic-denervated rats. *Am. J. Physiol.* **258**, R596-R601.

Overton, J. M., Davis-Gorman, G., and Fisher, L. A. (1990b). Central nervous effects of CRF and angiotensin II on cardiac output in conscious rats. *J. Appl. Physiol.*, in press.

Palkovits, M., Brownstein, M. J., and Vale, W. (1983). Corticotropin releasing factor (CRF) immunoreactivity in hypothalamic and extrahypothalamic nuclei of sheep brain. *Neuroendocrinology* **37**, 302–305.

Palkovits, M., Brownstein, M. J., and Vale, W. (1985). Distribution of corticotropin-releasing factor in rat brain. *Fed. Proc. Fed. Am. Soc. Exp. Biol.* **44**, 215–219.

Plotsky, P. M. (1986). Opioid inhibition of immunoreactive corticotropin-releasing factor secretion into the hypophysial-portal circulation of rats. *Regul. Pept.* **16**, 235–242.

Rennels, M. L., Gregory, T. F., Blaumanis, O. R., Fujimoto, K., and Grady, P. A. (1985). Evidence for a "paravascular" fluid circulation in the mammalian central nervous system, provided by the rapid distribution of tracer protein throughout the brain from the subarachnoid space. *Brain Res.* **326**, 47–63.

Roth, K. A., Weber, E., Barchas, J. D., Chang, D., and Chang, J.-K. (1983). Immunoreactive dynorphin-(1-8) and corticotropin-releasing factor in subpopulation of hypothalamic neurons. *Science* **219**, 189–191.

Sakanaka, M., Shibasaki, T., and Lederis, K. (1986). Distribution and efferent projections of corticotropin-releasing factor-like immunoreactivity in the rat amygdaloid complex. *Brain Res.* **382**, 213–238.

Saunders, W. S., and Thornhill, J. A. (1986). Pressor, tachycardic and behavioral excitatory responses in conscious rats following icv administration of ACTH and CRF are blocked by naloxone pretreatment. *Peptides (N.Y.)* **7**, 597–601.

Sawchenko, P. E. (1987). Adrenalectomy-induced enhancement of CRF and vasopressin immunoreactivity in parvocellular neurosecretory neurons: Anatomic, peptide and steroid specificity. *J. Neurosci.* **7**, 1093–1106.

Schipper, J., Steinbusch, H. W. M., Vermes, I., and Tilders, F. J. H. (1983). Mapping of CRF-immunoreactive nerve fibers in the medulla oblongata and spinal cord of the rat. *Brain Res.* **267**, 145–150.

Scoggins, B. A., Coghlan, J. P., Denton, D. A., Fei, D. W., Nelson, M. A., Tregear, G. W., Tresham, J., and Wang, X. (1984). Intracerebroventricular infusions of corticotropin releasing factor (CRF) and ACTH (1-24) raise blood pressure in sheep. *Clin. Exp. Pharmacol. Physiol.* **11**, 365–368.

Silverman, A.-J., Hou-Yu, A., and Chen, W.-P. (1989). Corticotropin-releasing factor synapses within the paraventricular nucleus of the hypothalamus. *Neuroendocrinology* **49**, 291–299.

Skofitsch, G., and Jacobowitz, D. M. (1985). Distribution of corticotropin releasing factor-like immunoreactivity in the rat brain by immunohistochemistry and radioimmunoassay: Comparison and characterization of ovine and rat/human CRF antisera. *Peptides (N.Y.)* **6**, 319–336.

Suda, T., Tozawa, F., Mouri, T., Demura, H., and Shizume, K. (1983). Presence of immunoreactive corticotropin-releasing factor in human cerebrospinal fluid. *J. Clin. Endocrinol. Metab.* **57**, 225–226.

Suda, T., Tomori, N., Tozawa, F., Mouri, T., Demura, H., and Shizume, K. (1984). Effect of dexamethasone on immunoreactive corticotropin-releasing factor in the rat median eminence and intermediate-posterior pituitary. *Endocrinology (Baltimore)* **114**, 851–854.

Suemaru, S., Hashimoto, K., Hattori, T., Inoue, H., Kageyama, J., and Ota, Z. (1986). Starvation-induced changes in rat brain corticotropin-releasing factor (CRF) and pituitary-adrenocortical response. *Life Sci.* **39**, 1161–1166.

Swanson, L. W., Sawchenko, P. E., Rivier, J., and Vale, W. W. (1983). Organization of ovine corticotropin-releasing factor immunoreactive cells and fibers in the rat brain: An immunohistochemical study. *Neuroendocrinology* **36**, 165–186.

Szemeredi, K., Bagdy, G., Stull, R., Calogero, A. E., Kopin, I. J., and Goldstein, D. S. (1988). Sympathoadrenomedullary inhibition by chronic glucocorticoid treatment in conscious rats. *Endocrinology (Baltimore)* **123**, 2585–2590.

Tofler, G. H., Brezinski, D., Schafer, A. I., Czeisler, C. A., Rutherford, J. D., Willich, S. N., Gleason, R. E., Williams, G. H., and Muller, J. E. (1987). Concurrent morning increase in platelet aggregability and the risk of myocardial infarction and sudden cardiac death. *N. Engl. J. Med.* **316**, 1514–1518.

Udelsman, R., Harwood, J. P., Millan, M. A., Chrousos, G. P., Goldstein, D. S., Zimlichman, R., Catt, K. J., and Aguilera, G. (1986). Functional corticotropin releasing factor receptors in the primate peripheral sympathetic nervous system. *Nature (London)* **319**, 147–150.

Valentino, R. J., and Wehby, R. G. (1988). Corticotropin-releasing factor: Evidence for a neurotransmitter role in the locus ceruleus during hemodynamic stress. *Neuroendocrinology* **48**, 674–677.

Wynn, P. C., Hauger, R. L., Holmes, M. C., Millan, M. A., Catt, K. J., and Aguilera, G. (1984). Brain and pituitary receptors for corticotropin releasing factor: Localization and differential regulation after adrenalectomy. *Peptides (N.Y.)* **5**, 1077–1084.

Yajima, F. Suda, T., Tomori, N., Sumitomo, T., Nakagami, Y., Ushiyama, T., Demura, H., and Shizume, K. (1986). Effects of opioid peptides on immunoreactive corticotropin-releasing factor release from the rat hypothalamus in vitro. *Life Sci.* **39**, 181–186.

Young, W. S., III (1986). Corticotropin-releasing factor mRNA in the hypothalamus is affected differently by drinking saline and by dehydration. *FEBS Lett.* **208**, 158–162.

Young, W. S., III, Walker, L. C., Powers, R. E., De Souza, E. B., and Price, D. L. (1986). Corticotropin-releasing factor mRNA is expressed in the inferior olives of rodents and primates. *Mol. Brain Res.* **1**, 189–192.

Zhang, T.-X., and Ciriello, J. (1985). Effect of paraventricular nucleus lesions on arterial pressure and heart rate after aortic barorecptor denervation in the rat. *Brain Res.* **341**, 101–109.

7

Corticotropin-Releasing Factor, Stress, and Animal Behavior

Belinda J. Cole
Department of Neuropsychopharmacology
Schering AG
West Berlin, Federal Republic of Germany

George F. Koob
Department of Neuropharmacology
Research Institute of Scripps Clinic
La Jolla, California 92037

I. Introduction

Although corticotropin-releasing factor (CRF) was originally isolated and characterized on the basis of its ability to induce adrenocorticotropin hormone (ACTH) release from the anterior pituitary (Vale *et al.*, 1981), a large body of evidence suggests that this neuropeptide also has a direct neurotropic action in the central nervous system. Thus neuroanatomical studies have demonstrated the existence of CRF-immunoreactive neurons and fibers outside the hypothalamus (Swanson *et al.*, 1983), and receptor binding studies have shown CRF binding sites widely distributed throughout the CNS (De Souza, 1987). At the cellular level, electrophysiological studies have shown that CRF produces a pronounced depolarization and excitation of hippocampal neurons (Aldenhoff *et al.*, 1983), and increases the firing rate of norepinephrine-containing neurons in the nucleus locus ceruleus (Valentino *et al.*, 1983). In addition, a recent study has demonstrated the depolarization-induced release of CRF from the amygdala (Smith *et al.*, 1986).

Theoretically, it has been widely hypothesized that extrahypothalamic

CRF serves a homologous function to CRF in the hypothalamic–pituitary–adrenal axis (Koob and Bloom, 1985). Specifically, since activation of the hypothalamic–pituitary axis is classically defined as "the stress response," extrahypothalamic CRF is also thought to be involved in responses to stressors in the central nervous system. Such a hypothesis is consistent with the neuroanatomical distribution of CRF (Swanson et al., 1983) and the ability of CRF to stimulate autonomic activity (Brown et al., 1982; Brown and Fisher, 1983; Fisher et al., 1982). In addition, as discussed in this chapter, a substantial body of evidence also implicates extrahypothalamic CRF in behavioral response to stressors.

This chapter will start by evaluating the extent to which the behavioral effects of centrally administered CRF support the hypothesis that this peptide is critically involved in initiating behavioral responses to stressful stimuli. More recent evidence concerning the behavioral effects of the CRF antagonist will then be discussed.

II. Centrally Administered CRF

A. Behavioral Activation

CRF has behaviorally activating properties when infused directly into the central nervous system. Administered intracerebroventricularly (icv), it produces a marked, dose-dependent (0.1–10.0 μg) increase in behavioral activation, as measured by locomotor activity in a familiar environment (Sutton et al., 1982; Koob et al., 1984; Kalivas et al., 1987). As CRF can stimulate both the hypothalamic–pituitary–adrenal axis (Vale et al., 1981) and the autonomic nervous system (Brown et al., 1982), one obvious question is whether either of these physiological effects of the peptide underlies its ability to produce locomotor hyperactivity. Activation of the hypothalamic–pituitary axis has been shown to be neither sufficient nor necessary for this behavioral effect of CRF, suggesting that the locomotor hyperactivity results from a direct action of CRF in the central nervous system. Thus it has been shown that systemic administration of CRF does not produce hyperactivity (Sutton et al., 1982), and that neither pretreatment with dexamethasone (K. T. Britton et al., 1986; D. R. Britton et al. 1986) nor hypohysectomy (Eaves et al., 1985) attenuates the behavioral activation induced by icv administration of CRF.

The role of the autonomic nervous system in this behavioral effect of CRF has received less attention. However, systemic administration of the beta-adrenoceptor antagonist propranolol potentiates the locomotor hyperactivity produced by central administration of CRF (Cole and Koob, 1988) at doses that do not themselves affect locomotor activity. In contrast, it should be noted that Britton and Indyk (1989) have shown that the ganglionic blocking drug chlorisondamine can attenuate CRF-induced hyperactivity. Although these authors reported that the dose of chlorisondamine studied (3.0 mg/kg) does not itself affect locomotor activity, our own studies (B. J. Cole and G. F. Koob, unpublished observations) have shown that the same dose of chlorisondamine has marked sedative properties on operant responding. It should also be noted that it is difficult to show sedative effects of drugs on locomotor activity in a familiar environment, because the spontaneous activity of rats is extremely low, unless tested in the dark component of the light-dark cycle. Taken together, these observations therefore suggest that CRF produces behavioral activation through a direct action in the central nervous system, and independently of its effects on the hypothalamic–pituitary–adrenal axis and the autonomic nervous system.

Several studies have also examined potential neurochemical and neuroanatomical substrates of this CRF-induced hyperactivity. These studies have so far suggested that CRF acts on different neurochemical systems than other, more widely studied stimulants (e.g., amphetamine and heroin) to induce locomotor hyperactivity. Thus while dopamine-receptor anatagonists and dopamine-depleting lesions of the nucleus accumbens attenuate the locomotor stimulating effects of indirect sympathomimetics, such as amphetamine and cocaine (Kelly and Iversen, 1976), neither of these treatments specifically affects CRF-induced hyperactivity (Koob et al., 1984; Swerdlow and Koob, 1985; Kalivas et al., 1987). Similarly, while systemic administration of the opiate antagonist naloxone blocks the behavioral activation produced by opioids (Segal et al., 1979), it does not affect CRF-induced hyperactivity (Koob et al., 1984). Finally, while infusions of the gamma-aminobutyric acid (GABA) agonist muscimol into the substantia inominata/lateral preoptic (SI/LPO) region severely attenuate the stimulant effects of both amphetamine and heroin, such infusions do not affect CRF-induced locomotor hyperactivity (Swerdlow and Koob, 1985). These results therefore suggest that CRF-induced locomotor hyperactivity is independent of both dopamine and opiate systems.

Studies of potential neuroanatomical substrates of CRF-induced hyperactivity have revealed that CRF-induced hyperactivity depends upon forebrain CRF receptors, although the critical substrates have not been precisely localized. The initial evidence for the importance of the forebrain in the stimulant effects of CRF came from a study performed by Tazi et al. (1987b). In this experiment, CRF was injected into either the lateral ventricle or the cisterna magna, after the cerebral aqueduct had been blocked by a cold-cream plug. This experiment revealed that under these conditions, only CRF infused into the lateral ventricle, and not the cisterna magna, produced hyperactivity. A further study also attempted to characterize the critical neural substrates in the forebrain in more detail. Consequently, CRF was infused directly into several forebrain structures, including the frontal cortex, nucleus accumbens, and the SI/LPO region. This study revealed that the magnitude of the CRF-induced locomotor activity was inversely related to the distance of the injection site from the SI/LPO region. In addition, only SI/LPO injection sites yielded activation levels greater than that produced by icv CRF infusions (Tazi *et al.*, 1987b). Although these results suggest some neuroanatomical specificity for the neural substrates of CRF-induced behavioral activation, another sensitive site, the ventral tegmental area, has since been found (Kalivas *et al.*, 1987).

The effects of repeated administration of CRF on locomotor activity have also recently begun to be studied. In this experiment, rats were initially habituated to photocell cages overnight, and then injected icv with CRF on 5 consecutive days. This experiment revealed that there is a striking differ-

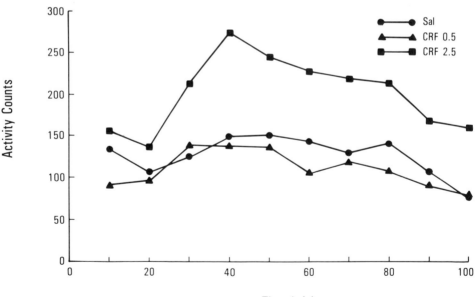

Figure 1 Effects of pretreatment with CRF (5 icv infusions) on the locomotor response to an sc injection of 0.75 mg/kg D-amphetamine, tested in wire mesh photocell cages, 9 days after the last CRF infusion.

ence between the effects of repeated administration of a low dose of CRF
(0.5 μg) and those of a high dose (2.5 μg). While on the first day of testing
there was no significant difference between the locomotor hyperactivity
produced by 0.5 and 2.5 μg CRF, on subsequent days the response to 0.5
μg showed rapid tolerance, while the response to 2.5 μg actually became
larger. This rapid tolerance to a low dose of CRF is similar to that seen
with repeated administration of caffeine (Holtzman and Finn, 1988), while
the increase seen with the high dose is more like the sensitization seen with
repeated administration of psychomotor stimulants, such as amphetamine
or cocaine (Robinson and Becker, 1986). Interestingly, the repeated administration of 2.5 μg CRF also produced an enhanced locomotor response
to a low dose of amphetamine tested 9 days later, whereas the repeated
administration of the low dose did not (see Figure 1) (M. Cador, B. J. Cole,
G. F. Koob, L. Stinus, M. Le Moal, unpublished observation). The results
therefore suggest that different mechanisms may be involved in the locomotor stimulant effects of low and high doses of CRF, with the low-dose effects
resembling those produced by caffeine, and the higher-dose effects perhaps
containing a dopamine-mediated component.

B. Behavioral Responses to Aversive Stimuli

1. Novelty

Although icv administration of CRF produces marked behavioral activation
in a familiar environment, identical doses of CRF produce behavioral inhibition in a novel, presumably stressful environment (Sutton et al., 1982).
More specifically, Sutton et al. (1982) showed that while typical saline-
treated control rats initially circle the outer squares of an open field rapidly
and then begin to explore the center, CRF-treated rats only move extremely
hesitantly in the outer squares. However, the specific role of novelty in these
different effects of CRF is questioned by the findings of Takahashi et al.
(1989). These authors showed that the effects of CRF on behavior in an
open field were not altered by preexposing rats to the test environment,
suggesting that it is some other factor, such as the size of the test chamber
or the intensity of illumination, that is the critical factor in determining
these differential effects of CRF. A specific reduction of exploratory behavior in mice has also been demonstrated by Berridge and Dunn (1986), using
a multiple-compartment chamber containing novel objects for the animals
to explore. CRF (0.075 μg) caused a reduction in the mean time per contact
with the novel stimuli, without affecting locomotor activity. Similarly, Britton et al. (1982) have shown that icv administration of CRF increases food
neophobia, tested in a novel environment. In this behavioral paradigm,
mildly food-deprived rats are placed into a novel open field where food is

available. While control rats enter the center of the open field to consume the food, CRF-treated rats show a marked decrease in exploration and ingestive behavior, and remain close to the edge of the open field. D. R. Britton et al. (1986) have also shown that this effect of CRF is not attenuated by blockade of the hypothalamic–pituitary–adrenal axis with dexamethasone. Although CRF has also been shown to reduce both food deprivation and pharmacologically induced feeding (Levine et al., 1983; Morley and Levine, 1983), it should be noted that it increases food neophobia at much lower doses.

2. Displacement Behavior

In addition to inhibiting feeding, icv administration of CRF simultaneously induces grooming behavior (Sutton et al., 1982; Morley and Levine, 1983). Since grooming is often observed in novel or other mildly stressful environments, it is considered a displacement activity. To examine the generality of the ability of CRF to facilitate displacement activities, the effects of CRF on several other experimental analogues of displacement behavior have been examined.

Tail-pinch-induced eating, schedule-induced polydipsia, and foot-shock-induced fighting have all been suggested to belong to a class of behaviors that are experimental analogues of displacement activities, or "coping" responses (Hennessy and Foy, 1987). These behaviors are thought to serve as adaptive responses to stressful stimuli because their performance reduces an aversive state of high arousal. In schedule-induced polydipsia, a food- but not water-deprived rat is typically exposed to a schedule in which small amounts of food are delivered intermittently. Such schedules result in the development of excessive drinking during the intervals between food delivery, and the performance of this behavioral response attenuates increases in plasma corticosterone levels caused by the schedule (Brett and Levine, 1979). The hypothesis that shock-induced fighting is a coping response is also based on the observation that rats shocked in pairs and allowed to fight show lower levels of circulating ACTH than rats shocked alone (Conner et al., 1971). The performance of tail-pinch-induced eating has not been specifically shown to attenuate plasma corticosterone or ACTH levels. However, tail-pinch-induced behaviors do appear to be reinforcing, since rats with their tails pinched, but not unpinched controls, will learn to run a maze for the opportunity to gnaw on wood (Koob et al., 1976).

ICV administration of CRF (0.1 and 0.5 μg) attenuates the performance of schedule-induced polydipsia (B. J. Cole, K. T. Britton, A. Tazi, C. Rivier, J. Rivier, W. Vale, and G. F. Koob, unpublished observations, 1989), but potentiates footshock-induced fighting at the same doses (Tazi et al., 1987a). Recent evidence has also shown that CRF dramatically attenuates the development of tail-pinch-induced eating (B. J. Cole and G. F. Koob, unpublished observations, 1989). In this behavioral paradigm, a non-food-deprived rat is placed into a familiar testing environment with a paper clip attached to its tail, so that the clip exerts a mild, constant pressure. The mild pressure reliably elicits eating in control rats, which increases in duration with repeated testing. As shown in Figure 2, the saline-treated controls showed the expected increase in the duration of eating with repeated testing. CRF, infused icv at extremely low doses (0.02, 0.1, and 0.5 µg), significantly attenuated the development of tail-pinch-induced eating (see Figure 2). In fact, none of the rats treated with 0.5 µg CRF ate at all, during any of the 5-min tests. Instead, the CRF-treated rats were signifi-

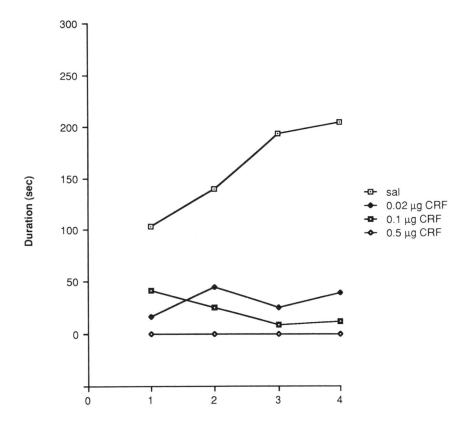

Session

Figure 2 Effects of icv infusions of CRF on the acquisition of tail-pinch-induced eating, as measured by the duration of eating. Each session duration was 5 min.

cantly more active than the saline-treated controls, and also spent more time in paper-clip- or tail-oriented behavior. Thus central administration of CRF does not globally enhance the performance of all displacement activities.

3. Conditioned Behavior

Two operant paradigms that are sensitive to anxiolytic drugs, namely, a Geller–Seifter conflict test and a conditioned suppression schedule, have also been used to examine the effects of CRF. In the former of these paradigms, the presentation of a reinforcing stimulus (food) is paired with an aversive stimulus (footshock) for part of each session. Britton et al. (Thatcher-Britton et al., 1985) have shown that CRF (0.5 and 1 μg) produces a significant decrease in both punished and unpunished responding in an operant conflict paradigm with incremental footshock, although the percent decrease in unpunished responding is greater than the percent decrease in punished responding. This decrease in punished responding is opposite to that produced by benzodiazepine agonists (Cook and Sepinwall, 1975).

In the conditioned suppression schedule, rats are initially trained to respond on a lever for food reinforcement. Once a stable level of responding has been obtained, a conditioned stimulus (CS) is presented prior to the delivery of a brief inescapable footshock (UCS), while the animal is responding on the baseline schedule. This procedure results in a reduction in food-reinforced responding during the presence of the CS. Central administration of CRF causes a dose-dependent reduction in both CS and pre-CS responding in this paradigm. However, the reduction in CS responding is more sensitive to CRF, occurring at lower doses (0.02 and 0.1 μg) than the reduction in pre-CS responding (0.5 μg), suggesting that this paradigm is more sensitive to the effects of CRF than the operant conflict paradigm (Cole et al.,1987). This pattern of sensitivity in the operant conflict paradigm and the conditioned suppression schedule is opposite to that seen with benzodiazepine agonists (e.g., chlordiazepoxide), which are more effective at alleviating response suppression in a conflict than a conditioned suppression paradigm (Dantzer, 1987), although the precise role of rate dependency in this dissociation is still controversial.

At the psychological level, it is not entirely clear what any differences in sensitivity between these two paradigms may reflect. However, of particular significance may be the fact that in an operant conflict paradigm, footshock delivery is entirely under the control of the animal, so that if the animal chooses not to respond during the conflict component of this schedule, it would not receive any footshock. In contrast, footshock presentation in the conditioned suppression schedule is entirely response-independent and uncontrollable by the animal. Interestingly, in the operant conflict paradigm with incremental footshock, the intensity of footshock that the animals choose to receive is often much greater than what will produce severe response inhibition in the conditioned suppression paradigm.

Another behavioral test frequently used to assess the effects of anxiolytic and anxiogenic drugs is the acoustic startle response. This reflex is an easily quantified muscular contraction in response to an intense acoustic stimulus. Like other anxiogenic treatments (see Davis, 1980, for review), CRF (1 μg) produces a marked increase in acoustic startle amplitude (Swerdlow *et al.*,1986).

4. Interpretation of the Behavioral Effects of Centrally Administered CRF on Behavioral Responses to Aversive Stimuli

Taken together, these results provide general support for the hypothesis that CRF potentiates behavioral responses to stressful (aversive) stimuli. However, it should be noted that in most of these stress-related behavioral paradigms (with the exception of the operant conflict paradigm and the food neophobia test), the behavioral effects of CRF have not been demonstrated to be mediated directly by the central nervous system, as opposed to the hypothalamic–pituitary–adrenal axis. In addition, there are some minor problems raised by these data for the hypothesis that CRF potentiates behavioral responses to stressful stimuli that deserve comment. First, it should be noted that the behavioral effects of CRF have only been examined in stress-related paradigms. If amphetamine had been tested *only* in the behavioral paradigms outlined above, it also would probably be concluded to potentiate the behavioral response to aversive stimuli. Consequently, it is important that the effects of CRF in other, non-stress-related paradigms be assessed (e.g., brain-stimulation reward threshold) (see Kornetsky and Esposito, 1981). Similarly, it is not known whether central administration of CRF is itself an aversive (or appetitive) event. Although high doses of CRF (5 μg) have been shown to produce a conditioned taste aversion in both one- and two-bottled tests (Gosnell *et al.*, 1983; P. Meuller, B. J. Cole, and G. F. Koob, unpublished observations), such demonstrations do not necessarily indicate that even a high dose of CRF is aversive (Hunt and Amit, 1987). Whether lower doses of CRF produce a conditioned place preference (or aversion) and a conditioned taste aversion is not known, but would be of considerable theoretical interest, particularly since all stimulants studied to date have produced a conditioned place preference, and are thus assumed to have rewarding properties (for review, see Swerdlow *et al.*, 1989). In addition, it should be remembered that CRF has been detected in the interneurons of the cerebral cortex (Swanson *et al.*, 1983). It seems somewhat unlikely that these CRF-containing interneurons are involved in the anxiogenic effects of CRF, but their behavioral significance has received extremely little attention, even though abnormalities have been detected in their function in senile dementia (De Souza et al., 1986).

The second problem with these results relates to the effects of CRF on tail-pinch-induced eating and schedule-induced polydipsia. Since both of these behaviors have been considered as coping responses to reduce aversive states of high arousal, it might be expected that CRF would potentiate their performance. This issue will be addressed in a later section, after the effects of the CRF antagonist in these pardigms have been discussed. The third problem is related to the effects of CRF in operant measures of anxiety, where this peptide has been shown not only to reduce responding in the conflict or CS component of conflict and conditioned suppression schedules, respectively, but also baseline response rates. The fourth and more general problem relates to the pharmacological specificity of the effects of CRF in these behavioral paradigms.

The ability of CRF to reduce responding in both the punished and the unpunished components of a conflict schedule could be interpreted as a general reduction in operant responding, perhaps related to the ability of CRF to suppress appetitive motivation (Levine et al., 1983), rather than as an enhanced response to aversive stimuli. This interpretation is supported to some extent by the fact that the percent reduction in baseline responding is greater than the percent reduction in conflict responding. However, against this hypothesis is the evidence that responding on a food-reinforced, random-interval, 60-s operant schedule is not attenuated by doses of CRF below 2.5 µg (B. J. Cole, K. T. Britton, A. Tazi, C. Rivier, J. Rivier, W. Vale, and G. F. Koob, unpublished observations, 1989). This dose is significantly higher than that required to reduce baseline response rates in either the conflict schedule or the conditioned suppression schedule (0.5 µg). One potential explanation for this lack of behavioral specificity may be the ability of CRF to reveal "latent anxiety," which generalizes from the punished to the otherwise nonfearful component of the behavioral paradigm. In support of such a hypothesis is the demonstration that increasing the level of foot-shock used in a conditioned suppression paradigm produces decrements not only in CS, but also pre-CS response rates (Hurwitz and Davis, 1983). Similar experiments with the operant conflict paradigm used by Britton et al. (Thatcher-Britton et al., 1985) cannot easily be performed, since the paradigm incorporates incremental footshock levels. In addition, it should be noted that a similar lack of behavioral specificity in operant measures of anxiety has been found with other purported "anxiogenic" agents, such as the benzodiazepine partial inverse agonist FG 7142 (Koob et al., 1986; Cole and Koob, 1988), although other drugs, such as picrotoxin and bicuculline, have been reported to produce specific reductions in punished responding in a slightly different conflict test, the water-lick test (Corda and Biggio, 1986).

The final, and perhaps most important, question relates to whether the behavioral paradigms in which CRF has been tested specifically detect anxiogenic effects of drugs. Unfortunately, where the data are known, this appears not to be the case. Many of the behavioral tests in which CRF has been tested were developed as screening procedures for anxiolytic-like benzodiazepine agonist compounds, and in this respect they appear to have considerable pharmacological specificity. For example, neuroleptics, stimulants, and antidepressants all produce behavioral effects in these paradigms different from those produced by benzodiazepine agonists (see Cook and Sepinwall, 1975, for review). In particular, the operant conflict paradigm and the food neophobia test have been suggested to be sensitive only to anxiolytic compounds (Cook and Sepinwall, 1975; Britton and Britton, 1981). Unfortunately, these behavioral paradigms do not appear to possess the same degree of specificity concerning potential anxiogenic compounds. For example, most stimulants, including amphetamine (Cook and Sepinwall, 1975), produce "anxiogenic-like" effects in an operant conflict paradigm, although it should be noted that these drugs have also been suggested to produce anxiogenic effects in humans.

The ability of most stimulants to produce "anxiogenic-like" effects in animal models of anxiety raises perhaps one of the most important questions concerning the purported stress-producing effects of CRF. Are these effects produced simply because CRF is a stimulant? Alternatively, are the "anxiogenic" and the "activating" effects of CRF-mediated by different neuroanatomical and neurochemical substrates? Since high levels of arousal have been argued to be aversive (Berlyne, 1960), and arousal appears to be a crucial determinant of emotions (Schachter and Singer, 1962), this latter hypothesis is extremely plausible. This question can be answered by comparing either the neuroanatomical or the neuropharmacological substrates of the activating and the anxiogenic effects of CRF.

5. Neuroanatomical and Neurochemical Substrates of Enhanced Behavioral Responses to Aversive Stimuli Produced by CRF

Recent experiments indicate that the anxiogenic and the activating behavioral effects of CRF are actually mediated by neuropharmacologically distinct substrates. For example, the benzodiazepine antagonist RO-15-1788 has been shown to attenuate the decrease in punished responding produced by CRF in an operant conflict test, but not to affect CRF-induced locomotor hyperactivity (Britton et al., 1988). However, the effects of RO-15-1788 on the CRF-induced reduction in punished responding may reflect two opposite drug effects, rather than a specific pharmacological interaction, since

RO-15-1788 was also shown to attenuate the reduction in punished responding caused by amphetamine. In addition, it should be noted that a benzodiazepine agonist, chlordiazepoxide, can reverse both the proconflict effects of CRF (Thatcher-Britton *et al.*, 1985) and CRF-potentiated startle (Swerdlow *et al.*, 1986). However, since benzodiazepines themselves have anxiolytic effects in these paradigms (Dantzer, 1987), both of these effects also probably result from two opposite drug effects, rather than a specific pharmacological interaction.

More recently, in the conditioned suppression paradigm, propranolol, a beta-adrenoceptor antagonist, was shown to reverse the anxiogenic effects of CRF (0.5 µg), but not those of the benzodiazepine partial inverse agonist FG 7142 (Cole and Koob, 1988). In addition, as discussed previously, propranolol (at the same doses) actually potentiates CRF-induced hyperactivity. These results therefore suggest that either the central or the peripheral noradrenergic (NE) systems are involved in the anxiogenic effects of CRF, but not its activating effects.

To dissociate the potential roles of central and peripheral NE in the enhanced conditioned fear produced by CRF, this work has been extended by using a charged analogue of clonidine, ST-91. This drug is a selective alpha-2 agonist that does not cross the blood–brain barrier. Alpha-2 agonists act in the central nervous system at presynaptic alpha-2 receptors to inhibit the firing rate of NE containing neurons (Cedarbaum and Aghajanian, 1978), but also in the periphery to prevent the release of NE (Langer, 1981). These experiments have shown that while central administration of ST-91, at doses that have previously been demonstrated to inhibit the firing rate of the NE containing nucleus locus ceruleus (Valentino *et al.*, 1986), does not affect performance of conditioned suppression itself, it does attenuate the enhanced response suppression produced by 0.5 µg of CRF during the CS presentation (see Figure 3a). In addition, these experiments showed that systemic administration of ST-91 produces a mild anxiolytic effect itself in the conditioned suppression paradigm, and at extremely low doses (1 µg/kg) also produces partial antagonism of the effects of CRF (Figure 3b). However, this effect is not dose-dependent. These results have also been extended to the operant conflict paradigm, and here the central administration of ST-91 can again attenuate the proconflict effects of CRF, although in this paradigm, systemic administration is ineffective. These results therefore suggest that activation of central NE systems may be critical for the "anxiogenic-like" effects of centrally administered CRF.

To address the pharmacological specificity of drugs that interact with NE systems to antagonize the anxiogenic effects of CRF, the interaction between CRF and methysergide, a nonspecific serotonin antagonist, in the operant conflict paradigm and the conditioned suppression schedule was

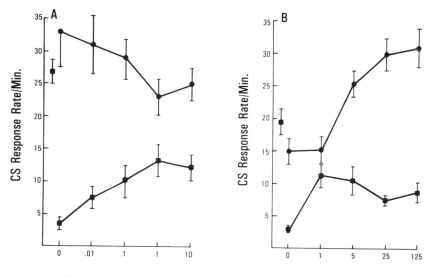

Figure 3 Effects of (A) icv and (B) sc injections of ST-91, alone and in combination with an icv infusion of 0.5 μg CRF (•) on the performance of a conditioned emotional response (CER). The data point on the far left of both panels shows the performance of the CRF-infused group when drug-free.

also examined. These experiments revealed that methysergide itself (1.25, 2.5, 5.0, and 10.0 mg/kg, ip) has extremely weak anxiolytic properties in both of these behavioral paradigms, and also does not reverse the effects of CRF. In addition, Kalivas *et al.* (1987) have shown that administration of CRF directly into the ventral tegmental area does not produce anxiogenic effects in an open field test, suggesting that the forebrain mesocorticolimbic dopamine systems are also not involved in the stress-enhancing effects of CRF.

It is important to emphasize that CRF does not appear to simply act like an alpha-2 antagonist (e.g., yohimbine) to produce its "anxiogenic-like" effects, as there are marked differences between the behavioral effects of CRF and alpha-2 antagonists. Although yohimbine has been reported to produce anxiogenic effects in both humans (Holmberg and Gershon, 1961) and monkeys (Redmond and Huang, 1979), the systemic administration of yohimbine does not produce "anxiogenic-like" effects in the conditioned suppression paradigm (B. J. Cole and G. F. Koob, unpublished results). Instead, at a low dose (1.25 mg/kg), this drug actually produced a mild anxiolytic effect, while a higher dose (5.0 mg/kg) produced a general reduction in the rate of responding that was greater during the pre-CS than the CS period (B. J. Cole and G. F. Koob, unpublished observations). K. T. Britton (unpublished observations) has also observed similar effects of yohimbine in the operant conflict test.

The hypothesis that central NE systems are involved in the "anxiogenic-like" but not the activating effects of CRF is also supported by the findings of Butler et al. (1988). Furthermore, these experiments performed by Butler et al. suggest that the NE-containing nucleus locus ceruleus may be the critical neuroanatomical substrate for the interaction between CRF and NE. These authors have shown that infusions of CRF directly into the region of the NE containing nucleus locus ceruleus increase the time an animal spends struggling in a forced swim test (an animal model of depression), increase the latency of an animal to emerge from a small dark container into a large, brightly illuminated open field, but do not affect spontaneous locomotor activity.

The behavioral evidence for a functional interaction between CRF and the NE-containing nucleus locus ceruleus in responses to aversive stimuli is also compatible with the results of several anatomical, electrophysiological, and biochemical studies. For example, Swanson et al. (1983) have demonstrated CRF-like immunoreactive neurons and fibers in the region of the locus ceruleus, and Cummings et al. (1983) have suggested that CRF terminals innervate the locus ceruleus. At the electrophysiological level, Valentino et al. (1983) have shown that central administration of CRF increases the firing rate of locus ceruleus neurons, and more importantly, that central administration of a CRF antagonist blocks stress-induced increase in their firing rate (Valentino and Wehby, 1988). These electrophysiological findings are paralleled by the biochemical studies of Dunn and Berridge (1987), who showed that central administration of CRF increases NE turnover in several forebrain regions. In addition, Chappell et al. (1986) have shown that both acute and chronic stress produce a neuroanatomically selective increase in the concentration of CRF in the region of the locus coeruleus. Given the evidence outlined above, this finding is obviously of significant interest. However, this change could reflect either an increase in CRF synthesis or a decrease in CRF release (or a combination of these events).

In summary, central administration of CRF has been shown to produce behavioral activation in familiar environments and behavioral responses that are compatible with the hypothesis that CRF potentiates behavioral responses to stressful stimuli in more aversive situations. In addition, the neuropharmacological substrates of these two effects of CRF appear to be different, with the central NE systems being involved in the anxiogenic but not the activating effects. While this evidence that exogenously administered CRF potentiates behavioral responses to stressful stimuli is interesting, the hypothesis that behavioral responses to stressful stimuli critically depend upon activation of endogenous CRF systems would be significantly strengthened by evidence of stress-protective effects of an antagonist to CRF.

III. Role of Endogenous CRF in Behavior

The relatively recent synthesis of a peptide antagonist to CRF, alpha-helical CRF (9–41) (Rivier et al., 1984) has provided an extremely useful tool for examining the functional significance of endogenous CRF systems in behavior. This peptide antagonist is, however, 10 times less potent than CRF itself in binding to central nervous system CRF receptors (De Souza, 1987).

A. Behavioral Activation

Since central administration of CRF produces locomotor hyperactivity (Sutton et al., 1982), endogenous CRF systems might be hypothesized to be involved in behavioral arousal. An initial experiment examining the effects of alpha-helical CRF on locomotor activity was performed in photocell cages overnight. In addition, the rats were not habituated to the photocell cages, so they would have been a novel, and therefore presumably stressful, environment. This experiment revealed that over a wide range of doses (6.25, 12.5, and 25 μg), the CRF antagonist has no effect on locomotor activity in these conditions (B. J. Cole and G. F. Koob, unpublished results). The same doses of the antagonist also did not alter food-deprivation (48 h) induced locomotor hyperactivity (B. J. Cole and G. F. Koob, unpublished results).

In contrast, the antagonist does have effects on the behavioral activation induced in two other, probably more stressful behavioral paradigms, namely, tail-pinch-induced eating and schedule-induced polydipsia. The performance of both of these behaviors appears to critically depend upon the production of behavioral activation (Robbins and Fray, 1980; Robbins and Koob, 1980), and is also related to an intermediate level of stress (Antelman et al., 1975; Brett and Levine, 1979). In these experiments, central administration of low doses of the CRF antagonist (1–5 μg) facilitated the acquisition of both tail-pinch-induced eating and schedule-induced polydipsia, while a higher dose (25 μg) produced a severe impairment in their development (see Figure 4). However, the same doses of the antagonist did not affect preestablished behavior in either paradigm (B. J. Cole and G. F. Koob, unpublished observations, 1989).

The most parsimonious explanation of these results is that there is an

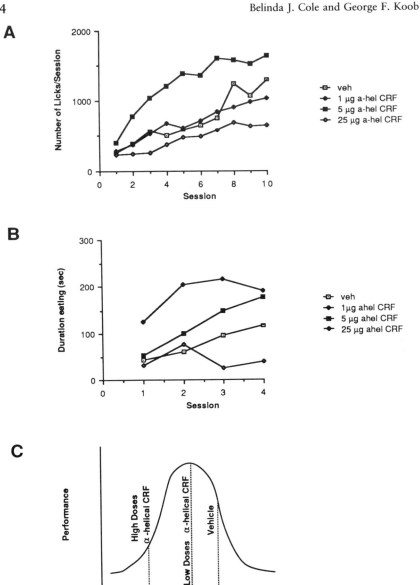

Figure 4 (A) Effects of icv infusions of alpha-helical CRF on the acquisition of schedule-induced polydipsia (SIP). The data show the mean number of licks/session for each group. (B) Effects of icv infusions of alpha-helical CRF on the acquisition of tail-pinch-induced eating. The data show the mean duration of eating/5-min session for each group. (C) Schematic diagram showing the hypothetic induced U-shaped relationship between arousal and performance.

inverted U-shaped relationship between arousal level and the acquisition of these behaviors. Thus the facilitation seen with low doses of the antagonist may result from the reduction of a supraoptimal arousal level to a more optimal level. The impairment seen with a high dose of the antagonist may result from an alpha-helical CRF-induced suboptimal arousal level, while the impairment seen with central administration of CRF (see earlier section) can be considered as resulting from overarousal (Figure 4c). However, the most important conclusion from these experiments is that although the CRF antagonist does not produce a neuroleptic-like decrease in all behavior, in certain more stressful conditions it can produce effects on behavioral arousal.

B. Behavioral Responses to Aversive Stimuli

1. Novelty

As central administration of CRF produces "anxiogenic-like" effects in a wide range of behavioral paradigms, it might be expected that the CRF antagonist would produce the opposite, namely "anxiolytic-like" or "stress-reduction-like" effects in the same paradigms. In some instances, this indeed appears to be the case, although in many cases negative results have been found. For example, while CRF reliably increases food neophobia tested in a novel environment, the CRF antagonist (1–25 μg) appears to be devoid of behavioral effects in this paradigm (K.T. Britton and G. F. Koob unpublished observations; B. J. Cole and G. F. Koob, unpublished observations). However, a slightly different behavioral paradigm for measuring behavioral responses to novelty has revealed effects of the CRF antagonist. In this paradigm, rats are placed into a small dark container, and their latency to emerge into a large, novel open field is recorded. Takahashi et al. (1989) have shown that central administration of the CRF antagonist reduces the latency for rats to emerge from the dark container into the open field. The reason for the discrepancy between these two measures of the response to novelty is unclear. It appears unlikely, in the face of the negative results on tests of food neophobia, that alpha-helical CRF attenuates the behavioral inhibition generally produced by novel stimuli. In addition, it should be remembered that central administration of CRF also appears not to specifically affect the behavioral response to a novel environment (Takahashi et al., 1989).

2. Restraint Stress

More robust effects of the CRF antagonist have been reported in behavioral paradigms utilizing restraint stress. For example, Krahn et al. (1986) have shown that central administration of the CRF antagonist (50 μg) prior to

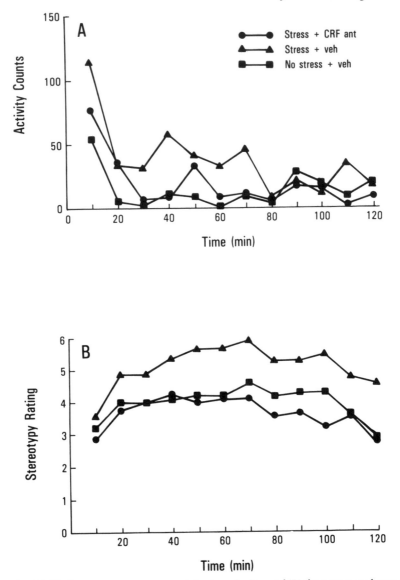

Figure 5 (A) The locomotor response to sc injection of saline and (B) the stereotyped response to sc injection of 3.0 mg/kg AMPH during the 2-h test sessions for the three separate groups. Values represent mean locomotor response and mean stereotypy rating for each 10 min epoch (N = 9), stress + CRF ant; N = 10, stress + veh; N = 10, no stress + veh).

restraint stress partially antagonizes the reduction in feeding caused by restraint. However, the antagonist did not affect food-deprivation-induced feeding. Similarly, Berridge and Dunn (1987) have shown that icv infusions of alpha-helical CRF attenuate the restraint-induced reduction of exploratory behavior in a multiple compartment chamber. These authors also showed that in unrestrained mice, the CRF antagonist does not affect exploratory behavior in this apparatus. The effects of the CRF antagonist on restraint-stress-induced sensitization of the behavioral response to amphetamine have also recently been explored. In this experiment, one group of rats was injected icv with the CRF antagonist (25 µg) prior to each of 5 90-min periods of restraint. A separate group of rats was injected with vehicle prior to restraint, and a third group served as unrestrained, vehicle-treated controls. Seven days after the last restraint period, the rats were tested for their locomotor response to saline, in prehabituated photocell cages. In this test, the vehicle-treated restrained rats were significantly more active than the two other groups, who did not differ (see Figure 5a). Four days later the same rats were tested for their response to 3.0 mg/kg d-amphetamine (sc), since stress has been previously shown to sensitize amphetamine-induced stereotyped behavior (Antelman et al., 1980). As shown in Figure 5b, the vehicle-treated restrained rats showed significantly more intense stereotyped behavior than the two other groups, who did not differ (Cole et al., 1990). Taken together, these results therefore suggest that endogenous CRF may be involved in several of the behavioral consequences of restraint stress, both immediate and long term. However, it should be noted that none of these experiments have controlled for the effects of alpha-helical CRF on the release of ACTH and corticosterone, so it is not yet clear whether these results are caused by an antagonism of central CRF systems or the hypothalamic–pituitary–adrenal axis.

3. Paradigms Utilizing Footshock

The effects of alpha-helical CRF in operant tests of anxiety have generally failed to reveal anxiolytic effects of this antagonist. For example, K. T. Britton et al. (1986; unpublished observations) have shown that alpha-helical CRF (1–50 µg) does not release punished responding in an operant conflict paradigm. Similarly, Cole et al. (1987) have shown that the antagonist (1–50 µg) does not affect performance of conditioned suppression. In contrast, Swerdlow et al. (1989) have shown that central administration of the CRF antagonist dose-dependently attenuates fear-potentiated startle. In this behavioral paradigm, the magnitude of the startle response is augmented by presenting the acoustic stimulus in the presence of a CS that has previously been paired with inescapable footshock.

Although central administration of alpha-helical CRF does not affect

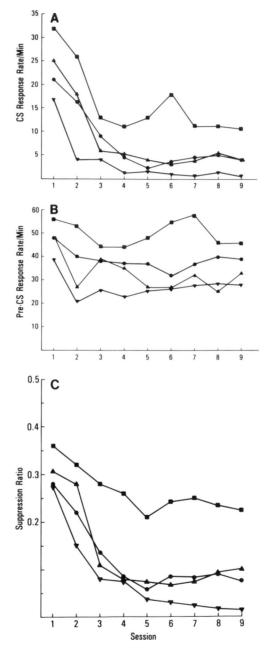

Figure 6 Effects of icv infusions of alpha-helical CRF on the acquistion of a conditioned emotional response. (A) Mean CS response rate/min; (B) mean pre-CS response rate/min; (C) mean suppression ratios on the right of each panel.

performance of preestablished conditioned suppression, it does attenuate the development of conditioned fear (see Figure 6). In this experiment, separate groups of rats were administered different doses of the antagonist prior to all of the nine acquisition sessions. While the vehicle-treated rats rapidly acquire the conditioned fear, as indexed by a reduction in response rates during the CS presentation, this acquisition is attenuated by alpha-helical CRF in a dose (1, 5, and 25 μg) dependent manner (Cole et al., 1987). Additionally, neither intravenous administration of a high dose (250 μg) of the antagonist (sufficient to attenuate plasma corticosterone levels) nor blockade of the hypothalamic–pituitary–adrenal axis with dexamathasone altered the acquisition of conditioned suppression. However, an extremely low dose (25 μg) of the antagonist (insufficient to alter plasma corticosterone levels) administered intravenously also impaired the development of conditioned fear. These results suggest that the ability of alpha-helical CRF to attenuate the development of conditioned fear is independent of its action on the hypothalamic–pituitary–adrenal axis, but also suggest a possible role for peripheral CRF in the development of conditioned fear.

There are two potential, but not mutually exclusive, explanations for these results. Firstly, it is possible that the CRF antagonist specifically impairs learning. Consistent with this hypothesis, icv administration of CRF has been shown to facilitate the acquisition of both a visual discrimination in a T maze and two-way active avoidance (Koob and Bloom, 1985). Alternatively, Kalin et al. (1988) have shown that central administration of alpha-helical CRF attenuates footshock-induced freezing in rats. It is possible that freezing occurs only toward the beginning of the acquisition of conditioned fear, and that this underlies the specific effect of alpha-helical CRF on the development of conditioned suppression. Other evidence supporting the hypothesis that alpha-helical CRF modulates the behavioral response to footshock, as opposed to learning, is the demonstration by Tazi et al. (1987a) that central administration of alpha-helical CRF dose dependently attenuates footshock induced fighting.

4. Interpretation of the Behavioral Effects of Alpha-Helical CRF

Taken together, these results show that endogenous CRF systems are involved in some, but not all, behavioral responses to stressful stimuli and suggest that the CRF antagonist has a different behavioral profile from classical anxiolytic drugs, such as benzodiazepine agonists (e.g., chlordiazepoxide and diazepam), and major tranquilizers (e.g., neuroleptics). Since the behavioral effects of the CRF antagonist obviously do not fit the profile of either a classical anxiolytic or sedative drug, the major question is how the behavioral effects of the CRF antagonist can best be characterized. In the following discussion, this question will be considered as two separate, but obviously related issues: first, under what experimental conditions does alpha-helical CRF affect behavior; and second, what is the nature of the behavioral alterations produced by alpha-helical CRF?

a. What Experimental Conditions Reveal Behavioral Effects of Alpha-Helical CRF? Alpha-helical CRF produces behavioral effects in a significantly more limited number of behavioral paradigms than either benzodiazepines or neuroleptics. These findings suggest that in a standard laboratory rat, endogenous CRF is not continuously released, and may only be released in response to highly specific stimuli. Although it must be recognized that other paradigms will undoubtedly be shown to be sensitive to the CRF antagonist in the future, the present results do cast doubt on the hypothesis that endogenous CRF systems are globally involved in all behavioral responses to all stressors. However, it should be noted that it is in the paradigms that elicit a relatively minor stress response, such as food-deprivation-induced eating (Krahn *et al.,* 1986) and food-deprivation-induced locomotor activity (B. J. Cole and G. F. Koob, unpublished observations, 1989), that the CRF antagonist most reliably fails to produce behavioral effects.

One conclusion suggested by these data is that the antagonist has dissociable effects on the development and maintenance of certain behaviors. Thus alpha-helical CRF does not affect the performance of an operant conflict paradigm (Thatcher-Britton *et al.,* 1986), a conditioned suppression schedule (Cole *et al.,* 1987), schedule-induced polydipsia, or tail-pinch-induced eating (B. J. Cole and G. F. Koob, unpublished observations, 1989), but does have marked effects on the development of the three latter behaviors. These results therefore suggest that once a behavioral response to a stressful stimulus is well established, its performance may become independent of endogenous brain CRF, even though these systems may have been important for the initial development of the behavioral response.

The CRF antagonist appears to produce particularly robust effects on the behavioral sequelae of two particular stressors, namely, restraint (Krahn *et al.,* 1986; Berridge and Dunn, 1987) and footshock (Tazi *et al.,* 1987a; Kalin *et al.,* 1989; B. J. Cole, K. T. Britton, A. Tazi, C. Rivier, J. Rivier, W. Vale, and G. F. Koob, unpublished observations, 1989). In contrast, it generally fails to affect the behavioral response to novelty. Since exposure to novel stimuli produces a peripheral stress response, it is presumably a stressful event for a rat. However, three different experiments have shown no effects of alpha-helical CRF on behavioral responses to novel stimuli, namely exploration in a multiple-compartment chamber (Berridge and Dunn, 1987; food neophobia, K. T. Britton and G. F. Koob, unpublished observations, 1989; locomotor activity in novel environment, B. J. Cole and G. F. Koob, unpublished observations, 1989). In contrast, Takahashi *et al.* (1989) have shown that alpha-helical CRF reduces the latency for a rat to emerge into a novel, illuminated open field from a small dark container. Given that several studies have failed to show an effect of the antagonist on behavior in a novel environment, it is obviously worth considering whether some other aspect of the particular test environment used by Takahaski *et al.* (1989) caused this dissociation. For example, perhaps these authors used particularly bright overhead lighting, or an exceptionally large open field. Alternatively, these authors may have found an effect of the antagonist in a novel environment simply because they used a different behavioral measure than the other paradigms. However, as discussed below, this hypothesis is somewhat unlikely, since the antagonist appears to have global effects on behavioral responses to other stressors.

It is not clear why the CRF antagonist has relatively robust and widespread effects on the behavioral consequences of restraint and footshock, but is somewhat ineffective at altering behavioral responses to novelty. One possibility is that CRF in the central nervous system is only released by relatively severe stressors. Such a hypothesis can obviously not be systematically evaluated in the context of the existing data, since no physiological indices (such as plasma corticosterone levels) of the intensity of the elicited stress response have been reported in any of these experiments. Alternatively, endogenous CRF may only be released by a particular class of stressors, whose nature is at present unclear. However, it is worth noting that all of the stressors that have so far been shown to be sensitive to the effects of the antagonist produce considerable behavioral activation, while novelty tends to inhibit ongoing behavior. Thus both restraint and footshock elicit strenuous struggling and escape attempts, while tail pinch and schedule-induced polydipsia both produce more general, but also strong, increases in behavioral activation.

b. What Is the Nature of the Behavioral Alterations Produced by Alpha-Helical CRF? Benzodiazepines have been suggested to specifically attenuate the behavioral inhibition induced by certain classes of aversive stimuli (namely, signals of punishment and nonreward, and novel and innate fear-inducing stimuli; see Gray, 1982). In this respect, the behavioral effects of the CRF antagonist again appear to differ significantly from those induced by benzodiazepines. Thus the antagonist can attenuate not only footshock-induced fighting but also footshock-induced freezing, and footshock-motivated acquisition of condition suppression. How can these widely ranging behavioral effects best be characterized? It is obvious that no simple classification, such as a selective inhibition of active or passive behavioral responses to the stressor, will suffice. Instead, it appears that the antagonist produces a much more global effect, perhaps related to attenuating the arousal induced by the stressor. As such, in contrast to benzodiazepines, CRF may be involved in the generation of the particular motivational state induced by certain aversive stimuli.

In conclusion, CRF in the central nervous system may be crucially involved in the generation of arousal by aversive (stressful) stimuli. Although such a hypothesis can explain *post hoc* the reported behavioral effects of the CRF antagonist, it is recognized that its generality severely limits its predictive power. In addition, it is not possible, on the basis of the existing data, to predict which stressors will produce CRF antagonist reversible behavioral effects. A more specific hypothesis must await further data on the effects of the antagonist in more wide-ranging behavioral paradigms.

IV. Suggestions for Future Research

Throughout this chapter, several instances have been discussed where important data for evaluating the hypothesis that CRF is crucially involved in initiating behavioral responses to stress are missing. In particular, it has been suggested that it is important to evaluate the behavioral effects of CRF in other, non-stress-related behavioral paradigms, to discover whether the effects of CRF are dissociable from other classes of stimulant drugs. However, this section will be focused primarily on suggestions for future research on three particular topics. First, more systematic behavioral studies with the CRF antagonist are necessary to evaluate the extent to which endogenous CRF is involved in initiating *all* behavioral responses to *all* stressors, and second, experiments attempting to unite the preclinical studies (discussed above), which suggest a role for CRF in initiating behavioral responses to stressors, and clinical studies (see Gold *et al.*, 1988a,b, for review), suggesting a role for CRF in the psychopathology of depression, are warranted. Third, since a large number of neurochemical systems, including CRF, opiates (Morley *et al.*, 1989), NE (Glavin, 1985), and benzodiazepines (Trullas *et al.*, 1988), have been implicated in behavioral responses to aversive stimuli, it is important to examine whether these different neurochemical systems mediate dissociable behavioral responses to stressors.

Related to the first of these points, information concerning the specificity of the stress-protective effects of alpha-helical CRF could easily be obtained by comparing the effects of the antagonist on one particular behavioral end point, following various stressors. For example, following the work of Krahn *et al.* (1986), who showed that alpha-helical CRF partially antagonizes the inhibition of feeding produced by restraint stress, it could be examined whether the CRF antagonist also attenuates the inhibition of feeding produced by other stressors, such as footshock, social defeat, cold-water swims, and lithium chloride. This data, if combined with neuroendocrine indices of the severity of the stressors, could then indicate whether CRF is a peptide generally involved in the behavioral responses to all stressors, or whether it has a more specific and less global role. Using a similar approach, a systematic study of whether a CRF antagonist protects against all of the behavioral consequences of a particular stressor could also be performed. In this case, the ability of the CRF antagonist to protect against several different behavioral consequences of one particular stressor could be systematically examined. Such an approach could also be combined with attempts to link the preclinical and clinical studies, by examining the effects of the CRF antagonist on stress induced behavioral effects that have been suggested to mimic the behavioral symptoms of affective disorders (see Anisman and Zacharko, 1982). For example, the ability of the antagonist to protect against the alterations produced in active behavior (Weiss *et al.*, 1982), intracranial self-stimulation (ICSS) (Zacharko *et al.*, 1984), and anxiety (Katz, 1981) induced by exposure to one particular stressor, such as restraint or cold-water swims, would again enable a more systematic examination of the hypothesis that CNS CRF is critically involved in initiating behavioral responses to stressors, and would also potentially provide a link between the preclinical and clinical studies.

References

Aldenhoff, J. B., Gruol, D. L., Rivier, J., Vale, W., and Siggins, G. R. (1983). Corticotropin releasing factor decreases port-burst hyperpolarizations and excites hippocampal pyramidal neurons in vitro. *Science* **221**, 875–876.

Anisman, H., and Zacharko, R. M. (1982). Depression: The predisposing influence of stress. *Behav. Brain Sci.* **5**, 89–137.

Antelman, S. M., Szechtman, H., Chin, P., and Fisher, A. E. (1975). Tail pinch-induced eating, gnawing and licking behavior in rats: Dependence on the nigrostriatal dopamine system. *Brain Res.* **99**, 319–337.

Antelman, S. M., Eichler, A. J., Black, C. A., and Kocan, D. (1980). Interchangeability between stress and amphetamine in sensitization. *Science* **207**, 329–331.

Berlyne, D. E. (1960). "Conflict Arousal and Curiosity." McGraw-Hill, New York.

Berridge, C. W., and Dunn, A. J. (1986). Corticotropin-releasing factor elicits naloxone sensitive stress-like alterations in exploratory behavior in mice. *Regul. Pept.* **16**, 83–93.

Berridge, C. W., and Dunn, A. J. (1987). A corticotropin-releasing factor antagonist reverses the stress-induced changes of exploratory behavior in mice. *Horm. Behav.* **21**, 393–401.

Brett, L. P., and Levine, S. (1979). Schedule-induced polydipsia suppresses pituitary-adrenal activity in rats. *J. Comp. Physiol. Psychol.* **93**, 946–956.

Britton, D. R., and Britton, K. T. (1981). A sensitive open field measure of analytic drug activity. *Pharmacol., Biochem. Behav.* **15**, 577–582.

Britton, D. R., and Indyk, E. (1989). Effects of ganglionic blocking agents on behavioral responses to centrally administered CRF. *Brain Res.* **478**(2), 205–210.

Britton, D. R., Koob, G. F., Rivier, J., and Vale, W. (1982). Intraventricular corticotropin-releasing factor enhances behavioral effects of novelty. *Life Sci.* **31**, 363–367.

Britton, D. R., Varela, M., Garcia, A., and Rivier, J. (1986). Dexamethasone suppresses pituitary-adrenal but not behavioral effects of centrally administered CRF. *Life Sci.* **38**, 211–216.

Britton, K. T., Lee, G., Dana, R., Risch, S. C., and Koob, G. F. (1986). Activating and "anxiogenic" effects of CRF are not inhibited by blockade of the pituitary-adrenal system with dexamethasone. *Life Sci.* **39**, 1281–1286.

Britton, K. T., Lee, G., and Koob, G. F. (1988). Corticotropin releasing factor and amphetamine exaggerate partial agonist properties of benzodiazepine antagonist, RO 15-1788 in the conflict test. *Psychopharmacology (Berlin)* **94**, 306–311.

Brown, M. R., and Fisher, L. A. (1983). Central nervous system effects of corticotropin releasing factor in the dog. *Brain Res.* **280**, 75–79.

Brown, M. R., Fisher, L. A., Spiess, J., Rivier, C., and Vale, W. (1982). Corticotropin-releasing factor: Actions on the sympathetic nervous system and metabolism. *Endocrinology (Baltimore)* **111**, 928.

Butler, P. D., Weiss, J. M., Stout, J. C., Kilts, C. D., Cook, L. L., and Nemeroff, C. B. (1988). Corticotropin-releasing factor produces anxiogentic and behavioral activating effects following microinfusion into the locus coeruleus. *Neurosci. Abstr.* **14**, 288.

Cedarbaum, J. M., and Aghajanian, G. K. (1978). Activation of locus coeruleus neurons by peripheral stimuli: Modulation by collateral inhibitory mechanism. *Life Sci.* **23**, 1383–1392.

Chappell, P. B., Smith, M. A., Hilts, C. D., Bissette, G., Ritchie, J., Andersen, C., and Nemeroff, J. (1986). Alterations in corticotropin-releasing factor-line immunoreactivity in discrete rat brain regions after acute and chronic stress. *J. Neurosci.* **10**, 2908–2916.

Cole, B. J., and Koob, G. F. (1988). Propranolol antagonizes the enhanced conditioned fear produced by corticotropin releasing factor. *J. Pharmacol. Exp. Ther.* **247**, 902–910.

Cole, B. J., Britton, K. T., and Koob, G. F. (1987). Central administration of alpha-helical corticotropin-releasing factor attenuates the acquisition of a conditioned emotional response. *Neurosci. Abstr.* **13**, 427.

Cole, B. J., Cador, M., Stinus, L., Rivier, J. Vale, W., Koob, G. F. and Le Moal, M. (1990). Central administration of a CRF antagonist blocks the development of stress-induced behavioral sensitization. *Brain Res.* **512**, 343–346.

Conner, R., Vernikos-Danellis, J., and Levine, S. (1971). Stress, fighting and neuroendocrine function. *Nature (London)* **234**, 564–566.

Cook, L., and Sepinwall, J. (1975). Behavioral analysis of the effects and mechanism of action of benzodiazepines. *In* "Mechanisms of Action of Benzodiazepines" (E. Costa and P. Greengard, eds.), p. 1. Raven Press, New York.

Corda, M. G., and Biggio, G. (1986). Stress and GABAergic transmission: Biochemical and behavioural studies. *Adv. Biochem. Psychopharmacol.* **41**, 121–136.

Cummings, S., Elde, R., Ells, J., and Lindall, A. (1983). Corticotropin-releasing factor immunoreactivity is widely distributed within the central nervous system of the rat: An immunohistochemical study. *J. Neurosci.* **3**, 1355–1368.

Dantzer, R. (1987). Behavioral analysis of anxiolytic drug action. *In* "Experimental Psychopharmacology" (A. J. Greenshaw and C. T. Dourish, eds.), p. 263. Humana Press, Clifton, New Jersey.

Davis, M. (1980). Neurochemical modulation of sensory-motor reactivity: Acoustic and tactile startle reflexes. *Neurosci. Biobehav. Rev.* **4**, 241–263.

De Souza, E. B. (1987). Corticotropin releasing factor receptors in the rat central nervous system: Characterization and regional distribution. *J. Neurosci.* **7**, 88–100.

De Souza, E. B., Whitehouse, P. J., Kuhar, M. J., Price, D. L., and Vale, W. W. (1986). Reciprocal changes in corticotropin-releasing factor (CRF)-like immunoreactivity and CRF receptors in cerebral cortex of Alzheimer's disease. *Nature (London)* **319**, 593–595.

Dunn, A. J., and Berridge, C. W. (1987). Corticotropin-releasing factor administration elicits a stress-like activation of cerebral catecholaminergic systems. *Pharmacol., Biochem. Behav.* **27**, 685–691.

Eaves, M., Britton, K. T., Rivier, J., Vale, W., and Koob, G. F. (1985). Effects of corticotropin releasing factor on locomotor activity in hypophysectomized rats. *Peptides (N.Y.)* **6**, 923–926.

Fisher, L. A., Rivier, J., Rivier, C., Spiess, J., Vale, W., and Brown, M. (1982). Corticotropin-releasing factor (CRF): Central effects on mean arterial pressure and heart rate in rats. *Endocrinology (Baltimore)* **110**, 2222–2224.

Glavin, G. B. (1985). Stress and brain noradrenaline: A review. *Neurosci. Biobehav. Rev.* **9**, 233–243.

Gold, P. W., Goodwin, F. K., and Chrousos, G. P. (1988a). Clinical and biochemical manifestations of depressions: Relation to the neurobiology of stress (first of two parts). *N. Engl. J. Med.* **319**, 348–353.

Gold, P. W., Goodwin, F. K., and Chrousos, G. P. (1988b). Clinical and biochemical manifestations of depression: Relation to the neurobiology of stress (second of two parts). *N. Engl. J. Med.* **319**, 413–420.

Gosnell, B. A., Morley, J. E., and Levine, A. S. (1983). A comparison of the effects of corticotropin releasing factor and sauvagine on food intake. *Pharmacol., Biochem, Behav.* **19**, 771–775.

Gray, J. A. (1982). "The Neuropsychology of Anxiety." Oxford Univ. Press, London and New York.

Hennessy, M. B., and Foy, T. (1987). Nonedible material elicits chewing and reduces the plasma corticosterone response during novelty exposure in mice. *Behav. Neurosci.* **101**, 237–245.

Holmberg, G., and Gershon, S. (1961). Autonomic and psychiatric effects of yohimbine hydrochloride. *Psychopharmacologia* **2**, 93–106.

Holtzman, S. G., and Finn, I. B. (1988). Tolerance to behavioral effects of caffeine in rats. *Pharmacol., Biochem. Behav.* **29**, 411–418.

Hunt, T., and Amit, Z. (1987). Conditioned taste aversion induced by self-administered drugs: Paradox revisited. *Neurosci. Biobehav. Rev.* **11**(1), 107–130.

Hurwitz, H. M. B., and Davis, H. (1983). The description and analysis of conditioned suppression: A critique of the conventional suppression ratio. *Anim. Learn. Behav.* **11**, 383–390.

Kalin, N. H., Sherman, J. E., and Takahashi, L. K. (1988). Antagonism of endogenous CRH systems attenuates stress-induced freezing behavior in rats. *Brain Res.* **457**, 130–135.

Kalivas, P. W., Latimer, L. G., and Duffy, P. (1987). Behavioral and neurochemical effects of corticotropin-releasing factor in the A10 dopamine region. *J. Pharmacol. Exp. Ther.* **242**, 757–763.

Katz, R. J. (1981). Animal models and human depressive disorders. *Neurosci. Biobehav. Rev.* 5, 231–246.

Kelly, P. H., and Iversen, S. D. (1976). Selective 6-OHDA induced destruction of mesolimbic dopamine neurons: Abolition of psychostimulant induced locomotor activity in rats. *Eur. J. Pharmacol.* 40, 45–56.

Koob, G. F., and Bloom, F. E. (1985). Corticotropin releasing factor and behavior. *Fed. Proc. Fed. Am. Soc. Exp. Biol.* 44, 259–263.

Koob, G. F., Fray, P. J., and Iversen, S. D. (1976). Tail-pinch stimulation: A sufficient motivation for learning. *Science* 194, 637–639.

Koob, G. F., Swerdlow, N., Seeligson, M., Eaves, M., Sutton, R., Rivier, J., and Vale, W. (1984). Effects of alpha-fluphenthixol and naloxone on CRF-induced locomotor activation. *Neuroendocrinology* 39, 459–464.

Koob, G. F., Braestrup, C., and Thatcher-Britton, K. (1986). The effects of FG 7142 and RO 15-1788 on the release of punished responding produced by chlordiazepoxide and ethanol in the rat. *Psychopharmacology (Berlin)* 90, 173–178.

Kornetsky, C., and Esposito, R. U. (1981). Reward and detection thresholds for brain stimulation: Dissociative effects of cocaine. *Brain Res.* 209, 496–500.

Krahn, D. D., Gosnell, B. A., Grace, M., and Levine, A. S. (1986). CRF antagonist partially reverses CRF- and stress-induced effects on feeding. *Brain Res. Bull.* 17, 285–289.

Langer, S. Z. (1981). Presynaptic regulation of the release of catecholamines. *Pharmacol. Rev.* 32, 337–362.

Levine, A. S., Rogers, B., Kneip, J., Grace, M., and Morley, J. E. (1983). Effect of centrally administered corticotropin releasing factor (CRF) on multiple feeding paradigms. *Neuropharmocology* 22, 337–339.

Morley, J. E., and Levine, A. S. (1983). Corticotropin-releasing factor, grooming and ingestive behavior. *Life Sci.* 81, 1459–1464.

Morley, J. E., Kay, N., and Solomon, G. F. (1989). Opioid peptides, stress, and immune function. *In* "Neuropeptides and Stress" (Y. Tache, J. E. Morley, and M. R. Brown eds.), p. 222. Springer-Verlag, Berlin and New York.

Redmond, D. E., Jr., and Huang, Y. H. (1979). Current concepts. 2. New evidence for a locus ceruleus-norepinephrine connection with anxiety. *Life Sci.* 25, 2149–2162.

Rivier, J., Rivier, C., and Vale, W. (1984). Synthetic competitive antagonists of corticotropin-releasing factor: Effect on ACTH secretion in the rat. *Science* 224, 889–891.

Robbins, T. W., and Fray, P. J. (1980). Stress-induced eating: Fact, fiction or misunderstanding. *Appetite* 1, 103–133.

Robbins, T. W., and Koob, G. F. (1980). Selective disruption of displacement behavior by lesions of the mesolimbic dopamine system. *Nature (London)* 285, 409–412.

Robinson, T. E., and Becker, J. B. (1986). Enduring changes in brain and behavior produced by chronic amphetamine administration: A review and evaluation of animal models of amphetamine psychosis. *Brain Res. Rev.* 11, 157–198.

Schachter, S., and Singer, J. E. (1962). Cognitive, social and psysiological determinants of emotional state. *Psychol. Rev.* 69, 379–399.

Segal, D. S., Browne, R. G., Arnsten, A., Derrington, D. C., Bloom, F. E., Guillemin, R., and Ling, N. (1979). Characteristics of β-endorphin-induced behavioral activation and immobilization. *In* "Endorphins in Mental Health Research" (E. Usdin, W. E. Bunney, and N. S. Kline, eds.), p. 307. Macmillan, London.

Siggins, G. R., Gruol, D., Aldenhoff, J., and Pittman, Q. (1985). Electrophysiological actions of corticotropin-releasing factor in the central nervous system. *Fed. Proc., Fed. Am. Soc. Exp. Biol.* 44, 237–242.

Smith, M. A., Bissette, G., Slotkin, T. A., Knight, D. L., and Nemeroff, C. B. (1986). Release of corticotropin-releasing factor from rat brain regions in vitro. *Endocrinology (Baltimore)* **118**, 1997–2001.

Sutton, R. E., Koob, G. F., Le Moal, M., Rivier, J., and Vale, W. (1982). Corticotropin releasing factor (CRF) produces behavioral activation in rats. *Nature (London)* **297**, 331–333.

Swanson, L. W., Sawchenko, P. E., Rivier, J., and Vale, W. (1983). The organization of ovine corticotropin releasing factor (CRF) immunoreactive cells and fibres in the rat brain: Immunohistochemical study. *Neuroendocrinology* **36**, 165–186.

Swerdlow, N. R., and Koob, G. F. (1985). Separate neural substrates of the locomotor-activating properties of amphetamine, caffeine and corticotropin releasing factor (CRF) in the rat. *Pharmacol., Biochem. Behav.* **23**, 303–307.

Swerdlow, N. R., Geyer, M. A., Vale, W. W., and Koob, G. F. (1986). Corticotropin releasing factor potentiates acoustic startle in rats: Blockade by chlordiazepoxide. *Psychopharmacology (Berlin)* **88**, 142–152.

Swerdlow, N. R., Britton, K. T., and Koob G. F. (1989). Potentiation of acoustic startle by corticotropin-releasing factor (CRF) and by fear are both reversed by alpha-helical CRF. *Neuropsychopharmacology* **2**, 285–292.

Swerdlow, N. R., Gilbert, O., and Koob, G. F. (1989). Conditioned drug effects on spatial preference: critical evaluation *In:* Neuromethods: vol 13, psychopharmacology I. (A. A. Boulton, G. B. Baker, and A. J. Greenshaw, eds), p. 399. Humana Press, Clifton, New Jersey.

Takahashi, L. K., Kalin, N. H., Vandenburgt, J. A., and Sherman, J. E. (1989). Corticotropin-releasing factor blocks defensive withdrawal and reverses inhibition associated with a novel environment. *Behav. Neurosci.* **103**, 648–654.

Tazi, A., Dantzer, R., Le Moal, M., Rivier, J., Vale, W., and Koob, G. F. (1987a). Corticotropin releasing factor antagonist blocks stress-induced fighting in rats. *Regul. Pept.* **18**, 37–42.

Tazi, A., Swerdlow, N. R., Le Moal, M., Rivier, J., Vale, W., and Koob, G. F. (1987b). Behavioral activation of CRF: Evidence for the involvement of the ventral forebrain. *Life Sci.* **41**, 41–50.

Thatcher-Britton, K., Morgan, J., Rivier, J., Vale, W., and Koob, G. F. (1985). Chlordiazepoxide attenuates CRF-induced responses suppression in the conflict test. *Psychopharmacology (Berlin)* **86**, 170–174.

Thatcher-Britton, K., Lee, G., Vale, W., Rivier, J., and Koob, G. F. (1986). Corticotropin releasing factor antagonists blocks activating and "anxiogenic" actions of CRF in the rat. *Brain Res.* **369**, 303–306.

Trullas, R., Havoundjian, H., and Skolnick, P. (1988). Is the benzodiazepine/GABA receptor chloride ionophore complex involved in physical and emotional stress. *Adv. Exp. Med. Biol.* **245**, 183–200.

Vale, W., Spiess, J., Rivier, C., and Rivier, J. (1981). Characterization of a 41 residue ovine hypothalamic peptide that stimulates the secretion of corticotropin and beta-endorphin. *Science* **213**, 1394–1397.

Valentino, R. J., and Wehby, R. G. (1988). Corticotropin-releasing factor: Evidence for a neurotransmitter role in the locus ceruleus during hemodynamic stress. *Neuroendocrinology* **48**(6), 674–677.

Valentino, R. J., Foote, S. L., and Aston-Jones, G. (1983). Corticotropin-releasing factor activates noradrenergic neurons of the locus coeruleus. *Brain Res.* **270**, 363–367.

Valentino, R. J., Martin, D. L., and Suzuki, M. (1986). Dissociation of locus coeruleus activity and blood pressure: Effects of clonidine and corticotropin-releasing factor. *Neurophar-macology* 25, 603–610.

Weiss, J. M., Bailey, W. H., Goodman, P. A., Hoffman, L. J., Ambrose, M. J., Salman, S., and Charry, J. M. (1982). A model for neurochemical study of depression. *In* "Behavioral Models and the Analysis of Drug Action" (M. Y. Spiegelstein and A. Levy, eds.), p. 195. Elsevier, Amsterdam.

Zacharko, R. M., Bowers, W. J., Kelley, M. S., and Anisman, H. (1984). Prevention of stressor-induced disturbances of self-stimulation by desmethyl imipramine. *Brain Res.* 321, 175–179.

8

Methods of Measuring Neuropeptides and Their Metabolism

Thomas P. Davis

Laboratory of Analytical Chemistry and Mass Spectrometry
Department of Pharmacology
College of Medicine
University of Arizona
Tucson, Arizona 85724

I. Introduction

The number of neuropeptides whose presence has been demonstrated or inferred in neurons and nerve terminals of the mammalian nervous system has grown substantially in the past decade. A major factor that stimulated this large growth in neuropeptide research was the development of highly sensitive techniques to measure/detect these important molecules. This chapter will review the development of these techniques and their application to the measurement of neuropeptides and their metabolism.

One of the first detection techniques to be applied to the measurement of peptides was radioimmunoassay. Radioimmunoassays for measuring peptide hormone levels in tissue extracts and in blood contributed significantly to our understanding of hormonal control mechanisms in the central nervous system and periphery. However, as with most analytical methods, there was a need for modification and improvement, particularly in the area of specificity. Since it was known that antisera could cross-react with several biologically active molecules, it was necessary to develop high-resolution chromatographic separation techniques that would complement the inherent sensitivity of radioimmunoassay detection.

Chromatographic techniques have been available for over 75 years, but the application to the separation of neuropeptides has been a recent development (Burgus and Rivier, 1976; Fledman et al., 1978; Regnier and Gooding, 1980; Davis et al., 1982). Initial studies addressing the separation of neuropeptides used ion-exchange materials because most of the classical amino acid analyses had used ion-exchange chromatography (Spackman et al., 1960). Although efforts were made to advance gas chromatography for the analysis of small peptides (Lakings and Gehrke, 1971), the preeminent chromatographic technique available until 1970 was ion-exchange chromatography. Commercial high-performance liquid chromatography (HPLC) instruments made their debut from 1970 to 1975, and the use of HPLC increased to the point where instruments are now commonplace in most neuroscience research laboratories. If one were to trace the development of neuropeptide research and high-performance liquid chromatographic techniques one would observe a parallelism that is not a coincidence. Since neuropeptides are biologically active at the picogram to nanogram level and amino acid sequences are quite conserved, it is critical to employ a selective, high-resolution technique to separate the molecules prior to detection. Reversed-phase HPLC techniques offer the unique aspect of being nondestructive, high-resolution, analytical tools. Any chromatographically separated peptide can be isolated, collected, and characterized for biological testing. This technique is uniquely appropriate for the biological scientist (Robinson, 1979).

As further advancements are made in neuropeptide research, analysts must continue to improve the specificity and sensitivity of analytical procedures. Since HPLC is a separation technique, it remains dependent on specific detectors with adequate sensitivity to detect very low levels of neuropeptides. The most sensitive and specific detection technique used in analytical chemistry has been mass spectrometry. However, the use of mass spectrometry (MS) for routine peptide analysis has been limited (Cooks et al., 1983). Liquid chromatography interfaces for the mass spectrometer have been a welcome addition, and several studies describing detection of neuropeptides in biological matrices have been published. Most of these applications are used in only a few laboratories, and much work is still ongoing in the area of liquid chromatography/mass spectrometry (LC/MS) analysis of neuropeptides (Worthy, 1983).

If the past 10 years was the decade of high-performance liquid chromatography, then the next 10 years may very well be the decade of capillary electrophoresis of neuropeptides. Electrophoresis has been used for several decades for analyzing proteins, but its application to the separation of neuropeptides has been limited to only a few studies. However, with the onset of capillary zone electrophoresis, the ability to separate and detect picogram to nanogram levels is now possible. While the high-resolution capabilities of HPLC are advantageous, the instrumentation is still quite expensive, and capillary zone electrophoresis may very well be a technique which laboratories will investigate.

Since analytical techniques are only of value to the neuroscientist if they can be applied to biological/biochemical problems, this chapter will conclude with a discussion of peptide metabolism where high-resolution separations are a requirement. It is well documented that the process of peptide metabolism is not merely a catabolic event leading to peptide inactivation, but a process that can lead to biologically active fragments. The potential number of fragments that can be formed from a given neuropeptide is dependent on the number of susceptible amino acid bonds in the sequence. Therefore, any analytical technique used must be capable of high-resolution separation. High-performance liquid chromatography offers the required high resolution and is the technique of choice for studies of peptide metabolism and processing. By combining high-resolution separation techniques with "state-of-the-art" detection, the peptide researcher is now able to describe the fate of many biologically active peptides.

II. Chromatographic Methods

A. High-Performance Liquid Chromatography

1. Separation Conditions

The effect of mobile-phase conditions (i.e., buffers) on liquid chromatographic separations of peptides has been under study for over a decade. Beginning with the early work of Hancock and Bishop (1976) where select peptides were analyzed underivatized after elution in methanol and water on C18-corasil and phenyl-corasil columns, it was shown that as low as 0.25–10.0 ng of peptide could be detected at 212–218 nm. While the resultant elution profiles were not particularly high resolution, this was one of the first demonstrations that underivatized peptides could be analyzed in a rapid fashion with very sensitive detection.

Since the bonded phase used in HPLC is itself a hydrophobic surface and despite secondary derivatization or end-capping procedures used by manufacturers to ensure maximal coverage, there are sufficient active silanol groups remaining to provide a surface to which peptides may adsorb. This adsorption can result in variable peptide recovery problems, long retention times, poor peak symmetry, and poor reproducibility of retention times. Adding an ionic component to the mobile phase (which is frequently an acid) acts to "salt out" silanol groups and does decrease adsorption, leading to improved resolution and separation. There are numerous ionic buffers that can be used, such as sodium dihydrogen phosphate, phosphoric acid, trifluoroacetic acid, triethylamine, and ammonium phosphate, but most laboratories adopt only one or two. The first of these is trialkyl ammonium phosphate (TAAP), which was reviewed by Rivier (1978) in a study on several neuropeptides using a variety of different analytical columns. The TAAP buffer system is compatible with reversed-phase HPLC packing materials and will yield high recoveries. Another advantage to using phosphate-based buffers is that the ultraviolet (UV) transparency is very good at peptide bond wavelengths. The only noticeable problem with this buffer is peak resolution. A complex separation of 20–30 similar peptides may be difficult using TAAP. The second buffer used by many laboratories is trifluoroacetate in the form of trifluoroacetic acid (Acharya et al., 1983). The advantage of trifluoroacetic acid is that it can be lyophilized from the peptide mixture and does not interfere with amino acid analysis, but it does suffer from very high background at 200–220 nm. Many of these UV-absorbing contaminants cannot be redistilled off. The relative effectiveness of trifluoroacetic acid and other perfluoronated carboxylic acids in the HPLC analysis of peptides was described by Bennett et al. (1980) on 12 standard peptides and proteins loaded onto several reversed-phase HPLC columns. These peptides were subjected to linear gradients of acetonitrile with each perfluoronated carboxylic acid. The retention times of peptide standards were different in each solvent system tested and progressed from trifluoroacetic acid to pentafluoropropanoic acid to heptafluorobutyric acid and then to undecafluorocaproic acid where all the peptides showed a greater retention time. This type of selectivity of mobile-phase counterion is not unusual and has been commented on by several authors in the literature (Molnar and Horvath, 1977; Rivier, 1978; Meek, 1980; Regnier and Gooding, 1980; Wilson et al., 1981; Davis and Culling-Berglund, 1985). This detailed and methodological approach to studies of perfluoronated carboxylic acids provides an excellent review on the effect of adding ionic components to the HPLC solvent system.

The peptide literature is replete with methods utilizing trifluoroacetic acid and TAAP buffers in the separation of neuropeptides with few laboratories utilizing sodium dihydrogen phosphate acidified with phosphoric acid. The author's laboratory is one of the few that uses sodium dihydrogen phosphate in the separation of neuropeptides ranging from Met-enkephalin to epidermal growth factor (Davis *et al.*, 1982, 1983, 1985, 1986, 1987, 1989). The advantage of dihydrogen phosphate is the low inherent absorbance at 200–220 nm and the predictability of elution times (i.e., retention time) when using amino acid hydrophobicity parameters (Molnar and Horvath, 1977; Meek, 1980; Wilson *et al.*, 1981). However, each peptide contributes its own unique hydrophobic and secondary structure characteristics to a separation, and the selection of the appropriate mobile phase must be made carefully. An excellent review on the subject of peptide solvent and column interaction was presented by Regnier and Gooding (1980) where the separation of a large series of peptides and proteins was presented in various mobile phases across several solid supports. This study demonstrates that a large number of factors determine a good separation and that all answers to the complex chemistry of separation are not known.

The driving force of any neuropeptide separation is the hydrophobicity of the peptide. Since the reversed-phase columns are hydrophobic supports it is not surprising that the separation would depend on hydrophobic interaction. Estimates of hydrophobicity based on octanol/water partition coefficients exist for many, but not all, of the amino acids (Molnar and Horvath, 1977). Therefore, if one were able to determine the retention coefficient of each amino acid on a particular reversed-phase column, one should be able to predict peptide retention. In a study by Meek (1980), the retention times of 20 different peptides were measured on a Lichrosorb RP-18 column using both fluorescence and absorbance detection. When these measured retention times were compared to predicted retention times quantitated from retention coefficients, the errors were small, yielding a correlation of 0.9996. This work was accomplished using a gradient of acetonitrile and perchlorate. It may not be predictable for all peptides, but it does provide interesting and valuable data for developing peptide separations.

While chromatographic retention is strongly dependent on hydrophobic interaction with the solid support, it is also determined by a relatively small number of amino acids located in the chromatographic contact region on the surface of the peptide (Regnier and Gooding, 1980). This may be why it is not always possible to predict the retention time of a given peptide based on hydrophobicity constants, as the number of amino acids binding to the "active site" of the versed-phase column varies. Furthermore, secondary structural changes in the peptide can occur in the mobile phase that contribute to variations in the chromatographic contact region. In summary, chromatographic retention time is not only based on hydrophobicity, but also on the secondary structure of the peptide in the buffer of the mobile phase (Wilson *et al.*, 1981; Regnier, 1987).

When describing the potential for conformational change and the effect this has on chromatographic behavior it is tempting to correlate this interaction to what occurs on a membrane receptor. Whether the receptor is part of a proteolytic enzyme or a postsynaptic neuron, the correlation of chromatographic behavior with membrane receptor binding is intriguing. As we attempt to develop models for studying the interaction of peptide drugs with surface properties associated with biological membranes, HPLC solid-support studies may prove valuable. Similar studies on the interaction of nonpeptide drugs have shown that the hydrophobic characteristics of solid supports provide good models for drug/membrane interaction (Crommen, 1979).

2. Detection

The primary method of detection for peptides is absorbance (ultraviolet detection) of either the peptide bond or aromatic amino acids. In 1951, Goldfarb et al. determined that peptides absorb light in the vicinity of 190 nm. Due to interferences in light absorption by commonly used solvents, no use of this wavelength was made. Since 191–194 nm is characteristic of the peptide bond, several manufacturers of organic solvents for liquid chromatographic analyses altered their distillation techniques to produce high-purity solvents that lacked significant levels of U.V. absorbable materials. The most significant analytical advantage of using lower wavelengths for peptide analysis is improved sensitivity. There is approximately 40- to 80-fold more sensitivity at 200–210 nm than in analyses performed at 280 nm. When utilizing wavelengths at or near the absorption maxima of the peptide bond, the specific absorbance values of different peptides vary much less than absorbance at 280 nm. In many cases absorbance at 190–210 nm is quite predictable for a given peptide because it is based on the number of peptide bonds in a given neuropeptide (Mayer and Miller, 1970).

The classic derivatization reagents used for fluorescence detection of peptides have been o-phthalaldehyde and fluorescamine (Joys and Kim, 1979). o-Phthaladehyde was first used with precolumn derivitization to measure biogenic amines (Davis et al., 1978). The advantage of using fluorescence detection of peptides is that sensitivity is enhanced over ultraviolet detection (Rubinstein et al., 1979). A disadvantage of fluorescence detection is that many biological materials other than the desired analyte will also fluoresce. When derivatizing postcolumn with either o-phthalaldehyde or fluorescamine one must be aware of the potential for increased background due to derivatization of all primary amines eluting from the HPLC column. However, if the researcher is studying a purified mixture of peptides, fluorescence techniques are ideal for sensitive detection (Frei et al., 1976; Schiltz et al., 1977).

A third detection technique that has been applied to the measurement of neuropeptides is electrochemical detection. Electrochemical detection (EC) takes advantage of the oxidation of amino acids in the peptide sequence after HPLC separation. Electrochemical detection has evolved as a simple and reliable technique for the determination of classical neurotransmitters such as catecholamines (Kissinger *et al.*, 1973, 1975) but has not been as predictable for measuring neuropeptides (Mousa and Couri, 1983; Bennett *et al.*, 1986; Fleming and Reynolds, 1986). While the technique is applicable to low-level determinations of low-molecular-weight peptides (where good oxidation potentials can be reached) it suffers from baseline instability, a need for high oxidation potentials if the peptide has significant secondary structure, and a requirement for extensive sample cleanup. Since the EC detector is not specific (due to oxidation of many molecules), one should confirm the identity of the analyte using another technique. Detectors have been recently designed that are not as sensitive to laboratory electrical interferences, but most EC detectors remain sensitive to gradient changes in mobile-phase organic solvents where electronic background induced by these changes can obscure the analyte signal (Mousa and Couri, 1983). Advances in analyte chemistry including derivatization with *o*-phthaladehyde followed by EC/LC are forthcoming. These advances will enhance sensitivity while improving the signal to noise ratio of the analyte.

3. Radioimmunoassay/HPLC

As stated earlier, radioimmunoassay techniques have added significantly to the advancement of neuropeptide biology. By coupling radioimmunoassay (RIA) with HPLC, major developments in the area of peptide quantitation and metabolism have occurred. Rossier *et al.* (1977) describe what occurs when there is significant cross reactivity of antisera for Leu-enkephalin and Met-enkephalin. To avoid misleading the reader, the authors found it necessary to express the results of the RIA in terms of an "arbitrary enkephalin unit" since they did not utilize a high-resolution chromatographic technique to separate the enkephalins prior to RIA. By combining high-performance liquid chromatography and radioimmunoassay (HPLC/RIA) one can develop a powerful tool for measuring several structurally similar neuropeptides in a single biological sample. By applying the technique to a study of several endorphins, Loeber *et al.* (1979) provided evidence that there is a specific regional distribution in the brain. This was accomplished by using an antisera that cross-reacted significantly with a large number of peptide fragments. By combining the antisera with a selective HPLC separation, the authors were able to measure each peptide separately. Further applications of combining RIA of enkephalins with octadecasilyl (C-18) separations of cerebral spinal fluid (CSF) samples provided evidence that the level of Met-enkephalin in CSF was three to four times lower than that found in human plasma and that CSF Met-enkephalin was not of pituitary origin nor a breakdown product of β-endorphin (Clement-Jones *et al.*, 1980). By using reversed-phase HPLC/RIA, researchers were also able to describe several variables associated with neuropeptide measurement including the effect of oxidation and enzymatic proteolysis during sample preparation (Buck *et al.*, 1983). If RIA is not used in conjunction with a selective chromatographic technique, the problems of cross-reactivity complicate the results and conclusions of the experiment. In the case of substance P, several peptide fragments, including fragments of substance P, physalaemin, and eledoisin, showed significant cross-reactivity. Upon analysis of dorsal root ganglia and spinal cord, as high as 200–1500 pg of substance P oxide was detected by HPLC/RIA (Buck *et al.*, 1983). This would have been missed without the use of HPLC. The process of RIA validation has also been used by several investigators to determine if tissue samples in question contain more than one immunoreactive species of peptide (Akil *et al.*, 1981; Vuolteenaho *et al.*, 1981; Weber *et al.*, 1982; Boarder *et al.*, 1983; Brinton *et al.*, 1983; Yang *et al.*, 1983).

When subjecting samples to reversed-phase HPLC for isolating specific neuropeptides for RIA detection, one must be aware of the extraction efficiencies and recovery of the original peptide mass (Bennett *et al.*, 1978; Jessop *et al.*, 1987). This is an important quality control procedure in the laboratory (Kirschbaum *et al.*, 1984). If the analyst does not use a chromatographic isolation procedure with RIA it is possible that the complete sequence of the peptide is not being measured due to enzymatic proteolysis. This can be checked by adding intact peptide at the beginning of the experiment and measuring recovery by HPLC at different stages of sample extraction. If this is not done then the analyst may be measuring a variable percent of endogenous peptide and not the intact peptide mass (Davis and Culling-Berglund, 1985).

III. Mass Spectrometric Methods

Mass spectrometry (MS) analysis of neuropeptides began with sequencing permethylated peptides after their separation in a gas–liquid chromatograph (GC) coupled to a mass spectrometer (GC/MS) (Priddle *et al.*, 1976). Since MS is inherently the most specific procedure for the analysis of any organic chemical, it is not surprising that both the electron impact (EI) and chemical ionization (CI) modes were used to obtain fragmentation patterns from which the amino acid sequences of the permethylated peptides were deduced. The gas chromatography of high-molecular-weight peptides as opposed to derivatives of di- and tripeptides has received little attention. This has been due to the need for derivatization of side-chain polar groups followed by separation on GC columns. Since early mass spectrometers were limited to a 1000 atomic mass unit (amu) span, most of the peptides analyzed were less than 1000 molecular weight. However, sequence analysis of peptides was routinely available in mid 1970s (Engelfried and Koenig, 1976; Ling et al., 1976; Priddle et al., 1976). Working with underivatized peptides related to substance P, Anderson et al. (1977) obtained conventional EI spectra using sample vaporization from a tungsten wire, the technique of rapid heating, proton transfer ionization using ammonia, and photoplate recording of the spectra. Characteristic sequence ions of hexapeptide amides and heptapeptide amides were also possible. Surprising was the lack of complexity in the spectra resulting from losses of small molecules that are typically observed in underivatized spectra.

The rapid development of field desorption mass spectrometry (FD/MS) where mass spectra of polar compounds of very low volatility can be analyzed, has led to sequencing of several neuropeptides (Desiderio et al., 1980). The limitation of FD/MS has been in the area of peptides with a molecular weight greater than 1000. Since FD/MS will permit direct analysis of peptides with relatively few ions formed, the analyst can enhance sensitivity through the application of selective ion monitoring in the EI mode (Frick et al., 1977). In the CI mode 45 different peptides between two and five residues long were measured using isobutane FD/MS. Although the peptides were derivatized at the 10-nM level, sequence information from the CI spectra was relatively clean (Mudgett et al., 1977).

The development of liquid chromatography coupled to mass spectrometry (LC/MS) is recent, due to inherent problems with volatility of peptides. By using a moving belt interface where the organic solvent is vaporized prior to entering the MS source, HPLC effluent can be analyzed in a routine manner. However, the moving belt does provide problems with build-up of mobile-phase contaminants. By using microbore columns the amount of organic solvent necessary to be vaporized is limited and the spectra are quite clean, leading to unambiguous peptide sequencing (Cooks et al., 1983; Worthy, 1983). Since MS is a detection technique and liquid chromatography is a separation technique, a combination of these two "state-of-the-art" procedures can lead to excellent sensitivity and accuracy (Desiderio et al., 1980). The development of tandem mass spectrometry (MS-MS) has enabled the analyst to enhance the dynamic range of MS analysis to 3000 amu. Since many peptides are less than 3000 amu, peptide sequencing by MS-MS is an excellent approach (Cooks et al., 1983). The most recent development of LC/MS interfacing is thermospray liquid chromatography. The thermospray LC/MS interface can tolerate liquid solutions flowing at rates of up to 2 ml/min and therefore does not require the use of microbore columns. The entire eluent stream from the column can be delivered into the MS ion source without splitting and losing detection sensitivity (Pilosof et al., 1984).

Another "soft analysis" technique developed for MS was fast atom bombardment mass spectrometry (FAB/MS). FAB/MS compliments other soft ionization techniques such as CI/MS and FD/MS fragmenting underivatized peptides to all sequential amino acids. Using free peptides in the 1–10 mg level, positive ion FAB/MS spectra of peptides of met-enkephalin and leu-enkephalin out to 16 amino acid sequences such as alpha-endorphin have been described (Morris and Panico, 1981). Further studies on dynorphin 1–8 in human placenta have also been published, showing human placenta villus tissue to contain both opioid receptors and peptides. These dynorphin peptides were extracted from the villus tissue and fractionated using reversed-phase HPLC followed by FAB/MS (Ahmed et al., 1987). Using a double-focusing, forward-geometry mass spectrometer with an FAB source, the peptide solutions were deposited on the FAB probe tip, the methanol was evaporated, and several hundred nanoliters of glycerol were added as a polar matrix. This resulted in excellent sensitivity and resolution of each characteristic amino acid from the octapeptide.

FAB/MS also complements the neuroscience laboratory in providing confirmation of neuropeptide structure and sequence after solid-phase synthesis and HPLC separation (Davis et al., 1989). Additionally, FAB/MS for the identification of unknown peptides from protein digests is a powerful technique. The ability to analyze protein digests by following radiolabeled oxygen throughout the separation permitted assignment of C-terminal peptides. This was important for experiments related to the metabolism of insulin produced by expression of recombinant DNA procedures (Rose et al., 1988).

In summary, developments in the area of mass spectrometry for the analysis of neuropeptides have been as significant as developments in HPLC. With the onset of "soft ionization" techniques such as fast atom bombardment and field desorption, the analysis of neuropeptides from 400 to 3000 amu is now possible. By combining high-resolution capabilities of liquid chromatography with a thermospray interface (Pilosof et al., 1984) researchers can sequence unknown peptides from proteolytic digests and determine biosynthetic mechanisms (May et al., 1982). While the instrumentation is quite costly and sophisticated, the potential for important advances in the neurosciences is without limit (Cooks et al., 1983; Cody et al., 1985).

IV. Capillary Electrophoresis

Electrophoresis has been an efficient method to separate proteins for many years. The use of capillaries in electrophoresis has led to high-resolution separations that can produce less current than wider tubes (for a given mobile phase), whereby temperature control is more efficient (Guzman *et al.*, 1989). By combining capillary electrophoretic separations with UV or fluorescence detection, enhancements in sensitivity have been impressive. Separations of myoglobin ranging from molecular weight 2500 to 17,000 have been accomplished in a relatively short period of time using capillary electrophoretic procedures (Cohen and Karger, 1987). Peptides from two to three amino acid residues up to 51 amino acids (insulin) can also be analyzed by capillary electrophoresis (Firestone *et al.*, 1987; Nielsen *et al.*, 1989). Although it is a destructive technique, capillary zone electrophoresis enables the analyst to separate trace levels of peptides ranging from 200 to proteins of 17,000 molecular weight. This wide dynamic range is not possible with single-column reversed-phase HPLC. Capillary zone electrophoresis can also be applied to large mixtures of peptides and proteins, thus providing an important analytical tool for the study of peptide biochemistry (Grossman *et al.*, 1989). It must be emphasized that the analysis is still dependent on the sensitivity of the detector after the separation. In this area, several detectors have been developed for capillary electrophoresis, including mass spectrometry (Smith *et al.*, 1988; Lee *et al.*, 1988). The electrospray ionization interface mass spectra of leu-enkephalin and vasotocin obtained by continuous electromigration are very impressive when the analyst realizes the detection capabilities are in the femtomole range (Smith *et al.*, 1988). Further application of capillary zone electrophoresis/mass spectrometry and capillary zone electrophoresis/tandem mass spectrometry with ionization at atmospheric pressure for the analysis of dynorphin peptides has also been accomplished (Lee *et al.*, 1988). Since capillary zone electrophoresis applications to neuropeptides are a very recent development, the technique offers future promise for studies of peptide metabolism/processing where the structure of the fragments is unknown and the need for sequence information is critical. With the development of automated instrumentation for analytical capillary electrophoresis the potential for routine peptide metabolism experiments being carried out with electrophoretic separations and mass spectrometry or fluorescence detection is promising (Brownlee and Compton, 1988).

Most of the capillary electrophoresis studies in the literature have concentrated on very few peptides from pure sources (i.e., standards), leaving the question of biological matrix interferences open. However, the separation of complex mixtures of peptides by capillary electrophoresis in a manner of seconds with ultraviolet or fluorescence detection is very appealing and may have a role in the routine laboratory if the sample matrix effects are not prohibitive. When one compares the enhanced sensitivity of capillary electrophoresis (20- to 100-fold over HPLC), it may be possible to measure peptide release from neuronal cultures by this technique (McCormick, 1988). As a powerful analytical technique, which is characterized by high efficiency and tremendous sensitivity, high-performance capillary electrophoresis may even replace RIA (Firestone *et al.*, 1987; Grossman *et al.*, 1988, 1989; Guzman *et al.*, 1989). Capillary electrophoretic instrumentation is still in its infancy, and the ideal instrument should provide predictable and reproducible results with excellent sensitivity. The analyst can look forward to advances in instrumentation so that the practice of capillary electrophoresis will become routine in the biochemical laboratory.

V. Application to Measurements of Neuropeptide Metabolism

A. Tissue Homogenates

The largest number of studies of neuropeptide metabolism has occurred since the discovery of enkephalins in 1975 (Hughes *et al.*, 1975). Most of the initial studies described the susceptibility of the Tyr–Gly bond of met-enkephalin to cleavage by aminopeptidases (Turner *et al.*, 1987). Brain homogenates rapidly hydrolyze the Tyr–Gly bond, with most of the aminopeptidase activity localized in the cytosolic fraction, which is only expressed in tissue homogenates when the cells are lysed. When Pert *et al.* (1976) described that the replacement of the glycyl residue by D-alanine (in position two of met-enkephalin) led to a long-acting analgesic it was obvious that aminopeptidases were important to enkephalin metabolism. Much later the membrane-bound form of the enzyme was shown to be aminopeptidase N and was found to be very important for enkephalin degradation (Matsas *et al.*, 1984). It also became obvious that there was cleavage at the Gly–Phe bond in perfused rat brain (Craves *et al.*, 1978) and mouse striatal membranes (Malfroy *et al.*, 1978). The assumption that this enzyme is unique and specific to enkephalin was based on the study of enkephalin only and lead to the problematic/confusing terminology "enkephalinase." This term has recently been shown to be erroneous in several articles because the enzyme is not specific (Schwartz *et al.*, 1981; Schwartz, 1983; Turner *et al.*, 1985; Hersh, 1985; McKelvy and Blumberg, 1986). The actual enzyme found to be responsible for endopeptidase cleavage of met-enkephalin at the Gly–Phe bond was neutral endopeptidase 3.4.24.11. It was only after misidentification of this enzyme as peptidyl dipeptidase A that the correct enzyme was found to be 3.4.24.11.

Endopeptidase 3.4.24.11 is primarily membrane bound, cleaves peptides at the amino side of hydrophobic amino acids, has preference for peptide substrates with a free COOH-terminal carboxyl group, has a pH optimum of 7.0–8.8, and is inhibited by phosphoramidon ($k_i = 3.4 \times 10^{-9}M$). Several groups have shown that hydrolysis of enkephalin by synaptic membranes can be inhibited by nanomolar levels of phosphoramidon, and reversed-phase HPLC was used to characterize the site of enzymatic cleavage. The conclusion that this new enkephalinase was synaptic membrane bound has led to many studies addressing the role E.C. 3.4.24.11 plays in regulating metabolism/degradation at the synaptic membrane of several biologically active peptides (Matsas et al., 1983; Turner et al., 1985, 1987, 1989; Hooper et al., 1985; Barnes et al., 1988; Bunnett et al., 1988a,b).

Together with studies on the metabolism of enkephalin using whole-brain homogenates, Marks et al. (1974) studied peptide hydrolases in rat hypothalamus and pituitary homogenates using reversed-phase HPLC. They provided evidence that rat brain homogenates contain a broad spectrum of enzymes capable of cleaving a variety of neuropeptides. This original work was followed by studies on somatostatin that described the probable enzymatic cleavage sites of somatostatin 14 by crude, rat brain homogenates (Marks and Stern, 1975). By forming rat brain homogenate extracts, several nonspecific enzymes were liberated that could act on many of the amino acid bonds in the somatostatin sequence. Furthermore, the "neutral endopeptidase" cleavage of somatostatin was similar to what the authors had found earlier for bradykinin, luteinizing hormone releasing hormone (LHRH), and substance P using HPLC procedures. This was the first study describing the cleavage of somatostatin (at several peptide bonds) by rat brain homogenates leading to a partial characterization of the enzymes involved. The same authors (Marks et al., 1976) described the correlation between the biological potency and the degradation of somatostatin. After testing somatostatin and a D-Trp analogue in rat brain homogenates, the authors described the potential of developing peptide analogues of somatostatin that are less rapidly inactivated. It is interesting to note that the hypothesis that somatostatin biological activity can be correlated with a change in biodegradation was active several years ago (Brown et al., 1976; Marks et al., 1976).

Studies on the central metabolism of enkephalins and endorphins continued with the observation that peptide fragments formed after the degradation of β-endorphin (β-E 1-31) were themselves biologically active (Guillemin et al., 1977; de Wied, 1978). These endorphin fragments, termed alpha-(β-E 1-16) and gamma-(β-E 1-17) endorphin, were formed by endopeptidase cleavage at the Leu–Phe bond (Burbach *et al.*, 1979, 1981, 1984; Burbach and de Kloet, 1982). Additional cleavage of endorphin by brain aminopeptidase activity leading to the formation of des-tyrosine endorphins was described by Hersh *et al.* (1980). These studies provided evidence that enzymatic metabolism of neuropeptides in brain homogenates could lead to the deactivation of the parent peptide and the formation of biologically active fragments. Further studies on the metabolism of des-tyrosine-gamma-endorphin (β-E (2-17); DTτE) in rat brain homogenates showed that the major metabolite formed was β-endorphin-6-17 (des-enkephalin-τ-endorphin; DEτE). This observation was made possible by the development of improved reversed-phase HPLC methods, which could separate the fragments formed from the incubation of DTτE with rat brain homogenates (Schoemaker *et al.*, 1982a,b). However, neurotransmitter receptor binding experiments showed that DEτE was inactive at central dopaminergic, serotonergic, muscarinic, benzodiazepine, and opiate receptors measured *in vitro*. Therefore, like DTτE, DEτE differs from classical neuroleptics in that it does not inhibit *in vitro* spiperon binding in the corpus striatum, frontal cortex, or mesolimbic areas of the rat brain (Schoemaker *et al.*, 1982b).

A comprehensive review describing the action of proteolytic enzymes on various lipotropins and endorphins was published by Burbach (1984). This review describes the pharmacokinetics of β-endorphin, including half-life in various tissues and biological fluids using HPLC/RIA methodology. Additional reviews on the specificity of neuropeptide peptidases have described several enzymes that act on specific amino acid sites (Schwartz *et al.*, 1981; Checler *et al.*, 1982; Matsas *et al.*, 1983; Schwartz, 1983; Turner *et al.*, 1985, 1987, 1989). These studies have generally focused on one or more specific peptides and have described the specific peptide bond that is hydrolyzed. After reviewing these manuscripts, it is evident that peptidases are indeed not specific to a particular peptide. This is apparent when studying brain homogenates with different peptide substrates (Davis *et al.*, 1982, 1983, 1984a,b, 1985, 1987), where metabolism of a given peptide may lead to inactivation or formation of biologically active fragments with varying receptor affinity (Davis *et al.*, 1987). Regulation of peptide metabolism is of interest to many neuroscientists, and it is now appreciated that a limited number of membrane peptidases acting in concert can terminate or modify the biological actions of most neuropeptides. Maintaining a balance in these peptidases is critical to maintain central homeostasis (Matsas *et al.*, 1984; Hooper *et al.*, 1985; Turner *et al.*, 1985).

An example of an imbalance of peptidases leading to an alteration in the accumulation of behaviorally active endorphins was noted in a study of postmortem tissues from patients diagnosed with schizophrenia (Schoemaker and Davis, 1984; Davis *et al.*, 1986). On the basis of the putative antipsychotic-like effects of τ-type endorphins, the authors investigated if β-endorphin metabolism was altered in postmortem brains from patients diagnosed with schizophrenia versus sex- and age-matched controls. When studying the *in vitro* metabolism of β-endorphin by twice-washed, regional homogenates a significant difference was noted in the accumulation of the putative neuroleptic peptide DEτE. As with many postmortem studies it is difficult to distinguish etiological factors related to the pathological conditions of the study from antemortem parameters, the most important being prior drug treatment. In particular, neuroleptic drug treatment is an often encountered complicating variable in schizophrenia research.

Given the profound pharmacological effects of different neuropeptides, characterizing their effectiveness in human pathological states is of prominent importance. To determine if the β-endorphin metabolic alterations that were noted in postmortem tissues were due to antemortem drug treatment, studies on the effect of neuroleptic drugs on β-endorphin metabolism were designed. By using osmotic minipumps haloperidol and chlorpromazine were administered to Sprague-Dawley rats over a period of 8 days. Animals were sacrificed and the brains removed for *in vitro* β-endorphin metabolism experiments using reversed-phase HPLC. Results from these studies showed that haloperidol (3 mg/kg/day) causes significant increases in the accumulation of the τ-type endorphin fragment DEτE. Chlorpromazine (4.2 mg/kg/day) also significantly increased accumulation. However, phenobarbital (20 mg/kg/day) had no effect. From these studies it became apparent that neuroleptic drugs can alter the accumulation of behaviorally active endorphin fragments by rat brain homogenates (Davis *et al.*, 1984a).

B. Synaptic Membranes

Since purified synaptic membrane (pSPM) preparations restrict potential interference of contaminating peptidases that may be present when using brain homogenates, pSPM preparations have been used to determine if centrally acting drugs alter synaptic membrane peptide metabolism (Davis and Culling-Berglund, 1987).

Using pSPM the effect of neuroleptic drug treatment on *in vitro* central metabolism of neurotensin was studied. Neurotensin is found in high concentrations in areas of the brain that involve behavior such as the nucleus accumbens, amygdala, locus ceruleus, periaqueductal gray, habenula, and several hypothalamic nuclei. Neurotensin has also been implicated as being an endogenous neuroleptic (Nemeroff, 1980). To determine if neuroleptic drugs alter the half-life and metabolism of neurotensin in the brain, pSPM from drug-treated rats were isolated and time-course incubated with neurotensin. All samples were analyzed by reversed-phase HPLC. Both haloperidol and chlorpromazine caused an increase in neurotensin metabolism at the pSPM. Although an increase in neurotensin metabolism would result in a loss of biological activity, a significant accumulation of the biologically active fragment neurotensin (9–13) was noted that had been previously shown to bind to the neurotensin receptor.

Studies on the hydrolysis and the metabolism of peptides using high-resolution HPLC techniques have yielded important clues as to the mechanism of enzymatic control of several other neuropeptides. Atrial natriuretic factor (ANF) is metabolized into several fragments with biological activity and recently has been shown to be metabolized actively at the renal brush border (Olins et al., 1987). Substance P and neurotensin are metabolized specifically by neutral endopeptidase 3.4.24.11 and angiotensin-coverting enzyme 3.4.15.1, respectively. The importance of these two enzymes in the hydrolysis of substance P and neurotensin is apparent when one appreciates the wide distribution of 3.4.24.11 in the organism. Using reversed-phase HPLC for the separation of the cleavage products of substance P and neurotensin, Skidgel et al. (1984) described the sequence of enzymatic hydrolysis events and proposed the potential binding site of angiotensin converting enzyme with substance P. However, not all peptides are metabolized in a predicted manner. Neurokinin B can be hydrolyzed by neutral endopeptidase 24.11 but not by angiotensin-converting enzyme. Using pSPM, Hooper and Turner (1985) described the cleavage sites of neurokinin B showing that there is an inherent specificity of action by enzymes on their substrates.

Based on earlier metabolism studies with the opioid peptide β-endorphin, our laboratory became interested in using reversed-phase HPLC to determine the specificity of enzymatic proteolysis for other opioid peptides. The proenkephalin A peptide, peptide E, contains one copy of met-enkephalin at the amino terminus, one copy of leu-enkephalin at the carboxy terminus, and several other important fragments. This substrate could be cleaved into two different enkephalins and several other endogenous peptides such as metorphamide, met-enkephalin-arg-arg, met-enkephalin-arg, and the bovine adrenal medullary (BAM) peptides (Figure 1). To study the metabolism of peptide E, reversed-phase HPLC analysis was used as shown in Figure 2. High-resolution separations were necessary because of the large potential number of fragments that could be formed after enzymatic cleavage. In describing peptide E metabolism it was obvious that several of the fragments formed had been previously localized in the brain by other laboratories (Mizuno et al., 1980a,b; Weber et al., 1983). Studies were designed to determine if these fragments were biologically active in vivo. By combining HPLC studies of peptide E metabolism with biological assays, the authors

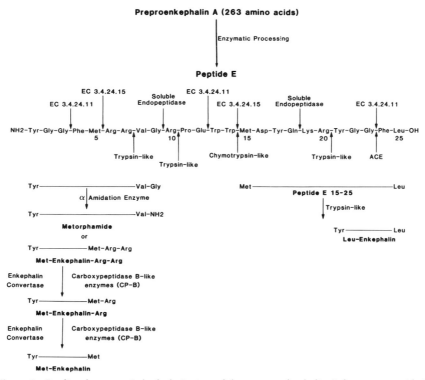

Figure 1 Predicted enzymatic hydrolysis sites of the preproenkephalin A fragment peptide E describing specific enzymes and showing the metabolic formation of known biologically active peptide fragments.

determined that many of the fragments formed by pSPM enzyme proteolysis were indeed centrally active (Dray and Davis, 1985; Davis *et al.*, 1985). Additionally, a unique fragment was discovered and synthesized that turned out to be a C-terminally extended enkephalin, peptide E 15–25, which was formed from the incubation of peptide E with pSPM (Davis *et al.*, 1987). When the stability of peptide E 15–25 was studied with synaptic plasma membranes for further *in vivo* characterization, it readily formed leu-enkephalin, as shown in Figure 3. Based on the predicted enzymatic cleavage sites it was apparent that peptide E 15–25 could be formed by either direct chymotrypsin-like cleavage, trypsin-like cleavage followed by metalloendopeptidase 3.4.24.15 hydrolysis, or cleavage by neutral endopeptidase 3.4.24.11 followed by 3.4.24.15 hydrolysis (Figure 1). To inhibit proteolysis of peptide E 15–25, an aminopeptidase inhibitor, bestatin, and an inhibi-

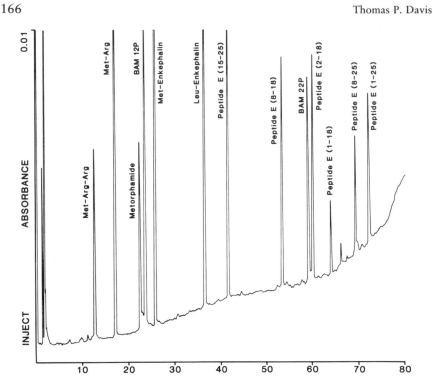

Figure 2 Reversed-phase HPLC chromatogram of peptide E (1–25) and 12 related fragments. Peptides were separated on an ultrasphere-ODS 5 μm column (25 cm × 4 mm) using a series of curvilinear gradients of filtered, degassed acetonitrile (18–45%) against 0.1 M NaH$_2$PO$_4$ (pH 2.4) over 80 min at 37°C. Each peak represents 300 ng of peptide on column. All HPLC peaks shown were confirmed by amino acid analysis of hydrolyzed samples.

tor of neutral endopeptidase 3.4.24.11, thiorphan, were studied. Shown in Figure 4 is the effect of these inhibitors on the incubation of peptide E 15–25 with rat brain pSPM. Note that several of the unknown fragments of Figure 3 are no longer apparent, but the appearance of leu-enkephalin is still present at a retention time of 27 min. By using reversed-phase HPLC the authors were able to further characterize which inhibitor "cocktail" would be appropriate to inhibit proteolysis of peptide E 15–25.

C. Brain Slices

One of the first studies of β-endorphin metabolism using rat striatal slices was described by Smyth and Snell (1977a,b). They concluded that β-endor-

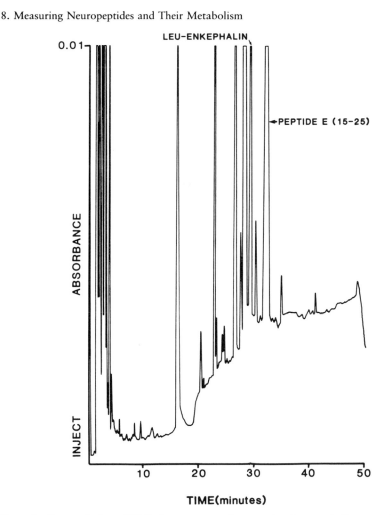

Figure 3 Reversed-phase HPLC chromatogram from an *in vitro* metabolism experiment of peptide E (15–25) with purified, rat brain synaptic membranes (60-min incubation). Peptides were separated on a Supelco LC-18 column (15 cm × 4.6 mm) using a linear gradient of filtered, degassed acetonitrile (5–22%) against 0.1 M NaH$_2$PO$_4$ (pH 2.4) over 40 min at 37°C. Approximately 122 μg of total synaptic membrane protein was injected on-column for analysis. Both leu-enkephalin and peptide E (15–25) were confirmed by amino acid analysis of collected HPLC peaks.

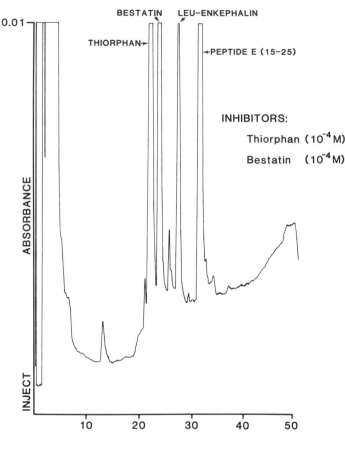

Figure 4 Reversed-phase HPLC chromatogram from an *in vitro* metabolism experiment of peptide E (15–25) with purified, rat brain synaptic membranes in the presence of protease inhibitors. Approximately 43.5 μg of protein was injected on column for analysis. All other conditions were the same as for Figure 3.

phin had a half-life of 3.2 h in striatal slices, whereas the half-life of gamma-endorphin was much shorter (1.1 h). Bacitracin did not effect the proteoly-sis of β-endorphin, but increased the half-life of τ-endorphin (3.6 h). Therefore, the amino terminus of β-endorphin was more resistent to proteo-lytic attack than the amino terminus of τ-endorphin. These investigators also demonstrated that the metabolic fragments were formed extracellularly in the slice preparation and that there was no evidence of active uptake by the tissue. Using a similar approach, our laboratory described the metabolic breakdown of des-tyrosine-τ-endorphin. The metabolic pattern of fragments formed after a 120-min incubation with striatal slices was compared to the metabolic pattern upon incubation of des-tyrosine-gamma-endorphin with homogenates of human caudate nucleus and homogenates from whole rat brain. No major differences were noted between the three tissue preparations studied, and the major fragment formed in each study was DEτE (β-E 6–17) (Schoemaker *et al.*, 1982a).

Since the slice technique does not require the homogenization of the tissue and the release of nonspecific, contaminating peptidases, a rapid incubation protocol using discrete 2 mm × 250 μm slices from specific regions of the rat brain has been developed (Li *et al.*, 1988). Incubating β-endorphin with rat brain slices from several regions has provided evidence for a regional specificity of enzymatic proteolysis. Further studies have also shown that β-endorphin half-life can vary over fivefold and is dependent on the region of brain studied (Li *et al.*, 1988). By using the brain slice technique with *in vitro* neuropeptide incubations coupled to reversed-phase HPLC separations, several important brain regions can be studied simultaneously. Requiring only 2-mm biopsies, several slices from a specific brain region can be time-course incubated to determine the effect of specific centrally acting drugs on regional metabolism of a given peptide. The slice technique is a much better approach for studying peptide metabolism because it offers several advantages, including (1) control of extracellular fluid composition, temperature, and pH to express or inhibit the activity of specific extracellular proteases; (2) slices contain complete neurons and processes that can be recorded from during the metabolism experiment; and (3) the possibility of non-specific/lysosomal enzymatic events is diminished if the tissue is not homogenized. We plan to continue using the regional brain slice technique coupled to high-resolution chromatography for studies of peptide metabolism in future experiments because the regional brain slice is functionally closer to the intact brain than is a homogenate (Li *et al.*, 1990).

VI. Conclusions

As stated above, there have been several recent advances in the analytical chemistry of peptides enabling neuroscientists to detect endogenous levels in tissues and blood. Since all neuropeptides are sequences of amino acids that can undergo both posttranslational modifications and metabolic peptidase cleavage, it is critically important to isolate and measure the particular peptide of interest. HPLC techniques offer the necessary resolution and specificity to separate complex mixtures of structurally similar peptides in a single analysis. While HPLC may not be as sensitive as capillary electrophoresis, you can recover the peptide for further biological testing. This is most important to the neuroscientist who is interested in isolating and characterizing peptides for determining structure–activity relationships.

Peptides offer a unique challenge to both the biologist and the chemist because of their inherent structural similarities. As neuroscientists continue to study mechanisms associated with neuropeptide interactions in the central nervous system, they must also be aware of ongoing advancements in analytical separations and detection. By improving analytical techniques and applying them to studies of peptide biology and biochemistry, we can look forward to continued growth in neuroscience research.

Acknowledgments

Research from the author's laboratory referred to here was supported by U.S. Public Health Service grants MH42600 from the National Institute of Mental Health, DK36289 from the National Institute of Diabetes, Digestive and Kidney Diseases, CA44869 from the National Cancer Institute, and DA06284 from the National Institute on Drug Abuse. The author thanks Terrence Gillesie, M.S., for assistance with proteolytic enzyme cleavage predictions, Alison Culling-Berglund, M.S., for Peptide E chromatography, and SarahAnne Jackson for assistance with typing the manuscript.

References

Acharya, A. S., DiDonato, A., Manjula, B. N., Fishetti, V. A., and Manning, J. M. (1983). Influence of trifluoroacetic acid on retention time of histidine-containing tryptic peptides in reverse phase HPLC. *Int. J. Pept. Protein Res.* **22**, 78–82.

Ahmed, M. S., Randall, L. W., Sibai, B., Dass, C., Fridland, G., Desiderio, D. M., and Tolun, E. (1987). Identification of dynorphin 1-8 in human placenta by mass spectrometry. *Life Sci.* **40**, 2067–2076.

Akil, H., Ueda, Y., Lin, H. L., and Watson, S. J. (1981). A sensitive coupled HPLC/RIA technique for separation of endorphins: Multiple forms of β-endorphin in rat pituitary intermediate vs. anterior lobe. *Neuropeptides (Edinburgh)* **1**, 429–446.

Anderson, W. R., Jr., Frick, W., Daves, G. D., Jr., Barofsky, D. F., Yamaguchi, I., Chang, D., Folkers, K., and Rosell, S. (1977). Mass spectra of underivatized peptide amides related to substance P. *Biochem. Biophys. Res. Commun.* **78**, 372–376.

Barnes, K., Turner, A. J., and Kenny, A. J. (1988). Electronmicroscopic immunocytochemistry of pig brain shows that endopeptidase-24.11 is localized in neuronal membranes. *Neurosci. Lett.* **94**, 64–69.

Bennett, G. W., Johnson, J. V., and Marsden, C. A. (1986). HPLC/ECD of neuropeptides in neural and endocrine tissues. *In* "Monitoring Neurotransmitter Release During Behavior" M. H. Joseph, M. Filleny, I. A. MacDonald, and C. A. Marsden, eds.), Part 4, p. 244. VCH, Chichester, England.

Bennett, H. P. J., Hudson, A. M., Kelly, L., McMartin, C., and Purdon, G. E. (1978). A rapid method, using octadecasilyl-silica, for the extraction of certain peptides from tissues. *Biochem. J.* **175**, 1139–1141.

Bennett, H. P. J., Browne, C. A., and Solomon, S. (1980). The use of perfluorinated carboxylic acids in the reversed-phase HPLC of peptides. *J. Liq. Chromatogr.* 3(9), 1353–1365.

Boarder, M. R., Weber, E., Evans, C. J., Erdelyi, E., and Barchas, J. D. (1983). Measurement of total opioid peptides in rat brain and pituitary by radioimmunoassay directed at the α-N-acetyl derivative. *J. Neurochem.* 40(6), 1517–1522.

Brinton, R. E., Deshmukh, P. P., Chen, A., Davis, T. P., Hsiao, A., and Yamamura, H. I. (1983). A nonequilibrium 24-hour vasopressin radioimmunoassay: Development and basal levels in the rat brain. *Brain Res.* 266, 344–347.

Brown, M., Rivier, J., and Vale, W. (1976). Somatostatin analogs with selected biologic activities. *Metab., Clin. Exp.* 24, Suppl. 1, 1501–1503.

Brownlee, R. G., and Compton, S. W. (1988). Automated instrumentation for analytical capillary electrophoresis. *Am. Biotech. Lab.* 6, 10–17.

Buck, S. H., Walsh, J. H., Davis, T. P., Brown, M. R., Yamamura, H. I., and Burks, T. F. (1983). Characterization of the peptide and sensory neurotoxic effects of capsaicin in the guinea pig. *J. Neurosci.* 3(10), 2064–2074.

Bunnett, N. W., Debas, H. T., Turner, A. J., Kobayashi, R., and Walsh, J. H. (1988a). Metabolism of gastrin and cholecystokinin by endopeptidase 24.11 from the pig stomach. *Am. J. Physiol.* 255, G676–G684.

Bunnett, N. W., Turner, A. J., Hryszko, J., Kobayashi, R., and Walsh, J. H. (1988b). Isolation of endopeptidase-24.11 (EC 3.4.24.11, "Enkephalinase") from the pig stomach. *Gastroenterology* 95, 952–957.

Burbach, J. P. H. (1984). Action of proteolytic enzymes on lipotropins and endorphins: Biosynthesis biotransformation and fate. *Pharmacol. Ther.* 24, 321–354.

Burbach, J. P. H., and de Kloet, E. R. (1982). Proteolysis of β-endorphin in brain tissue. *Peptides (N.Y.)* 3, 451–453.

Burbach, J. P. H., Loeber, J. G., Verhoef, J., de Kloet, E. R., and de Wied, D. 1979). Biotransformation of endorphins by a synaptosomal plasma membrane preparation of rat brain and by human serum. *Biochem. Biophys. Res. Commun.* 86(4), 1296–1303.

Burbach, J. P. H., de Kloet, E. R., Schotman, P., and de Wied, D. (1981). Proteolytic conversion of β-endorphin by brain synaptic membranes. *J. Biol. Chem.* 256(23), 12463–12469.

Burbach, J. P. H., Lebouille, J. L. M., and Wang, X.-C. (1984). Proteolytic conversion of neuropeptides into active fragments. *Proc. Meet. Eur. Soc. Neurochem. 5th*, Budapest, Hungary, pp. 237–246.

Burgus, R., and Rivier, J. (1976). Use of high pressure liquid chromatography in the purification of peptides *Pept., Pro. Eur. Pept. Symp.*, *14th, 1976*, pp. 85–94.

Checler, F., Kitabgi, P., and Vincent, J.-P. (1982). Degradation of neurotensin by brain synaptic membranes. *Ann. N. Y. Acad. Sci.* 400, 413–414.

Clement-Jones, V., Lowry, P. J., Rees, L. H., and Besser, G. M. (1980). Development of a specific extracted radioimmunoassay for methionine enkephalin in human plasma and cerebrospinal fluid. *J. Endocrinol.* 86, 231–243.

Cody, R. B., Jr., Amster, I. J., and McLafferty, F. W. (1985). Peptide mixture sequencing by tandem Fourier-transform mass spectrometry. *Proc. Natl. Acad. Sci. U.S.A.* 82, 6367–6370.

Cohen, A. S., and Karger, B. L. (1987). High-performance sodium dodecyl sulfate polyacrylamide gel capillary electrophoresis of peptides and proteins. *J. Chromatogr.* 397, 409–417.

Cooks, R. G., Busch, K. L., and Glish, G. L. (1983). Mass spectrometry: Analytical capabilities and potentials. *Science* 222, 273–291.

Craves, F. B., Law, P. Y., Hunt, C. A., and Loh, H. H. (1978). The metabolic disposition of radiolabelled enkephalins *in vitro* and *in situ*. *J. Pharmacol. Exp. Ther.* 206, 492–506.

Crommen, J. (1979). Reversed-phase ion-pair high-performance liquid chromatography of drugs and related compounds using underivatized silica as the stationary phase. *J. Chromatogr.* **186**, 705–724.

Davis, T. P., and Culling-Berglund, A. J. (1985). High-performance liquid chromatographic analysis of in vitro central neuropeptide processing. *J. Chromatogr.* **327**, 279–292.

Davis, T. P., and Culling-Berglund, A. J. (1987). Neuroleptic drug treatment alters in vitro central neurotensin metabolism. *Psychoneuroendocrinology* **12**(4), 253–260.

Davis, T. P., Gehrke, C. W., Gehrke, C. W., Jr., Cunningham, T. D., Kuo, K. C., Gerhardt, K. O., Johnson, H. D., and Williams, C. H. (1978). High performance liquid chromatographic separation and fluorescence measurement of biogenic amines in plasma, urine and tissue. *Clin. Chem. (Winston-Salem, N. C.)* **24**, 1317–1324.

Davis, T. P., Chen, A., and Yamamura, H. I. (1982). High performance liquid chromatography of pharmacologically active amines and peptides in biological materials. *Life Sci.* **30**, 971–987.

Davis, T. P., Culling, A. J., Schoemaker, H., and Galligan, J. J. (1983). β-Endorphin and its metabolites stimulate motility of the dog small intestine. *J. Pharmacol. Exp. Ther.* **227**(2), 499–507.

Davis, T. P., Schoemaker, H., and Culling, A. J. (1984a). Centrally acting drugs alters in vitro β-endorphin processing in the rat. *Eur. J. Pharmacol.* **100**, 249–251.

Davis, T. P., Schoemaker, H., and Culling-Berglund, A. J. (1984b). Characterization of in vitro proteolytic processing of β-endorphin by reversed-phase HPLC. *Peptides (N.Y.)* **5**, 1037–1042.

Davis, T. P., Porreca, F., Burks, T. F., and Dray, A. (1985). The proenkephalin A fragment, peptide E: central processing and CNS activity in vivo. *Eur. J. Pharmacol.* **111**(2), 177–184.

Davis, T. P., Culling-Berglund, A. J., and Schoemaker, H. (1986). Specific regional differences of in vitro β-endorphin metabolism in schizophrenics. *Life Sci.* **39**, 2601–2609.

Davis, T. P., Shook, J. E., Gillespie, T. J., Culling-Berglund, A. J., Papietro, H. M., and Porreca, F. (1987). The proenkephalin A fragment peptide E is metabolized centrally to a novel peptide with opioid activity. *Proc. West. Pharmacol. Soc.* **30**, 321–325.

Davis, T. P., Gillespie, T. J., and Porreca, F. (1989). Peptide fragments derived from the β-chain of hemoglobin (hemorphins) are centrally active in vivo. *Peptides (N.Y.)* **10**(3), 552–557.

Desiderio, D. M., Stein, J. L., Cunningham, M. D., and Sabbatini, J. Z. (1980). High pressure (performance) liquid chromatography and field desorption mass spectrometry of hypothalamic oligopeptides. *J. Chromatogr.* **195**, 369–377.

de Wied, D. (1978). Psychopathology as a neuropeptide dysfunction. *In* "Characteristics and Function of Opioid" (J. M. Van Ree and L. Terenius, eds.), pp. 113–122. Elsevier/North-Holland, Amsterdam.

Dou, L., Mazzeo, J., and I. S. Krull. (1990). Determination of amino acids, peptides and proteins by HPLC combined with electrochemical detection. *Biochromatography* **5**(2). 74–96.

Dray, A., and Davis, T. P. (1985). The proenkephalin A fragment metorphamide shows supraspinal and spinal opioid activity in vivo. *Peptides (N.Y.)* **6**, 217–221.

Engelfried, C., and Koenig, W. A. (1976). Mass spectrometric investigation of peptide amides. *Biomed Mass Spectrom.* **3**, 241–244.

Feldman, A. J., Cohn, M. L., and Blair, D. (1978). Neuroendocrine peptides—analysis by reversed-phase high performance liquid chromatography. *J. Liq. Chromatogr.* **1**(6), 833–848.

Firestone, M. A., Michaud, J.-P., Carter, R.H., and Thormann, W. (1987). Capillary zone electrophoresis and isotachophoresis as alternatives to chromatographic methods for purity control of synthetic peptides. *J. Chromatogr.* **407,** 363–368.

Fleming, L. H., and Reynolds, N. C. (1986). Separation and detection of closely related endorphins by liquid chromatography–electrochemistry. *J. Chromatogr.* 375(1), 65–73.

Frei, R. W., Michel, L., and Santi, W. (1976). Post-column fluorescence derivation of peptides problems and potential in high-performance liquid chromatography. *J. Chromatogr.* **126,** 665–677.

Frick, W., Daves, G. D., Jr., Barofsky, D. F., Barofsky, E., Fisher, G. H., Chang, D., and Folkers, K. (1977). Sample derivatization and structure analysis by field desorption mass spectrometry peptide methylation-methanolysis. *Biomed. Mass Spectrom.* 4(3), 152–154.

Goldfarb, A. R., Saidel, L. J., and Mosovich, E. (1951). The ultraviolet absorption spectra of proteins. *J. Biol. Chem.* **193,** 397–404.

Grossman, P. D., Wilson, K. J., Petrie, G., and Lauer, H. H. (1988). Effect of buffer pH and peptide composition on the selectivity of peptide separations by capillary zone electrophoresis. *Anal. Biochem,* **173,** 265–270.

Grossman, P. D., Colburn, J. C., Lauer, H. H., Nielsen, R. G., Riggin, R. M., Sittampalam, G. S., and Rickard, E. C. (1989). Application of free-solution capillary electrophoresis to the analytical scale separation of proteins and peptides. *Anal. Chem.* **61,** 1186–1194.

Guillemin, R., Ling, N., Burgus, R., Bloom, F., and Segal, D. (1977). Characterization of the endorphins, novel hypothalamic and neurohypophysial peptides with opiate-like activity. Evidence that they induce profound behavioral changes. *Psychoneuroendocrinology* **2,** 59–62.

Guzman, N. A., Hernandez, L., and Hoebel, B. G. (1989). Capillary electrophoresis: A new era in microseparations. *Biopharmacology* **2,** 22–37.

Hancock, W. S., and Bishop, C. A. (1976). High pressure liquid chromatography in the analysis of underivatized peptides using a sensitive and rapid procedure. *FEBS Lett.* **72,** 139–142.

Hersh, L. B. (1985). Characterization of membrane-bound aminopeptidases from rat brain: Identification of the enkephalin-degrading aminopeptidase. *J. Neurochem.* **44,**(5), 1427–1435.

Hersh, L. B., Smith, T. E., and McKelvy, J. F. (1980). Cleavage of endorphins to des-Tyr endorphins by homogeneous bovine brain aminopeptidase. *Nature (London)* **286,** 160–162.

Hooper, N. M., and Turner, A. J. (1985). Neurokinin B is hydrolyzed by synaptic membranes and by endopeptidase-24.11 ("enkephalinase") but not by angiotensin converting enzyme. *FEBS Lett.* **190,** 133–136.

Hooper, N. M., Kenny, A. J., and Turner, A. J. (1985). Neurokinin A (substance K) is a substrate for endopeptidase-24.11 but not for peptidyl dipeptidase A (angiotensin-converting enzyme). *Biochem. J.* **231,** 357–361.

Hughes, J., Smith, T. W., Kosterlitz, H. W., Fothergic, L. A., Morgan, B. A., and Morris, H. R. (1975). Identification of two related pentapeptides from the brain with potent opiate agonist activity. *Nature (London)* **258,** 577–579.

Jessop, D. S., Patience, R. L., Cunnah, D., and Rees, L. D. (1987). The use of reversed-phase high-performance liquid chromatography to detect proteolytic activity from human pancreas in a radioimmunoassay for corticotrophin-releasing factor. *J. Endocrinol.* **114,** 147–151.

Joys, T. M., and Kim, H. (1979). o-Phthaladehyde and the fluorogenic detection of peptides. *Anal. Biochem.* **94,** 371–377.

Kirschbaum, J., Perlman, S., Joseph, J., and Adamovics, J. (1984). Ensuring accuracy of HPLC assays. *J. Chromatogr. Sci.* **22**, 27–30.

Kissinger, P. T., Refshauge, C., Dreiling, R., and Adams, R. N. (1973). An electrochemical detector for liquid chromatography with picogram sensitivity. *Anal. Lett.* **6**, 465.

Kissinger, P. T., Riggin, R. M., Alcorn, R. L., and Rau, L.-D. (1975). Estimation of catecholamines in urine by high performance liquid chromatography with electrochemical detection. *Biochem. Med.* **13**, 299–306.

Lakings, D. B., and Gehrke, C. W. (1971). Analysis of base composition of RNA and DNA hydrolysates by gas-liquid chromatography. *J. Chromatogr.* **62**, 347–367.

Lee, E. D., Muck, W., Henion, J. D., and Covey, T. (1988). On-line capillary zone electrophoresis-ion spray tandem mass spectrometry for the determination of dynorphins. *J. Chromatogr.* **458**, 313–321.

Li, Z. W., Brendel, K., Culling-Berglund, A. J., and Davis, T. P. (1988). Regional specificity of β-endorphin metabolism in brain slices of the rat. *Proc. West. Pharmacol. Soc.* **31**, 67–70.

Li, Z. W., Brendel, U., Biijl, W., van Nispen, J., and Davis, T. P. (1990). Neuropeptide processing in regional brain slices: Effect of conformation and sequence. *J. Pharm. Exp. Ther.* **253**(2) 851–857.

Ling, B., Burgus, R., and Guillemin, R. (1976). Isolation, primary structure and synthesis of α-endorphin and τ-endorphin, two peptides of hypothalamic–hypophysial origin with morphinomimetic activity. *Proc. Natl. Acad. Sci. U.S.A.* **73**, 3942–3946.

Loeber, J. G., Verhoef, J., Burbach, J. P. H., and Witter, A. (1979). Combination of high pressure liquid chromatography and radioimmunoassay is a powerful tool for the specific and quantitative determination of endorphins and related peptides. *Biochem. Biophys. Res. Commun.* **86**(4), 1288–1295.

Malfroy, B., Smerts, J. P., Guyon, A., Roques, B. P., and Schwartz, J. C. (1978). High affinity enkephalin-degrading peptidase in brain is increased after morphine. *Nature (London)* **276**, 523–526.

Marks, N., and Stern, F. (1975). Inactivation of somatostatin (GH-RIH) and its analogs by crude and partially purified rat brain extracts. *FEBS Lett.* **55**, 220–223.

Marks, N., Galoyan, A., Grynbaum, A., and Lajtha, A. (1974). Protein and peptide hydrolases of the rat hypothalamus and pituitary. *J. Neurochem.* **22**, 735–739.

Marks, N., Stern, F., and Benuck, M. (1976). Correlation between biological potency and biodegradation of a somatostatin analogue. *Nature (London)* **261**, 511–512.

Matsas, R., Fulcher, I. S., Kenny, A. J., and Turner, A. J. (1983). Substance P and [Leu]enkephalin are hydrolyzed by an enzyme in pig caudate synaptic membranes that is identical with the endopeptidase of kidney microvilli. *Proc. Natl. Acad. Sci. U.S.A.* **80**, 3111–3115.

Matsas, R., Kenny, A. J., and Turner, A. J. (1984). The hydrolysis of peptides, including enkephalins, tachykinins and their analogues by endopeptidase-24.11. *Biochem. J.* **223**, 433–440.

May, H. E., Tanzer, F. S., Fridland, G. H., Wakelyn, C., and Desiderio, D. M. (1982). High performance liquid chromatography and proteolytic enzyme characterization of peptides in tooth pulp extracts. *J. Liq. Chromatogr.* **5**(11), 2135–2154.

Mayer, M. M., and Miller, J. A. (1970). Photometric analysis of proteins and peptides at 191-194nm. *Anal. Biochem.* **36**, 91–100.

McCormick, R. M. (1988). Capillary zone electrophoresis separation of peptides and proteins using low pH buffers in modified silica capillaries. *Anal. Chem.* **60**, 2322–2328.

McKelvy, J. F., and Blumberg, S. (1986). Inactivation and metabolism of neuropeptides. *Annu. Rev. Neurosci.* **9**, 415–434.

Meek, J. L. (1980). Prediction of peptide retention times in high-pressure liquid chromatography on the basis of amino acid composition. *Proc. Natl. Acad. Sci. U.S.A.* **77**(3), 1632–1636.

Mizuno, K., Minamino, N., Kangawa, K., and Matsuo, K. (1980a). A new endogenous opioid peptide from bovine adrenal medulla: Isolation and amino acid sequence of a dodecapeptide (BAM-12P). *Biochem. Biophys. Res. Commun.* **95**, 1482.

Mizuno, K., Minamino, N., Kangawa, K., and Matsuo, K. (1980b). A new family of endogenous "big" met-enkephalins from bovine adrenal medulla: purification and structure of docosa-(BAM-22P) and eicosapeptide (BAM-20P) with very potent opiate activity. *Biochem. Biophys. Res. Commun.* **97**, 1283.

Molnar, I., and Horvath, C. (1977). Separation of amino acids and peptides on non-polar stationary phases by high-performance liquid chromatography. *J. Chromatogr.* **142**, 623–640.

Morris, H. R., and Panico, M. (1981). Fast atom bombardment: A new mass spectrometric method for peptide sequence analysis. *Biochem. Biophy. Res. Commun.* **101**(2), 623–631.

Mousa, S., and Couri, D. (1983). Analysis of enkephalins, β-endorphins and small peptides in their sequences by highly sensitive high-performance liquid chromatography with electrochemical detection: Implication is opioid peptide metabolism. *J. Chromatogr.* **267**, 191–198.

Mudgett, M., Bowen, D. V., Field, F. H., and Kindt, T. J. (1977). Peptide sequencing: The utility of chemical ionization mass spectrometry. *Biomed. Mass Spectrom.* **4**(3), 159–171.

Nemeroff, C. B. (1980). Neurotensin: Perchance an endogenous neuroleptic? *Biol. Psychiatry* **15**, 283–302.

Nielsen, R. G., Sittampalam, G. S., and Rickard, E. C. (1989). Capillary zone electrophoresis of insulin and growth hormone. *Ana. Biochem.* **177**, 20–26.

Olins, G. M., Spear, K. L., Siegel, N. R., and Zurcher-Neely, H. A. (1987). Inactivation of atrial natriuretic factor by the renal brush border. *Biochim. Biophys. Acta* **901**, 97–100.

Pert, C. B., Pert, A., Chang, J. K., and Fong, B. T. (1976). [D-Ala]-met-enkephalinamide: A potent long-lasting synthetic pentapeptide analgesic. *Science* **194**, 330–332.

Pilosof, D., Kim, H.-Y., Vestal, M. L., and Dyckes, D. F. (1984). Direct monitoring of sequential enzymatic hydrolysis of peptides by thermospray mass spectrometry. *Biomed. Mass Spectrom.* **11**(8), 403–407.

Priddle, J. D., Rose, K., and Offord, R. E. (1976). The separation and sequencing of permethylated peptides by mass spectrometry directly coupled to gas-liquid chromatography. *Biochem. J.* **157**, 777–780.

Regnier, F. E. (1987). The role of protein structure in chromatographic behavior. *Science* **238**, 319–323.

Regnier, F. E., and Gooding, K. M. (1980). High-performance liquid chromatography of proteins. *Anal. Biochem.* **103**, 1–25.

Rivier, J. (1978). Use of trialkyl ammonium phosphate (TAAP) buffers in reverse-phase HPLC for high resolution and high recovery of peptides and proteins. *J. Liq. Chromatogr.* **1**(3), 343–366.

Robinson, A. L. (1979). HPLC: The new king of analytical chemistry? *Science* **203**, 1329–1332.

Rose, K., Savoy, L.-A., Simona, M. G., Offord, R. E., and Wingfield, P. (1988). C-Terminal peptide identification by fast atom bombardment mass spectrometry. *Biochem. J.* **250**, 253–259.

Rossier, J., Bayon, A., Vargo, T. M., Ling, N., Guillemin, R., and Bloom, F. (1977). Radio-immunoassay of brain peptides: Evaluation of a methodology for the assay of β-endorphin and enkephalin. *Life Sci.* **21**, 847–852.

Rubinstein, M., Chen-Kiang, S., Stein, S., and Udenfriend, S. (1979). Characterization of proteins and peptides by high-performance liquid chromatography and fluorescence monitoring of their tryptic digests. *Anal. Biochem.* **95**, 117–121.

Schiltz, E., Schnackerz, K. D., and Gracy, R. W. (1977). Comparison of ninhydrin, fluorescamine and o-phthaldialdehyde for the detection of amino acids and peptides and their effects on the recovery and composition of peptides from thin layer fingerprints. *Anal. Biochem.* **79**, 33–41.

Schoemaker, H., and Davis, T. P. (1984). Differential in vitro metabolism of β-endorphin in schizophrenia. *Peptides (N.Y.)* **5**, 1049–1054.

Schoemaker, H., Chen, A., Davis, T. P., and Yamamura, H. I. (1982a). A study of the metabolism of des-Tyrosine-τ-endorphin using an improved HPLC system. *Psychopharmacol. Bull.* **18**(4), 144–148.

Schoemaker, H., Davis, T. P., Pedigo, N. W., Chen, A., Berens, E. S., Ragan, P., Ling, N. C., and Yamamura, H. I. (1982b). Identification of β-endorphins-(6–17) as the principal metabolite of des-Tyrosine-τ-endorphin (DTτE) in vitro and assessment of its activity in neurotransmitter receptor binding assays. *Eur. J. Pharmacol.* **81**, 459–468.

Schwartz, J.-C. (1983). Metabolism of enkephalinase and the inactivating neuropeptidase concept. *Trends Neurosci.* **6**, 45–48.

Schwartz, J.-C., Malfroy, B., and de la Baume, S. (1981). Biological inactivation of enkephalin and the role of enkephalin-dipeptidyl-carboxypeptidase ("enkephalinase") as neuropeptidase. *Life Sci.* **29**, 1715–1740.

Skidgel, R. A., Engelbrecht, S., Johnson, A. R., and Erdos, E. G. (1984). Hydrolysis of substance P and neurotensin by converting enzyme and neutral endopeptidase. *Peptides (N.Y.)* **5**, 769–776.

Smith, R. D., Olivares, J. A., Nguyen, N. T., and Udseth, H. R. (1988). Capillary zone electrophoresis-mass spectrometry using an electrospray ionization interface. *Anal. Chem.* **60**, 436–441.

Symth, D. G., and Snell, C. R. (1977a). Metabolism of the analgesic peptide lipotropin C-fragment in rat striatal slices. *FEBS Lett.* **78**, 225–227.

Smyth, D. G., and Snell, C. R. (1977b). Proteolysis of lipotropin C-fragment takes place extracellularly to form τ-endorphin and (methionine) enkephalin. *Biochem. Soc. Trans.* **5**, 1397–1399.

Spackman, D. H., Stein, W. H., and Moore, S. (1960). The disulfide bonds of ribonuclease. *J. Biol. Chem.* **235**, 648–659.

Turner, A. J., Matsas, R., and Kenny, A. J. (1985). Are there neuropeptide-specific peptidases? *Biochem. Pharmacol.* **34**(9), 1347–1356.

Turner, A. J., Hooper, N. M., and Kenny, A. J. (1987). Metabolism of neuropeptides. In "Mammalian Ectoenzymes" pp. 211–247. Am. Elsevier, New York.

Turner, A. J., Hooper, N. M. and Kenny, A. J. (1989). Neuropeptide-degrading enzymes. In "Neuropeptides: A Methodology" (G. Fink, and A. J. Harmar, eds.), Chapter 8, pp. 189–223. Wiley, New York.

Vuolteenaho, O., Leppaluoto, J., Vakkuri, O., Karppinen, J. Hoyhtya, M., and Ling, N. (1981). Development and validation of a radioimmunoassay for beta-endorphin-related peptides. *Acta Physiol. Scand.* **112**, 313–321.

Weber, E., Evans, C. J., Chang, J.-K., and Barchas, J. D. (1982). Brain distributions of α-neoendorphin and β-neo-endorphin: Evidence for regional processing differences. *Biochem. Biophys. Res. Commun.* **108**(1), 81–88.

Weber, E., Esch, F. S., Bohlen, P., Paterson, S., Corbettt, A. D., McKnight, A. T., Kosterlitz, H. W., Barchas, J. D., and Evans, C. J. (1983). Metorphamide: Isolation, structure, and biological activity of an amidated opioid octapeptide from bovine brain. *Proc. Natl. Acad. Sci. U.S.A.* **80,** 7362–7366.

Wilson, K. J., Honegger, A., Stotzel, R. P., and Hughes, G. J. (1981). The behaviour of peptides on reverse-phase supports during high-pressure liquid chromatography. *Biochem. J.* **199,** 31–41.

Worthy, W. (1983). Progress in coupling systems boosts LC/MS prospects. *Chem. Eng. News,* **9,** 19–20.

Yang, H.-Y. T., Panula, P., Tang, J., and Costa, E. (1983). Characterization and location of Met^5-enkephalin-Arg^6-Phe^7 stored in various rat brain regions. *J. Neurochem.* **40**(4), 969–976.

II

Endocrine
Regulation

9

Stress, the Hypothalamic–Pituitary– Adrenal Axis, and Depression

James C. Ritchie
Departments of Psychiatry and
Pharmacology
Duke University Medical Center
Durham, North Carolina

Charles B. Nemeroff
Departments of Psychiatry and
Pharmacology
Duke University Medical Center
Durham, North Carolina

I. Introduction

Control of the hypothalamic–pituitary–adrenal (HPA) axis is a multistep integrated process involving several central nervous system sites (cerebral cortex, amygdala, locus ceruleus, hippocampus, etc.). Most, but perhaps not all, of these central inputs are eventually channeled to the hypothalamus. In the hypothalamus these signals are transduced to humoral-type messages, release and release-inhibiting hormones, that are then released from nerve terminals in the eminence, the site of the primary plexus of the hypothalamo–hypophyseal–portal system. These hypothalamic hypophysiotrophic hormones released from the hypothalamus travel a short distance to the anterior pituitary, where the signal is amplified and converted by the release of pituitary trophic hormones. The adrenohypophyseal hormones are then released into the general circulation, travel to their appropriate target organs, and effect a multitude of specific organ system responses. These responses are known to have major influences on blood pressure regulation, reproductive function, and energy mobilization. In addition to the central control mentioned above, the various neuroendocrine axes are also influenced by a variety of "feedback" control loops. These feedback controls can be of both a fast and slow nature and are known to involve both central and peripheral sites.

Corticotropin-releasing factor (CRF), a recently described 41-amino-acid-containing peptide (Vale *et al.*, 1981), is the hypothalamic releasing hormone that controls HPA axis activity. It is primarily found at a pivotal location in the HPA axis, that is, where the CNS portions of the axis interact with the peripheral members of the axis. As such, it is uniquely qualified to modulate HPA axis activity. Additionally, there is accumulating evidence that CRF is synthesized in neurons at several extrahypothalamic sites within the central nervous system (CNS), and in the periphery. In the CNS, preclinical data from various disciplines provide additional evidence that CRF acts as a neurotransmitter. In the peripheral plasma the function(s) of CRF is unknown but concentration changes have been noted during acute hemorrhage (Bruhn *et al.*, 1987), insulin-induced hypoglycemia (Sasaki *et al.*, 1987b), and pregnancy (Sasaki *et al.*, 1984). Thus a burgeoning data base suggests a role for this peptide beyond that of a hypothalamic releasing hormone. In this chapter we will examine the available data concerning the involvement of CRF in both the stress response and the pathophysiology of depression, often hypothesized to be the pathological manifestation of an aberrant stress response. It is hoped that this discussion will lead the reader to a better understanding of the postulated connection between the stress response and major affective illness, which underlies the stress–diathesis model of depression, and the unique role of CRF in this relationship.

II. CRF and the Stress Response

Stress increases plasma ACTH and glucocorticoid concentrations. Apparently the activation of the HPA axis by stress is due to the release of several neuromodulators including CRF, arginine, vasopressin (AVP), oxytocin (OT), angiotensin II, vasoactive intestinal peptide (VIP), epinephrine, and norepinephrine. Although this plethora of modulators of the stress response contributed greatly to the immense difficulty in the initial isolation and characterization of CRF, it is now clear that CRF is *the* major physiological regulator of ACTH secretion during stress. Evidence for this assertion is provided by the finding that stress-induced ACTH release can be almost completely abolished by pretreatment with a CRF antiserum or the CRF antagonist, alpha-helical $oCRF_{9-41}$ (Linton *et al.*, 1985; C. Rivier *et al.*, 1982; J. Rivier *et al.*, 1984). Additionally, CRF concentrations have been measured in hypophyseal portal plasma of pentobarbital-anesthetized rats. Gibbs and Vale (1982) found CRF concentrations of approximately 100 pM under these conditions and a basal secretory rate of 1.6 pg/min that was not affected by dexamethasone. Hemorrhage (15% decrease of total blood volume, a severe physiologic stress) resulted in a twofold rise in CRF concentration under similar conditions (Plotsky and Vale, 1984). This rise was abolished by dexamethasone pretreatment. Both intravenous and intracerebroventricular (icv) CRF injection cause ACTH and beta-endorphin release from the adrenohypophysis, and this effect is attenuated by dexamethasone pretreatment (Donald et al., 1983). CRF has also been shown to increase the rate of synthesis of ACTH as determined by increases in pro-opiomelanocortin (POMC) mRNA concentrations. Additionally, long-term administration of CRF has been shown to increase the actual number of pituitary corticotrophs (Gertz et al., 1987), an effect exhibiting the trophic nature of CRF.

As noted above, several studies have shown that glucocorticoids can attenuate both CRF and ACTH secretion. The mechanisms of this negative feedback are multiple, complex, and poorly understood. Negative feedback loops have been characterized by their latency period into a fast and slow component. The fast feedback loop acts within minutes at the level of the anterior pituitary to reduce ACTH secretion and does not seem to be mediated through neural mechanisms. It most probably results from an alteration of calcium flux that stabilizes the corticotroph membrane and thus inhibits ACTH release in the presence of high glucocorticoid concentrations (Gagner and Drouin, 1985; Widmaier and Dallman, 1984). The slow or delayed feedback has a longer latency period and is believed to be mediated at the level of the hippocampus, hypothalamus, and POMC transcription in the pituitary. This delayed feedback most probably represents inhibition of both ACTH synthesis and release (Jones and Hillhouse, 1976). Plasma corticosterone concentrations of 8–12 μg/dl suppress the increase in portal plasma CRF concentrations induced by nitroprusside (a hypotensive stressor), whereas corticosterone concentrations of 40 μg/dl are necessary to reduce basal portal plasma CRF concentrations (Plotsky et al., 1985).

The effects of CRF on ACTH release can be potentiated by a number of other, weaker ACTH secretagogues. The consistent detection of residual ACTH release above baseline values in stressed rats injected with anti-CRF serum is concordant with this finding (Rivier and Vale, 1983a). Treatment with the ganglionic blocking agent chlorisondamine or a V_1 vasopressin receptor antagonist partially prevents the normal elevation of plasma ACTH in stressed rats; when given in conjunction with anti-CRF serum it completely abolishes this rise (Rivier and Vale, 1983a). These results strongly indicate that, even though CRF represents a major regulator of ACTH release in response to stress, other factors are involved (i.e., peripheral catecholamines, vasopressin, etc). The mechanism here most probably involves the synergistic interactions observed between CRF, catecholamines, and AVP *in vitro* and *in vivo* (Vale *et al.*, 1983; Rivier and Vale, 1983a). These synergisms may in fact involve interactions at the pituitary CRF receptor not unlike those of the benzodiazepines and barbituates at the GABA receptor.

CRF has also been proposed to be a CNS regulator with integrative properties coordinating the organism's biological functions following stress (Axelrod and Reisine, 1984). When injected icv or directly into the CNS, CRF produces effects that are clearly not mediated by modulation of the HPA axis. Administration in this manner of as little as 19 nmol of CRF produces physiological changes very much like those observed during the stress response. Intracerebroventricular CRF increases heart rate, oxygen consumption, mean arterial pressure, and blood glucose and catecholamine concentrations. All of the above appear to be mediated by increased central sympathetic outflow (Brown *et al.*, 1982; Fisher and Brown, 1984). It is important to note that after icv injection into the third ventricle of conscious dogs, the concentration of CRF has been measured in the peripheral circulation. No increase in plasma CRF was observed, suggesting that CRF did not leak into the periphery and initiate the above changes (Lenz *et al.*, 1985).

Microinjection studies have been performed in an attempt to localize the CNS site of action of CRF. These studies indicate that no single brain area is responsible for the observed responses to exogenous CRF injection (Brown, 1986). Recently, it has been reported that the increases in heart rate, mean arterial pressure, and locomotion following icv CRF can be blocked by pretreatment with iv naloxone (Saunders and Thornhill, 1986). This suggests that the increased sympathetic activation, caused by icv CRF administration may be under endogenous opioid control. Valentino *et al.* (1986) have reported increases in both HPA and locus ceruleus (LC) activity following icv CRF, with no concomitant changes in blood pressure. It has also been demonstrated that icv, but not iv, CRF suppresses gastrointestinal motor activity, an effect that is observed in stressed animals (Bueno and Fioramonti, 1986), and moreover that CNS CRF administration acts to inhibit gastric acid secretion through vagal and adrenal mechanisms, which are not mediated by activation of the HPA axis (Tache *et al.*, 1983).

The central administration of exogenous CRF produces a variety of behavioral effects. Intracerebroventricular CRF decreases food intake after food deprivation (Morley and Levine, 1982). When infused into the arcuate–ventromedial hypothalamus and the mesencephalic gray, CRF suppresses sexual receptivity in the female rat (Sirinathsinghji *et al.*, 1983). CRF given icv in the home environment produces a dose-dependent locomotor activation in rats that cannot be reproduced by iv injection of the peptide (Sutton *et al.*, 1982). CRF also increases grooming behavior and changes the frequency of behaviors normally elicited in response to a novel environment (Britton *et al.*, 1982). These behavioral responses are generally insensitive to dexamethasone administration (Britton *et al.*, 1986a), are not abolished by hypophysectomy, and appear to be receptor mediated (Britton *et al.*, 1986b). The changes in locomotor activity caused by CRF are not mediated by the mesolimbic and mesocortical dopamine systems (Kalivas *et al.*, 1987). This suggests that the stress-like behavioral effects of CRF are neurochemically different from those produced by more common stressors, like footshock or restraint. Also, there is no evidence that icv CRF produces analgesia which is well known to occur after stress (Sherman and Kalin, 1986).

In summary, it should be emphasized that icv administration of CRF produces behavioral changes generally consistent with increased emotionality and arousal (states generally elicited by most stressors). These changes include increased locomotion, grooming, rearing, vocalization, sniffing, and decreased feeding. CRF also appears to potentiate the effects of exposure to a novel environment. These anxiogenic effects of CRF are opposite to those of most anxiolytics. Thus, these data lend support to the hypothesis that CRF, endogenous to the CNS, acts in a nonendocrine fashion as a modulator of the stress response.

Another line of investigation relevant to the role of CRF in the stress response concerns the CNS distribution of CRF and the changes that occur in CRF concentration in response to stressful stimuli. Using micropunch dissection techniques coupled with a sensitive and specific CRF radioimmunoassay, we have determined the distribution of CRF in 32 rat brain nuclei. Measurable concentrations of CRF were found in all the areas studied (Chappell *et al.*, 1986), and the pattern of distribution generally parallels that visualized by immunohistochemical techniques. Functional roles for chemical messengers in the CNS can often be inferred from neuroanatomic localization. Thus, given its role as a hypothalamic releasing factor, CRF was found in highest concentration in the pariventricular nucleus (PVN) and median eminence. Relatively high concentrations of CRF were also discovered in the amygdala, the bed nucleus of the stria terminalis, and the raphe nuclei. High CRF concentrations were also noted in brain regions containing major perikarya for the catecholamine and indoleamine neurotransmitters. Thus CRF seems strategically located to influence the activity of the monoamine containing systems of the CNS.

The heterogeneous distribution of CRF is in agreement with its putative role as a neurotransmitter or neuromodulator in the CNS. Indeed, studies have shown that CRF fulfills several of the requisite criteria to be considered a CNS neurotransmitter. Our group was the first to demonstrate potassium-induced, calcium-dependent release of CRF from slices of hypothalamus, amygdala, midbrain, striatum, and cortex (Smith *et al.*, 1986;

Owens *et al.*, 1987). Electrophysiological studies have revealed that microinfusion of CRF alters the firing rate of CNS neurons in the locus ceruleus (LC) (Valentino *et al.*, 1983). The LC contains the major noradrenergic cell population that projects to the forebrain. This circuit has been implicated in the pathogenesis of both depression and anxiety (Svensson, 1987). CRF has also been shown to alter firing rates in the hippocampus and causes EEG changes suggestive of increased arousal in the hippocampus and cortex (Ehlers *et al.*, 1983; Aldenhoff *et al.*, 1983).

To further investigate the effects of stress on endogenous CRF, we (Chappell *et al.*, 1986) also measured CRF concentrations in 36 microdissected rat brain regions following either acute stress (immobilization for 3 h at 4°C) or chronic stress (series of unpredictable stressors for 13 days). Because stress is known to activate the HPA axis, a reduction in CRF concentration in the median eminence of the hypothalamus was predicted. A 50% reduction was, in fact, observed in both the acute and chronic stress groups. Also of interest was the twofold rise of CRF concentrations in the LC in both the acute and chronic stress groups. Chronically stressed rats also exhibited increased CRF concentrations in the anterior hypothalamic and periventricular nuclei and decreased CRF concentration in the dorsal vagal complex. Thus it appears that in chronically stressed rats the rate of CRF synthesis in neurons that project to the median eminence is unable to keep pace with its release. Measurement of concentrations alone cannot distinguish between alterations in synthesis, release, or degradation. It is, however, interesting to note that the LC was one of the few regions to exhibit a stress-related change in this experiment, especially in light of the data, discussed above, demonstrating the ability of CRF to alter neuronal firing rates in this brain area.

The concantenation of findings presented above strongly suggests that CRF functions as the major physiological integrator of the stress response. In this regard CRF is now recognized to function as both a hormone (in the endocrine system) and a neurotransmitter.

III. CRF and Depression

Because CRF plays a preeminent role in the HPA axis, is a major neurotransmitter peptide in the CNS, mediates the stress response, and finally because it is well established that drug-free patients who fulfill criteria for major depression are as a group hypercortisolemic, it was logical to investigate whether CRF hypersecretion was responsible for this HPA axis hyperactivity. In reviewing the data concerning the possible linkage of CRF to major depression, two salient facts must be kept in mind. First, direct CNS experimentation cannot, for the most part, be performed on humans. Thus, researchers are forced to rely on indirect techniques, which often fail to provide indisputable proof of their hypotheses. Second, in an organism as complicated as the human, virtually no deviation in homeostasis goes uncompensated. Major depression quite likely represents a state in which several compensatory alterations have been made, perhaps before psychopathology is evident.

To directly test the hypothesis that CRF is hypersecreted in depression, our group, in a series of studies, measured the concentration of CRF in cerebrospinal fluid (CSF) using a sensitive and specific radioimmunoassay (Nemeroff *et al.*, 1984). In our first study, the concentration of CRF in CSF was found to be elevated in drug-free depressed patients compared to normal controls, schizophrenics, or patients with senile dementia. Eleven of the 23 depressed patients exhibited CRF CSF concentrations greater than that of the highest control. In a second study (Banki *et al.*, 1987) we measured CSF CRF concentrations in a large number of depressed and schizophrenic, as well as control, subjects. The depressed patients showed an almost twofold elevation versus the control group. The schizophrenic patients had a small but significant elevation in their CSF CRF concentrations, largely because of high levels in three patients. We have also recently reported on CSF CRF concentrations in patients with chronic pain (France *et al.*, 1988). Chronic pain patients, with or without major depression, do not exhibit the elevated CSF CRF concentrations observed in the depressed patients.

The nonnormal distribution of CSF CRF concentrations observed in these studies suggests that there may be a subgroup of depressed patients with elevated CSF CRF concentrations. In all of the above studies CSF CRF concentrations were not correlated with dexamethasone suppression test (DST) results. However, Roy and his colleagues (1987), though unable to reproduce our finding of increased CSF CRF concentrations in the depressed group as a whole, found DST nonsuppressors to have significantly higher CSF concentrations of CRF than DST suppressors. Recently Risch *et al.* (1989) confirmed the increase in CSF CRF concentrations in drug-free depressed patients.

In a very recent study (Arato *et al.*, 1989) we obtained cisternal and lumbar CSF from completed suicide victims and sudden death controls. Again we observed marked elevations in CRF concentrations in the CSF of the suicide victims, some of whom certainly were depressed. By obtaining both cisternal and lumbar CSF in this study, we were also able to demonstrate a rostral–caudal gradient for CRF in CSF. This was interpreted as indicating a supraspinal source for the peptide. The exact neuroanatomical source of CRF in CSF remains a subject for future investigation.

The above data led us to hypothesize that chronic hypersecretion of

CRF in the CNS would lead to a reduction in the number of CRF binding sites (downregulation) in the CNS of depressed individuals. This hypothesis is based upon the well-established phenomenon in pharmacology, neurobiology, and endocrinology that chronic exposure to an agonist results in a compensatory decrease in the number of postsynaptic receptor binding sites. Our group therefore measured the affinity and number of CRF binding sites in the frontal cortex of a group suicide victims and age- and sex-matched, sudden death controls (Nemeroff et al., 1988). Scatchard analysis of the data over a wide range of concentrations revealed no difference in the affinity of the radioligand for its receptor. There was, however, a 23% decrease in the receptor density (Bmax) in the suicide group. No significant correlations were found between receptor density and sex, age, or postmortem delay. These findings are taken as additional evidence of CRF hypersecretion in suicide victims, and, by extension, possibly major depression.

In a recent study (Nemeroff et al., 1990), the concentration of CRF in CSF was measured in a group of depressed patients prior to electroconvulsive theraphy (ECT) and 24 h after receiving their final treatment. There was a significant reduction in CSF CRF concentrations after the ECT regimen and concomitant clinical improvement. This indicates that elevated concentrations of CSF CRF in depressed patients, like hypercortisolemia, may represent a state, rather than a trait marker of depression.

Myriad studies in normal volunteers as well as in patients with a variety of endocrine and psychiatric disorders have shown that intravenously administered CRF increases the secretion of ACTH and other POMC products from the anterior pituitary. The CRF-induced increase in plasma ACTH and cortisol concentrations is clearly dose dependent. In human subjects, ovine CRF produces a more robust response that rat/human CRF owing to its longer plasma half-life. Schulte et al. (1985) continously administered ovine CRF to human volunteers for 8–24 h. This resulted in an increase in plasma ACTH and cortisol concentrations in a pattern similar to that seen in depressed patients. Despite the high constant level of CRF maintained throughout this study, a persistent circadian rhythm of ACTH was observed. Thus the circadian variations of HPA axis activity cannot be completely explained merely by a circadian periodicity in CRF release. The availability of synthetic CRF lead to the development of a CRF stimulation test (Gold et al., 1984; Holsboer et al., 1984). This testing paradigm has been used quite successfully in the differential diagnosis of the two types of ACTH-dependent Cushing's syndrome (pituitary-dependent versus ectopic ACTH syndrome). The CRF stimulation test has also been studied in patients with psychiatric disorders. As a group, patients with major depression exhibit a blunted ACTH response to CRF when compared to normal controls. This finding has been replicated in other laboratories (Amsterdam *et al.*, 1988) and by our group in DST nonsuppressors (C. B. Nemeroff, K. R. R. Krishnan, J. C. Ritchie, and B. J. Carroll, unpublished observations). Whether the blunted ACTH response is secondary to the negative feedback of cortisol on the anterior pituitary or is due to the downregulation of CRF receptors on the corticotrophs caused by chronic CRF hypersecretion is currently unknown. In an effort to clarify this issue von Bardeleben and Holsboer (1989) reported on a combined dexamethasone–CRF challenge test. These researchers performed the standard CRF stimulation test while their subjects were under the influence of high glucocorticoid feedback. If ACTH blunting in depressed patients were due solely to high negative glucocorticoid feedback, one would predict that blunting would be seen both in the normal controls and the depressed patients. Unfortunately, ACTH concentrations were not reported in this study. However, plasma cortisol concentrations were completely blunted by dexamethasone pretreatment, but in the control group only. Interestingly, the depressed group exhibited a marked cortisol rise after CRF under these circumstances. These data indicate that hypercortisolemia per se is not responsible for the blunted ACTH response to CRF in depression. These authors also speculate that "synergistic factors" such as AVP are probably involved here, emphasizing again the partially compensated nature of the depressed state.

It should be noted that similar HPA responses (i.e., ACTH blunting) have been shown to occur in patients with panic disorder, alcoholism, and anorexia nervosia (Holsboer *et al.*, 1987; Hotta *et al.*, 1986). Because all of these states are characterized by a hypercortisolemia, these findings do little to clarify the current controversy.

Measurement of peripheral plasma CRF-like immunoreactivity was first accomplished by Suda *et al.* (1985) using immunoaffinity chromatography and RIA technology. They reported basal plasma CRF concentrations of 6 ± 0.5 pg/ml. Plasma CRF concentrations were reportedly altered by stress and negative glucorticoid feedback and exhibited a circadian rhythm. Additionally, plasma CRF concentrations were increased in Addison's disease and were low but detectable in Cushing's syndrome. These results suggest that a major component of plasma CRF is of hypothalamic origin. The authors also stated that other extrahypothalamic sources could not be ruled out as a minor source of plasma CRF. In the same year Cunnah *et al.* (1985) reported in a similar study, using a different RIA, that normal plasma CRF concentrations ranged from 20 to 108 pg/ml did not change with insulin hypoglycemia, were unaffected by dexamethasone pretreatment, were elevated in Cushing's syndrome, and were extremely high (550–9300 pg/ml) in plasma from pregnant women in the third trimester. They concluded that the principle source of plasma CRF was not the hypothalamus. The following year two groups published the first plasma CRF measurements in psychiatric patients (Charlton *et al.*, 1986; Widerlov *et al.*, 1986). The English group used a direct two-site immunoradiometric assay (IRMA) and was unable to show any diurnal variation in CRF plasma levels or any difference between depressed and control individuals. Widerlov *et al.* used a conventional RIA and found CRF concentrations to be significantly higher in the depressed group. To date, several more studies have appeared concerning plasma CRF and its possible sources (Stalla *et al.*, 1987; Sasaki *et al.*, 1987a; Yokoe *et al.*, 1988; Sumitomo *et al.*, 1987). These studies seem evenly divided over the issue of the ultimate source of CRF in peripheral plasma. The situation is not unlike the current debate surrounding the monoamine metabolite 3-methoxy-4-hydroxyphenethyleneglycol (MHPG) and its sources. The problem is complex because, like MHPG, several peripheral tissue sources of CRF have been identified (i.e., pancreas, testes, adrenal medulla, placenta). Also, not unlike MHPG, the percentage of CRF in the periphery due to hypothalamic sources may vary based on the status of the organism. CRF immunoreactivity has also recently been described in urine (Maser-Gluth and Vecsei, 1989). If this observation is confirmed, the measurement of 24-h excretion patterns of CRF may prove more useful than isolated plasma concentrations. We are unaware of any other recent studies of plasma CRF in psychiatric patients.

Recently a plasma binding protein for CRF has been described (Orth and Mount, 1987; Linton *et al.*, 1988; Ellis *et al.*, 1988). Although this protein has not been completely characterized, it is thought to be of approximately 40,000 molecular weight and to not bind ovine CRF. The binding protein does not appear to be present in sheep or rat plasma, and binding requires both the N-terminal and C-terminal sequences of human CRF_{1-41}. The plasma binding protein does not appear to be related to either of the putative CRF receptors, central or pituitary (Errol DeSousa, personal communication). These findings indicate that the direct RIA of human CRF in unextracted plasma leads to spurious results and may explain the discrepancies in CRF concentrations observed using affinity-purified RIAs or direct IRMAs. Additionally, it is tempting to speculate on why CRF is protected in the periphery, if in fact that is the purpose of the carrier molecule. Does this imply a function for CRF in the periphery, or is coupling to the binding protein necessary to prevent the passage of peripheral CRF into the CNS? Further research will obviously be necessary to solve these intriguing questions.

Special mention must also be made of the high concentrations of CRF found in maternal plasma in the last trimester of pregnancy. Sasaki *et al.*,

(1984) published the first study concerning plasma CRF concentrations during pregnancy. These workers found high concentrations of CRF in maternal plasma during the third trimester of pregnancy. CRF concentrations were undetectable (<10 pg/ml) during the first and second trimester, 1 day postpartum, and in nonpregnant women. Since the original observation, several additional studies have been published (Goland et al., 1986; Maser-Gluth et al., 1987; Loatikainen et al., 1987; Sasaki et al., 1987a; Campbell et al., 1987). All confirm the original findings and show a direct correlation between maternal CRF plasma levels and gestational age. Linton et al. (1988) demonstrated that the bulk of CRF in maternal plasma is bound to the binding protein and exhibits reduced bioactivity. Frim et al. (1988) conclusively showed that the source of CRF in late pregancy plasma is the placenta itself. Using molecular biology techniques these researchers were able to demonstrate that placental CRF mRNA was identical to that of hypothalamic CRF mRNA. Also, placental CRF mRNA content increased in parallel with the rise in CRF concentration. Campbell et al. (1987) also found low CRF levels in umbilical cord plasma. This implies a limited transfer of placental CRF to the fetus and suggests a limited role for it within the fetus. Thus a physiological purpose for the late rise of CRF during pregnancy has yet to be ascertained. The identification of yet another hypothalamic releasing hormone in the placenta may just be another indicator of the totipotent nature of the placenta. It is interesting to postulate that perhaps CRF plays a paracrine role in regulating protein expression and secretion from the placenta, or perhaps its role is to ready the maternal physiology for the stress of labor and delivery. It is also possible that the precipitous fall in CRF, ACTH, and cortisol levels in the maternal plasma, at the time of delivery, leaves the HPA axis in a totally uncompensated state and may be involved in the development of a postpartum depression.

The possible mechanisms involving CRF and the pathogenesis of depression are numerous. If the blunted ACTH response to infused CRF in depressed patients is due to increased CRF secretion from the CNS, one may postulate mechanisms involving defective second messenger systems in the pituitary, increased noradrenergic drive to the hypothalamus from overdriven CRF-sensitive neurons in the LC or amygdala, or altered degradation of CRF by peptidases. If the CRF infusion findings are due to increased feedback at glucocorticoid pituitary receptors, one is tempted to recall the seminal work of Sapolsky and colleagues (1987), concerning age-associated decreases in stress responsiveness and the neurodegenerative properties of high glucocorticoid concentrations on the hippocampus. Further research initiatives will be necessary to elucidate the complete role of CRF in the etiology of depression.

IV. Summary

We have attempted to present a thorough topical review of current studies linking CRF to the stress response and major depression. This view is rendered plausible by both the clinical studies and the preclinical studies in which centrally administered CRF in animals produced behavioral effects similar to those seen in depressed patients. It seems likely from the studies described above that the activity of certain CRF-containing neurons is altered in major depression. The exact nature of the alteration(s) remains obscure. In major depression, CRF is most likely hypersecreted, resulting in increased CRF concentrations and downregulation of CRF receptors in the frontal cortex. The increased CRF secretion may be responsible, at least in part, for the activation of the HPA axis commonly observed in depressed patients. It remains unclear, however, which, CRF-responsive or -containing neurons are hyperactive in depression. No data are currently available concerning CRF biosynthesis rates in brain tissue as assessed, for example, by *in situ* hybridization techniques. Similarly, we are ignorant regarding the exact source of CRF in CSF or in plasma. Finally, virtually nothing is known about the regulation of the processing of CRF from its prohormone or of the peptidases responsible for its degradation. Nevertheless, the bulk of current findings is concordant with the view that CRF plays a role in the final common pathway of the stress response. The development of new pharmacological treatments for the affective disorders, based on these and future studies, may prove benefical to those patients who do not respond to traditional treatments.

Acknowledgments

This work was supported by NIMH grants MH-42510, MH-42088, and MH-40159. We are grateful to Andrea Laws for the preparation of this manuscript.

References

Aldenhoff, J. B., Giul, P. L., Rivier, J., Vale, W., and Siggins, G. R. (1983). Corticotropin-releasing factor decreases postburst hyperpolarizations and excites hippocampal neurons. *Science* **221**, 875–877.

Amsterdam, J. D., Maeslin, G., Winokur, A., Berioisly, N., Kling, M., and Gold, P. W. (1988). The oCRH stimulation test before and after clinical recovery from depression. *J. Affective Disord.* **14**, 213–222.

Arato, M., Banki, C. M., Bissette, G., and Nemeroff, C. B. (1989). Elevated cerebrospinal fluid concentrations of corticotropin-releasing factor in suicide victims. *Biol. Psychiatry* **25**, 355–359.

Axelrod, J., and Reisine, T. D. (1984). Stress hormones: Their interaction and regulation. *Science* **224**, 452–459.

Banki, C. M., Bissette, G., Arato, M. O'Connor, L., and Nemeroff, C. B. (1987). Cerebrospinal fluid corticotropin-releasing factor-like immunoreactivity in depression and schizophrenia. *Am. J. Psychiatry* **144**, 873–877.

Britton, D. R., Koob, G. F., Rivier, J., and Vale, W. (1982). Intraventricular corticotropin-releasing factor enhances behavioral effects of novelty. *Life Sci.* **31**, 363–367.

Britton, K. T., Lee, G., Dana, R., Risch, S. C., and Koob, G. F. (1986a). Activating and "anxiogenic" effects of corticotropin-releasing factor are not inhibited by blockade of the pituitary-adrenal system with dexamethasone. *Life Sci.* **39**, 1281–1286.

Britton, K. T., Lee, G., Vale, W., Rivier, J., and Koob, G. F. (1986b). Corticotropin releasing factor (CRF) receptor antagonist blocks activating and anxiogenic actions of CRF in the rat. *Brain Res.* **369**, 303–306.

Brown, M. (1986). Corticotropin releasing factor: Central nervous system sites of action. *Brain Res.* **399**, 10–14.

Brown, M. R., Risher, L. A., Rivier, J., Spiess, J., Rivier, C., and Vale, W. (1982). Corticotropin-releasing factor: Effects on the sympathetic nervous system and oxygen consumption. *Life Sci.* **30**, 207–210.

Bruhn, T. O., Engeland, W. C., Anthony, E. L. P., Gann, D. S., and Jackson, I. M. D. (1987). Corticotropin-releasing factor in dog adrenal medulla is secreted in response to hemmorrhage. *Endocrinology (Baltimore)* **120**, 25–33.

Bueno, L., and Fioramonti, J. (1986). Effects of corticotropin-releasing factor, corticotropin, and cortisol on gastrointestinal motility in dogs. *Peptides (N.Y.)* **7**, 73–77.

Campbell, E. A., Linton, E. A., Wolfe, C. D. A., Scraggs, P. R., Jones, M. T., and Lowry P. J. (1987). Plasma corticotropin-releasing hormone concentrations during pregnancy and parturition. *J. Clin. Endocrinol. Metab.* **64**, 1054–1059.

Chappell, P. B., Smith, M. A., Kilts, C. D., Bissette, G., Ritchie, J., Anderson, C., and Nemeroff, C. B. (1986). Alterations in CRF-like immunoreactivity in discrete brain regions after acute and chronic stress. *J. Neurosci.* **6**, 2908–2914.

Charlton, B. G., Leake, A., Ferrier, I. N., Linton, E. A., and Lowry, P. J. (1986). Corticotropin-releasing factor in plasma of depressed patients and controls. *Lancet* 161–162.

Cunnah, D., Jessop, D. S., Perry, L. Afshar, F., Setchell, M., and Rees, L. H. (1985). Measurement of plasma and cerebrospinal fluid levels of human corticotropin-releasing factor. *J. Endocrinol., Suppl.* **107**, 18, Abstr. 31, 649.

Donald, R. A., Redekopp, C., Cameron, V., Nicholls, M. G., Bolton, J., Livesey, J., Espiner, E. A., Rivier, J., and Vale, W. (1983). The hormonal actions of corticotropin-releasing factor in sheep: Effect of intravenous and intracerebroventricular injection. *Endocrinology (Baltimore)* **113**, 886–870.

Ehlers, C. L., Henriksen, S. J., Wang, M., Rivier, J., Vale, W., and Bloom, F. E. (1983). Corticotropin releasing factor produces increases in brain excitability and convulsive seizures in rats. *Brain Res.* **278**, 332–337.

Ellis, M. J., Livesey, J. H., and Donald, R. A. (1988). Circulating plasma corticotropin-releasing factor-like immunoreactivity. *J. Endocr.* **227**, 299–307.

Fisher, L. A., and Brown, M. R. (1984). Corticotropin-releasing factor and angeotensin II: Comparison of CNS actions to influence neuroendocrine and cardiovascular function. *Brain Res.* **296**, 41–47.

France, R. D., Urban, B., Krishnan, K. R. R., Bissette, G., Banki, C. M., Nemeroff, C. B., and

Speilman, F. J. (1988). Corticotropin-releasing factor-like immunoreactivity in chronic pain patients with and without major depression. *Biol. Psychiatry* **23**, 86–88.

Frim, D. M., Emanuel, R. L., Robinson, B. G., Smas, C. M., Adler, G. K., and Majzoub, J. A. (1988). Characterization and gestational regulation of corticotropin-releasing hormone messenger RNA in human placenta. *J. Clin. Invest.* **88**, 287–292.

Gagner, J. P., and Drouin, J. (1985). Opposite regulation of pro-opiomelanocortin gene transcription by glucocorticoids and CRH. *Mol. Cell. Endocrinol.* **40**, 25–32.

Gertz, B. J., Contreras, L. N., McComb, D. J., Kovacs, K., Tyrrell, J. B., and Dallman, M. F. (1987). Chronic administration of corticotropin-releasing factors increases pituitary corticotroph number. *Endocrinology (Baltimore)* **120**, 381–388.

Gibbs, D. M., and Vale, W. (1982). Presence of corticotropin-releasing factor-like immunoreactivity in hypophysial portal blood. *Endocrinology (Baltimore)* **111**, 1418–1420.

Goland, R. S., Wardlaw, S. L., Stark, R. I., Brown, L. S., and Frantz, A. G. (1986). High levels of corticotropin-releasing hormone immunoactivity in maternal and fetal plasma during pregnancy. *J. Clin. Endocrinol. Metab.* **63**, 1199–1203.

Gold, P. W., Chrousos, G., Kellner, C., Post, R., Augerinos, P., Schulte, H., Oldfield, E., and Loriaux, D. L. (1984). Psychiatric implications of basic and clinical studies with corticotropin-releasing factor. *Am. J. Psychiatry* **141**, 619–627.

Holsboer, F., Bardeleben, U. V., Gerken, A., Stalla, G. K., and Muller, D. A. (1984). Blunted corticotropin and normal cortisol response to human corticotropin releasing factor in depression. *N. Engl. J. Med.* **311**, 1127–1130.

Holsboer, F., Bardelaben, U. V., Butler, R., Heuser, I., and Steiger, A. (1987). Stimulation response to corticotropin-releasing hormone (CRH) in patients with depression, alcoholism, and panic disorder. *Horm. Metab. Res., Suppl.* **16**, 80–88.

Hotta, M., Shibasaki, T., Masuda, A., Imaki, T., Demura, H., Ling, N., and Shizume, K. (1986). The responses of plasma adrenocorticotrophin and cortisol to corticotrophin-releasing hormone (CRH) and cerebrospinal fluid immunoreactive CRF in anorexia nervosa patients. *J. Clin. Endocrinol. Metab.* **62**, 319–324.

Jones, M. T., and Hillhouse, E. W. (1976). Structure-activity relationship and the mode of action of corticosteroid feedback on the secretion of corticotropin-releasing factor (corticoliberin). *J. Steroid Biochem.* **7**, 1189–1202.

Kalivas, P. W., Duffy, P., Latimer, L. G. (1987). Neurochemical and behavioral effects of corticotropin-releasing factor in the ventral tegmental area of the rat. *J. Pharmacol. Exp. Ther.* **242**, 757–764.

Lenz, H. J., Fisher, L. A., Vale, W. W., and Brown, M. R. (1985). Corticortopin-releasing factor, sauvagine, urotensin-I: Effects on blood flow. *Am. J. Physiol.* **249** (Regul. Integr. Comp. Physiol. 18), R85–R90.

Linton, E. A., Tilders, F. J. H., Hodgkinson, S., Berkenbosch, F., Vermes, I., and Lowry, P. J. (1985). Stress induced secretion of adrenocorticotropin in rats is inhibited by administration of antisera to ovine corticotropin-releasing factor and vasopressin. *Endocrinology (Baltimore)* **116**, 966–969.

Linton, E. A., Wolfe, C. D. A., Behan, D. P., and Lowry, P. J. (1988). A specific carrier substance for human corticotropin releasing factor in late gestational maternal plasma which could mask the ACTH-releasing activity. *Clin. Endocrinol. (Oxford)* **28**, 315–324.

Loatikainen, T., Virtanen, T., Raisanen, I., and Salminen, K. (1987). Immunoreactive corticotropin-releasing factor and corticotropin during pregnancy, labor and puerperium. *Neuropeptides (Edinburgh)* **10**, 343–353.

Maser-Gluth, C., and Vecsei, P. (1989). Corticotropin-releasing factor-like immunoreactivity in human 24 H urine. *Clin. Endocrinol. (Oxford)* **30**, 405–412.

Maser-Gluth, C., Lorenz, U., and Vecsei, P. (1987). In pregnancy corticotropin-releasing-factor in maternal blood and aminiotic fluid correlates with gestational age. *Horm. Metab. Res., Suppl.* **16,** 42–46.

Morley, J. E., and Levine, A. S. (1982). Corticotropin releasing factor, grooming and ingestive behavior. *Life Sci.* **31,** 1459–1464.

Nemeroff, C. B., Widerlov, E., Bissette, G., Walleus, H., Karlsson, I., Kilts, C. D., Vale, W., and Loosen, P. T. (1984). Elevated concentrations of CSF corticotropin-releasing factor-like immunoreactivity in depressed patients. *Science* **226,** 1342–1344.

Nemeroff, C. B., Owens, M. J., Bissette, G., Andorn, A. C., and Stanley, M. (1988). Reduced corticotropin-releasing factor (CRF) binding sites in the frontal cortex of suicides. *Arch. Gen. Psychiatry* **45,** 577–579.

Nemeroff, C. B., Bissette, G., Akil, H., and Fink, M. (1990). Cerebrospinal fluid neuropeptides in depressed patients treated with ECT: Corticotropin-releasing factor, β-endorphin, and somatostatin. *Br. J. Psychiatry* (in press).

Orth, D. N., and Mount, C. D. (1987). Specific high-affinity binding protein for human corticotropin-releasing hormone in normal human plasma. *Biochem. Biophys. Res. Commun.* **143**(2), 411–417.

Owens, J. J., Maynor, B., and Nemeroff, C. B. (1987). Release of corticotropin-releasing factor (CRF) from rat prefrontal cortex *in vitro. Soc. Neurosci. Abstr.* **13,** 1110.

Plotsky, P. M., and Vale, W. (1984). Hemorrhage-induced secretion of corticotropin releasing factor like immunoreactivity into the rat hypophysial portal circulation and its inhibition by glucocorticoids. *Endocrinology (Baltimore)* **114,** 164–169.

Plotsky, P. M., Otto, S., and Sapolsky, R. M. (1985). Inhibition of immunoreactive corticotropin releasing factor secretion into the hypophysial portal circulation by delayed glucocorticoid feedback. *Endocrinology (Baltimore)* **119,** 1126–1130.

Risch, S. C., Lewine, R. J., Jewart, R. D., Pollard, W. E., Kalin, N. H., Stipetic, M., Risby, E. D., and Brummer, M. (1989). The relationship between lateral ventricle size and CSF peptides and neurotransmitters in depressed patients and normal controls. *Proc. 28th Annu. Meet. Am. Coll. Neuropsychopharmacol.,* p. 205.

Rivier, C., and Vale, W. (1983a). Modulation of stress-induced ACTH release by corticotropin-releasing factor, catecholamines, and vasopressin. *Nature (London)* **305,** 325–327.

Rivier, C., and Vale, W. (1983b). Interaction of corticotropin-releasing factor and arginine vasopressin on adrenocorticotropin secretion *in vivo. Endocrinology (Baltimore)* **113,** 939–942.

Rivier, C., Rivier, J., and Vale, W. (1982). Inhibition of adrenocorticotropic hormone secretion in the rat by immunoneutralization of corticotropin-releasing factor. *Science* **218,** 377–379.

Rivier, J., Rivier, C., and Vale, W. (1984). Synt etic competitive antagonists of corticotropin-releasing factor: Effect on ACTH secretion in the rat. *Science* **224,** 889–891.

Roy, A., Pickar, D., Paul, S., Doran, A., Chrousos, G. P., and Gold, P. W. (1987). CSF corticotropin-releasing hormone in depressed patients and normal control subjects. *Am. J. Psychiatry* **144,** 641–645.

Sapolsky, R., Armanine, M., and Packan, M. A. (1987). Stress and glucocorticoids in aging. *Endocrinol. Metab. Clin.* **16,** 965–980.

Sasaki, A., Liotta, A. S., Luckey, M. M., Margioris, A. N., Suda, T., and Krieger, D. T. (1984). Immunoreactive corticotropin-releasing factor is present in human maternal plasma during the third trimester of pregnancy. *J. Clin. Endocrinol. Metab.* **59**(4), 812–814.

Sasaki, A., Sato, S., Murakami, O., Go, M., Inoue, M., Shimizu, Y., Hanew, K., Andoh, N., Sato, I., Sasano, N., and Yoshinaga, K. (1987a). Immunoreactive corticotropin-releasing hormone present in human plasma may be derived from both hypothalamic and extrahypothalamic sources. *J. Clin. Endocrinol. Metab.* **65**, 176–181.

Sasaki, A., Shinkawa, O., Margioris, A. N., Liotta, A. S., Sato, S., Murakami, O., Go, M., Shimizu, Y., and Hanew, K. (1987b). Immunoreactive corticotropin releasing hormone in human plasma during pregnancy, labor, and delivery. *J. Clin. Endocrinol. Metab.* **64**, 224–229.

Saunders, W. S., and Thornhill, J. A. (1986). Pressor, tachycardic, and behavioral excitatory responses in conscious rats following ICV administration of ACTH and CRF are blocked by naloxone pretreatment. *Peptides (N.Y.)* **7**, 597–601.

Schulte, H. M., Chrousos, G. P., Gold, P. W., Booth, J. D., Oldfield, E. H., Cutler, G. B., and Loriaux, D. L. (1985). Continous administration of synthetic ovine corticotropin-releasing factor in man. *J. Clin. Invest.* **75**, 781–785.

Sherman, J. E., and Kalin, N. H. (1986). ICV-CRH potently affects behavior without altering antinociceptive responding. *Life Sci.* **39**, 433–441.

Sirinathsinghji, D. J. S., Rees, L. H., Rivier, J., and Vale, W. (1983). Corticotropin-releasing factor is a potent inhibitor of sexual receptivity in the female rat. *Nature (London)* **305**, 232–235.

Smith, M. A., Bissette, G., Slotkin, T. A., Knight, D. L., and Nemeroff, C. B. (1986). Release of corticotropin-releasing factor from rat brain regions *in vitro*. *Endocrinology (Baltimore)* **118**, 1997–2004.

Stalla, G. K., Stalla J., von Werder, K., Muller, O. A., Ludecke, D. K., Schrell, U., and Fahlbusch, R. (1987). Corticotropin releasing hormone in plasma of patients with Cushing's disease. *Klin. Wochenschr.* **65**, 529–530.

Suda, T., Tomori, N., Yajima, F., Sumitoma, T., Nakagami, Y., Ushiyama, T., Demura, H., and Shizume, K. (1985). Immunoreactive corticotropin-releasing factor in human plasma. *J. Clin. Invest.* **76**, 2026–2029

Sumitomo, T., Suda, T., Tomori, N., Yajima, F., Nakagami, Y., Ushiyama, T., Demura, H., and Shizume, K. (1987). Immunoreactive corticotropin-releasing factor in rat plasma. *Endocrinology (Baltimore)* **120**, 1391–1396.

Sutton, R. E., Koob, G. F., Lemoal, M., Rivier, J., and Vale, W. W. (1982). Corticotropin releasing factor produces behavioral activation in rats. *Nature (London)* **297**, 331–333.

Svensson, T. H. (1987). Peripheral, autonomic regulation of locus coeruleus noradrenergic neurons in brain: Putative implications for psychiatry and psychopharmacology. *Psychopharmacology (Berlin)* **92**, 1–15.

Tache, Y., Goto, Y., Gunion, M. W., Vale, W., Rivier, J., and Brown, M. (1983). Inhibition of gastric acid secretion in rats by intercerebral injection of corticotropin-releasing factor. *Science* **222**, 935–937.

Vale, W., Spiess, C., Rivier, C., and Rivier, J. (1981). Characterization of a 41-residue ovine hypothalamic peptide that stimulates secretion of corticotropin and β-endorpin. *Science* **213**, 1394–1397.

Vale, W., Vaughan, J., Smith, M., Yamamoto, G., Rivier, J., and Rivier, C. (1983). Effects of synthetic ovine corticotropin releasing factor, glucocorticoids, catecholamines, neurohypophysial peptides, and other substances on cultured corticotropic cells. *Endocrinology (Baltimore)* **113**, 1121–1131.

Valentino, R. J., Foote, S. L., and Aston-Jones, G. (1983). Corticotropin-releasing factor activates noradrenergic neurons of the locus coeruleus. *Brain Res.* **270**, 363–366.

Valentino, R. J., Martin, D. L., and Suzuki, M. (1986). Dissociation of locus coeruleus activity and blood pressure: Effects of clonidine and corticotropin-releasing factor. *Neuropharmacology* **25**, 603–610.

von Bardeleben, U., and Holsboer, F. (1989). Cortisol response to a combined dexamethasone-human corticotrophin-releasing hormone challenge in patients with depression. *J. Neuroendocrinol.* **1**(6), 485–488.

Widerlov, E., Wahlestedt, C., Hakanson, R., and Ekmar, R. (1986). Altered brain neuropeptide function in psychiatric illnesses with special emphasis on NPV and CRF in major depression. *Clin. Neuropharmacol.* **9**, Suppl. 4, 572–575.

Widmaier, E. P., and Dallman, M. F. (1984). The effects of corticotropin-releasing factor on adrenocorticotropin secretion from perifused pituitaries *in vitro:* Rapid inhibition by glucocorticoids. *Endocrinology (Baltimore)* **115**, 2368–2374.

Yokoe, T., Audhya, T., Brown, C., Hutchinson, B., Passarelli, J., and Hollander, C. S. (1988). Corticotropin-releasing factor levels in the peripheral plasma and hypothalamus of the rat vary in parallel with changes in the pituitary-adrenal axis. *Endocrinology (Baltimore)* **123**, 1348–1354.

10

Use of Neuroendocrine Tests in the Psychiatric Assessment of the Medically Ill Patient

Diana O. Perkins
Department of Psychiatry
University of North Carolina
School of Medicine
Chapel Hill, North Carolina 27599-7160

Robert A. Stern
Department of Psychiatry
University of North Carolina
School of Medicine
Chapel Hill, North Carolina 27599-7160

Robert N. Golden
Department of Psychiatry
University of North Carolina
School of Medicine
Chapel Hill, North Carolina 27599-7160

*Helen L. Miller**
Department of Psychiatry
University of North Carolina
School of Medicine
Chapel Hill, North Carolina 27599-7160

Dwight L. Evans
Departments of Psychiatry & Medicine
University of North Carolina
School of Medicine
Chapel Hill, North Carolina 27599-7160

I. Introduction
II. Neuroendocrine Challenge Tests in Mood Disorders
III. Neuroendocrine Findings in Patients with Medical Illness and Mood Disorders
   A. Neuroendocrine Challenge Tests in Cancer
   B. Neuroendocrine Challenge Tests in Chronic Pain
   C. Neuroendocrine Challenge Tests in Neurological Diseases
   D. Neuroendocrine Challenge Tests in Thyroid Disease and Vitamin B_{12} Deficiency
   E. Neuroendocrine Challenge Tests in Other Medical Conditions
IV. Summary and Conclusions
   References

*Present address: Department of Psychiatry, Yale University School of Medicine, West Haven, Connecticut 06516.

I. Introduction

Diagnosing clinical depression is especially challenging in patients with medical illness. Symptoms and signs of depression, such as weight loss, apathy, insomnia, and low energy, may result either from the medical condition or as a complication of medical treatment. For this reason, an objective biological marker for clinical depression in the medically ill patient would have great value, as this could facilitate accurate diagnosis and effective treatment planning. Neuroendocrine challenge tests, in particular the dexamethasone suppression test (DST) and the thyrotropin-releasing hormone (TRH) stimulation test, have shown promise in this regard. These tests have been developed and extensively studied in psychiatric populations. The DST detects dysregulation in the hypothalamic–pituitary–adrenal (HPA) axis, while the TRH stimulation test detects dysregulation in the hypothalamic–pituitary–thyroid (HPT) axis.

While a substantial literature documents the occurrence of HPA and HPT axis dysregulation in many psychiatric patients with primary mood disorders (Golden and Potter, 1986), less is known about the biology of mood disorders associated with or caused by medical illness. Such depressive episodes often have many clinical similarities with major depressive episodes that occur in the psychiatric population. These similarities may be coincidental, or may reflect similar underlying biological alterations such as dysregulation in the HPA or HPT axes. The DST and the TRH stimulation tests thus have value as research tools for examining the function and status of the HPA and HPT axes in medically ill patients with major depression.

In a limited number of medical illnesses the DST and/or the TRH stimulation tests have been applied to patients with coexistent mood disorders. After summarizing the application of these neuroendocrine tests in psychiatric patients with primary mood disorders, we will review the diagnostic value and research uses of these neuroendocrine challenge tests in patients with cancer, chronic pain, a variety of neurological disorders such as dementia, stroke, Parkinson's disease, and multiple sclerosis, and in organic mood disorders secondary to vitamin B_{12} deficiency and thyroid disease.

II. Neuroendocrine Challenge Tests in Mood Disorders

Neuroendocrine challenge tests can provide insight into biological alterations associated with mood disorders. Patients with major depression frequently exhibit dysregulation of the HPA axis, as detected by nonsuppression of serum cortisol following administration of the synthetic glucocorticoid dexamethasone according to a standardized procedure (Carroll *et al.*, 1981). For example, in our previously reported study of hospitalized psychiatric patients, 63% of those meeting Diagnostic and Statistical Manual of Mental Disorders (DSM-III) criteria for a major depressive episode exhibited nonsuppression of serum cortisol at either 4 p.m. or 11 p.m. following the administration of a standard dexamethasone challenge. This percentage was significantly greater than in our control group, where only 14% of psychiatric inpatients not meeting criteria for a major mood disorder, but with depressive symptoms, exhibited cortisol nonsuppression (Evans and Nemeroff, 1987).

HPA axis hyperactivity as measured by the DST appears to be a state-related phenomenon. Normalization of HPA axis regulation (i.e., suppression of cortisol following dexamethasone administration) is associated with clinical improvement following antidepressant treatment. Furthermore, normalization of response may be correlated with decreased risk of relapse (Nemeroff and Evans, 1984). To the extent that cortisol nonsuppression following dexamethasone represents a "state" marker for depression, the DST may play a role in the clinical management of depressed patients (Evans and Golden, 1987).

The proportion of patients exhibiting cortisol nonsuppression following dexamethasone varies according to the subtype of mood disorder. In our study, the majority of patients suffering from the melancholic or psychotic subtypes of major depression exhibit nonsuppression (78% and 95%, respectively), whereas a lower proportion (48%) of patients with the nonpsychotic, nonmelancholic subtype exhibit nonsuppression (Evans and Nemeroff, 1987). Serum cortisol concentrations following dexamethasone similarly vary with the subtype of mood disorder, with higher postdexamethasone cortisol levels in patients with melancholic or psychotic subtypes when compared to major depressed patients without these features (Evans and Nemeroff, 1987). Others have reported similar findings (Schatzberg *et al.*, 1983). Thus, cortisol nonsuppression following dexamethasone challenge may be a marker for severity of affective illness, or may define a biologically distinct group of mood disorder patients (Evans and Nemeroff, 1987).

The sensitivity and specificity of the DST in detecting major depression have been studied extensively. In a review of the literature pooling data from 128 studies with 5111 subjects from both inpatient and outpatient settings, Arana *et al.* (1985) found the overall sensitivity of the DST to be 44%. In this same review the sensitivity for melancholic or endogenous subtypes was 50% and for psychotic depression 67%. Similarly, we found the sensitivity of the DST to be 63% for hospitalized patients with major depression (Evans and Nemeroff, 1987). Arana *et al.* (1985) also reviewed the specificity of the DST. When healthy subjects were utilized as the comparison group, the specificity was 93%; with nondepressed psychiatric patients as controls, the specificity was 77%. Thus, the DST has been found to have moderate sensitivity and a high specificity for major depression, in particular for the more severe melancholic and psychotic subtypes. As is true for diagnostic tests in general, the positive predictive value of the DST varies depending on the prevalence of major depression, and is higher in populations with a high prevalence of major depression, such as psychiatric inpatient units.

Dysregulation of the HPT axis also occurs in patients with major depression. Several researchers have reported a blunted thyroid-stimulating hormone (TSH) response to TRH administration in approximately 25% of patients with major depression (Loosen, 1985; Loosen and Prange, 1982; Gold *et al.*, 1982). False positive results may occur in patients taking lithium, or who have renal failure, severe weight loss, or thyroid disease (Loosen and Prange, 1982). Positive DST and TRH stimulation test results have not been shown to be related in depressed patients (Extein *et al.*, 1981; Haggerty *et al.*, 1987). However, we have found an elevated basal TSH level in patients with major depression. This elevation is correlated with cortisol nonsuppression following dexamethasone (Haggerty *et al.*, 1987). Although hypercortisolemia can affect TSH release, this alone was insufficient to explain the blunted TSH response to TRH (Loosen and Prange, 1982). Thus, further research is needed to determine if a relationship exists between dysregulation of the HPA and HPT axes in major mood disorders (see Nemeroff and Evans, 1989, for review).

III. Neuroendocrine Findings in Patients with Medical Illness and Mood Disorder

Many medical conditions have behavioral or mood disturbance as a prominent feature. These psychiatric symptoms may be the direct result of central nervous system (CNS) dysfunction, as with thyroid disease, vitamin B_{12} deficiency, or a variety of neurological conditions. Alternatively, the behavioral or mood symptoms may be a more general phenomenon, as in secondary depression in the cancer patient. Complicating the assessment of depression in the medically ill is the overlap between the signs and symptoms of depression and debilitating physical illness, such as anorexia, weight loss, insomnia, and decreased energy. A biological marker for depression would be invaluable in the assessment of depressive symptoms in patients with cancer, stroke, or other debilitating medical illnesses. Thus, neuroendocrine challenge tests have been investigated for use as an adjunct in the diagnosis of mood disorders in patients with coexisting medical illness.

A. Neuroendocrine Challenge Tests in Cancer

Depressive symptoms frequently occur in cancer patients, and may be underrecognized and undertreated by physicians (Petty and Noyes, 1981; Levine *et al.*, 1978). A biological marker for major depression would be a welcome adjunct to traditional clinical assessment in these patients whose physical illness may often obscure a treatable major depression.

We studied 83 patients with recently diagnosed nonovarian gynecological cancer in order to investigate the clinical and neuroendocrine features of depressive symptoms in this population (Evans *et al.*, 1986). Almost half (39 patients) had significant depression, with 19 (23%) meeting DSM-III criteria for major depression, and 20 (24%) meeting criteria for dysthymic disorder or adjustment disorder with depressed mood. Another 6 patients (7%) met criteria for other psychiatric diagnoses, and the remaining 38 (46%) patients did not meet the diagnostic criteria for a DSM-III psychiatric disorder.

We studied the HPA and HPT axes in these cancer patients, utilizing the DST and TRH stimulation tests, respectively. Forty percent of 15 patients with major depression had positive DST results. This proportion is similar to the 48% nonsuppression seen in hospitalized psychiatric patients meeting DSM-III criteria for a nonpsychotic, nonmelancholic, major depressive episode. Postdexamethasone serum cortisol levels in the depressed cancer patients were also similar to the nonpsychotic, nonmelancholic, depressed psychiatric patients (Evans *et al.*, 1986; Evans and Nemeroff, 1987). The sensitivity of the DST for the diagnosis of major depression in this cancer study was 40%, and the specificity was 88%, similar to the sensitivity and specificity of the DST in the psychiatric population (Arana *et al.*, 1985).

Although the sample size was small, a blunted TSH response to TRH was found in 29% of cancer patients with a major depressive episode, and in 8% of those with no psychiatric diagnosis. This is similar to findings reported by others in studies of depressed psychiatric patients (Loosen and Prange, 1982).

In summary, these neuroendocrine and clinical findings in cancer patients suggest that depression secondary to cancer is similar to the spectrum of depressive illness seen in psychiatric patients (see Evans *et al.*, 1990a,b, for reviews). The usefulness of the DST as an aid to clinical diagnosis of major depression in patients with cancer is limited by the relatively frequent occurrence of factors associated with false positive test results. In our study 28 out of 111 screened subjects were excluded because of at least one potentially confounding condition, such as toxic or infectious illness, or use of certain medications. We believe that further research examining neuroendocrine aspects of depression in cancer patients is warranted, although it would be premature to routinely use these tests in clinical practice.

B. Neuroendocrine Challenge Tests in Chronic Pain

Chronic pain disorder is often associated with depressive symptoms (Krishnan and France, 1987; Large, 1980). Controversy exists over the nature of chronic pain disorder, with some arguing that chronic pain disorder is simply a somatic expression of depression (Blumer *et al.*, 1982). Endocrine challenge tests may thus shed light on the relationship between chronic pain and major depressive disorders. The DST is also a potential adjunct for the diagnosis of major depression in this population.

Several studies have examined HPA axis function in the chronic pain population. In a meta-analysis of several studies, the DST has been found to have moderate sensitivity and high specificity, similar to that reported for the detection of major depression in the psychiatric population (Arana *et al.*, 1987). France *et al.* (1984) studied 42 patients with chronic low back pain. Of the 22 patients who met DSM-III criteria for major depression, 41% exhibited abnormal cortisol response to dexamethasone. None of the 20 patients without major depression (10 patients diagnosed with dysthymia, 10 with adjustment disorder with depressed mood) had abnormal DST results. In subsequent studies France and Krishnan (1985) and France *et al.* (1987) have replicated this finding of significantly higher proportions of a positive DST result in chronic pain patients with major depression compared to chronic patients without major depression. Furthermore, France *et al.* (1987) found the mean postdexamethasone plasma cortisol level to be significantly higher in depressed chronic pain patients compared to those without depression. Atkinson *et al.* (1986a,b) also found that the proportions of patients with positive DST were significantly different between chronic pain patients meeting Research Diagnostic Criteria (RDC) for major depression (41.7%) compared to chronic pain patients without a psychiatric illness (8.3%).

The DST has also been studied in chronic daily headache. Martignoni *et al.* (1986) found that 29% of chronic daily headache patients exhibited cortisol nonsuppression (as detected by 4 p.m. serum cortisol only) following dexamethasone administration. Elevated values for the MMPI Depression Scale were correlated with positive DST result, but scores on the Hamilton Rating Scale for Depression were equally distributed between DST positive and DST negative subjects. Systematic clinical psychiatric assessment of subjects was not done, so that psychiatric diagnoses were not reported.

One study did not find an association between depression and DST nonsuppression (Blumer *et al.*, 1982). In this study there was no difference in Hamilton Depression Rating Scale scores between chronic pain patients with positive DST compared with patients with negative DST results. Once again, however, systematic psychiatric diagnostic assessment was not done. Hamilton Depression Rating Scale scores may be elevated in the chronic pain population because of the high frequency of somatic complaints, and thus may not be highly correlated with clinical depression. In contrast, Krishnan *et al.* (1985) found depression, as measured with the Hamilton Depression Scale and the Montgomery–Asberg Depression Rating Scale, to be highly correlated with positive DST results in chronic pain patients, while anxiety, as measured by the Hamilton Anxiety Scale, was not.

HPA axis function has been studied in the nondepressed chronic pain population as well. Magni *et al.* (1989) studied a group of 63 nondepressed patients with chronic pain disorder. Cortisol nonsuppression was found in 17%. No significant differences were detected between patients whose pain had an organic etiology versus a nonorganic etiology. There has been one study with the DST in a series of 23 patients with fibrositis, a rheumatic disorder diagnosed by chronic unexplained generalized aches and pains in multiple sites, multiple pain "trigger points," and the presence of six or more nonspecific symptoms including variation of symptoms by weather, activity, or stress, insomnia, fatigue, anxiety, chronic headache, irritable bowel syndrome, swelling, and numbness (Hudson *et al.*, 1984). While there may be some evidence of a relationship between fibrositis and depression (Hudson *et al.*, 1984), none of these patients met DSM-III criteria for a major depressive episode, and only one fibrositis patient exhibited cortisol nonsuppression; none of 22 normal controls had positive DST results. These results indicate that chronic pain alone does not result in HPA axis hyperactivity as detected by the DST.

The HPT axis has been studied less extensively in the chronic pain population. France *et al.* (1986) found no significant difference in TSH response to TRH between chronic patients with and without DSM-III major depression. Overall, 18% had a blunted TSH response. We are not aware of other published reports examining the TRH stimulation test in patients with chronic pain.

While preliminary, these studies suggest that the DST may be useful in distinguishing syndromal major depression in the chronic pain patient. Furthermore, the major depression that occurs in the chronic pain population may share certain biological factors with that which occurs in the psychiatric population. Further research is indicated to clarify the relationship between HPA axis dysregulation and chronic pain disorder, and to determine the diagnostic usefulness of the DST in the chronic pain patient.

C. Neuroendocrine Challenge Tests in Neurological Diseases

Differential diagnosis of depressive illness in patients with disorders of the CNS is a difficult but important task for the clinician. Appropriate antidepressant treatment, based on accurate diagnosis, may lead to improved rehabilitation and, in some cases, reversal of the cognitive and motor deficits thought to be directly associated with the neurological illness. The difficulty in diagnosis is due, in part, to the finding that symptoms and signs associated with the neurological disorder may mask (e.g., aphasia, anosognosia) or mimic (e.g., apathy, abulia, bradykinesia, emotional lability) the depressive symptomatology evidenced by psychiatric patients without known neurological illness. Because of these difficulties, clinicians and researchers have attempted to employ biological markers of mood disorder, such as neuroendocrine challenge tests, rather than rely solely on the traditional interview and self-report instruments designed for psychiatric populations.

1. Stroke

Depressive symptomatology occurs in approximately 50% of stroke patients (Sinyor *et al.*, 1986; Starkstein *et al.*, 1988; Stern and Bachman, 1989). Severity of physical disability is not typically related to severity of depressive symptoms, suggesting that mood disorders following stroke are not merely an expected grief reaction to loss of function. Furthermore, poststroke mood disorders have been found to be associated with specific lesion loci (Robinson *et al.*, 1983; Stern and Bachman, 1989). Accurate diagnosis of poststroke depression is critical because depression can significantly reduce the speed and success of stroke rehabilitation outcome (Sundet *et al.*, 1988), and many depressed stroke patients respond favorably to pharmacotherapy (Lipsey *et al.*, 1984; Reding *et al.*, 1986). However, traditional standardized measures of depressive symptomatology require intact verbal abilities as well as accurate emotional expression, functions frequently disturbed following cerebral lesions. Consequently, Ross and Rush (1981) have proposed the use of the DST to assist in the diagnosis of poststroke mood disorders.

Recent reviews of the use of the DST in poststroke depression have described its limitations (Evans and Golden, 1987; Evans *et al.*, 1990a). DST sensitivity has ranged from 47 to 80%, while specificity has ranged from 70 to 95%. This variability may be due to several factors. For example, diagnostic criteria have varied from study to study, but typically rely on DSM-III or RDC criteria for psychiatric depressive disorders. Rather than relying on psychiatric criteria, some authors have argued that DST sensitivity and specificity in poststroke patients would improve if diagnostic criteria were modified specifically for this population of neurologically ill patients (Ross *et al.*, 1986).

An additional limitation has been the employment of a 5-μg/dl post-dexamethasone cortisol cut off criterion in predominantly older patients. As pointed out by Fogel (1986), this traditional cutoff for a positive DST was not intended for use in elderly populations. There is growing evidence to indicate that postdexamethasone cortisol levels are significantly correlated with age in both psychiatric and medically ill populations (Fogel and Satel, 1985; Fogel et al., 1985). Therefore, the employment of the 5-μg/dl cortisol cutoff in stroke patients, as well as in older patients with other neurological illnesses (e.g., dementia, Parkinson's disease), may result in inflated sensitivity rates and poor specificity.

Another important issue with regard to the interpretation of DST results in stroke patients is the possibility that the neurological damage may directly affect neuroendocrine regulation without concomitant development of depressive symptomatology (Bauer et al., 1983). For example, the location and size of the lesion have been found to alter DST results, without necessarily leading to depressive symptomatology (Evans and Nemeroff, 1985; Feibel et al., 1983; Lipsey et al., 1985).

To date, there have not been reports of other neuroendocrine challenge tests, such as the TRH test, in the diagnosis of depression in stroke patients. Although potentially useful, the same limitations as described for the DST might apply for these other tests.

2. Dementia

The relationship between mood changes and dementing illnesses has also received a great deal of attention in recent years. One of the reasons for the abundance of literature on this topic is the recognition that major depression and other mood disorders can result in cognitive changes that mimic dementing illnesses, such as Alzheimer's disease (AD). This "pseudodementia" frequently makes differential diagnosis of cognitive decline in the elderly a difficult task (Haggerty et al., 1988). It has been suggested that the DST be used as a possible tool in improving the differential diagnosis of dementia and depression (Grunhaus et al., 1983). Research findings to date, however, have been inconsistent.

The incidence of DST nonsuppression in patients with primary degenerative dementia has been reported to range from 0 to 57%. Sensitivity and specificity rates of the DST in identifying patients with depressive symptomatology have been similarly varied. As in the poststroke literature, this variability is likely due to a number of factors, including (1) the effects of age and/or concurrent medical illness on DST abnormality, (2) vague or inconsistent diagnostic criteria for dementia and/or depression, (3) inappropriate cortisol cutoff criteria, and (4) small sample size.

Although some early investigations reported low false positive rates in the use of the DST in demented, nondepressed patients (e.g., Carnes *et al.*, 1983a), other studies have yielded a high number of false positives (e.g., Spar and Gerner, 1982; Greenwald *et al.*, 1986). For example, in a study by Balldin and colleagues (1983), 57% of patients with AD and 73% of multi-infarct dementia patients were nonsuppressors. The abnormal DST results were not related to either age or depression severity. In a more recent investigation by Serby *et al.* (1988), there was a 56% incidence of DST nonsupression in a sample of 34 male inpatients and outpatients with progressive degenerative dementia, but without depression. An interesting finding of this study was a U-shaped pattern of DST nonsuppression. That is, patients early and late in the course of dementia had higher postdexamethasone cortisol levels than patients with moderately severe dementia.

Differential diagnosis of dementia and depression is especially crucial in the early stages of dementia. Jenike and Albert (1984) found that the DST was clinically useful in mildly impaired AD patients, but demonstrated poor specificity in the more impaired patients. In contrast, De Leo and co-workers (1988) recently reported a high number of false positive DST results (37.5%) in a group of nondepressed patients in the early stages of AD.

In studies comparing demented patients with and without depression to depressed, nondemented, elderly patients, the findings have also been inconsistent. Some investigators have found that abnormal DST results are related to the presence of depressive symptomatology and not merely to the underlying dementing illness (e.g., Carnes *et al.*, 1983b; Katona and Aldridge, 1985; Evans, 1988). Other studies have found that nonsuppression resulted in patients with dementia without concurrent depression (Georgotas *et al.*, 1986; Gierl *et al.*, 1987).

Recent studies comparing patients with depressive "pseudodementia" to patients with both dementia and depression have also yielded conflicting results. For example, Alexopoulos and colleagues (1985) found that demented patients without depression had a significantly lower incidence of abnormal DST than comparison groups of elderly depressed patients with or without cognitive dysfunction. However, there was no significant difference in abnormal DST results between patients with depression and reversible dementia (i.e., those whose cognitive dysfunction diminished after successful antidepressant treatment) and patients with both depression and dementia (i.e., those whose cognitive dysfunction remained after antidepressant treatment).

More recently, the TRH stimulation test has been investigated in demented patients, with results similar to those observed in the DST–dementia literature. For example, false positive results (i.e., TSH blunting) have been reported in nondepressed, AD patients (e.g., Sunderland *et al.*, 1985; McAllister and Hays, 1987). Other studies, however, have not found increased TSH blunting in AD subjects compared to controls (e.g., Peabody *et al.*, 1986). A recent report by Lampe and colleagues (1988) also failed to find overall significant differences in TSH response to TRH in non-depressed AD patients compared to controls. The AD patients, however, did not show an expected dose-response difference in TSH response when given different TRH doses.

3. Parkinson's Disease

Depressive symptomatology is frequently observed in patients with Parkinson's disease (PD) (Taylor *et al.*, 1986), a disorder thought to be due to degeneration of dopaminergic neurons in nigrostriatal pathways. The mood disorders accompanying PD occur in patients both with and without dementia. As in other CNS disorders, accurate diagnosis of depression in PD is important as well as difficult. The literature on the utility of neuroendocrine challenge tests in the diagnosis of depression in PD is not as extensive as in Alzheimer's disease and other dementing illnesses. The results of existing studies, however, are as equivocal. For example, Mayeux *et al.* (1986) found a 45% rate of nonsuppression in a group of 49 PD patients. Existence of depressive symptomatology was not associated with abnormal DST results. Similar results were found in a small study by Kawamura and colleagues (1987). In contrast, other reports have indicated moderate sensitivity (43–57%) and high specificity (84–96%) (Pfeiffer *et al.*, 1986; Frochtengarten *et al.*, 1987).

Few studies of the TRH test in PD patients have been conducted, and none have addressed the utility of the test in diagnosing depressive disorders.

4. Multiple Sclerosis

Patients with multiple sclerosis (MS) have long been known to exhibit behavioral disorders, including depressive symptomatology (Schiffer and Babigian, 1984). Similar to other neurological disorders, accurate diagnosis of depression can be hampered due to the signs and symptoms of the neurological illness masking or mimicking depression. Unlike stroke, dementia, and Parkinson's disease, the utility of the DST has not received much investigation in MS.

Gaughan and Popkin (1985) reported a case of a 29-year-old female with a long history of severe MS and recent depressive symptomatology. Following an abnormal DST, antidepressant medication was initiated. Subsequently, depressive symptomatology dramatically diminished and a repeat DST was normal.

Reder and colleagues (1987) recently reported a prospective study of the relationship between DST, depressive symptomatology, and ACTH treatment response in MS. They found a 47% incidence of DST nonsuppression in their active MS group, which was significantly greater than their control group (11%), but similar to a comparison group of non-MS patients with major depression (45%). Depression severity was not correlated with DST results in the MS group, and the MS patients' depression scores were, for the most part, in the normal range. In contrast, postdexamethasone suppression of cortisol was significantly associated with neurological improvement following 1 week of ACTH therapy. The authors concluded that while DST nonsuppression does not appear to be related to depression in MS, the DST may be a useful test of glucocorticoid sensitivity in this population.

In summary, although MS is known to be associated with affective disturbance, there have been too few studies to date to assess the utility of the DST in diagnosing depression in this population. Furthermore, there have been no reports to date on the utility of other neuroendocrine tests, such as the TRH test, in the diagnosis of depression in MS.

5. Summary

The utility of neuroendocrine challenge tests in the diagnosis of mood disorders in neurological illness remains unclear. Methodological problems, such as the confounding effects of age and medical illness, varied and overinclusive diagnostic criteria for both depression and dementia, inappropriate DST cutoff criteria, and small sample sizes, have all contributed to the conflicting reports. In addition, neuroendocrine markers of depression may be directly affected by some of the medications used to treat these neurological disorders, such as dopaminergic agonists in PD, or ACTH in MS. Medication effects have not routinely been addressed. Another salient factor involves the neurochemical alterations directly caused by the disease, such as disruption of catecholamine pathways following stroke, degeneration of cholinergic neurons in AD, destruction of dopaminergic pathways in PD, and demyelination of hypothalamic neurons in MS. Each of these neurotransmitter systems has been linked to affective illness (Golden and Janowsky, 1990) as well as to alterations of the HPA and HPT axes (Janowsky *et al.*, 1988). It is possible, therefore, that an abnormal neuroendocrine challenge test result may be a marker of the CNS lesion, itself, rather than a useful aid in differentiating depressive illness from neurological disease. Still, the DST and other neuroendocrine challenge tests may thus serve to increase our understanding of the biology of CNS disorders, as well as the biology of depression in this population.

D. Neuroendocrine Challenge Tests in Thyroid Disease and Vitamin B_{12} Deficiency

Patients with an organic mood syndrome may have HPA axis dysregulation similar to patients with primary major depressive disorder. In a small series of patients with organic affective syndrome secondary to vitamin B_{12} deficiency, thyroid disease, or both, four out of six subjects were found to exhibit cortisol nonsuppression following dexamethasone administration (Evans and Nemeroff, 1984). The cortisol nonsuppressors in this series included two vitamin B_{12} deficient patients, one case of hypothyroidism, and one patient with combined vitamin B_{12} and thyroxine deficiency. The two patients that exhibited a normal cortisol response to dexamethasone challenge included one case of hyperthyroidism and one case of combined vitamin B_{12} and thyroxine deficiency.

There is one other case study of neuroendocrine testing in a patient with vitamin B_{12} deficiency. The patient presented with symptoms of a major depression with melancholia and was subsequently found to have a vitamin B_{12} deficiency (James et al., 1986). She had cortisol nonsuppression that normalized after vitamin B_{12} replacement, although her mood disorder did not resolve.

In a report of 33 patients with newly diagnosed thyrotoxicosis, 10 met DSM-III criteria for organic affective syndrome, but only one nondepressed subject exhibited cortisol nonsuppression (Kathol et al., 1985). These findings are difficult to interpret, however, because blood samples were drawn at 8 a.m. instead of at 4 p.m. and 11 p.m., and thus the sensitivity and specificity of the DST could have been affected (Carroll et al., 1981).

There are two case studies reporting DST results in patients with hyperthyroidism. One describes a case of apathetic thyrotoxicosis presenting as a psychotic depression (Kronfol et al., 1982). While the patient had markedly elevated nocturnal plasma cortisol levels, she exhibited normal suppression of cortisol following dexamethasone. A similar case reports another patient with apathetic thyrotoxicosis, who also exhibited normal cortisol suppression (Martin and Waltz, 1984).

Patients with an underlying subclinical thyroid disorder may exhibit behavioral or mood symptoms as the only manifestation of the thyroid dysfunction. We have measured antithyroid antibody titers in 45 patients with significant depressive symptoms consecutively admitted to a psychiatric inpatient unit (Nemeroff et al., 1985). In 20% of the patients, antithyroid antibodies were detected, compared to the 5–10% expected from normal population data. Thyroid antibody status was not, however, correlated with cortisol nonsuppression detected by the DST.

TRH stimulation tests cannot be used to study affective disorders in patients with clinical thyroid disease, since any abnormalities of the HPT axis will reflect the primary disease process. We are not aware of any studies of the HPT axis in vitamin B_{12}-deficient patients.

In summary, the majority of vitamin B_{12}-deficient patients with major depression reported have abnormal dexamethasone suppression tests that normalize after vitamin B_{12} replacement. In addition, there are data to suggest that thyroxine deficiencies may be associated with cortisol nonsuppression. Fahs (1985) pointed out that the incidence of cortisol nonsuppression in vitamin B_{12}-deficient patients without affective symptoms is not known. Therefore, one cannot say with certainty whether the vitamin B_{12} deficiency itself or the affective disorder is responsible for the HPA axis dysregulation. With regard to thyrotoxicosis, the limited data suggest that depression is not associated with cortisol nonsuppression following dexamethasone challenge. Further research is needed to clarify the relationship between neuro-endocrine abnormalities and organic mood syndromes, and to explore the clinical significance of these findings.

E. Neuroendocrine Challenge Tests in Other Medical Conditions

Several medical illnesses, physical symptoms, and commonly prescribed medications have been associated with cortisol nonsuppression following dexamethasone administration, independent of any psychiatric illness (see American Psychiatric Association Task Force on Laboratory Tests in Psychiatry, 1987, for review). Acute medical conditions, such as congestive heart failure, uncontrolled hypertension, and severe toxic or infectious processes, may result in HPA hyperactivity as detected through cortisol nonsuppression following dexamethasone. Severe weight loss and dehydration may also result in positive DST results. However, less severe medical illness has not been associated with abnormal DST results (Carnes *et al.*, 1983b; Fogel and Satel, 1985). As expected, diseases of the neuroendocrine system, such as Cushing's syndrome, also may lead to HPA axis hyperactivity. Diabetes mellitus, both controlled and uncontrolled, has been associated with positive DST. Pregnancy and high-dose estrogens (but not normal-dose estrogen as in oral contraceptives) have been associated with positive DST. Finally, a severe, debilitating disease, such as advanced renal disease, hepatic disease, or advanced malignancy, may lead to HPA axis dysfunction.

Any drug that induces hepatic microsomal enzymes will increase the rate of dexamethasone metabolism, potentially resulting in a false positive DST. Such drugs include certain anticonvulsants (phenytoin, carbamezapine), sedative hypnotics (barbiturates, meprobamate, glutethimide, methaqualone), alcohol in large quantities, and possibly narcotics and reserpine.

Thus, many medical conditions, in particular severe, acute illness, may lead to HPA axis hyperactivity, and thus a positive DST. In addition, many drugs may produce false positive DST results. Clinical diagnostic application of the DST to the diagnosis of mood disorders in the medically ill will be limited by the relative prevalence of these potential confounders.

IV. Summary and Conclusions

Two neuroendocrine challenge tests, the DST and the TRH stimulation test, have been applied to the study of secondary mood disorders in patients with coexistent medical conditions, specifically cancer, chronic pain, vitamin B_{12} deficiency, thyroid disorders, and several neurological disorders. The potential value of this research lies in (1) developing a biological marker to use as a diagnostic adjunct to clinical assessment of mood disorders in this population and (2) developing and understanding of HPA and HPT dysfunction in patients with secondary mood disorders and organic mood disorders, especially in comparison to such dysfunction in primary mood disorders.

Small sample sizes, limited numbers of studies, and several methodological problems contribute to variable study outcomes, and limit the conclusions that can be made from this research. For several medical illnesses, including cancer, chronic pain disorder, and dementia, preliminary studies suggest a potential role for the DST as a diagnostic adjunct to clinical assessment. However, clinical application of the DST or TRH stimulation test for routine diagnostic assessment is not warranted at this point. Further research to clarify the useful applications of the DST or TRH stimulation test is needed. Understanding neuroendocrine aspects of secondary depression in patients with medical illness may lead to improved understanding of the pathophysiology of secondary depression and organic mood disorders.

References

Alexopoulos, G. S., Young, R. C., Haycox, J. A., Shamoian, C. A., and Blass, J. P. (1985). Dexamethasone suppression test in depression with reversible dementia. *Psychiatr. Res.* 16, 277–285.

American Psychiatric Association Task Force on Laboratory Tests in Psychiatry (1987). The dexamethasone suppression test: an overview of its current status in psychiatry. *Am. J. Psychiatry* 144(10), 1253–1262.

Arana, G. W., Baldessarini, R. J., and Ornsteen, M. (1985). The dexamethasone suppression test for diagnosis and prognosis in psychiatry. *Arch. Gen. Psychiatry* 42, 1193–1204.

Arana, G. W., Teicher, M. H., and Baldessarini, M. H. (1987). The utility of the dexamethasone suppression test: Reply. *Arch. Gen. Psychiatry* 44, 95–96.

Atkinson, J. H., Jr., Kremer, E. F., Risch, S. C., and Janowsky, D. S. (1986a). Basal and post-dexamethasone cortisol and prolactin concentrations in depressed and non-depressed patients with chronic pain syndromes. *Pain* 25(1), 23–24.

Atkinson, J. H., Jr., Kremer, E. F., Risch, S. C., Dana, R., and Janowsky, D. S. (1986b). Neuroendocrine responses in psychiatric and pain patients with major depression. *Biol. Psychiatry* 21(7), 612–620.

Balldin, J., Gottfries, C. G., Karlsson, I., Lindstedt, G., Langstrom, G., and Walinder, J. (1983). Dexamethasone suppression test and serum prolactin in dementia disorders. *Br. J. Psychiatry* 143, 277–281.

Bauer, M., Gans, J. S., Harley, J. P., and Cobb, W. (1983). Dexamethasone Suppression Test and depression in a rehabilitation setting. *Arch. Phys. Med. Rehabil.* **64**, 421–422.

Blumer, D., Zorick, F., Heilbronn, M., and Roth, T. (1982). Biological markers for depression in chronic pain. *J. Nerv. Ment. Dis.* **170**(7), 425–428.

Carnes, M., Smith, J. C., Kalin, N. H., and Bauwens, S. F. (1983a). The dexamethasone suppression test in demented outpatients with and without depression. *Psychiatr. Res.* **9**, 337–344.

Carnes, M., Smith, J. C., Kalin, N. H., and Bauwens, S. F. (1983b). Effects of chronic medical illness and dementia on the dexamethasone suppression test. *J. Am. Geriatr. Soc.* **31**, 269–271.

Carroll, B. J., Feinberg, M., Greden, J. F., Tarika, J., Albala, A. A., Haskett, R. F., James, N. M., Kronfol, Z., Lohr, N., Steiner, M., de Vigne, J. P., and Young, E. (1981). A specific laboratory test for the diagnosis of melancholia. *Arch. Gen. Psychiatry* **38**, 15–22.

De Leo, D., Schifano, F., and Magni, G. (1988). Results of dexamethasone suppression test in early Alzheimer's dementia. *Eur. Arch. Psychiatr. Neurol. Sci.* **238**, 19–21.

Evans, D. L. (1988). Use of the dexamethasone suppression test in clinical psychiatry. *In* "Recent Advances in the Hypothalamic-Pituitary-Adrenal Axis" (C. B. Nemeroff and A. S. Schatzburg, eds.), pp. 133–155. Raven Press, New York.

Evans, D. L., and Golden, R. N. (1987). The dexamethasone suppression test—A review. *In* "Handbook of Clinical Psychoneuroendocrinology" (C. B. Nemeroff and P. T. Loosen, eds.), pp. 313–335. Guilford Press, New York.

Evans, D. L., and Nemeroff, C. B. (1984). The dexamethasone suppression test in organic affective syndrome. *Am. J. Psychiatry* **141**(11), 1465–1467.

Evans, D. L., and Nemeroff, C. B. (1985). The DST and organic affective disorder: Reply. *Am. J. Psychiatry* **141**, 146–147.

Evans, D. L., and Nemeroff, C. B. (1987). The clinical use of the dexamethasone suppression test in DSM-III affective disorders: Correlation with the severe depressive subtypes of melancholia and psychosis. *J. Psychiatr. Res.* **21**(2), 185–194.

Evans, D. L., McCartney, C. F., Nemeroff, C. B., Raft, D., Quade, D., Golden, R. N., Haggerty, J., Jr., Holmes, V., Simon, J. S., Droba, M., Mason, G. A., and Fowler, W. C. (1986). Depression in women treated for gynecological cancer: Clinical and neuroendocrine assessment. *Am. J. Psychiatry* **143**, 447–451.

Evans, D. L., Stern, R. A., Golden, R. N., Haggerty, J., Jr., Perkins, D. O., Simon, J. S., and Nemeroff, C. B. (1990a). Neuroendocrine and peptide challenge tests in primary and secondary depression. *In* "Neuropeptides in Psychiatry" (C. B. Nemeroff, ed.). American Psychiatric Press, Washington, D.C. In press.

Evans, D. L., Golden, R. N., Nemeroff, C. B., Pedersen, C. A., McCartney, C. F., Haggerty, J., Jr., Simon, J. S., and Raft, D. (1990b). Clinical aspects of neuropeptide research. *In* "Neuropsychopharmacology" (W. E. Bunney, Jr., H. Hippins, G. Laakmann, and M. Schmauss, eds.). Springer-Verlag, Berlin and New York. In press.

Extein, I., Potash, A. L. C., and Gold, M. S. (1981). Relationship of TRH test and dexamethasone suppression test abnormalities in unipolar depression. *Psychiatr. Res.* **4**, 49–53.

Fahs, J. J. (1985). The DST and organic affective disorder. *Am. J. Psychiatry* **142**, 991–002.

Feibel, J., Kelly, M., Lee, L., *et al.* (1983). Loss of adrenocorticol suppression after acute brain injury: Role of increased intracranial pressure and brain stem function. *J. Clin. Endocrinol. Metab.* **57**, 1245–1250.

Fogel, B. S. (1986). The Dexamethasone Suppression Test in stroke. *Arch. Neurol. (Chicago)* **43**, 105.

Fogel, B. S., and Satel, S. L. (1985). Age, medical illness, and the DST in depressed general hospital inpatients. *J. Clin. Psychiatry* **46**, 95–97.

Fogel, B. S., Satel, S. L., and Levy, S. (1985). Occurrence of high concentrations of post dexamethasone cortisol in elderly psychiatric inpatients. *Psychiatr. Res.* **15**, 85–90.

France, R. D., and Krishnan, K. R. (1985). The dexamethasone suppression test as a biologic marker of depression in chronic pain. *Pain* **21**, 49–55.

France, R. D., Krishnan, K. R., Houpt, J. L., and Maltbie, A. A. (1984). Differentiation of depression from chronic pain with the dexamethasone suppression test in DSM-III. *Am. J. Psychiatry* **141**(12), 1577–1579.

France, R. D., Krishnan, K. R., Goli, V., Manepalli, A. N., and Dickson, L. (1986). Preliminary study of thyrotropin releasing hormone stimulation test in chronic low back pain patients. *Pain* **27**, 51–55.

France, R. D., Krishnan, K. R., Trainor, M., and Pelton, S. (1987a). Chronic pain and depression. IV. DST as a discriminator between chronic pain and depression. *Pain* **28**(1), 39–44.

Frochtengarten, M. L., Villares, J. C. B., Maluf, E., and Carlini, E. A. (1987). Depressive symptoms and the dexamethasone suppression test in parkinsonian patients. *Biol. Psychiatry* **22**, 386–389.

Gaughan, T. J., and Popkin, M. K. (1985). The utility of the dexamethasone suppression test in affective disorder associated with multiple sclerosis. *Psychiatr. Med.* **2**, 323–327.

Georgotas, A., McCue, R. E., Kim, O. M., Hapworth, W. E., Reisbert, B., Stoll, P. M., Sinaiko, E., Fanelli, C., and Stokes, P. E. (1986). Dexamethasone suppression in dementia, depression, and normal aging. *Am. J. Psychiatry* **143**, 452–456.

Gierl, B., Groves, L., and Lazarus, L. W. (1987). Use of the Dexamethasone Suppression Test with depressed and demented elderly. *J. Am. Geriatr. Soc.* **35**, 115–120.

Gold, M. S., Pottash, A. L. C., and Extein, I. (1982). "Symptomless" autoimmune thyroiditis in depression. *Psychiatr. Res.* **6**, 261–269.

Golden, R. N., and Janowsky, D. S. (1990). Biologic theories of depression. *In* "Affective Disorders: Facts, Theories, and Treatment Methods" (B. Wolman and D. Stricker, eds.). Wiley, New York (in press).

Golden, R. N., and Potter, R. N. (1986). Neurochemical and neuroendocrine dysregulation in affective disorders. *Psychiatr. Clin. North Am.* **9**, 313–327.

Greenwald, B. S., Mathé, A. A., Mohs, R. C., Levy, M. I., Johns, C. A., and Davis, K. L. (1986). Cortisol and Alzheimer's Disease. II. Dexamethasone suppression, dementia severity, and affective symptoms. *Am. J. Psychiatry* **143**, 442–446.

Grunhaus, L., Dilsaver, S., Greden, J. F., and Carroll, B. J. (1983). Depressive pseudodementia: A suggested diagnostic profile. *Biol. Psychiatry* **2**, 215–225.

Haggerty, J., Jr., Simon, J. S., and Evans, D. L., and Nemeroff, C. B. (1987). Relationship of serum TSH concentration and antithyroid antibodies and DST response in psychiatric inpatients. *Am. J. Psychiatry* **144**(11), 1491–1493.

Haggerty, J., Jr., Golden, R. N., Evans, D. L., and Janowsky, D. S. (1988). The differential diagnosis pseudodementia in the elderly. *Am. J. Med.* **43**, 61–74.

Hudson, J. I., Pliner, L. F., Hudson, M. S., Goldenberg, D. L., and Melby, J. C. (1984). The dexamethasone suppression test in fibrositis. *Biol. Psychiatry* **19**(10), 1489–1493.

James, S. P., Golden, R. N., and Sack, D. A. (1986). Vitamin B_{12} deficiency and the dexamethasone suppression test. *J. Nerv. Ment. Dis.* **174**(2), 560–561

Janowsky, D. S., Golden, R. N., Rapaport, M., Cain, J. J., and Gillin, J. C. (1988). Neurochemistry of depression and mania. *In* "Depression and Mania" (A. Georgotas and R. Cancro, eds.), pp. 244–264. Am. Elsevier, New York.

Jenike, M. A., and Albert, M. S. (1984). The dexamethasone suppression test in patients with presenile and senile dementia of the Alzheimer's type. *J. Am. Geriatr. Soc.* **32**, 441–444.

Kathol, R. G., Delahunt, J. W., and Cooke, R. (1985). Urinary free cortisol levels and dexamethasone suppression testing in organic affective disorder associated with hyperthyroidism. *Am. J. Psychiatry* **142**(10), 1193–1195.

Katona, C. L. E., and Aldridge, C. R. (1985). The dexamethasone suppression test and depressive signs in dementia. *J. Affective Disord.* **8**, 83–89.

Kawamura, T., Kinoshita, M., and Nemoto, H. (1987). Low-dose dexamethasone suppression test in Japanese patients with Parkinson's Disease. *J. Neurol.* **234**, 264–265.

Krishnan, K. R., and France, R. D. (1987). Chronic pain and depression. *South. Med. J.* **80**(5), 558–561.

Krishnan, K. R., France, R. D., Pelton, S., and McCann, V. D. (1985). What does the dexamethasone suppression test identify? *Biol. Psychiatry* **20**(9), 957–964.

Kronfol, Z., Greden, J. P., Condon, M., Feinberg, M., and Carroll, B. J. (1982). Application of biological markers in depression secondary to thyrotoxicosis. *Am. J. Psychiatry* **139**, 1319–1322.

Lampe, T. H., Plymate, S. R., Risse, S. C., Kopeikin, H., Cubberley, L., and Raskind, M. A. (1988). TSH responses to two TRH doses in men with Alzheimer's disease. *Psychoneuroendocrinology* **13**, 245–254.

Large, R. (1980). The psychiatrist and the chronic pain patients: 172 anecdotes. *Pain* **9**, 253–263.

Levine, P. M., Silverfarb, P. M., and Lipowski, Z. J. (1978). Mental disorders in cancer patients. *Cancer (Philadelphia)* **42**, 1385–1391.

Lipsey, J. R., Robinson, R. G., Pearlson, G. D., Rao, K., and Price, T. R. (1984). Nortriptyline treatment of post-stroke depression: A double-blind study. *Lancet* **1**, 287–300.

Lipsey, J. R., Robinson, R. G., Pearlson, G. D., Rao, K., and Price, T. R. (1985). The Dexamethasone Suppression Test and mood following stroke. *Am. J. Psychiatry* **142**, 318–323.

Loosen, P. T. (1985). The TRH-induced TSH response in psychiatric patients: A possible neuroendocrine marker. *Psychoneuroendocrinology* **10**(3), 237–260.

Loosen, P. T., and Prange, A. J. (1982). Serum thyrotropin response to thyrotropin-releasing hormone in psychiatric patients: A review. *Am. J. Psychiatry* **139**, 405–416.

Magni, G., Talamo, R. R., Stella, A., Mottaran, R., and Salar, G. (1989). DST in chronic pain patients not suffering from major depression. *Pharmopsychiatry* **22**(1), 8–10.

Martignoni, E., Facchinetti, F., Manzoni, G. C., Petraglia, F., Nappi, G., and Genazzani A. R. (1986). Abnormal dexamethasone suppression test in daily chronic headache sufferers. *Psychiatr. Res.* **19**(1), 51–57.

Martin, R. S., and Waltz, G. W. (1984). DST not affected by conditions producing secondary depressions. *Am. J. Psychiatry* **141**, 1.

Mayeux, R., Stern, Y., Williams, J. B. W., Cote, L., Frantz, A., and Dyrenfurth, I. (1986). Clinical and biochemical features of depression in Parkinson's Disease. *Am. J. Psychiatry* **143**, 756–759.

McAllister, T. W., and Hays, L. R. (1987). TRH Test, DST, and response to desipramine in primary degenerative dementia. *Biol. Psychiatry* **22**, 189–193.

Nemeroff, C. B., and Evans, D. L. (1984). Correlation between the dexamethasone suppression test in depressed patients and clinical response. *Am. J. Psychiatry* **141**, 247–249.

Nemeroff, C. B., and Evans, D. L. (1989). Thyrotropin releasing hormone (TRH). *Ann. N. Y. Acad. Sci.* **533**, 304–310.

Nemeroff, C. B., Simon, J. S., Haggerty, J., Jr., and Evans, D. L. (1985). Anti-thyroid antibodies in depressed patients. *Am. J. Psychiatry* **142**(7), 840–843.

Peabody, C. A., Thornton, J. E., and Tinklenberg, J. R. (1986). Progressive dementia associated with thyroid disease. *Am. J. Psychiatry* **47**, 100.

Petty, F., and Noyes, R., Jr. (1981). Depression in cancer. *Biol. Psychiatry* **16**, 1203–1221.

Pfeiffer, R. F., Hsieh, H. H., Diercks, M. J., Glaeske, C., Jefferson, A., and Cheng, S. (1986). Dexamethasone suppression test in Parkinson's disease. *Adv. Neurol.* **45**, 439–442.

Reder, A. T., Lowy, M. T., Meltzer, H. Y., and Antel, J. P. (1987). Dexamethasone suppression test abnormalities in multiple sclerosis: Relation to ACTH therapy. *Neurology* **37**, 840–853.

Reding, M. J., Orto, L. A., Winter, S. W., Fortuna, I. M., Di Ponte, P., and McDowell, F. H. (1986). Antidepressant therapy after stroke: A double-blind trial. *Arch. Neurol. (Chicago)* **43**, 763–765.

Robinson, R. G., Kubos, K. L., Starr, L. B., Rao, K., and Price, T. R. (1983). Mood changes in stroke patients: Relationship to lesion location. *Compr. Psychiatry* **24**, 555–566.

Ross, E. D., and Rush, A. J. (1981). Diagnosis and neuroanatomical correlates of depression in brain-damaged patients: Implications for a neurology of depression. *Arch. Gen. Psychiatry* **38**,. 1344–1354.

Ross, E. D., Gordon, W. A., Hibbard, M., and Egelko, S. (1986). The Dexamethasone Suppression Test, post-stroke depression, and the validity of DSM-III diagnostic criteria. *Am. J. Psychiatry* **143**, 1200–1201.

Schatzberg, A. F., Rothchild, A. J., Stahl, J. B., Bond, T. C., Rosenbaum, A. H., Lofgren, S. B., MacLaughlin, R. A., Sullivan, M. A., and Cole, J. O. (1983). The dexamethasone suppression test: Identification of subtypes of depression. *Am. J. Psychiatry* **140**, 88–91.

Schiffer, R. B., and Babigian, H. M. (1984). Behavioral disorders in multiple sclerosis, temporal lobe epilepsy, and amyotrophic lateral sclerosis. *Arch. Neurol. (Chicago)* **41**, 1067–1069.

Serby, M., Zucker, D., Kaufman, M., Franssen, E., Duvvi, K., Rypma, B., and Rotrosen, R. (1988). Clinical stages of dementia and the dexamethasone suppression test. *Prog. Neuro-Psychopharmacol. Biol. Psychiatry* **12**, 833–836.

Sinyor, D., Jacques, P., Kaloupek, D. G., Becker, R., Goldenberg, M., and Coopersmith, H. (1986). Poststroke depression and lesion location: An attempted replication. *Brain* **109**, 537–546.

Spar, J. E., and Gerner, R. (1982). Does the dexamethasone suppression test distinguish dementia from depression? *Am. J. Psychiatry* **139**, 238–240.

Starkstein, S. E., Robinson, R. G., and Price, T. R. (1988). Comparison of patients with and without poststroke major depression matched for size and location of lesion. *Arch. Gen. Psychiatry* **45**, 247–252.

Stern, R. A., and Bachman, D. L. (1989). Dysphoric mood and vegetative disturbance following stroke: Patterns of lesion localization. *J. Clin. Exp. Neuropsychol.* **11**, 97–98 (abstr.).

Sunderland, T., Tariot, P. N., Mueller, E. A., Newhouse, P. A., Murphy, D. L., and Cohen, R. M. (1985). TRH stimulation test in dementia of the Alzheimer type and elderly controls. *Psychiatr. Res.* **16**, 269–275.

Sundet, K., Finset, A., and Reinvang, I. (1988). Neuropsychological predictors in stroke rehabilitation. *J. Clin. Exp. Neuropsychol.* **10**, 363–379.

Taylor, A. E., Saint-Cyr, J. A., Lang, A. E., and Kenny, F. T. (1986). Parkinson's Disease and depression: A critical re-evaluation. *Brain* **109**, 279–292.

III
Immune Function

11

The Role of Stress and Opioids as Regulators of the Immune Response

John. E. Morley
Geriatric Research, Education and
Clinical Center
St. Louis Veterans Administration
Medical Center
St. Louis, Missouri, and
Division of Geriatric Medicine
St. Louis University School of Medicine
St. Louis, Missouri 63104

Donna Benton
Geriatric Research, Education and
Clinical Center
Sepulveda Veterans Administration
Medical Center
Sepulveda, California 91303

George F. Solomon
Geriatric Research, Education and Clinical Center
Sepulveda Veterans Administration Medical Center
Sepulveda, California 91303, and
Department of Psychiatry
University of California
Los Angeles, California

I. Introduction

II. *In Vitro* Effect of Opioids on the Immune System
   A. Natural Killer (NK) Function
   B. Chemotaxis
   C. Macrophages
   D. Superoxide Production
   E. T-Cell Rosettes
   F. Mast Cells
   G. Complement System
   H. Interferon
   I. Lymphocytes
   J. Thymocytes

III. Do Immune Cells Produce Opioids?
   A. Opioids and the Immune System
   B. Opioid Receptors and the Immune System

I. Introduction

In recent years there has been increasing evidence that the immune system is regulated by the central nervous system and that, in turn, central nervous system function may be modulated by peptides produced by the immune system (Morley *et al.*, 1987). The concept of the mind modulating the immune system is not new, however. Galen had suggested that melancholy women were more prone to cancer than sanguine women. Oliver Wendell Holmes remarked on the better recovery from battle wounds seen in victorious soldiers compared to the conquered ones. Sir William Osler felt that in the preantibiotic era the recovery from tuberculosis was determined more by psychological factors than by the chest pathology. In the 1920s immunity was demonstrated to be capable of being modulated by clinical Pavlovian conditioning. Ader and Cohen demonstrated that after saccharin was paired with cyclophosphamide, it was capable of reducing antibody responses when given alone. These findings, and others, have led to the establishment and growth of the now well-recognized field of psychoneuroimmunology.

Stress is a term that is readily recognized by everyone but defies a rigorous scientific definition. It is widely thought of as the emotional and biologic responses to novel or threatening situations. In humans, however, the term "distress" may be preferable, more clearly defining the fact that it is the response that is being referred to, rather than the stimulus. Distress has been postulated to be capable of precipitating an overt illness when it occurs coincidentally with an incipient infection or neoplasm (Riley, 1981). In addition, it is recognized that the responses to stress may be protective of the organism, particularly when the stress is short-lived, the so-called "eustress" state. There is increasing evidence that early responses to stress enhance the immune system, while prolonged stress leads to suppression of immunity. Increasingly, it also appears that immune system responses to stress may at first activate the central nervous system to help ward off the stress, but when the stressor is prolonged, may decrease the psychic trauma by depressing central nervous system function.

The classical response to stress, as conceived by Hans Selye, is the activation of the hypothalmic–pituitary–adrenal axis. The rise in corticosteroids is a relatively late event and on the whole leads to suppression of immune function. On the other hand, stress activation of corticotropin-releasing factor leads to the release of ACTH and beta-endorphin from the pituitary. While ACTH is "carrying its message to the adrenal to dump cortisol into the bloodstream," beta-endorphin has its opportunity to circulate in the bloodstream and carry its message to its target organ(s). Until recently there was little information concerning the target organ(s) affected by the hormone beta-endorphin. However, recent studies have suggested that the immune system may represent an important target organ for beta-endorphin. Not only does stress cause the release of beta-endorphin from the pituitary, but it also activates the adrenal medulla, resulting in the release of the methionine- and leucine-enkephalin precursor into the circulation. Fragments from this precursor could also play a role in immunomodulation.

This chapter will provide an overview of current knowledge on the role of opioid peptides as immunomodulators. We will first review the effects of opioid peptides *in vitro* and then discuss the emerging evidence that opioid peptides acutely modulate natural killer (NK) cell activity in humans *in vivo*. Effects of morphine treatment on the immune system in animals will then be addressed. Finally, the possible role of the immune system in the development of opiate addiction will be discussed.

II. *In Vitro* Effects of Opioids on the Immune System

Opioid peptides have been demonstrated to produce a variety of effects on the immune system *in vitro*. These effects are summarized in Table I.

A. Natural Killer Function

Natural killer (NK) cells are thought to play an important role as tumor cell scavengers and also in transplant rejection. In 1983 Matthews *et al.* reported that beta-endorphin enhanced natural cytotoxicity *in vitro*. This finding was confirmed by two other groups in the following year (Faith *et al.*, 1984; Kay *et al.*, 1984). These studies demonstrated that beta-endorphin enhanced NK cell activity at concentrations of 10^{-7} to $10^{-8} M$. The dose response showed an inverted U-shaped dose response. There was individual variation in the responsiveness to beta-endorphin, with clear-cut responses being demonstrated in less than half of the subjects studied (Kay *et al.*, 1984). In responders the response is stable and can be reelicited when tested in their peripheral blood lymphocytes on multiple occasions. Besides beta-endorphin, a number of other opioid peptides, including methionine-enkephalin dynorphin (1–13), D-(Ser^2)-leucine-enkephalin-Thr (DSLET), and [D-Ala^2, N-Me-Phe^4, Gly-01 5]-enkephalin (DAGO) have been shown

Table I
Effects of Opioid Peptides on the Immune System *In Vitro*

Natural killer cells
  Enhanced, naloxone reversible
  Des-Tyr-endorphins more potent
Monocytes
  Increased chemotaxis, stereospecific
Macrophages
  Increased Na$^+$ and Ca^{2+} uptake
  Increased superoxide production
Mast cells
  Increased histamine release
  Antagonizes prostaglandin inhibition of serotonin release
Lymphocytes
  Increased T-cell rosette formation
  Biphasic effects on mitogen-induced proliferation of lymphocytes
  Enhanced proliferation of autologous mixed lymphocyte reaction
Thymocytes
  Stimulates calcium uptake into thymocytes
  Non-opioid-mediated effect
Complement
  Beta-endorphin binds to terminal complexes of SC5h-9 and C5h-9
Interferon and interleukin
  Increases or decreases gamma-interferon production
  Increases interleukin-2 production

to have variable effects on human NK activity (Oleson and Johnson, 1988). It has been suggested that when the cytolytic capacity is low, NK activity is enhanced by endogenous opioids while high basal NK activity is suppressed by endogenous opioids. This would be in keeping with our *in vivo* studies, which have suggested that stressors lead to downregulation of the *in vitro* responsiveness to beta-endorphin *(vide infra)*. Thus, it may be that the *in vitro* response is determined by the subject's internal response to an external stressor, such as blood drawing.

In a series of studies we have attempted to define the structural characteristics necessary to elicit the NK response to beta-endorphin (Kay *et al.*, 1987). A number of Des-Tyr-endorphin fragments (2–16, 2–17, 6–17, and 1–9) potently stimulated NK activity at concentrations as low as 10^{-15} M. The fragments (10–16) and (14–16) showed no activity. These studies are compatible with the concept that the ability of the endorphins to stimulate NK activity rests predominantly in the (6–9) amino acid fragment. This is the alpha-helical portion of the molecule. However, the nonopioid endorphin fragment's ability to enhance NK activity is reversed by the opioid antagonist naloxone. This suggests a role for the opioid portion of the molecule in the stimulation of NK activity. One possible explanation is that the receptor site is of the double-lock variety with the (6–9) portion acting as a key to allow access to the opioid receptor. A similar double-lock receptor confirmation has previously been reported for the dynorphin molecule (Chanvin and Goldstein, 1981; Morley and Levine, 1983).

Recently, Williamson *et al.* (1987) reported that while beta-endorphin increased NK activity over the dose range of 10^{-7} to 10^{-11} *M*, sequences that bind only to nonopiate receptors reduced NK activity. It is possible that they failed to go to low enough concentrations and thus were only demonstrating an effect on the left-hand side of the inverted-U dose response.

In our early studies, we noticed a particularly interesting phenomenon; namely, that interferon- and interleukin-2-stimulated NK cell activity is inhibited by the opiate antagonist naloxone (Kay *et al.*, 1984, 1987). This suggested to us a close linkage between interleukin-2 and beta-endorphin stimulation of NK cell activity. This could be due to an interaction at the level of the receptors or at a post-receptor site. Our preliminary studies *(vide infra)* have suggested that this interaction occurs at the receptor level.

B. Chemotaxis

In 1984 Van Epps and Saland found that both beta-endorphin and methionine-enkephalin are chemotactic for human monocytes, although this response was present in only 70% of subjects. Neutrophils were less responsive. Neutrophil migration toward fMLP is enhanced by beta-endorphin (Simpkins *et al.*, 1984). This effect is reversed by L- but not D-naloxone demonstrating stereospecificity (Ruff *et al.*, 1985).

Wheat gluten hydrosylates have opioid-like, that is, exorphin, activity (Morley, 1982). Alpha-gliadin inhibits leukocyte migration in patients with celiac disease. This effect of gliadin on leukocyte migration is inhibited by naloxone, suggesting a possible role for exorphins in the pathogenesis of celiac disease (Horvath *et al.*, 1985).

C. Macrophages

Methionine-enkephalin enhanced lysis of antibody-coated target cells by rat peritoneal macrophages (Solomon *et al.*, 1987). These macrophages demonstrated increased sodium and calcium ion uptake and superoxide production. Methionine enkephalin enhanced cyclic GMP and cyclic AMP levels, though the effect on cyclic GMP occurred at much lower concentrations.

Both delta and kappa opioid receptors have been identified on a macrophage cell line.

D. Superoxide Production

Both dynorphin and beta-endorphin stimulated superoxide radical production from polymorphonuclear leukocytes (Sharp *et al.*, 1985). This effect we inhibited by L- and D-naloxone, suggesting that it was a non-opioid-mediated effect (Simpkins *et al.*, 1985). We have previously suggested that the ability of beta-endorphin to stimulate free radical production may be a link between stress and accelerated aging, with free radical generation producing tissue damage (Morley *et al.*, 1989a).

E. T-Cell Rosettes

Both morphine and beta-morphine enhance the number of rosettes formed by human peripheral blood lymphocytes when they are exposed to sheep red blood cells (Wybran *et al.*, 1979). The effect is naloxone reversible.

F. Mast Cells

Morphine promotes histamine release from mast cells and thus may be a cause of flushing. Beta-endorphin antagonizes the prostaglandin E_1 (PGE_1) induced inhibition of immunoglobin E (IgE) mediated serotonin release from mast cells (Yamasaki *et al.*, 1982). This is a naloxone-reversible effect.

   Naloxone has been reported to decrease cyclical psychosis and flushing (Goldstein and Keiser, 1983). Nalamefene, a long-acting opioid antagonist, has been shown to block alcohol-induced oriental flushing (Ho *et al.*, 1988).

G. Complement System

The C-terminus of beta-endorphin binds to the terminal complexes of human complement SC5h-9 and C5h-9 (Schweigerer *et al.*, 1982). The significance of this finding is uncertain, but it may reflect a mechanism by which complement can be bound to immune system cells, thus enhancing local levels of complement.

H. Interferon

Beta-endorphin augments gamma-interferon and interleukin-2 production (Mandler *et al.*, 1986). Another study, however, found suppression of gamma interferon by beta-endorphin (Peterson *et al.*, 1987). This appears to be a classical opioid effect mediated by reactive oxygen intermediates and prostaglandin E_2.

I. Lymphocytes

Opioid peptides modulate mitogen-stimulated proliferation of lymphocytes (Gelman *et al.*, 1982). These effects are absent in older animals (Norman *et al.*, 1988). Beta-endorphin enhanced proliferation of the autologous mixed lymphocyte reaction (Froelich, 1987). This effect was partially blocked by naloxone. The effect of beta-endorphin was independent of increased interleukin secretion. Beta-endorphin reversed prostaglandin E_2 suppression of the autologous mixed-lymphocyte reaction.

In our studies we have shown that in PHA-stimulated lymphocytes, labeled interleukin-2 was displaced by naloxone, and that conversely tritiated naloxone was displaced by interleukin-2 (Morley *et al.*, 1989a). Beta-endorphin induced the TAC antigenic site. These studies suggest that in lymphocytes the low-affinity interleukin-2 binding site is modulated by opioids.

J. Thymocytes

Opioid peptides appear to play a role in the modulation of thymic function. Beta-endorphin has been shown to significantly stimulate calcium uptake into rate thymocytes (Hemmick and Bidlack, 1987). The effect was not naloxone reversible.

III. Do Immune Cells Produce Opioids?

A. Opioids and the Immune System

Stimulated T-helper lymphocytes have been shown to express the preproenkephalin mRNA sequence as well as to produce immunoreactive methionine enkephalin in the supernatants (Zurawski *et al.*, 1986). Similarly, leukocytes from a B-cell leukemia were shown to express enkephalin mRNA (Monstein *et al.*, 1986). Spleen and machrophages have been shown to express mRNA to pro-opiomelanocortin (POMC) and immunoreactive beta-endorphin (Lolart *et al.*, 1986). Corticotropin-releasing factor has been shown to stimulate immunoreactive beta-endorphin release from human peripheral blood lymphocytes (Smith *et al.*, 1986). Overall these studies support the contention that immune cells produce opioid peptides. This suggests that opioids may modulate the immune system in a paracrine manner.

B. Opioid Receptors and the Immune System

A number of studies have examined the potential ability of opioids to bind to immune system cells. These studies have suggested that some binding sites exist on lymphocytes, granulocytes, and monocytes (Sibinga and Goldstein, 1988). The data, however, is extremely incomplete. No study has clearly shown stereospecificity; although binding to both the N- and C-terminals of beta-endorphin has been suggested.

In our preliminary studies we have found that expression of opioid receptors requires the preincubation of lymphocytes for 48 h or their stimulation with phytohemagglutinin (PHA) (N. Kay and J. E. Morley, unpublished observations). This binding of [^{3}H]naloxone is displaced by interleukin-2, though not in a parallel fashion to beta-endorphin. [^{125}I]Interleukin-2 is displaced by naloxone and beta-endorphin. The method by which the opioid receptor on lymphocytes interacts with the interleukin-2 receptor remains to be determined.

IV. Physiological Regulation of NK Cells During Stress in Humans

Exercise in humans has been demonstrated to enhance NK cell activity (Brahmi *et al.*, 1985; Targan *et al.*, 1981; Fiatarone *et al.*, 1989). As beta-endorphin is released during acute exercise we have postulated that it represents a potential physiologic mechanism by which exercise activates NK cells. In our studies, eight young women completed a maximal bicycle ergometer test (Fiatarone *et al.*, 1988). Exercise lasted approximately $10\frac{1}{2}$ minutes with the subjects achieving a maximum mean heart rate of 145 beats/min. The subjects underwent the study twice, receiving naloxone (100ug/kg) and placebo in a randomized, blind, crossover study. Exercise parameters were not altered by naloxone infusion. The subjects demonstrated the predicted exercise increase in NK activity. Naloxone significantly attenuated the increase in NK activity seen with exercise. In addition to an increase in NK activity, exercise also increased the number of circulating NK cells as measured by the cellular markers Leu 11$^+$ and Leu 19$^+$, suggesting that opioids only modulate NK activity and not the increase in NK cell number (presumably due to release of lymphocytes from the spleen during acute exercise). Following acute exercise, beta-endorphin could no longer stimulate NK cell activity *in vitro*. This lack of effect was partially attenuated by naloxone infusion. These data further support the concept that the increase in NK activity during exercise is opioid mediated. These data do not allow us to distinguish whether these effects are mediated by pituitary beta-endorphin release or adrenal medullary enkephalin release.

Epidemiological studies have suggested an independent inverse correlation between physical activity and colon cancer in males (Gerhardson *et al.*, 1986) and between college athleticism and subsequent breast cancer and reproductive malignancies in women (Frisch *et al.*, 1985). In addition, animal studies showed that tumor growth can be limited by exercise (Rusch and Kline, 1944). Our study now provides a physiological mechanism by which exercise, through endogenous opioid release, enhances NK activity and thus would decrease carcinogenesis.

In published studies we have found that a mental stressor (mental arithmetic to metronome) leads to an increase in NK cell activity within 10 min (Naliboff, B. F. Solomon, D. Benton, and J. E. Morley, unpublished observations). The potential role of endogenous opioids in this effect is currently under study.

V. Conclusion

There is strong evidence for a functional effect of opioids on the immune system. Recent studies have extended the early *in vitro* studies to *in vivo* human studies, suggesting a physiological role for opioid peptides in the regulation of the human immune system. Present *in vitro* data support the concept that both opiate and nonopiate effects are produced by opioid peptides acting on the immune system. Opioid binding in the immune system is poorly characterized, but there is mounting evidence for a double-lock receptor system. Opioid peptides that modulate the immune system could originate from circulating opioid peptides produced by the pituitary or adrenal medulla, from opioid peptides synthesized and secreted from the immune system itself (autocrine), or from the nervous system. There is a need to apply more rigorous methodology to the study of opioids in the immune system to more fully define the role of these peptides in regulating the immune response ot stress.

References

Brahmi, Z., Thomas, J. E., Park, M., and Dowdeswell, J. R. G. (1985). The effect of acute exercise on natural killer cell activity of trained and sedentary human subject. *J. Clin. Immunol.* 5, 321–328.

230 John E. Morley *et al.*

Chanvin, C., and Goldstein, A. (1981). Specific receptor for the opioid peptide dynorphin: Structure activity relationships. *Proc. Natl. Acad. Sci. U.S.A.* **78**, 6543–6547.

Faith, R. E., Liang, J. H., Murgo, A. J., *et al.* (1984). Neuroimmunomodulation with enkephalins enhancement of natural killer (NK) cell activity in vitro. *Clin. Immunol. Immunopathol.* **31**, 412–418.

Fiatarone, M. A., Morley, J. E., Bloom, E. T., *et al.* (1988). Endogenous opioids and the exercise induced augmentation of natural killer cell activity. *J. Lab. Clin. Med.* **112**, 544–552.

Fiatarone, M. A., Morley, J. E., Bloom, E. T., *et al.* (1989). The effect of exercise on natural killer cell activity in young and old subjects. *Gerontology* **44**, M37–M45.

Frisch, R. E., Wyshak, G., Albright, N. L., *et al.* (1985). Lower prevalence of breast cancer and cancer of the reproductive system among former college athletes compared to nonathletes. *Br. J. Cancer* **52**, 885–891.

Froelich, C. J. (1987). Modulation of the autologous mixed lymphocyte reaction by beta-endorphin. *J. Neuroimmunol.* **17**, 1–10.

Gelman, S. C., Schwartz, J. M., Milner, R. J., *et al.* (1982). Beta-endorphin enhances lymphocyte proliferative responses. *Proc. Natl. Acad. Sci. U.S.A.* **79**, 4226–4230.

Gerhardson, M., Norell, S. E., Kiviranta, H., *et al.* (1986). Sedentary jobs and colon cancer. *Am. J. Epidemiol.* **123**, 775–780.

Goldstein, D. J., and Keiser, H. R. (1983). A case of episodic flushing and organic psychosis: Reversal by opiate antagonists. *Ann. Intern. Med.* **98**, 30–34.

Hemmick, L. M., and Bidlack, J. M. (1987). B-endorphin modulation of mitogen-stimulated calcium uptake by rat thymocytes. *Life Sci.* **41**, 1971–1978.

Ho, S., Allen, J. J., DeMaster, E. G., *et al.* (1988). The opiate antagonist malmefene inhibits ethanol-induced flushing in Asians: A preliminary study of alcoholism. *Clin. Exp. Res.* **12**, 705–712.

Horvath, K., Graf, L., Walcz, E., *et al.* (1985). Naloxone antagonizes effect of alpha-gliadin on leukocyte migration in patients with celiac disease. *Lancet* **2**, 180–185.

Kay, N., Allen, J., and Morley, J. E. (1984). Endorphins stimulate normal human peripheral blood lymphocyte natural killer activity. *Life Sci.* **35**, 53–59.

Kay, N., Morley, J. E., and van Rhee, J. A. (1987). Enhancement of human lymphocyte natural killing function by non-opioid fragments of beta-endorphin. *Life Sci.* **40**, 1083–1087.

Lolart, S. J., Clements, J. A., Markevick, A. J., *et al.* (1986). Pro-opiomelanocortin messenger ribonucleic acid and postranslational processing of beta endorphin in spleen macrophages. *J. Clin. Invest.* **77**, 1776–1784.

Mandler, R. N., Biddison, W. E., Mandler, R., *et al.* (1986). Beta-endorphin augments the cytolytic activity and interferon production of natural killer cells. *J. Immunol.* **136**, 934–393.

Matthews, P. M., Froelich, C. J., Sibbitt, W. C., *et al.* (1983). Enhancement of Natural cytotoxicity by beta-endorphin. *J. Immunol.* **130**, 1658–1662.

Monstein, J. J., Folkesson, R., and Terenius, L. (1986). Proeenkephalin A-like mRNA in human leukemia leukocytes and CNS-tissues. *Life Sci.* **39**, 2234–2241.

Morley, J. E. (1982). Food peptides: A new class of hormones? *JAMA, J. Am. Med. Assoc.* **247**, 2379–2380.

Morley, J. E., and Levine, A. S. (1983). Involvement of dynorphin and the Kappa opioid receptor in feeding. *Peptides (N.Y.)* **4**, 797–800.

Morley, J. E., Kay, N. E., Solomon, G. F., and Plotnikoff, N. P. (1987). Neuropeptides: Conductors of the immune orchestra. *Life Sci.* **41**, 527–544.

Morley, J. E., Kay, N., and Solomon, G. F. (1989a). Opioid peptides, stress and immune function. *In* "Neuropeptides and Stress" (Y. Tache, J. E. Morley, and M. R. Brown, eds.), pp. 222–234. Springer-Verlag, Berlin and New York.

Morley, J. E., Flood, J. F., and Silver, A. J. (1989b). The anorexia of the elderly. *Ann. N.Y. Acad. Sci.* 575:50–59.

Norman, D. C., Morley, J. E., and Chang, M. P. (1988). Aging decreases beta-endorphin enhancement of T-cell mitogenesis in mice. *Mech. Ageing Dev.* 46, 185–191.

Oleson, D. R., and Johnson, D. R. (1988). Regulation of human natural cytotoxicity by enkephalins and selective opiate agonists. *Brain, Behav, Immun.* 2, 171–186.

Peterson, P. K., Sharp, B., Gekker, G., *et al.* (1987). Opioid-mediated suppression of interferon-gamma production by cultured peripheral blood mononuclear cells. *J. Clin. Invest.* 80, 826–831.

Riley, V. (1981). Psychoneuroendocrine influences on immunocompetence and neoplasia. *Science* 212, 1100–1109.

Ruff, M. R., Wahl, S. M., Mesgenhagen, *et al.* (1985). Opiate receptor-mediated chemotaxis of human monocytes. *Neuropeptides (Edinburgh)* 5, 363–366.

Rusch, H. P., and Kline, B. E. (1944). The effect of exercise on the growth of a mouse tumor. *Cancer Res.* 4, 116–118.

Schweigerer, L., Bhakdi, S., and Teschemacher, H. (1982). Specific non-opiate binding sites for human beta-endorphin on the terminal complex of human complement. *Nature (London)* 296, 572–574.

Sharp, B. M., Keane, W. F., Suh, H. J., *et al.* (1985). Opioid peptides rapidly stimulate superoxide production by human polymorphonuclear leukocytes and macrophages. *Endocrinology (Baltimore)* 117, 793–795.

Sibinga, N. E., and Goldstein, A. (1988). Opioid peptides and opioid receptors in cells of the immune system. *Annu. Rev. Immunol.* 6, 219–249.

Simpkins, C. O., Dickey, C. A., and Fink, M. P. (1984). *Life Sci.* 34, 2251–2255.

Simpkins, C. O., Ives, N., Tate, E., *et al.* (1985). Naloxone inhibits superoxide release from human neurophils. *Life Sci.* 37, 1381–1386.

Smith, E. M., Morrill, A. C., Meyer, W. J., III, and Blalock, J. E. (1986). Corticotropin releasing factor induction of leukocyte-derived immunoreactive ACTH and endorphins. *Nature (London)* 3211, 881–884.

Solomon, A. S., Kay, N., and Morley, J. E. (1987). Endorphins: A link between personality, stress, emotions, immunity and disease. *In* "Enkephalins and Endorphins: Stress and the Immune System" (N. P. Plotnikoff, R. E. Faith, A. J. Murgo, and R. D. Good, eds.), pp. 129–144. Plenum, New York.

Targan, S., Britvan, L., and Dorey, F. (1981). Activation of human NKCC by moderate exercise: Increased frequency or NK cells with enhanced capability of effector-target lytic interactions. *Clin. Exp. Immunol.* 45, 352–360.

Van Epps, D. E., and Saland, L. (1984). Beta-endorphin and met-enkephalin stimulate human chemotaxis. *J. Immunol.* 132, 3066–3073.

Williamson, S. A., Knight, R. A., Lightman, S. L., and Hobbs, J. R. (1987). Differential effects of β-endorphin fragments on human natural killing. *Brain, Behav, Immun.* 1, 329–335.

Wybran, J., Appelboom, J., Famaey, J. P., and Govaerts, A. (1979). Suggestive evidence for receptors for morphine and methionine enkephalin on normal human blood T lymphocytes. *J. Immunol.* 123, 1068–1072.

Yamasaki, Y., Shimamura, O., Kizer, A. *et al.* (1982). IgE mediated ^{14}C-serotonin release from rat mast cells modulated by morphine and endorphins. *Life Sci.* 31, 471–478.

Zurawski, G., Benedik, M., Kamb, B. J., *et al.* (1986). Activation of mouse T-helper cells induces abundant preproenkephalin mRNA synthesis. *Science* 232, 772–774.

12

Corticotropin-Releasing Factor Receptors in the Brain–Pituitary–Immune Axis

Elizabeth L. Webster   *Dimitri E. Grigoriadis*
Errol B. De Souza
Laboratory of Neurobiology
Neuroscience Branch
National Institute on Drug Abuse
Addiction Research Center
Baltimore, Maryland 21224

I. Introduction

Recent evidence suggests that the endocrine, immune, and central nervous systems interact and respond to physiological and pharmacological stimuli in a coordinated manner. While the interactions between the brain and endocrine system have long been recognized, research has recently focused on the participation of the nervous and endocrine systems in the regulation of immune-related responses. In turn, the immune system influences neural activity and endocrine secretions. The bidirectional communication between the neuroendocrine and immune systems and between the immune and central nervous systems appears to be mediated by neurotransmitters, hormones, and receptors common to the three systems. Paracrine secretion, humoral pathways (see Blalock, 1989; Morley *et al.*, 1987), and direct innervation of lymphoid tissue by primary sensory (Payan and Goetzl, 1985) and sympathetic nerve (see Felten *et al.*, 1985) fibers provide modes for the nervous, immune, and endocrine systems to communicate with each other. The coordinated response of these three systems during stress provides a primary example of how the brain–pituitary–immune axis serves to integrate the homeostatic responses of the organism.

Stress, or disruptions of homeostasis, can result from physical and psychological as well as immunological challenges. As described by Selye (1976), stress elicits a wide spectrum of changes within the nervous, endocrine, and immune systems. A key neurohormone that plays a significant role in integrating the response to stress throughout the neuro–endocrine–immune axis is corticotropin-releasing factor (CRF). Studies examining nervous–immune system and endocrine–immune system interactions have demonstrated that CRF regulation of pro-opiomelanocortin- (POMC) derived peptide secretion and, conversely, glucocorticoid feedback control of CRF and POMC-derived peptides, is a common feature of all three systems. CRF appears to be the primary mediator of the stress response both in terms of activating the hypothalamic–pituitary–adrenocortical (HPA) axis and the sympatho-adrenomedullary system (see Chapters 2, 5, 6, and 9). The activation of the HPA axis resulting in the secretion of CRF from the hypothalamus and consequent release of pituitary adrenocorticotropin (ACTH) and adrenal cortisol or corticosterone is the primary stress-related response in the endocrine system. The classic stress-related response of the nervous system involves activation of the sympatho-adrenomedullary system. In concert with the sympatho-adrenomedullary system, hormones of the HPA axis prepare the organism for physical and mental exertion directed toward restoring homeostasis. In addition to these well-known effects of stress on the nervous and endocrine systems, stress alters immune functions, resulting in changes in both immunocompetence and exaggerated immunoresponsiveness as observed in allergic and autoimmune diseases. Stress-induced effects on the immune system appear to be primarily mediated through hormones of the HPA axis and autonomic outflow (Livnat *et al.*, 1985). Interactions between the immune system and the autonomic nervous system are evidenced both by anatomical studies demonstrating that sympathetic neurons innervate lymphoid tissue and establish synaptic-like contacts with immune cells (see Felten *et al.*, 1985) and by pharmacological studies demonstrating specific receptor-mediated effects of adrenergic compounds on specific immune cell responses (reviewed in Livnat *et al.*, 1985). Moreover, immune responses appear sensitive to modulations of the autonomic nervous system such as those observed during stress and those induced experimentally, such as chemical sympathectomy (Cross and Rozman, 1988). The presence of receptors for immune cell products and the modulation of neuronal activity elicited by antigenic stimulation and by immune cell products, particularly in hypothalamic nuclei concerned with regulating the autonomic nervous system, suggest that nervous–immune system interactions are reciprocal.

A complete regulatory circuit interconnects the HPA axis and the immune system (reviewed in Blalock, 1989). For example, CRF and immunostimulation induce and glucocorticoids suppress POMC-derived peptide secretion in human peripheral blood (Smith et al., 1986) and mouse splenic (Harbour et al., 1987) leukocytes. CRF has also been reported to directly suppress human peripheral blood natural killer cytolysis (Pawlikowski et al., 1988) and monocyte chemotaxis (Stepien et al., 1987) in vitro. In addition to direct actions of CRF on cellular immune responses and the production of POMC-derived peptides by leukocytes, the activation of the sympathetic nervous system and HPA axis by CRF also indirectly influences cellular and humoral immunity. Administration of CRF intracerebroventricularly (icv) has been reported to suppress rat splenic natural killer cell activity subsequently measured in vitro (Irwin et al., 1987, 1988). This centrally mediated action of CRF on natural killer activity appears to be due primarily to an activation of the sympathetic nervous system rather than the HPA axis (Irwin et al., 1987, 1988).

Thus, CRF plays a significant role in integrating the stress-related responses to immunological agents such as viruses, bacteria, or tumor cells, and by the more traditional physiological and psychological challenges throughout the neuro–endocrine–immune axis. Since the actions of CRF are mediated through membrane receptors, this chapter will summarize the characteristics of CRF receptors in the brain–pituitary–immune axis with respect to their kinetic, pharmacological, and biochemical profiles, molecular weights, and second messenger activity. Furthermore, the localization of CRF receptors in tissues of the brain–pituitary–immune axis will be described and their physiological roles will be discussed in the context of their distribution.

II. CRF Receptors in the Brain, Pituitary, and Spleen

A. Kinetics and Pharmacology

Radioligand binding studies in membrane homogenates and autoradiographic studies in slide-mounted tissue sections have identified and characterized CRF receptors in the brain–pituitary–immune axis using a variety of iodine-125-labeled analogs. The *in vitro* binding characteristics of CRF receptors in rat (De Souza, 1987) and human (De Souza *et al.*, 1986) brain homogenates was defined using ^{125}I-Tyr^0-rat/human CRF. Binding of ^{125}I-Tyr^0-CRF to brain homogenates was dependent on time and temperature, was sensitive to pH and ionic strength of the incubation buffer, and was linear with membrane protein concentration. Receptor binding was optimal in 50 m*M* Tris HCl buffer, pH 7.2, and was maximal for 90- to 180-min incubation periods at room temperature with minimal degradation of the radioiodinated peptide occurring under these conditions. Using these assay conditions, equilibrium binding of ^{125}I-Tyr^0-CRF to brain (Figure 1) (De Souza, 1987), anterior pituitary (Figure 1) (De Souza *et al.*, 1984a; Grigoriadis and De Souza, 1989a), neurointermediate pituitary (Grigoriadis and De Souza, 1989a), and spleen (Webster and De Souza, 1988) membranes

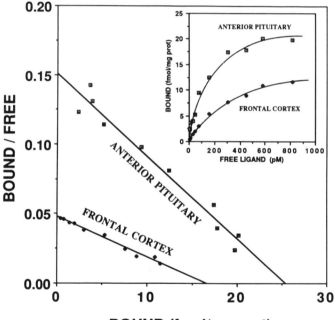

Figure 1 Saturation isotherms of ^{125}I-Tyr^0-oCRF binding to rat cortical and anterior pituitary membranes. Rat anterior pituitary and frontal cortex membranes were prepared and incubated with increasing concentrations of ^{125}I-Tyr^0-oCRF (0.05–1.0 n*M*). Direct saturation plots (see inset) indicate that binding was saturable, specific, and to a single homogeneous class of binding sites with apparent affinity values (K_D) of 200–400 p*M* as assessed by the nonlinear least-squares curve fitting program LIGAND (Munson and Rodbard, 1980). Specific binding was defined in both cases in the presence of 1 μ*M* unlabeled r/hCRF.

was both saturable and reversible. Scatchard analysis of the equilibrium binding of ^{125}I-Tyr^0-CRF in these tissues revealed a high-affinity binding site with an apparent K_D of 200–600 pM (Figure 1). The relative density of CRF binding sites was highest in the anterior and intermediate lobes of the pituitary, with moderate densities present in brain and low, but detectable, quantities of receptors present in spleen. Data from competition curves demonstrated that the CRF binding sites in these four tissues were comparable and exhibited a pharmacological specificity for CRF analogs and fragments that corresponded well with their intrinsic potency in stimulating or inhibiting anterior pituitary secretion of ACTH *in vitro* (Table I). These data indicate that the structural requirements for CRF activity are shared by brain, pituitary, and spleen receptors.

Table I

Pharmacological Specificity of CRF receptors in Brain, Pituitary, and Spleen[a]

Peptide	Brain K_i (nM)	Pituitary K_i (nM)	Spleen K_i (nM)
Nle^{21,38} r/hCRF	ND	ND	0.55 (2)
Nle^{21},Tyr^{32}oCRF	ND	2.8 ± 0.36 (4)	ND
r/h CRF	1.01 ± 0.05 (6)	0.88 ± 0.12 (4)	0.77 ± 0.05 (3)
oCRF	2.39 ± 0.11 (4)	1.43 ± 0.23 (3)	1.24 ± 0.09 (3)
α-helical oCRF	ND	ND	0.61 ± 0.07 (3)
α-helical oCRF(9–41)	16.73 ± 1.67 (3)	6.8 ± 1.56 (3)	11.03 ± 1.01 (3)
Ac oCRF (4–41)	0.47 ± 0.08 (3)	ND	ND
oCRF(7–41)	ND	104.0 ± 12.5 (3)	44.56 (2)
oCRF(1–39)	828.2 (2)	ND	164.40 (2)
oCRF(1–22)OH	ND	>1000 (3)	>1000 (3)
r/hCRF(1–20)	>1000 (3)	ND	>1000 (3)
r/hCRF(21–41)	>1000 (3)	ND	ND
r/hCRF(6–33)	>1000 (3)	ND	ND
VIP	>1000 (3)	>1000 (2)	>1000 (3)
AVP	>1000 (3)	>1000 (2)	>1000 (3)
Angiotensin II	>1000 (3)	ND	>1000 (3)
Substance P antagonist	ND (3)	>1000 (2)	>1000 (1)
Interleukin-1	ND (3)	ND	>1000 (2)
His^1,Nle^{27}GRF	>1000 (3)	ND	ND

[a]The pharmacological specificity of ^{125}I-Tyr^0-CRF binding to homogenates of brain, pituitary, or spleen membranes was characterized by the inhibition of various related and unrelated peptides. Membranes were incubated with 200–400 pM ^{125}I-Tyr^0-CRF in the presence or absence of the various peptides listed above (3–15 concentrations) and assessed for ^{125}I-Tyr^0-CRF binding. All assays were performed in triplicate with the number of experiments performed for any one peptide listed in parentheses. The K_i values were obtained by analyzing the data using LIGAND (Munson and Rodbard, 1980). Abreviations: r/hCRF, rat/human corticotropin-releasing factor; oCRF, ovine corticotropin-releasing factor; VIP, vasoactive intestinal peptide; AVP, arginine vasopressin, GRF, growth hormone releasing factor. ND, not determined. The data presented in the table are adapted from De Souza (1987) (brain), Grigoriadis and De Souza (1989a) (pituitary), and Webster and De Souza (1988) (spleen).

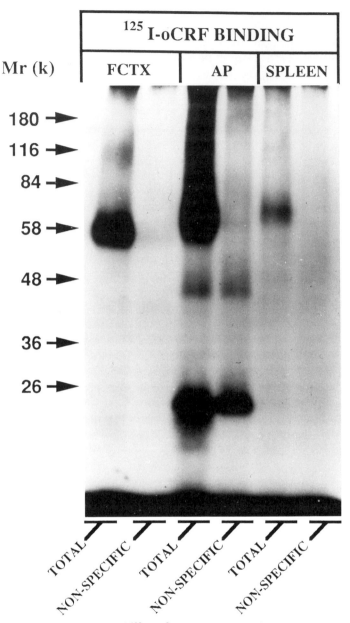

Figure 2 Covalent incorporation of ^{125}I-Tyr^0-oCRF into mouse brain, pituitary, and spleen homogenates. Labeling patterns of ^{125}I-Tyr^0-oCRF affinity cross-linked membranes (300–400 μg protein) from mouse demonstrate that the specific binding site, as defined in the presence of 1 μM unlabeled r/hCRF, in brain has a different apparent molecular weight from that in either pituitary or spleen. Mouse frontal cortex (FCX) exhibited a specific binding protein with an apparent molecular weight of 58,000 while anterior pituitary (AP) and spleen exhibited a

B. Identification of Molecular Weight and Structural Composition of CRF Receptors Using Chemical Affinity Cross-Linking Techniques

The ligand binding subunits of the CRF receptors in brain, pituitary, and spleen have been identified by chemical affinity cross-linking techniques. The details of the procedures are described elsewhere (Grigoriadis and De Souza, 1988, 1989a,b). Briefly, following equilibrium binding of ^{125}I-Tyr^0-CRF to crude membrane homogenates, the radioligand was irreversibly bound to the receptor using the homobifunctional cross-linking reagent disuccinimidyl suberate (DSS). Following the cross-linking procedure, the membrane pellets were washed twice in buffer, solubilized in sodium dodecyl sulfate (SDS) and subjected to SDS-polyacrylamide gel electrophoresis (SDS-PAGE), dried, and exposed to Kodak X-AR film in order to generate autoradiograms. Using these procedures, we and others have demonstrated that following affinity cross-linking of CRF to its receptor in anterior pituitary (Nishimura et al., 1987; Grigoriadis and De Souza, 1988, 1989a,b), neurointermediate lobe of the pituitary (Grigoriadis and De Souza, 1989a), and spleen (unpublished), the molecular weight of the CRF receptor as defined by SDS-PAGE is approximately 75,000 (Figure 2). In the mouse pituitary tumor cell line (AtT-20), however, the molecular weight of the CRF receptor appears to be approximately 66,000 (Rosendale et al., 1987). On the other hand, the CRF receptor in brain resides on a protein with an apparent molecular weight of 58,000 (Figure 2) (Grigoriadis and De Souza, 1988, 1989b). The pharmacological specificity of labeling was typical of the CRF binding site since both the brain- and pituitary/spleen-labeled proteins (i.e., molecular weight 58,000 and 75,000 proteins, respectively) exhibited the appropriate rank order profiles characteristic of the CRF receptor. Furthermore, the differences in the molecular weight of the CRF binding protein in brain versus the pituitary were present in a variety of species including rat, mouse, cow, pig, monkey, and human. The differences in the apparent molecular weight of central versus peripheral CRF receptors may possibly reflect different structural components of the CRF receptors that exist in these tissues. In order to compare the structural characteristics of the CRF receptor in brain and anterior pituitary, we first examined the hypothesis that the proteins themselves were identical but that the carbohy-

---

specifically labeled protein centered at approximately 75,000. In the presence of 1 μM unlabeled r/hCRF (nonspecific) the covalent incorporation could be inhibited in all tissues. In the absence of the cross-linking reagent DSS, no incorporation of ^{125}I-Tyr^0-oCRF could be observed (data not shown). Molecular weights of prestained protein markers are indicated on the left.

drate components of the receptors in the various tissues were different. These studies were carried out by subjecting cerebral cortical and anterior pituitary CRF receptors to various enzymatic deglycosylation treatments.

The data presented in Table II summarize the results obtained from a variety of affinity interactions and enzymatic treatments. CRF receptors in both brain and anterior pituitary are glycoproteins since they specifically adsorbed onto the immobilized lectins concanavalin A and wheat-germ agglutinin, and could be eluted off with the complimentary sugars. Concanavalin A (Con-A) binds molecules that contain alpha-D-mannopyranosyl or alpha-D-glucopyranosyl residues, and since both the cortical and anterior pituitary CRF receptors adsorbed to and specifically eluted from this lectin, the data suggest that these proteins contain some high-mannose derivatives in their carbohydrate chains. In addition, the demonstration that both forms of the CRF receptor specifically adsorbed to and eluted from wheatgerm agglutinin (which binds N-linked carbohydrates or terminal sialic acid residues) suggests that CRF receptors in both tissues also contain complex carbohydrate moieties. Furthermore, these data indicate that the carbohydrate composition of CRF receptors in both cerebral cortex and anterior pituitary is quite diverse in nature, containing both high-mannose derivatives and N-linked acetylglucosamine or terminal sialic acid residues.

Studies utilizing exoglycosidases and endoglycosidases confirm that both forms of the CRF receptor contain complex carbohydrate chains but to differing degrees, thus conferring unique structural characteristics to brain and pituitary CRF receptors (see Table II). Treatment of both cortical

Table II
Summary of the Biochemical Characteristics of Brain and Pituitary CRF Receptors[a]

Treatment	Brain	Pituitary
Wheat germ agglutinin	Adsorb	Adsorb
Concanavalin A	Adsorb	Adsorb
Neuraminidase	58k ⟶ 50k	75k ⟨ 70k / 58k
α-Mannosidase	58k ⟨ 60k / 50k	75k ⟶ 75k
N-Glycanase	58k ⟶ 40–45k	75k ⟶ 40–45k

[a]Data summarizing the glycosylation studies indicate that both the cortex and the anterior pituitary CRF receptors are glycosylated but contain different types of sugar residues. Values indicate apparent molecular masses (in daltons) as determined by SDS-polyacrylamide gel electrophoresis. (Reproduced with permission, Grigoriadis and De Souza, 1989b).

and pituitary CRF receptors with neuraminidase demonstrated that both forms of the receptor are sensitive to the effects of this exoglycosidase and provided additional evidence that these proteins are glycosylated. Since neuraminidase specifically cleaves only terminal sialic acid residues, the results suggest that both receptors are glycoproteins with carbohydrate chains containing some terminal sialic acid residues. Treatment of CRF receptors with the exoglycosidase alpha-mannosidase revealed differential sensitivity to this enzyme between cortical and anterior pituitary receptors. Specifically, the cortical CRF receptor was affected by the addition of alpha-mannosidase, while the pituitary CRF receptor remained largely unaffected. However, since anterior pituitary CRF receptors were able to interact with the lectin Con-A (suggesting the existence of mannose derivatives), the more pronounced effect of the enzyme in cerebral cortex than in anterior pituitary may be due, in part, to better accessibility of the mannose substrates to the enzyme. Consequently, the data indicate that both the cortical and pituitary CRF receptors contain some mannose side chains, but due to the heterogeneous nature of these carbohydrate chains, they appear to behave differently in the presence of the alpha-mannosidase enzyme or concanavalin A. Further studies utilizing sequential enzyme treatment of neuraminidase followed by alpha-mannosidase or alpha-mannosidase digestion in solubilized receptor preparations may be necessary to conclusively resolve these differences.

Endoglycosidase treatment of cortical and anterior pituitary CRF receptors produced drastic effects on the mobilities of both forms of the receptor (see Table II). N-Glycanase specifically hydrolyzes asparagine-linked oligosaccharides from glycoproteins and glycopeptides to yield free oligosaccharide and the peptide or protein containing aspartic acid residues. Following N-glycanase treatment, the mobilities of brain and pituitary CRF receptors were greatly increased and both forms of the receptor now migrated on SDS-PAGE with an apparent molecular weight of 40,000–45,000. This indicates that the major form of glycosylation in both CRF receptor types is N-linked through the asparagine residues on the protein backbone. Furthermore, the data suggest that the heterogeneity in the apparent molecular weights observed is due to differences in posttranslational modification of the CRF receptor in the brain and anterior pituitary. Further studies on the discrete components of glycosylation in central and peripheral CRF receptors are required to elucidate the differences in posttranslational glycosylation resulting in heterogeneous populations of CRF receptors.

In an attempt to determine whether the proteins of the anterior pituitary CRF receptor differ from those in the brain, we used proteases to specifically cleave the labeled receptor proteins into fragments that could be assessed by SDS-PAGE. We used the two proteases *Staphylococcus aureus* V8 and papain to perform limited proteolysis on the two receptor preparations. In performing the limited proteolysis experiments, it became apparent that these same proteases that were being used to cleave the CRF binding subunit would also cleave between specific amino acid residues on the CRF peptide, which was used to covalently label the receptor protein. During the course of the peptide mapping studies, this was indeed what was observed. Although the ^{125}I-Tyr^0-CRF peptide was being proteolyzed, there was sufficient incorporation of the label into peptide fragments that could be visualized, and the peptide maps of both the proteins, under conditions of proteolysis by two different proteases, appeared to be similar. Thus, in both anterior pituitary and cerebral cortex, the CRF ligand binding subunit appears to have the same enzyme cleavable sites. These data strongly suggest that CRF receptors in these two share structural similarities if not identity with each other.

From these biochemical studies, we have determined that the ligand binding subunits of the brain and pituitary CRF receptors reside on a polypeptide of 40,000–45,000. The heterogeneity between brain and pituitary CRF receptors appears to result from differential posttranslational glycosylation of the native protein and not from inherent differences in the protein structure. The glycosylation of these receptors is predominantly complex carbohydrate in nature and contains N-acetylglucosamine and/or terminal sialic acid residues. Both forms of the receptor also contain some high-mannose chains. Consequently, the molecular weights of the native affinity cross-linked receptor subunits are greatly overestimated due to this heavy glycosylation. The functional significance of the microheterogeneity observed in the carbohydrate moieties of brain and anterior pituitary CRF receptors remains to be determined.

C. Characterization of CRF Receptor-Mediated Second Messenger Activity

1. Evidence from Radioligand Binding Studies

Agonist binding to receptors mediating their effects through alterations in adenylate cyclase activity have been shown to be influenced by divalent cations and guanine nucleotides. Magnesium ions enhance agonist binding to receptors coupled to a guanine nucleotide regulatory protein by stabilizing the agonist high-affinity state of the receptor. In contrast, guanine nucleotides selectively decrease the affinity of agonists for their receptors by promoting the dissociation of the agonist high-affinity form of the receptor.

Consistent with CRF receptors being coupled to a guanine nucleotide regulatory protein, the binding of iodine-125-labeled analogs of CRF to pituitary (Perrin *et al.*, 1986), brain (De Souza, 1987; Webster and De Souza, 1988) and spleen (Webster and De Souza, 1988) homogenates was reciprocally modulated by divalent cations and guanine nucleotides. CRF binding was dependent on the presence of magnesium ions with linear increases in specific binding observed up to a concentration of 10 mM $MgCl_2$ (Figure 3). This effect was specific for magnesium, as only small increases in specific binding were observed in the presence of a comparable concentration of $CaCl_2$. In contrast to the effects of magnesium, the addition of increasing concentrations of guanosine 5′-triphosphate (GTP) to the incubation medium resulted in an inhibition of ^{125}I-Tyr^0-CRF binding in anterior (Aguilera *et al.*, 1988; Grigoriadis and De Souza, 1989a; Perrin *et al.*, 1986) and intermediate (Grigoriadis and De Souza, 1989a) lobes of pituitary, in brain (De Souza, 1987; Webster and De Souza, 1988), and in spleen (Webster and De Souza, 1988). The nonhydrolyzable GTP analogs, guanyl-5′-imidodiphosphate [Gpp(NH)p] and guanosine 5′-gamma-thiotriphosphate (GTP-γ-S), were more potent. This effect appeared to be specific to the guanine nucleotides, as similar experiments indicated that equimolar concentrations of adenosine 5′-triphosphate (ATP) had no effect on CRF binding.

While the data of these studies demonstrate similarities in the respective effects of Mg^{2+} and guanine nucleotides in regulating CRF receptors in pituitary, brain, and spleen, some subtle differences were observed in the sensitivity with which Mg^{2+} and guanine nucleotides regulate the specific binding of ^{125}I-Tyr^0-CRF to brain and spleen homogenates. For example, although Mg^{2+} produced a much greater increase (on a percentage basis) in ^{125}I-Tyr^0-CRF-specific binding in mouse brain than in mouse spleen, Mg^{2+} appeared to be more potent in increasing ^{125}I-Tyr^0-CRF binding to spleen than brain homogenates, since an approximately 10-fold lower EC_{50} was observed in spleen (Figure 3). Interestingly, the regulation of specific ^{125}I-Tyr^0-CRF binding in brain and spleen also exhibited some differences in terms of the magnitude of the effect and the species of guanine nucleotide. Whereas GTP inhibited the specific ^{125}I-Tyr^0-CRF binding to mouse brain to a greater extent than to spleen homogenates, Gpp(NH)p produced a greater percent suppression of ^{125}I-Tyr^0-CRF binding to mouse spleen than brain (Webster and De Souza, 1988). Thus, although there appear to be subtle differences in the sensitivity and guanine nucleotide specificity, the modulation of CRF receptor binding in pituitary, brain, and spleen by divalent cations and guanine nucleotides suggests that CRF receptors throughout the brain–pituitary–immune axis represent two-state receptors coupled through a guanine nucleotide binding protein to a second messenger system.

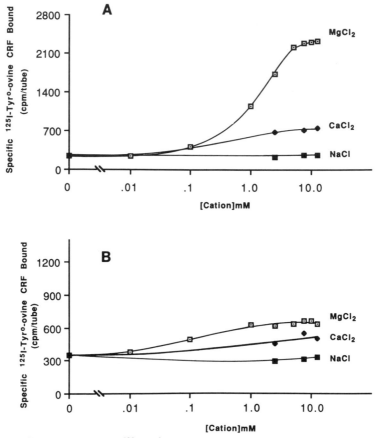

Figure 3 Effects of cations on ^{125}I-Tyr^0-oCRF binding to (A) mouse brain and (B) spleen homogenates. Parallel experiments were run in which spleen or whole brain homogenates were incubated with ^{125}I-Tyr^0-oCRF in 50 mM Tris containing 2 mM EGTA, 0.1% BSA, 100 μM bacitracin, 100 kIU/ml aprotonin, and varying concentrations of MgCl$_2$ hr, CaCl$_2$ hr, or NaCl, final pH 7.2. Each point is the average of three to four determinations. The data shown are from a representative experiment. In spleen, 10 mM MgCl$_2$ increased specific binding by approximately 90% while CaCl$_2$ maximally increased specific binding by approximately 60% at 7.5 mM CaCl$_2$; the EC$_{50}$ values for MgCl$_2$ and CaCl$_2$ were 0.13 and 2.1 mM, respectively. In brain, the specific binding of ^{125}I-Tyr^0-oCRF was increased by 850% at 12.5 mM MgCl$_2$ and 250% by 12.5 mM CaCl$_2$; EC$_{50}$ values for MgCl$_2$ and CaCl$_2$ were 1.4 and 1.5 mM, respectively. NaCl did not affect ^{125}I-Tyr^0-oCRF binding to spleen or brain homogenates in the range of concentrations (0–12.5 mM) tested. Reproduced with permission from Webster and De Souza (1988).

2. Characterization of CRF Receptor-Mediated Adenylate Cyclase Activity

Corticotropin-releasing factor stimulation of POMC-derived peptide secretion is mediated by the activation of adenylate cyclase in both the anterior (Giguere *et al.*, 1982; Bilezikjian and Vale, 1983) and neurointermediate (Meunier *et al.*, 1982) lobes of the pituitary. The stimulation of cAMP production and POMC secretion in anterior pituitary was dose-related and exhibited appropriate pharmacology (Aguilera *et al.*, 1983; Bilezikjian and Vale, 1983; Giguere *et al.*, 1982; Holmes *et al.*, 1984; Labrie *et al.*, 1982). CRF stimulation of cAMP and POMC-peptide secretion (Aguilera *et al.*, 1983; Bilezikjian and Vale, 1983; Giguere *et al.*, 1982; Holmes *et al.*, 1984; Labrie *et al.*, 1982; Meunier *et al.*, 1982), and activation of a cAMP-dependent protein kinase in anterior pituitary cells and in AtT-20 cells (Aguilera *et al.*, 1983; Litvin *et al.*, 1984) demonstrated comparable EC_{50} values in the nanomolar range. Thus, CRF initiates a cascade of enzymatic reactions in anterior pituitary cells beginning with the receptor-mediated stimulation of adenylate cyclase, which ultimately regulates POMC peptide secretion and possibly synthesis.

In a manner similar to that elucidated in pituitary, CRF stimulated adenylate cyclase activity in brain (Battaglia *et al.*, 1987; Chen *et al.*, 1986) and spleen (Webster *et al.*, 1989). Both basal and CRF-stimulated adenylate cyclase activity in rat brain (Battaglia *et al.*, 1987) and mouse spleen (Webster *et al.*, 1989) were dependent on time and tissue protein concentration. The pharmacological potency of various CRF analogs in stimulating adenylate cyclase activity in brain and spleen (Figure 4a) was consistent with their affinities for CRF receptors (Table III) and their potencies in eliciting POMC-derived peptide secretion from the pituitary. The CRF antagonist α-helical oCRF (9–41) competitively inhibited CRF stimulated adenylate cyclase in brain (Battaglia *et al.*, 1987; Chen *et al.*, 1986) and spleen (Figure 4b) (Webster *et al.*, 1989) homogenates. While the EC_{50} values for the various CRF peptides in stimulating cAMP production were comparable in brain, pituitary, and spleen, the V_{max} values were significantly lower in mouse spleen homogenates. The differences in the V_{max} values in the three tissues (Table III) probably reflect the higher concentration of CRF receptors in the pituitary and brain compared to the spleen.

Studies of the biochemical mechanisms of CRF receptor-mediated stimulation of cAMP production in pituitary, brain, and spleen indicate that CRF receptors are coupled through a guanine nucleotide protein to adenylate cyclase; however, these findings do not exclude the possibility that CRF receptors are coupled to other second-messenger systems as well. Evidence from studies in anterior pituitary and AtT-20 cells in culture indicate that CRF receptors are linked to other intracellular messenger systems by cAMP-

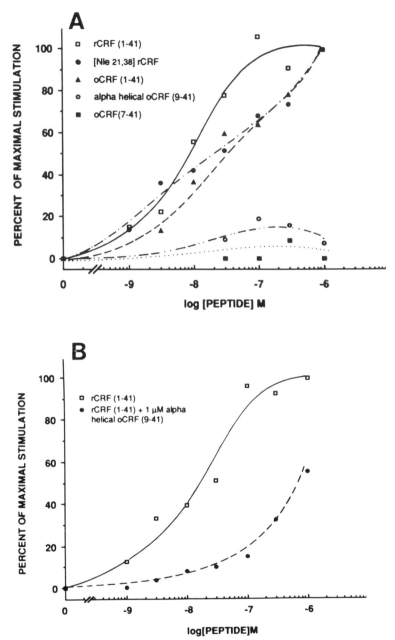

Figure 4 Pharmacological profile of CRF-receptor mediated stimulation of adenylate cyclase activity in mouse spleen. Mouse spleen homogenates were incubated with (A) varying concentrations of CRF related peptides or (B) varying concentrations of rat/human CRF in the presence (open squares) and absence (closed circles) of 1 μM of the receptor antagonist α-helical oCRF(9–41). Data are expressed as a percent of the maximal stimulation above basal activity elicited by the respective peptides or 1 μM r/hCRF for α-helical oCRF(9–41) and oCRF(7–

Table III

Stimulation of Adenylate Cyclase Activity in Brain and Spleen by Various CRF-Related and Unrelated Peptides[a]

Peptide	Brain		Spleen	
	EC_{50} (nM)	V_{max}	EC_{50} (nM)	V_{max}
Nle[21,38] r/hCRF	16 ± 5	110 ± 6	20.9 ± 8.9	18.6 ± 2.6
r/hCRF	36 ± 4	115 ± 7	13.2 ± 3.7	20.2 ± 2.7
oCRF	100 ± 21	121 ± 22	16.0 ± 3.5	19.1 ± 4.4
α-helical oCRF	43 ± 12	36 ± 7	ND	ND
Ac oCRF(4–41)	38 ± 2	98 ± 9	ND	ND
α-helical oCRF(9–41)	>1000	NS	>1000	NS
oCRF(7–41)	>1000	NS	>1000	NS
oCRF(1–39)	>1000	NS	ND	ND
AVP	ND	ND	>1000	NS
N-Formyl-methionyl-leucyl-phenylalanine	ND	ND	>1000	NS
Substance P	ND	ND	>1000	NS

[a]Data represent the mean ± SEM of values calculated from at least three independent concentration-response curves in which each concentration was determined in triplicate. NS indicates that there was no significant detectable stimulation of adenylate cyclase at peptide concentrations up to 1 μM. Basal activity (in the presence of 100 μM GTP) was approximately 100 pmol cAMP/min/mg protein in brain (rat fronto-parietal cortex) and 74 pmol cAMP/min/mg protein in mouse spleen. V_{max} values are calculated as pmol cAMP/min/mg protein and represent the stimulation above basal activity. ND, not determined. The data presented in the table are adapted from Battaglia et al. (1987) (brain) and Webster et al. (1989) (spleen).

dependent as well as cAMP-independent mechanisms (reviewed in Abou-Samra et al., 1987). Since CRF stimulated adenylate cyclase in the absence of Ca^{2+} and in the presence of EGTA in brain (Battaglia et al., 1987; Chen et al., 1986), pituitary (Holmes et al., 1984; Labrie et al., 1982) and spleen (Webster et al., 1989) homogenates, CRF-receptor-mediated stimulation of cAMP production does not appear to involve a Ca^{2+}/calmodulin mechanism. However, as has been demonstrated for a number of other stimulus–secretion hormone and transmitter systems, the stimulation of ACTH release by CRF and other agents does require Ca^{2+} (reviewed in Abou-Samra et al., 1987). Corticotropin-releasing factor appeared to elevate cytosolic Ca^{2+} in AtT-20 cells through a receptor-mediated mechanism linked to cAMP-dependent protein kinase (Guild and Reisine, 1987; Luini et al., 1985). Other signal transduction mechanisms involving methyltransferases

41). Basal activity (activity in the presence of 100 μM GTP) was approximately 74 pmol cAMP/min/mg protein. Each point represents the mean data from three to eight independent experiments in which each concentration was determined in triplicate. EC_{50} and V_{max} values from the pooled experiments are presented in Table III. Reproduced with permission from Webster et al. (1989).

also appear to be linked to CRF receptors, as CRF has been shown to increase ACTH secretion, protein carboxylmethylation, and phospholipid methylation in AtT-20 cells (Heisler *et al.*, 1983; Hook *et al.*, 1982). The stimulation of both protein carboxylmethylation and phospholipid methylation by CRF was dose dependent and exhibited an appropriate pharmacology for the CRF receptor (Heisler *et al.*, 1983; Hook *et al.*, 1982). Preliminary evidence suggests that CRF also may regulate cellular responses through products of arachidonic acid metabolism (Abou-Samra *et al.*, 1986, 1987). CRF increased the release of [^{3}H]arachidonic acid from prelabeled pituitary cells. Furthermore, inhibition of the cyclooxygenase metabolic pathway by indomethacin augmented, while inhibitors of the lipoxygenase pathway suppressed, CRF-stimulated ACTH release (Abou-Samara *et al.*, 1986, 1987). Evidence in anterior pituitary cells suggests that CRF does not directly regulate phosphotidylinositol turnover or protein kinase C activity (Abou-Samara *et al.*, 1987; Guillon *et al.*, 1987). However, stimulation of protein kinase C either directly or by specific ligands (vasopressin or angiotensin II) enhanced CRF-stimulated adenylate cyclase activity, ACTH release, and inhibited phosphodiesterase activity (Abou-Samara *et al.*, 1987; Bilezikjian and Vale, 1987; Labrie *et al.*, 1987). In turn, CRF suppressed arginine vasopressin-stimulated inositol triphosphate levels in rat anterior pituitary cells (Bilezikjian and Vale, 1987). Thus, the effects of CRF on anterior pituitary cells and possibly in neurons and other cell types expressing CRF receptors are likely to involve complex interactions among intracellular second messenger systems.

D. Localization and Physiological Roles of CRF Receptors

The autoradiographic distribution of ^{125}I-Tyr^0-CRF binding sites in mouse pituitary, brain, and spleen is shown in Figure 5.

1. Pituitary

Mouse pituitary autoradiograms showed specific binding sites for ^{125}I-Tyr^0-CRF in anterior and intermediate lobes, while no specific binding sites for CRF were apparent in the posterior pituitary (Figure 5a). In agreement with previous autoradiographic studies in our laboratory in rat and human anterior pituitary (De Souza *et al.*, 1984a, 1985a,b; Grigoriadis and De Souza, 1989a), the autoradiographic localization of CRF receptors in mouse pituitary demonstrates a clustering of binding sites that corresponds to the distribution of corticotrophs. The intermediate lobe shows a uniform distribution of binding sites characteristic of the homogeneous population of POMC-producing cells in this lobe. The presence of CRF receptors on corticotroph cells was further confirmed by studies using biotin-conjugation

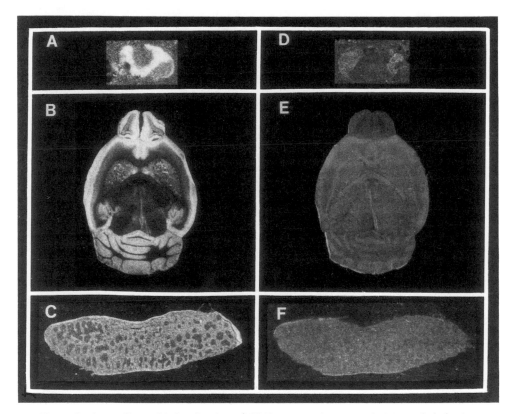

Figure 5 Autoradiographic localization of CRF receptors in mouse pituitary, whole brain, and spleen. Darkfield photomicrographs demonstrating the total distribution of ^{125}I-Tyr^0-oCRF binding sites in (A) mouse pituitary, (B) brain, and (C) spleen. In darkfield illumination, the bright areas represent high densities of CRF receptors. In (A) (horizontal section of pituitary), note the higher density of CRF receptors in the intermediate lobe of the pituitary compared to the anterior lobe as well as the conspicuous absence of CRF binding sites in the posterior lobe. In (B) (horizontal section of brain), note the higher densities of binding sites in cerebral cortex, olfactory bulb, cerebellum, and in a variety of limbic areas. In (C) (saggital section of spleen), note the diffuse density of CRF binding sites that are localized to the red pulp regions and the high density of CRF binding sites in the marginal zone surrounding the white pulp zone. There was a notable absence of CRF binding in the white pulp regions, which contain high concentrations of T and B lymphocytes. (D–F) Darkfield photomicrographs showing the absence of specific binding in adjacent sections of all three tissues in which 1 μM unlabeled r/hCRF was included in the incubation medium.

(Westlund *et al.*, 1984) and iodine-125-labeling (Leroux and Pelletier, 1984) in conjunction with immunocytochemical staining of corticotrophs using an ACTH antiserum. Thus, the distribution pattern of CRF receptors within the pituitary supports the functional role of CRF as the primary physiological regulator of POMC-derived peptide secretion from the anterior and intermediate lobes of the pituitary.

2. Central Nervous System

Receptor autoradiography and binding studies in different CNS regions in rat (De Souza, 1987; De Souza *et al.*, 1984b, 1985c; Wynn *et al.*, 1984) and primates (De Souza and Kuhar, 1986a,b; Millan *et al.*, 1986) demonstrated that, in general, the highest concentration of CRF binding sites was distributed in brain regions involved in cognitive function (cerebral cortex), in limbic areas involved in emotion and stress responses (amygdala, nucleus accumbens, and hippocampus), in brainstem regions regulating autonomic function (locus ceruleus and nucleus of the solitary tract), and in olfactory bulb (De Souza, 1987; De Souza *et al.*, 1984b, 1985c; Wynn *et al.*, 1984). In addition, there was a high density of CRF binding sites in the molecular layer of the cerebellar cortex (De Souza *et al.*, 1985c; Wynn *et al.*, 1984) and in the spinal cord, where the highest concentrations were present in the dorsal horn (Bell and De Souza, 1989; De Souza *et al.*, 1985c).

In support of a neurotransmitter role for CRF within the CNS, the densities and sites of localization of CRF receptors correspond well with the relative distribution of CRF-immunoreactive (CRF-ir) terminals in specific brain regions. For example, CRF cell bodies in the neocortex are concentrated in laminae II and III with projections to laminae I and IV (Olschowka *et al.*, 1982; Cummings *et al.*, 1983; Swanson *et al.*, 1983), which are areas rich in CRF receptors. Corticotropin-releasing factor mRNA and immunoreactivity have been identified in neurons of the inferior olive that project via climbing fibers to the cerebellum (Cummings *et al.*, 1988; Palkovits *et al.*, 1987; Powers *et al.*, 1987; Young *et al.*, 1986). The demonstration that CRF-ir appears to be present in climbing fibers in the molecular layer of the cerebellum (Cummings *et al.*, 1988; Palkovits *et al.*, 1987; Powers *et al.*, 1987; Young *et al.*, 1986), which contains high concentrations of CRF receptors (De Souza *et al.*, 1985c; Powers *et al.*, 1987), provides compelling evidence that CRF acts as a neurotransmitter in the olivocerebellar pathway. Other examples include the distribution of CRF-ir fibers in primary sensory neurons of the dorsal horn of the spinal cord (Skofitsch *et al.*, 1984; Merchenthaler *et al.*, 1983; Schipper *et al.*, 1983; Olschowka *et al.*, 1982), which coincides with the distribution of CRF receptors in adult (De Souza *et al.*, 1985c) and neonatal (Bell and De Souza, 1989) rat spinal cord. In addition, the distribution of CRF-ir nerve terminals corresponds to the distribution of CRF binding sites in olfactory tubercle, caudate-putamen, nucleus of the diagonal band of Broca, medial and lateral septal nuclei, the cranial nerve nuclei in brainstem, and in other brainstem regions including the central gray, inferior olive, reticular formation, and the parabrachial nuclei. While relatively low concentrations of CRF receptors are present in most of the hypothalamus, binding sites are present in the external layer of the median eminence, where the greatest concentration of CRF-ir fibers is found (Olschowka *et al.,* 1982; Cummings *et al.,* 1983; Swanson *et al.,* 1983). In addition, autoradiographic data have localized receptors in low to moderate concentrations in the paraventricular nucleus of the hypothalamus (De Souza *et al.,* 1985c), which may represent presynaptic autoreceptors and/or receptors for regulating peptide release not only in the median eminence but also in brainstem regions subserving autonomic functions.

Studies examining the effects of icv administration of CRF on glucose utilization and electrophysiological studies also indicate a high degree of correlation between CNS areas sensitive to CRF and the relative densities of CRF receptors in these regions. In general, CRF altered glucose utilization differentially in brain regions that have been implicated in mediating responses to stress. For example, high densities of CRF receptors are present in brain areas showing altered glucose utilization, including the cerebral cortex, nucleus accumbens, median eminence of the hypothalamus, spinal nucleus of the trigeminal nerve, cuneate nucleus, dorsal tegmental nucleus, locus ceruleus, and cerebellum (Sharkey *et al.,* 1989). While changes in glucose utilization in the hypothalamus following CRF reflect its neuroendocrine role, the observed changes in the locus ceruleus, prefrontal cortex, and nucleus accumbens support activation of cerebral noradrenergic and mesocortical dopaminergic systems (Sharkey *et al.,* 1989). Iontophoretic application of CRF caused increased spontaneous firing rates in the majority of neurons tested in the cortex and hippocampus, whereas the spontaneous activity of neurons in the thalamus and lateral septum was more frequently reduced (Eberly *et al.,* 1983). Direct application (via pressure ejection) of CRF to neurons of the locus ceruleus produced dose-related increases in spontaneous activity in both anesthetized and unanesthetized rats (Valentino *et al.,* 1983). In contrast, the spontaneous activity of neurons in the parvocellular region of the paraventricular nucleus and arcuate nucleus was depressed following superfusion of CRF in brain slice preparations (Siggins *et al.,* 1985).

The autoradiographic localization of CRF receptors provides an anatomical basis for some of the observed actions of CRF within the CNS corresponding to those changes produced by many forms of stress. The hypothalamus may represent a primary site of action for integrating some endocrine, autonomic, and behavioral effects of CRF. A role has been proposed for CRF in the control of food intake (Morley and Levine, 1982; Britton *et al.* 1982). Microinfusions of CRF into the hypothalamus have been shown to have antipyretic effects (Bernardini *et al.*, 1984) and to suppress sexual behavior (Sirinathsinghji *et al.*, 1983). In addition, icv injections of CRF have been shown to inhibit the release of growth hormone (Rivier and Vale, 1984a; Ono *et al.*, 1984), luteinizing hormone (Ono *et al.*, 1984; Rivier and Vale, 1984b), vasopressin, and oxytocin (Plotsky *et al.*, 1985) and to have deleterious effects on reproductive functions. CRF can also stimulate the secretion of somatostatin in cultured rat hypothalamic cells and cerebral cortical cells (Peterfreund and Vale, 1983).

The autonomic effects of CRF are evident in a variety of species and include increased plasma concentrations of epinephrine, norepinephrine, glucose, and glucagon (Brown *et al.*, 1982a,b), and cardiovascular parameters such as increased heart rate and mean arterial pressure (Fisher *et al.*, 1982), and decreased gastric acid secretion (Tache *et al.*, 1983) and gastric motility (Pappas *et al.*, 1987). CRF may produce some of its effects via receptors in the parabrachial nucleus, medullary reticular formation, nucleus of the solitary tract, or other brain regions known to participate in autonomic function. CRF binding sites are also present in several forebrain areas that exert a powerful influence on autonomic outflow. These regions include the hypothalamus, especially the paraventricular hypothalamus, bed nucleus of the stria terminalis, amygdala, septum, hippocampus, and cingulate cortex.

3. Spleen

In autoradiographic studies on slide-mounted sections of mouse spleen, ^{125}I-Tyr^0-CRF binding sites were primarily localized to the red pulp and marginal zones (Figure 5c). The localization of ^{125}I-Tyr^0-CRF binding sites in mouse spleen to regions known to have a high concentration of macrophages suggests that CRF receptors are present on splenic macrophages. In addition, the uptake pattern of India ink by phagocytic cells corresponded closely to the distribution of ^{125}I-Tyr^0-CRF binding sites in the same tissue section, which suggests that CRF receptors are present on phagocytes. The absence of specific ^{125}I-Tyr^0-CRF-binding sites in the periarteriole and peripheral follicular white pulp regions of the spleen suggests that neither T nor B lymphocytes have specific high-affinity CRF receptors comparable to those localized in the marginal zone and red pulp areas of the spleen (Webster and De Souza, 1988) or in slide-mounted sections of the pituitary (see Section II,D,1) and brain (see Section II,D,2). In order to further confirm the identity of the specific cell type(s) expressing CRF receptors, we evaluated specific ^{125}I-Tyr^0-CRF binding activity in various splenic cell populations separated on the basis of their physical and functional properties. While these results did not allow us to exclude the possibility that other cell types also account for some ^{125}I-Tyr^0-CRF binding, CRF receptors were expressed primarily on resident splenic macrophages. Interestingly, CRF receptors were not found on peritoneal macrophages or macrophage cell lines, suggesting that the expression of CRF receptors may be induced in macrophages by factors present in the splenic microenvironment (Webster *et al.*, 1990).

The demonstration of CRF receptors on mouse splenic macrophages further establishes that the interaction of monocytes/macrophages with the HPA axis may represent a significant component of the regulatory circuit interconnecting the immune system with the HPA axis. Glucocorticoids, CRF, and POMC-derived peptides regulate monocyte/macrophage responses, and in turn, monocyte/macrophage-derived products also influence the HPA axis. CRF and immunostimulation induce POMC-derived peptide secretion in human peripheral blood (Smith *et al.*, 1986) and mouse splenic (Harbour *et al.*, 1987) leukocytes. Kavelaars *et al.* (1989) have recently provided preliminary evidence that CRF stimulates human peripheral blood monocytes to secrete interleukin-1 (IL-1), which in turn stimulates B lymphocytes to secrete immunoreactive β-endorphin. Conversely, systemic injection of IL-1 increases serum ACTH and glucocorticoids in mice and rats (Besedovsky *et al.*, 1986). While IL-1 has been reported to directly stimulate ACTH release in AtT-20 cells (Woloski *et al.*, 1985) and to stimulate ACTH release (Bernton *et al.*, 1987; Brown *et al.*, 1987) and POMC mRNA (Brown *et al.*, 1987) in primary rat pituitary cultures, other studies have found that IL-1 stimulated pituitary ACTH release by a central action mediated by CRF (Berkenbosch *et al.*, 1987; Sapolsky *et al.*, 1987; Uehara *et al.*, 1987). The secretion of IL-1 by monocytes (Woloski *et al.*, 1985) and POMC-derived peptide secretion by human peripheral blood leukocytes (Smith *et al.*, 1986) are inhibited by glucocorticoids.

While the functional role of CRF in mouse spleen has not been defined, the presence of CRF immunoreactivity in primary sensory afferent nerves (Skofitsch *et al.*, 1984) and in human peripheral blood lymphocytes (Ritchie *et al.*, 1986) indicates that there are potential sources of CRF in spleen that could be released by neurosecretion or paracrine secretion from leukocytes, respectively. Thus, CRF from these putative sources may regulate IL-1 and/or POMC-derived peptide secretion. The regulatory actions of IL-1 on immune responses are well known. In addition, POMC-derived peptides have been demonstrated to have regulatory influences on cellular immune functions including lymphocyte proliferation, antibody formation, natural killer cell activity, macrophage activation, and chemotaxis (reviewed in Blalock, 1989). Both POMC-derived mRNA and POMC-derived peptides including β-endorphin have been localized in subpopulations of macrophages (Lolait *et al.*, 1984, 1986) and in Newcastle disease virus-infected leukocytes (Westley *et al.*, 1986) in mouse spleen. In addition, CRF may directly regulate some effector functions of macrophages such as chemotaxis, phagocytosis, cytotoxicity, and Ia expression that are suppressed by factors that activate cAMP production (Verghese and Synderman, 1983).

III. Summary

CRF is the primary physiological regulator of POMC-derived peptide secretion from the anterior pituitary gland. In addition to its endocrine effects, the widespread distribution of CRF-containing neurons and receptors in the CNS and the direct effects of CRF on autonomic function, behavior, and neuronal electrical activity in various regions suggest that endogenous CRF also functions as a neurotransmitter or neuromodulator. More recent evidence suggests that CRF may also play a significant role in integrating the response of the immune system to physiological, psychological, and immunological stressors. These findings suggest that CRF plays a fundamental role in integrating stress-related responses throughout the neuro–immuno–endocrine axis. The actions of CRF in the CNS, pituitary, and spleen are mediated by specific, high-affinity membrane receptors that show similar kinetic and pharmacological properties and regulation by divalent cations and guanine nucleotides (Table IV). Furthermore, CRF receptors in the

Table IV

Similarities and Differences in the *In Vitro* Characteristics of Corticotropin-Releasing Factor (CRF) Receptors in Brain, Pituitary, and Spleen

Characteristic	Brain	Pituitary Anterior	Pituitary Intermediate	Spleen
Affinity (K_D; pM)	200–400	200–400	200–400	200–400
Binding in the presence of divalent cations (e.g., Mg^{2+}	Increased	Increased	Increased	Increased
Binding in the presence of guanine nucleotides (e.g., GTP)	Decreased	Decreased	Decreased	Decreased
Second messenger (stimulation of adenylate cyclase activity)	Yes	Yes	Yes	Yes
Pharmacology comparable to CRF-stimulated ACTH secretion *in vitro*	Yes	Yes	Yes	Yes
Apparent molecular mass (Da)	58,000	75,000	75,000	75,000
Structural composition	Glycoprotein	Glycoprotein	Glycoprotein	Glycoprotein

brain, pituitary, and spleen are functionally linked to a guanine nucleotide binding protein mediating stimulation of adenylate cyclase. Chemical affinity cross-linking studies followed by SDS-PAGE and autoradiography demonstrated that the molecular weight of the CRF receptor binding protein is different in central versus peripheral tissues. Enzymatic digestion studies demonstrated that the CRF receptor is a glycoprotein and that the differences observed in the molecular weight are due to the microheterogeneity of the carbohydrate moieties on the receptors in the two types of tissues. Furthermore, limited proteolysis revealed that the CRF receptor binding protein in the brain or periphery contained the same proteolytic enzyme cleavage sites, suggesting that the protein backbone of the receptor is identical in all tissues.

References

Abou-Samra, A-B., Catt, K. J., and Aguilera, G. (1986). Role of arachadonic acid in the regulation of adrenocorticotropin release from rat anterior pituitary cells in culture. *Endocrinology (Baltimore)* **119**, 1427–1431.

Abou-Samra, A-B., Harwood, J. P., Catt, K. J., and Aguilera, G. (1987). Mechanisms of action of CRF and other regulators of ACTH release in pituitary corticotrophs. *Ann. N. Y. Acad. Sci.* **512**, 67–84.

Aguilera, G., Harwood, J. P., Wilson, J. X., Morell, J., Brown, J. H., and Catt, K. J. (1983). Mechanisms of action of corticotropin-releasing factor and other regulators of corticotropin release in rat pituitary cells. *J. Biol. Chem.* **258**, 8039–8044.

Aguilera, G., Abou-Samra, A. B., Harwood, J. P., and Catt, K. J. (1988). Corticotropin releasing factor receptors: Characterization and actions in the anterior pituitary gland. *Adv. Exp. Med. Biol.* **245**, 83–106.

Battaglia, G., Webster, E. L., and De Souza, E. B. (1987). Characterization of corticotropin-releasing factor (CRF) receptor-mediated adenylate cyclase activity in rat central nervous system. *Synapse* **1**, 572–581.

Bell, J. A., and De Souza, E. B. (1989). Functional corticotropin-releasing factor receptors in neonatal spinal cord. *Peptides (N.Y.)* **9**, 1317–1322.

Berkenbosch, F., Van Oers, J., Del Rey, A., Tilders, F., and Besedovsky, H. (1987). Corticotropin-releasing factor producing neurons in the rat activated by interleukin-1. *Science* **238**, 524–526.

Bernardini, G. L., Richards, D. B., and Lipton, J. M. (1984). Antipyretic effect of centrally administered CRF. *Peptides (N.Y.)* **5**, 57–59.

Bernton, E. W., Beach, J. E., Holaday, J. W., Smallridge, R. C., and Fein, H. G. (1987). Release of multiple hormones by a direct action of interleukin-1 on pituitary cells. **Science 238,** 519–521.

Besedovsky, H., Del Rey, A., Sorkin, E., and Dinarello, C. (1986). Immunoregulatory feedback between Interleukin-1 and glucocorticoids. *Science* **233**, 652–654.

Bilezikjian, L. M., and Vale, W. W. (1983). Glucocorticoids inhibit corticotropin-releasing factor-induced production of adenosine $3',5'$-monophosphate in cultured anterior pituitary cells. *Endocrinology (Baltimore)* **113**, 657–662.

Bilezikjian, L. M., and Vale, W. W. (1987). Regulation of ACTH secretion from corticotrophs: The interaction of vasopressin and CRF. *Ann. N. Y. Acad. Sci.* **512**, 85–96.

Blalock, J. E. (1989). A molecular basis for bidirectional communication between the immune and neuroendocrine systems. *Physiol. Rev.* **69,** 1–32.

Britton, D. R., Koob, G. F., Rivier, J., and Vale, W. (1982). Intraventricular corticotropin-releasing factor enhances behavioral effects of novelty. *Life Sci.* **31,** 363–367.

Brown, M. R., Fisher, L. A., Rivier, J., Spiess, J., Rivier, C., and Vale, W. (1982a). Corticotropin-releasing factor: Effects on the sympathetic nervous system and oxygen consumption. *Life Sci.* **30,** 201–210.

Brown, M. R., Fisher, L. A., Spiess, J., Rivier, C., Rivier, J., and Vale, W. (1982b). Corticotropin-releasing factor: Actions on the sympathetic nervous system and metabolism. *Endocrinology (Baltimore)* **111,** 928–931.

Brown, S. L., Smith, L. R., and Blalock, J. E. (1987). Interleukin 1 and interleukin 2 enhance proopiomelanocortin gene expression in pituitary cells. *J. Immunol.* **139,** 3181–3183.

Chen, F. M., Bilezikjian, L. M., Perrin, M. H., Rivier, J., and Vale, W. (1986). Corticotropin releasing factor receptor-mediated stimulation of adenylate cyclase activity in the rat brain. *Brain Res.* **381,** 49–57.

Cross, R. J., and Rozman, T. L. (1988). Central catecholamine depletion impairs *in vivo* immunity but not *in vitro* lymphocyte activation. *J. Neuroimmunol.* **19,** 33–45.

Cummings, S., Elde, R., Ells, J., and Lindvall, A. (1983). Corticotropin-releasing factor immunoreactivity is widely distributed within the central nervous system of the rat: An immunohistochemical study. *J. Neurosci.* **3,** 1355–1368.

Cummings, S., Sharp, B., and Elde, R. (1988). Corticotropin-releasing factor in cerebellar afferent systems: A combined immunohistochemistry and retrograde transport study. *J. Neurosci.* **8,** 543–554.

De Souza, E. B. (1987). Corticotropin-releasing factor receptors in the rat central nervous system: Characterization and regional distribution. *J. Neurosci.* **7,** 88–100.

De Souza, E. B., and Kuhar, M. J. (1986a). Corticotropin-releasing factor receptors in the pituitary gland and central nervous system: Methods and overview. *In* "Methods in Enzymology" (P. M. Conn, ed.), Vol. 124, pp. 560–590. Academic Press, Orlando, Florida.

De Souza, E. B., and Kuhar, M. J. (1986b). Corticotropin-releasing factor receptors: Autoradiographic identification. *In* "Neuropeptides in Neurologic and Psychiatric Disease" (J. B. Martin and J. Barchas, eds.), pp. 179–198. Raven Press, New York.

De Souza, E. B., Perrin, M. H., Rivier, J., Vale, W., and Kuhar, M. J. (1984a). Corticotropin-releasing factor receptors in rat pituitary gland: Autoradiographic localization. *Brain Res.* **296,** 202–207.

De Souza, E. B., Perrin, M. H., Insel, T. R., Rivier, J., Vale, W. W., and Kuhar, M. J. (1984b). Corticotropin-releasing factor receptors in rat forebrain: Autoradiographic identification. *Science* **244,** 1449–1451.

De Souza, E. B., Insel, T. R., Perrin, M. H., Rivier, J., Vale, W., and Kuhar, M. J. (1985a). Differential regulation of corticotropin-releasing factor receptors in anterior and intermediate lobes of pituitary and in brain following adrenalectomy in rats. *Neurosci. Lett.* **56,** 121–128.

De Souza, E. B., Perrin, M. H., Whitehouse, P. J., Rivier, J., Vale, W., and Kuhar, M. J. (1985b). Corticotropin-releasing factor receptors in human pituitary gland: Autoradiographic localization. *Neuroendocrinology* **41,** 419–422.

De Souza, E. B., Insel, T. R. Perrin, M. H., Rivier, J., Vale, W., and Kuhar, M. J. (1985c). Corticotropin-releasing factor receptors are widely distributed within the rat central nervous system: An autoradiographic study. *J. Neurosci.* **5,** 3189–3203.

De Souza, E. B., Whitehouse, P. J., Kuhar, M. J., Price, D. L., and Vale, W. (1986). Reciprocal changes in corticotropin-releasing factor (CRF)-like immunoreactivity and CRF receptors in cerebral cortex of Alzheimer's disease. *Nature (London)* **319,** 593–595.

Eberly, L. B., Dudley, C. A., and Moss, R. L. (1983). Iontophoretic mapping of corticotropin-releasing factor (CRF) sensitive neurons in the rat forebrain. *Peptides (N.Y.)* **4**, 837–841.

Felten, D. L., Felten, S. Y., Carlson, S. L., Olschowka, J. A., and Livnat, S. (1985). Noradrenergic and peptidergic innervation of lymphoid tissue. *J. Immunol.* **135**, 755s–765s.

Fisher, L. A. Rivier, J. Rivier, C., Spiess, J., Vale, W. W., and Brown, M. R. (1982). Corticotropin-releasing factor (CRF): Central effects on mean arterial pressure and heart rate in rats. *Endocrinology (Baltimore)* **110**, 2222–2224.

Giguere, V., Labrie, F., Cote, J., Coy, D. H., Sueiras-Diaz, J., and Schally, A. V. (1982). Stimulation of cyclic AMP accumulation and corticotropin release by synthetic ovine corticotropin-releasing factor in rat anterior pituitary cells: Site of glucocorticoid action. *Proc. Natl. Acad. Sci. U.S.A.* **79**, 3466–3469.

Grigoriadis, D. E., and De Souza, E. B. (1988). The brain corticotropin-releasing factor (CRF) receptor is of lower apparent molecular weight than the CRF receptor in anterior pituitary. *J. Biol. Chem.* **263**, 10927–10931.

Grigoriadis, D. E., and De Souza, E. B. (1989a). Corticotropin-releasing factor (CRF) receptors in intermediate lobe of the pituitary: Biochemical characterization and autoradiographic localization. *Peptides (N.Y.)* **10**, 179–188.

Grigoriadis, D. E., and De Souza, E. B. (1989b). Heterogeneity between brain and pituitary corticotropin releasing factor (CRF) receptors is due to different glycosylation. *Endocrinology (Baltimore)* **125**(4), 1877–1888.

Guild, S., and Reisine, T. (1987). Molecular mechanisms of corticotropin-releasing factor stimulation of calcium mobilization and adrenocorticotropin release from anterior pituitary tumor cells. *J. Pharmacol. Exp. Ther.* **241**, 125–130.

Guillon, G., Gaillard, R. L., Kehrer, P., Schoenenberg, P., Muller, A. F., and Jard, S. (1987). Vasopressin and angiotensin induce inositol lipid breakdown in rat adenohypophysial cells in primary culture. *Regul. Pep.* **18**, 119–129.

Harbour, D. V., Smith, E. M., and Blalock, J. E. (1987). Novel processing for proopiomelanocortin in lymphocytes: Endotoxin induction of a new prohormone-cleaving enzyme. *J. Neurosci. Res.* **18**, 95–101.

Heisler, S., Hook, V. Y. H., and Axelrod, J. (1983). Corticotropin-releasing factor stimulation of protein carboxylmethylation in mouse pituitary tumor cells. *Biochem. Pharmacol.* **32**, 1295–1299.

Holmes, M. C., Antoni, F. A., and Szentendrei, T. (1984). Pituitary receptors for corticotropin-releasing factor: No effect of vasopressin on binding or activation of adenylate cyclase. *Neuroendocrinology* **39**, 162–169.

Hook, V. Y. H., Heisler, S., and Axelrod, J. (1982). Corticotropin-releasing factor stimulates phospholipid methylation and corticotropin secretion in mouse pituitary tumor cells. *Proc. Natl. Acad. Sci. U.S.A.* **79**, 6220–6224.

Irwin, M. R., Vale, W., and Britton, K. T. (1987). Central corticotropin-releasing factor suppresses natural killer cell toxicity. *Brain, Behav., Immun.* **1**, 81–87.

Irwin, M. R., Hauger, R. L., Brown, M. R., and Britton, K. T. (1988). CRF activates autonomic nervous system and reduces natural killer cell cytotoxicity. *Am. J. Physiol.* **255**, R744–R747.

Kavelaars, A., Ballieux, R. E., and Heijnen, C. J. (1989). The role of IL-1 in the corticotropin-releasing factor and arginine vasopressin-induced secretion of immunoreactive β-endorphin by human peripheral blood mononuclear cells. *J. Immunol.* **142**, 2338–2342.

Labrie, F. Gagne, B., and Lefevre, G. (1982). Corticotropin-releasing factor stimulates adenylate cyclase activity in anterior pituitary. *Life Sci.* **31**, 1117–1121.

Labrie, F., Giguere, V., Meunier, H., Simard, J., Gussard, F., and Raymond, V. (1987). Multiple factors controlling ACTH secretion at the anterior pituitary level. *Ann. N.Y. Acad. Sci.* **512**, 97–114.

Leroux, P., and Pelletier, G. (1984). Radioautographic study of binding and internalization of corticotropin-releasing factor by rat anterior pituitary corticotrophs. *Endocrinology (Baltimore)* 114, 14–21.

Litvin, Y., Pasmantier, R., Fleischer, N., and Erlichman, J., (1984). Hormonal activation of the cAMP-dependent protein kinases in AtT-20 cells. *J. Biol. Chem.* 259, 10296–10302.

Livnat, S., Felten, S. Y., Carlson, S. L., Bellinger, D. L., and Felten, D. L. (1985). Involvement of central and peripheral catecholamine systems in neural-immune interactions. *J. Neuroimmunol.* 10, 5–30.

Lolait, S. J., Lim, A. T. W., Toh, B. H., and Funder, J. W. (1984). Immunoreactive beta-endorphin in a subpopulation of mouse spleen macrophages. *J. Clin. Invest.* 73, 277–280.

Lolait, S. J., Clements, J. A., Markwick, A. J., Cheng, C., McNally, M., Smith, A. I., and Funder, J. W. (1986). Pro-opiocortin messenger ribonucleic acid and posttranslational processing of beta endorphin in spleen macrophages. *J. Clin. Invest.* 77, 1776–1779.

Luini, A., Lewis, D., Guild, S., Corda, D., and Axelrod, J. (1985). Hormone secretagogues increase cytosolic calcium by increasing cAMP in corticotropin-secreting cells. *Proc. Natl. Acad. Sci. U.S.A.* 82, 8034–8038.

Merchenthaler, I., Hynes, M. A., Vigh, S., Schally, A. V., and Petrusz, P. (1983). Immunocytochemical localization of corticotropin-releasing factor (CRF) in the rat spinal cord. *Brain Res.* 275, 373–377.

Meunier, H., Lefevre, G., Dumont, G., and Labrie, F. (1982). CRF stimulates alpha-MSH secretion and cyclic AMP accumulation in rat pars intermedia cells. *Life Sci.* 31, 2129–2135.

Millan, M. A., Jacobowitz, D. M., Hauger, R. L., Catt, K. J., and Aguilera, G. (1986). Distribution of corticotropin-releasing factor receptors in primate brain. *Proc. Natl. Acad. Sci. U.S.A.* 83, 1921–1925.

Morley, J. E., and Levine, A. S. (1982). Corticotropin-releasing factor, grooming and ingestive behavior. *Life Sci.* 31, 1459–1464.

Morley, J. E., Kay, N. E., Solomon, G. F., and Plotnifkoff, N. P. (1987). Neuropeptides: Conductors of the immune orchestra. *Life Sci.* 41, 527–544.

Munson, P. J., and Rodbard, D. (1980). LIGAND: A versatile computerized approach for characterization of ligand binding systems. *Anal. Biochem.* 197, 220–239.

Nishimura, E., Billestrup, N., Perrin, M. H., and Vale, W. (1987). Identification and characterization of a pituitary corticotropin-releasing factor binding protein by chemical cross-linking. *J. Biol. Chem.* 262, 12893–12896.

Olschowka, J. A., O'Donohue, T. L., Mueller, G. P., and Jacobowitz, D. M. (1982). The distribution of corticotropin-releasing factor-like immunoreactive neurons in rat brain. *Peptides (N.Y.)* 3, 995–1015.

Ono, N., Lumpkin, M. D., Samson, W. K., McDonald, J. K., and McCann, S. M. (1984). Intrahypothalamic action of corticotropin-releasing factor (CRF) to inhibit growth hormone and LH release in the rat. *Life Sci.* 35, 1117–1123.

Palkovits, M., Leranth, C., Gores, T., Young, W. S., III (1987). Corticotropin-releasing factor in the olivocerebellar tract of rats: Demonstration by light and electron microscopic immunohistochemistry and in situ hybridization histochemistry. *Proc. Natl. Acad. Sci. U.S.A.* 84, 3911–3915.

Pappas, T. N., Welton, M., Debas, H. T., Rivier, J., and Tache, Y. (1987). Corticotropin-releasing factor inhibits gastric emptying in dogs: Studies on its mechanism of action. *Peptides (N.Y.)* 8, 1011–1014.

Pawlikowski, M., Zelazowski, P., Dohler, K. D., and Stepien, H. (1988). Effects of two neuropeptides: Somatolibrin (GRF) and corticolibrin (CRF) on human natural killer activity. *Brain, Behave., Immun.* 2, 50–56.

Payan, D. G., and Goetzl E. J. (1985). Modulation of lymphocyte function by sensory neuro-peptides. *J. Immunol.* **135**, 783s–785s.

Perrin, M. H., Haas, Y., Rivier, J. L., and Vale, W. W. (1986). Corticotropin-releasing factor binding to the anterior pituitary receptor is modulated by divalent cations and guanyl nucleotides. *Endocrinology (Baltimore)* **118**, 1171–1179.

Peterfreund, R. A., and Vale, W. W. (1983). Ovine corticotropin-releasing factor stimulates somatostatin secretion from cultured brain cells. *Endocrinology (Baltimore)* **112**, 1275–1278.

Plotsky, P. M., Bruhn, T. O., and Otto, S. (1985). Central modulation of immunoreactive arginine vasopressin and oxytocin secretion into the hypophysial-portal circulation by corticotropin-releasing factor. *Endocrinology (Baltimore)* **116**, 1669–1671.

Powers R. E., De Souza, E. B., Walker, L. C., Price, D. L., Vale, W. W., and Young, W. S., III (1987). Corticotropin-releasing factor as a transmitter in the human olivocerebellar pathway. *Brain Res.* **415**, 347–352.

Ritchie, J. C., Owens, M., O'Connor, L., and Nemeroff, C. B. (1986). Measurement of ACTH and CRF immunoreactivity in adrenal and lymphocytes. *Soc. Neurosci. Abstr.* **12**, 286.5.

Rivier, C., and Vale, W. (1984a). Corticotropin-releasing factor (CRF) acts centrally to inhibit growth hormone secretion in the rat. *Endocrinology (Baltimore)* **114**, 2409–2411.

Rivier, C., and Vale, W. (1984b). Effect of long term administration of CRF on the pituitary–adrenal and pituitary-gonadal axis in the male rat. *J. Clin. Invest.* **75**, 689–694.

Rosendale, B. E., Jarrett, D. B., and Robinson, A. G. (1987). Identification of a corticotropin-releasing factor-binding protein in the plasma membrane of AtT-20 mouse pituitary tumor cells and its regulation by dexamethasone. *Endocrinology (Baltimore)* **120**, 2357–2366.

Sapolsky, R., Rivier, C., Yamamoto, G., Plotsky, P., and Vale, W. (1987). Interleukin-1 stimu-lates the secretion of hypothalamic corticotropin-releasing factor. *Science* **238**, 522–523.

Schipper, J., Steinbusch, H. W. M., Vermes, I., and Tilders, F. J. H. (1983). Mapping of CRF-immunoreactive nerve fibers in the medulla oblongata and spinal cord of the rat. *Brain Res.* **267**, 145–150.

Selye, H. (1976). "The Stress of Life." McGraw-Hill, New York.

Sharkey, J., Appel, N. M., and De Souza, E. B. (1989). Alteration in local cerebral glucose utilization following central administration of corticotropin-releasing factor in rats. *Synapse* **4**, 80–87.

Siggins, G. R., Gruol, D., Aldenhoff, J., and Pittman, Q. (1985). Electrophysiological actions of corticotropin-releasing factor in the central nervous system. *Fed. Proc., Fed. Am. Soc. Exp. Biol.* **44**, 237–242.

Sirinathsinghji, D. J. S., Rees, L. H., Rivier, J., and Vale, W. (1983). Corticotropin-releasing factor is a potent inhibitor of sexual receptivity in the female rat. *Nature (London)* **305**, 232–235.

Skofitsch, G., Hamill, G. S., and Jacobowitz, D. M. (1984). Capsaicin depletes corticotropin-releasing factor-like immunoreactive neurons in the rat spinal cord and medulla oblon-gata. *Neuroendocrinology* **38**, 514–517.

Smith, E. M., Morrill, A. C., Meyer, W. J., III, and Blalock, J. E. (1986). Corticotropin releas-ing factor induction of leukocyte-derived immunoreactive ACTH and endorphins. *Na-ture (London)* **321**, 881–882.

Stepien, H., Zelazowski, P., Pawlikowski, M., and Dohler, K. P. (1987). Corticotropin-releas-ing factor (CRF) suppression of human peripheral blood leukocyte chemotaxis. *Neu-roendocrinol. Lett.* **9**, 225–230.

Swanson, L. W., Sawchenko, P. E., Rivier, J., and Vale, W. (1983). Organization of ovine Corticotropin-releasing factor immunoreactive cells and fibers in the rat brain: An immunohistochemical study. *Neuroendocrinology* 35, 165–186.

Tache, Y., Goto, Y., Gunion, M., Vale, W., Rivier, J., and Brown, M. R. (1983). Inhibition of gastric acid secretion in rats by intracerebral injection of corticotropin-releasing factor. *Science* 222, 935–937.

Uehara, A., Gottschall, P. C., Dahl, R. R., and Arimura, a. (1987). Interleukin-1 stimulates ACTH release by an indirect action which requires endogenous corticotropin-releasing factor. *Endocrinology (Baltimore)* 121, 1580–1582.

Valentino, R. J., Foote, S. L., and Aston-Jones, G. (1983). Corticotropin-releasing factor activates noradrenergic neurons of the locus ceruleus. *Brain Res.* 270, 363–367.

Verghese, M. W., and Snyderman, R. (1983). Hormonal activation of adenylate cyclase in macrophage membranes is regulated by guanine nucleotides. *J. Immunol.* 130, 869–873.

Webster, E. L., and De Souza, E. B. (1988). Corticotropin-releasing factor receptors in mouse spleen: Identification, autoradiographic localization, and regulation by divalent cations and guanine nucleotides. *Endocrinology (Baltimore)* 122, 609–617.

Webster, E. L., Battaglia, G., and De Souza, E. B. (1989). Functional corticotropin-releasing factor (CRF) receptors in mouse spleen: Evidence from adenylate cyclase studies. *Peptides (N.Y.)* 10, 395–401.

Webster, E. L., Tracey, D. E., Jutila, M., Wolfe, S. A., Jr., and De Souza, E. B. (1990). Corticotropin-releasing factor (CRF) receptors in mouse spleen: Identification of receptor-bearing cells as resident macrophages. *Endocrinology (Baltimore)* 127, 440–452.

Westley, H. J., Kleiss, A. J., Kelley, K. W., Wong, P. K. Y., and Yuen, P.-H. (1986). Newcastle disease virus-infected splenocytes express the proopiomelanocortin gene. *J. Exp. Med.* 163, 1589–1594.

Westlund, K. N., Wynn, P. C., Chmielowiec, S., Collins, T. J., and Childs, G. V. (1984). Characterization of a potent biotin-conjugated CRF analog and the response of anterior pituitary corticotrophs. *Peptides (N.Y.)* 5, 627–634.

Woloski, B. M. R. N. J., Smith, E. M., Meyer, W. J., III, Fuller, G. M., and Blalock, J. E. (1985). Corticotropin-releasing activity of monokines. *Science* 230, 1035–1037.

Wynn, P. C., Hauger. R. L., Holmes, M. C., Millan, M. A., Catt, K. J., and Aguilera, G. (1984). Brain and pituitary receptors for corticotropin-releasing factor: localization and differential regulation after adrenalectomy. *Peptides (N.Y.)* 5, 1077–1084

Young W. S., III, Walker, L. C., Powers, R. E., De Souza, E. B., and Price, D. L. (1986). Corticotropin-releasing factor mRNA is expressed in the inferior olives of rodents and primates. *Brain Res.* 387, 189–192.

13

Modulation of Immunity and Neoplasia by Neuropeptides Released by Stressors

Raz Yirmiya
Department of Psychology
The Hebrew University of Jerusalem
Mount Scopus, Jerusalem, Israel

Yehuda Shavit
Department of Psychology
The Hebrew University of Jerusalem
Mount Scopus, Jerusalem, Israel

Shamgar Ben-Eliyahu
Department of Psychology
University of California
Los Angeles, California

Robert P. Gale
Department of Medicine, Division of
Hematology and Oncology
University of California
Los Angeles, California

John C. Liebeskind
Department of Psychology
University of California
Los Angeles, California

Anna N. Taylor
Department of Anatomy and Cell Biology
University of California
Los Angeles, California
and West Los Angeles VA Medical Center
Brentwood Division
Los Angeles, California

Herbert Weiner
Department of Psychiatry and
Biobehavioral Sciences
University of California
Los Angeles, California

I. The Concept of Stress

The concept of stress flows directly from Darwin's formulation of natural selection. Despite the fact that credit for the concept is customarily accorded to Walter B. Cannon and Hans Selye, it is to Darwin that we owe a complete reassessment of the relationship between the organism and its environment, incorporated in the concept of natural selection. In his view, the environment is in constant change (seasonal, climatic, chemical, geological, etc.), or it is continually being altered by its inhabitants. In the organism's struggle for existence, the environment is potentially threatening or dangerous due to the withdrawal of resources, to the disruption of health by infection, starvation, heat or cold, and to the threat of predators or competitors. Thus, stressors are selective pressures that derive from the physical and social environment. The environment can be threatening to the survival, integrity, and reproductive success of individuals and of species. The environmental challenges, called stresses or stressors, elicit physiological, as well as behavioral and psychological, responses, which are specific and appropriate to the stressful situation.

This definition differs from the one provided by Hans Selye in 1970, who defined stress as "the non-specific response of the body to any demand made upon it." Three important aspects are missing from Selye's definition. The first is that specific stressors do produce specific patterns of hormonal and neurochemical responses, which depend on several factors including the ability of animals to cope with the stress (e.g., whether the stressor is escapable or inescapable) (Anisman *et al.*, 1980; Weiss, 1971), the physical and psychological consequences of the stress (Gibbs, 1986), and the social conditions (Thoa *et al.*, 1977), age (Ritter and Pelzer, 1978), and genetic makeup (Wimer *et al.*, 1974) of the animal. The second aspect is that stressors have bodily consequences, as well as behavioral psychological consequences. Animals have a variety of behavioral strategies for survival in dealing with the threat of predators. These behavioral responses must be appropriate to the threat if they are to succeed; were they random or indiscriminate (nonspecific), survival would not be assured. When the threat to survival is infection, the appropriate response is immunological. If the threat to reproductive success is competition among males for mates, the appropriate response is to fight the rival, submit to him, or flee from him to find another mating partner. The third aspect is that even if the physiological responses to stressors are with some exceptions similar in different species and genera, what differs between similar species is the interpretation of the threatening signal. It is not the physical form of this signal that is important for an advantageous response, but its "value as a predictor or correlate" (Levins and Lewontin, 1985).

In the following chapter we describe the effects of stress on immunity and neoplasia and also the immunomodulatory role of several neuropeptides and hypophyseal hormones that are released when an animal is exposed to various stressors. The previously mentioned aspects of the definition of stress should be kept in mind when interpreting the results of these studies since different stressors elicit different profiles of hormonal changes, which in turn result in differential immune competency and resistance to neoplasms. This possibility may help to explain at least some of the variability in results obtained in studies on stress, immunity, and neoplasia. Most of the work in this area has not tied the immunomodulatory effects of stressors with the mediators of the response. Additionally, the causal relationship between stressors, immunity, and neoplasia has not been established. Our work on the role of neuropeptides in mediating the effects of various stressors on immunity and neoplasia attempts to address these issues.

II. Stress, Immunity, and Cancer

The interactions among stressors, emotions, and susceptibility to infection have been studied for many years. Tobach and Bloch (1958) were among the first to study the relationship between stress and susceptibility to acute tuberculosis. Their data indicated that the stress of crowding significantly reduced survival time of mice challenged with the tubercule bacillus.

Pursuing this line of research, numerous stressors (such as handling, crowding, isolation, separation from the mother, loud noise, electric shock, forced swimming, and rotation) have been evaluated in behavioral epidemiological studies. Immune function was not directly measured in these early studies, but the effect of the stressors on the susceptibility to bacterial and viral infectious agents was studied across species ranging from fish to human beings. In general, stress has been found to reduce the resistance of animals to infectious agents. However, several reports found that stress had a protective effect against infection. The nature and chronicity of the stressor, the time at which the infectious agent is introduced relative to the stressor, and the housing and social conditions of the animals appear to be important factors in determining the outcome of this type of study (see Ader, 1981, for review).

Stressors are associated with alterations of humoral and cellular immune mechanisms in both laboratory animals and humans. Decreased response to mitogens and antigens, reduced lymphocyte-mediated cytotoxicity, reduced delayed hypersensitivity, diminished skin-graft rejection, graft-versus-host reactivity, and suppressed antibody responses have all been observed after exposure to stressful stimuli. Other studies, however, show that stressors can also augment immune function. Several of the same factors mentioned earlier were also found to play an important role in determining the effects of stressors on the immune system. For example, the chronicity of the stressor, the time between the application of the stressor and the measurement of the immune response, the intensity of the stressor, and its controllability all play a role in determining the outcome (for reviews, see Monjan, 1981; Solomon and Amkraut, 1981).

The literature on stressors and neoplasia allows the reader to arrive at the same conclusions. Stressors alter the incidence and development of experimental tumors in animals. In general, stressors appear to enhance tumor induction and development (although stress-induced retardation of tumor growth has also been reported). These inconsistent findings may be due to differences in the nature of the stressors, tumor lines, timing of the stress relative to tumor administration, and the species of the host in the different studies. Nevertheless, several major factors fundamental to determining the effects of stressors on neoplasia have been identified. These include (1) chronic versus acute stressors: chronic stressors reportedly retard tumor growth and acute stressors enhance it; (2) the coping ability of the animal: Animals given control over the stressor are less affected; and (3) housing conditions (for reviews, see Sklar and Anisman, 1981; Riley, 1981).

III. Modulation of Immunity of Neuropeptides and Pituitary Hormones Released by Stressors

In the last decade, many neuropeptides and hypophyseal hormones have been shown to modulate immune function. Some of these substances are known to be released by stressors and may mediate some of their effects on the immune system. In the following section, the effects of several of these "stress-related" substances on immunity are reviewed.

A. Arginine Vasopressin

Several lines of evidence suggest that arginine vasopressin (AVP) is involved in the hypothalamic modulation of the stress response: AVP is released by stressful stimuli (Mirsky *et al.*, 1954), potentiates the release of adrenocorticotropic hormone (ACTH) by corticotropin-releasing factor (CRF) (Gillies *et al.*, 1982), and is thus involved in modulating the activation of the hypothalamic–pituitary–adrenal (HPA) axis during stressful stimuli (Gibbs, 1986). Brattleboro (DI) rats, which are homozygous for diabetes insipidus (DI) because they cannot produce AVP, exhibit altered hormonal, physiological, and behavioral responses to stressors: Both an increase and a decrease in the response to stressors have been described. For example, DI rats show more stress-induced gastric erosion (Wideman and Murphy, 1985), but a reduced HPA axis activation (McCann *et al.*, 1966), and no stress-induced analgesia produced by swimming (Bodnar *et al.*, 1980).

Recent findings suggest an immunomodulatory role of AVP. Vasopressin levels in the brain and plasma are altered following immune system activation. For example, brain levels of immunoreactive AVP are elevated after the experimental induction of swelling and inflammation of the joints in rats (Millan *et al.*, 1985). Plasma AVP increases after the administration of bacterial endotoxin to rats (Kastin, 1986). These alterations in AVP levels may result from the accumulation of circulating endogenous and exogenous immunoglobulins in hypothalamic magnocellular neurons (possibly vasopressinergic) (Meeker *et al.*, 1987). AVP has also been found to promote the production of gamma-interferon in mitogen-stimulated lymphocytes, thus acting like interleukin-2 (Johnson *et al.*, 1982a), and AVP receptors on T-cells have been identified (Torres and Johnson, 1988). AVP stimulates prostaglandin synthesis and secretion by human mononuclear phagocytes (Locher *et al.*, 1983), and AVP immunoreactivity is found in lymphoid tissues such as the thymus (Markwick *et al.*, 1986) and lymph nodes (Aravich *et al.*, 1987).

We have compared the cytotoxic activity of natural killer (NK) cells of rats of the AVP-deficient, diabetes insipidus (DI), and normal Long–Evans (LE) strains (the former is derived from the latter). We also compared the effects of swimming stress, morphine administration, and AVP replacement on NK cell activity in these two strains (Yirmiya *et al.*, 1989b). In these experiments, the initial NK cell activity of DI rats was significantly higher than in LE rats (ranging between 149 and 189%). Both swim stress and morphine administration significantly suppressed NK activity in DI and LE rats, yet no difference in the degree of suppression between the two strains was observed. AVP replacement, effective in normalizing water intake in DI rats, had no significant effect on NK cell activity. DI rats exhibited lower plasma corticosterone levels, which did not increase with AVP replacement. These results suggest that AVP does not directly modulate NK cell activity. It is likely that other differences between DI and LE rats (e.g., lower plasma corticosterone levels) secondary to the AVP deficiency are responsible for the elevated baseline NK cell activity. Neither AVP nor other hormones affected by AVP deficiency seem to be involved in the effects of swim stress and morphine on NK cells.

We have tested the biological significance of the differential NK activity in DI and LE rats. Rats from both strains were injected into the tail vein with cells of the heterologous tumor MADB106 mammary adenocarcinoma. Two weeks later, lungs were removed and surface lung metastases were counted. Since we have showed that NK activity against MADB106 target cells *in vitro* is higher in DI than in LE rats, we expected DI rats to have fewer metastases. In contrast to our expectation, the number of metastases was significantly higher in DI than in LE rats. Moreover, administration of AVP to DI rats (via an osmotic minipump) for 2 days before and 12 days after tumor inoculation significantly reduced the number of metastases to that of control LE rats. These findings suggest the AVP may be involved in resistance to tumor metastases, regulating mechanisms other than NK activity.

B. Corticotropin-Releasing Factor and Adrenocorticotropic Hormone

In 1936, Selye reported that "diverse nocuous agents" resulted in adrenal hyperplasia. Later, many investigators observed that a variety of stressful stimuli cause the secretion of ACTH from the anterior pituitary gland, which in turn stimulates synthesis and release of corticosteroids from the adrenal cortex (Axelrod and Reisine, 1984). ACTH secretion is regulated by hypothalamic CRF (Vale *et al.*, 1981), which is believed to be secreted by paraventricular neurons following stressful stimuli (Axelrod and Reisine, 1984; Rivier *et al.*, 1982). Besides regulating the secretion of ACTH, CRF affects autonomic functions: It stimulates increases in plasma epinephrine, norepinephrine, neuropeptide-Y, glucagon, and glucose, and elevates arterial pressure, heart rate, and cardiac output (Brown and Fisher, 1989). Additionally, it suppresses gastric acid secretion, stimulates gastric contractions and pepsin secretion (Weiner *et al.*, 1989), and induces the pulsatile release of the gonadotropins (Rivier *et al.*, 1986).

Almost any aspect of the immune system can be modulated to some degree by glucocorticoids (Fauci, 1978). Although most of the effects of CRF and ACTH on immunity are mediated by the release of glucocorticoids, both peptides may act directly on the immune system. Both high- and low-affinity ACTH receptors have been described on lymphocytes (Johnson *et al.*, 1982b). Furthermore, an ACTH receptor on mouse and human mononuclear cells was found to be similar if not identical to the one found in the adrenal cortex (Blalock *et al.*, 1985). CRF receptors have also been identified in the mouse spleen (Webster and DeSouza, 1988).

Administration of ACTH to animals was shown to suppress several immune functions. For example, ACTH depresses antibody formation (Hayashida and Li, 1957), produces atrophy of lymphoid tissue (Dougherty, 1952), suppresses inflammation, and prolongs the survival of skin grafts (Osgood and Favour, 1951; Medawar and Sparrow, 1956). *In vitro* studies showed that ACTH inhibits antibody response to T-cell-dependent and -independent antigens and suppresses the mitogen-stimulated secretion of gamma-interferon by spleen cells (Johnson *et al.*, 1982b, 1984). Intraventricular administration of CRF suppresses NK cell activity (Irwin *et al.*, 1987, 1988), an effect that is antagonized by central (but not systemic) preadministration of the CRF antagonist alpha-helical CRF (Irwin *et al.*, 1987). Furthermore, pretreatment of animals with the ganglionic-blocking agent, chlorisondamine, completely abolishes the CRF-induced increase in plasma norepinephrine levels and the reduction in NK activity, without affecting ACTH and corticosterone levels (Irwin *et al.*, 1988), suggesting that these effects are mediated by the sympathetic nervous system. The physiological role of CRF in mediating the effects of stress on immunity was recently demonstrated by showing that central administration of CRF antibody completely antagonized footshock stress induced suppression of NK activity (Irwin *et al.*, in press). The finding that antibody treatment did not affect circulating levels of ACTH and corticosterone again demonstrates that CRF suppresses NK activity independently of pituitary–adrenal activation.

C. Growth Hormone

In rats, a decrease in plasma growth hormone (GH) levels follows both acute and prolonged stressful stimuli (Brown and Martin, 1974; Lenox *et al.*, 1980). This decrease appears to be mediated by CRF (Rivier and Vale, 1985). On the other hand, studies in rhesus and squirrel monkeys have demonstrated an increase in plasma GH levels during stress (Brown *et al.*, 1971). Humans may show elevated GH levels during psychological stress, particularly the more anxious and neurotic subjects (Miyabo *et al.*, 1979; Weiner, 1988).

Certain lymphoid cell lines and normal mouse thymocytes have been shown to express specific and high-affinity receptors for GH in some studies (Arrenbbrecht, 1974), but not in others (e.g., Nagy *et al.*, 1983a). Growth hormone was shown to slightly enhance antibody levels after immunization of rats with *Pasteurella pestis* extracts, and to antagonize the immunosuppressive effect of ACTH in that paradigm (Hayashida and Li, 1957). In old animals, injections of GH or implantation of GH- and prolactin-secreting pituitary adenoma cells completely reverse thymic atrophy, restore T-cell-dependent immune function, and enhance NK cell cytotoxicity (Kelly *et al.*, 1986; Davila *et al.*, 1987). In humans, nanogram concentrations of GH potentiate colony formation by normal T cells and induce lymphoproliferation (Mercola *et al.*, 1981; Kiess *et al.*, 1983). On the other hand, GH treatment in children with GH deficiency has been reported to decrease the percentage of B cells, the T helper/suppressor ratio, and mitogen responses (Rappaport *et al.*, 1986).

Hypophysectomy of rodents suppresses many immunological functions. Several of these functions can be restored by GH replacement. In mice, GH treatment reverses the depressed immune reactivity to antigens *in vitro* (Gisler and Schenkel-Hulliger, 1971) and restores reduced NK cell activity (Saxena *et al.*, 1982). In rats, the administration of GH after hypophysectomy counteracts cortisol-induced leukopenia (Chatterton *et al.*, 1973), and restores the normal production of precipitating antibodies and skin rejection responses (Comsa *et al.*, 1974; Comsa and Leonhardt, 1975). In a similar vein, NK cell activity in GH-deficient children is significantly reduced (Kiess *et al.*, 1986). These studies suggest that GH (and PRL, see next section) are tonically setting the operating level of several immune functions including NK cell activity. The role that these hormones have in modulating phasic immunological responses to stressors is less clear and should be studied further.

D. Prolactin (PRL)

Many types of physically or emotionally stressful stimuli induce PRL secretion. For example, ether anesthesia (Shin, 1979), cold (Jobin *et al.*, 1975) and immobilization stress (Riegel and Meites, 1976), footshock (Kant *et al.*, 1987), and surgery (Riegel and Meites, 1976) have all been reported to elevate plasma PRL levels. The release of PRL may be mediated by the PRL-releasing hormones (Shin, 1979), and regulated by other factors, such as endogenous opioid peptides (Rossier *et al.*, 1980).

Although several studies have failed to find PRL receptors on lymphoid tissue, other studies report the existence of PRL receptors on both lymphocytes and monocytes (Bellussi *et al.*, 1987). Daily PRL injections during immunization against sheep red blood cells (SRBC) increase antibody production against them (Spangelo *et al.*, 1984). PRL administration also enhances the lactogenic immune response, protecting neonates from enteric infections (Ijaz *et al.*, 1990). On the other hand, antibodies to PRL potently inhibit both murine and human lymphocyte proliferation in response to both T and B cell mitogens (Hartmann *et al.*, 1989). Under certain conditions, PRL dramatically increases the proliferative response of mouse splenocytes to Con A (Bernton *et al.*, 1988). Selective inhibition of PRL secretion by the dopamine agonist drug, bromocriptine (BRC), inhibits the development of the contact sensitivity reaction to dinitrochlorobenzene (DNCB), antibody formation against SRBC, and the development of adjuvant arthritis (Nagy *et al.*, 1983b; Berczi and Nagy, 1982). BRC also inhibits the *in vivo* tumoricidal activation of peritoneal macrophages, possibly by interfering with the production of macrophage activating factors by lymphocytes (Bernton et al., 1988). All of the effects of BRC can be reversed by PRL replacement.

Prolactin restores several impaired immune functions in hypophysectomized animals, including antibody response to SRBC, contact sensitivity to DNCB and the adjuvant arthritis response (Nagy *et al.*, 1983a; Berczi and Nagy, 1982). The minimum effective dose of PRL in these studies was approximately 10 times lower than the dose required for induction of lactation, and could be antagonized by the simultaneous administration of ACTH (Nagy *et al.*, 1983a,b; Berczi *et al.*, 1983).

E. Opioid Peptides

Exposure to many types of stressors releases endogenous opioid peptides, including β-endorphin (Guillemin *et al.*, 1977) and met-enkephalin (Owens *et al.*, 1988). Evidence from our laboratory and others suggests that exposure to stressors is associated with profound analgesia. By varying the parameters of footshock, different forms of "stress-induced analgesia" are produced, each with distinct neurochemical and hormonal correlates. Thus, a single stressor, inescapable footshock of constant intensity, can elicit analgesia via different mechanisms depending on the temporal parameters of its application. Exposure of rats to prolonged, intermittent footshock causes analgesia that is blocked by the opiate antagonist naloxone (Lewis *et al.*, 1980), develops tolerance with daily repetitions, and develops cross-tolerance with morphine administration. This analgesia is attenuated by hypophysectomy, adrenalectomy, and adrenal demedullation (Terman *et al.*, 1984), suggesting that it depends on the release of enkephalins from the adrenal medulla, and leads to a deficit in escape learning called "learned helplessness" (Maier *et al.*, 1983). In contrast, exposure to a brief, continuous footshock causes a comparable degree of analgesia, which is not blocked by naloxone (Lewis *et al.*, 1980), does not develop tolerance and cross-tolerance to morphine, and is unaffected by ablation of the pituitary or adrenal glands or associated with later learning deficits (Lewis *et al.*, 1980; Terman *et al.*, 1984).

These studies suggest that very specific forms of stressful procedures can trigger an analgesia mediated by opioid peptides. However, they also indicate that at least two forms of "stress analgesia" occur. We have, therefore, reasoned that this fact—that an opioid and nonopioid form of "stress analgesia" exist—might help account for the many discrepant reports on the effects of stressful procedures on immune function.

This hypothesis is particularly interesting, because the opiates and endogenous opioid peptides have been implicated in the regulation of the immune system. Human opiate addicts are more susceptible to infections and demonstrate deficits in immune function. Administration of opiates usually produces immunosuppression, demonstrated by reduced phagocytosis, antibody production, blastogenic responses to mitogens, cellular immunity, NK cell activity, and lymphokine production (Yahya and Watson, 1987; Sibinga and Goldstein, 1988). On the other hand, opioid peptides, including endorphins and enkephalins, have usually been found to enhance immune function. Yet some published reports describe the immunosuppressive effects of high doses of opioid peptides (for recent reviews, see Fischer, 1988; Sibinga and Goldstein, 1988).

Opiate agonists and antagonists have also been implicated in tumor development. The systemic administration of opiates, endogenous opioids, and opioid antagonists participates in the regulation of tumor growth (Zagon and McLaughlin, 1986). The intracerebral administration of β-endorphin into the nucleus raphe magnus enhances the rate of tumor metastasis (Simon *et al.*, 1984).

Whether opiates and opioid peptides act directly or indirectly upon immunocompetent cells remains to be determined. Nonetheless, evidence exists for opiate receptors on monocytes, granulocytes, lymphocytes, mast cells, and the terminal complexes of human complement (see Sibinga and Goldstein, 1988, for review). Blalock and his colleagues describe structural similarities between interferon, ACTH, and the endorphins. They have also shown that intracerebral administration of interferon induces a naloxone-sensitive analgesia and catatonia, and that lymphocytes can produce and secrete ACTH and endorphin-like peptides along with interferon (Weigent and Blalock, 1987).

In our laboratory we were particularly interested in the effects of opioids on NK cells, because they provide (along with cytotoxic T cells) protection against viral infections and neoplastic disease (Herberman and Ortaldo, 1981). NK cells are a subpopulation of lymphocytes that spontaneously recognize and kill certain target cells, and that have been implicated in immune surveillance against tumors, in particular against tumor metastasis (Herberman and Ortaldo, 1981). It is especially noteworthy in this context that NK activity was found to be markedly reduced by stressors such as starvation, cold-water swim, restraint, and examination (Saxena *et al.*, 1980; Aarsstad *et al.*, 1983; Okimura *et al.*, 1986; Glaser *et al.*, 1986). Several *in vitro* studies have shown that NK cells taken from human subjects and rats and incubated with physiological levels of both β-endorphin and met-enkephalin manifest enhanced activity that can be attenuated by opioid antagonists (Faith *et al.*, 1984; Mandler *et al.*, 1986; Matthews *et al.,* 1983). However, the effects of opioids *in vivo* on NK cells, especially in relation to stress, are not clear. Therefore, we have investigated the effect of opioid and nonopioid stress paradigms on NK activity.

1. Effects of Morphine and Opioid and Nonopioid Stress on NK Cell Cytotoxicity

In our initial studies we found that 4 daily exposures to the intermittent (opioid), but not to the continuous (nonopioid), form of footshock resulted in significant suppression of NK activity to 74% of control levels. This suppression was prevented by administration of the opioid antagonist naltrexone (10 mg/kg) 20 min before the intermittent stress sessions (Shavit *et al.,* 1984). Injections of naltrexone or saline alone had no significant effect on NK activity.

In a second experiment, rats were given morphine to determine whether it would mimic the effect of the intermittent (opioid) footshock. Daily injections of morphine for 4 days produced a dose-related suppression of NK activity (Shavit *et al.,* 1984); 10 mg/kg of morphine had no significant effect, but injections of either 30 or 50 mg/kg markedly suppressed NK activity to a degree comparable to that seen after intermittent footshock. These findings support the view that endogenous opioid peptides can suppress NK activity.

Later we reported that a single exposure to intermittent footshock stress or a single high dose of morphine (>20 mg/kg, sc) suppresses NK cell cytotoxicity (Shavit *et al.,* 1987). The suppression is evident 3 h after the end of the procedure. The activity of NK cells returns to normal within 24 h. Morphine-induced NK suppression occurs in cells derived simultaneously from the spleen, bone marrow, and peripheral blood, suggesting that it is not produced from selective egress of these cells from the spleen (Shavit *et al.,* 1987). We have extended these findings to two other narcotic agents commonly used in general anesthesia, fentanyl and sufentanil. Both significantly suppress NK cell activity in rats for up to 12 h, an effect that can be blocked by naltrexone. Pretreatment with poly I:C, an interferon inducer, significantly attenuates the suppressive effect of fentanyl on NK activity (Beilin *et al.,* 1989).

The involvement of opioid peptides in producing these results was further explored by examining whether tolerance and cross-tolerance would develop to the stress- and morphine-induced suppression of NK activity. We found that tolerance to the NK-suppressive effect of the intermittent footshock does not develop even after 30 daily sessions, whereas tolerance to morphine's effect does develop after 14 daily injections (Shavit *et al.,* 1986b). Suppression of NK activity both in morphine-naive and in morphine-tolerant rats still occurs after intermittent footshock, thus indicating that cross-tolerance does not occur between the effects of morphine and the shock procedure (Shavit *et al.*, 1986b).

The development of tolerance to the suppressive effect of morphine on NK activity suggests that this effect is mediated via opioid (possibly μ) receptors. Because rats do not become tolerant to intermittent footshock and no cross-tolerance with morphine occurs, it seems likely that the immune suppressive effects of stress and morphine are mediated by different mechanisms, perhaps by different opioid receptor types. These findings may have important clinical implications. Although a single, very high dose of an opiate drug might be expected to be immunosuppressive in man, these deleterious effects should show rapid tolerance as drug use is continued. Thus, morphine should prove safe to use in the long-term management of cancer pain, for example. In fact, failing to manage such pain adequately would be expected to cause pain and distress, the immunosuppressive and tumor enhancing consequences of which do not diminish over time.

Morphine injected into the lateral cerebral ventricles of rats (20 and 40 μg) suppresses NK cell activity to the same level as a 1000-fold higher systemic dose. The icv effect of morphine is blocked by naltrexone (Shavit *et al.*, 1986a). In contrast, NK activity is unaffected by systemic administration of N-methylmorphine, an analog of morphine that does not cross the blood–brain barrier (Shavit *et al.*, 1986a). These results again suggest that opiate receptors in the brain mediate the morphine-induced suppression of NK cell cytotoxicity.

The stereospecificity of opiate-induced NK cell suppression has also been studied by comparing the effect of the opiate alkaloid levorphanol with its opiate-inactive stereoisomer, dextrorphan: only the former (10 mg/kg, sc) significantly suppresses NK cell activity in the intact rat. *In vitro*, however, both opiates suppress NK cell activity at very high concentrations (Martin *et al.*, 1985). These results suggest that the *in vivo* effect of levorphanol is mediated by opiate receptors, whereas the *in vitro* effect is not. Furthermore, these results support our earlier hypothesis that opiate alkaloids, such as morphine and levorphanol, suppress NK cell activity by binding to brain opiate receptors, rather than acting directly upon NK cells. We next sought to determine the type of opiate receptor mediating the *in vivo* effect of opiates by using β-funaltrexamine (β-FNA), an irreversible antagonist of the μ-opiate receptor. When injected directly into the lateral cerebral ventricles, β-FNA significantly blocked morphine-induced NK suppression (Sohn *et al.*, 1986). Taken together, these data further support our hypothesis that morphine's effect on NK cells is mediated by opioid receptors in the brain.

However, we have recently found marked strain differences in the response of NK cell activity to morphine administration in mice. Three hours after a single injection of a high dose of morphine (100 mg/kg), but not of saline solution, NK cell activity is significantly suppressed in C57BL/6By mice but significantly enhanced in BALB/cBy. In members of both strains, the suppressive and enhancing effects of morphine are completely blocked by the administration of naltrexone 20 min before morphine injection (R. Yirmiya, F. Martin, Y. Shavit, and J. C. Liebeskind, unpublished). Not unexpectedly, morphine administration raises plasma corticosterone levels to equivalent levels (about 600 ng/ml) in both strains.

Several physiological mechanisms could account for our immunological findings. As previously mentioned, morphine and opioid peptides released by stressors might suppress immune function by acting directly on opiate receptors present on various cells of the immune system (Sibinga and Goldstein, 1988), or on brain opioid receptors. Alternatively, the effects of morphine and opioids on NK activity could involve modulation of the autonomic nervous system, which has recently been shown to innervate immune organs such as the spleen, thymus, and lymph nodes (Felten et al., 1985). Finally, opioids and morphine might affect NK cells by their effects on hormone release. For example, ACTH and corticosterone are well known to suppress various aspects of immune function, including NK activity (Hochman and Cudkowicz, 1978), and opioid peptides and morphine are known to cause release of ACTH (Morley, 1983). Our findings in mice, showing a strain-dependent suppressive or enhancing effect of morphine on NK cell activity, accompanied by a comparable elevation in plasma corticosterone, argue against an exclusive role for corticosteroids in mediating morphine's effect. The finding that the effects of morphine on metastases of the NK-sensitive tumor MADB106 are not affected by preadministration of the glucocorticoid antagonist RU38486 (see next section) supports this conclusion.

We have recently tested the generality of the hypothesis that the phenomenon of stress-induced suppression of NK activity is always opioid mediated. We found a stress paradigm, forced swimming, that induces NK suppression not blocked by the opioid antagonist naltrexone. This stressor also produces naltrexone-insensitive analgesia and elevated plasma corticosterone levels (Ben-Eliyahu et al., 1990), and it enhances tumor growth (see next section). These studies indicate that the suppression of NK cell cytotoxicity by stressors does not require mediation by opioid peptides.

2. Effects of Morphine and Opioid and Nonopioid Stress on Tumor Growth

Lewis et al. (1983b) found that rats subjected to the opioid, but not the nonopioid, form of footshock before being implanted with a rat mammary adenocarcinoma (MAT 13762B) had reduced median survival time and percent survival compared to nonstressed controls. Because the analgesia produced by intermittent footshock is prevented by opioid antagonists, the effects of this stressor on tumor progression were studied after preadministration with naltrexone. Naltrexone prevented the footshock-induced rapid tumor progression, whereas morphine (50 mg/kg), administered for 4 days before tumor implantation, enhanced it (Lewis *et al.*, 1983a,b). Furthermore, tolerance developed to the tumor-enhancing effect of morphine when administered for 14 days. Consistent with the findings of our NK experiments, the effects of intermittent footshock manifested neither tolerance after 14 daily stress exposures nor cross-tolerance in morphine-tolerant rats (Lewis *et al.*, 1983a,b). Thus, opioid peptides presumably released by intermittent footshock appear to be involved in the decreased resistance of rats to the mammary tumor as they appear to be involved in the suppression of NK cytotoxicity.

Several mechanisms by which opioids and morphine enhance tumor progression are possible: Some tumor cell lines carry surface opioid receptors, making it possible that opioids released by stressors directly affect tumor cells. However, it is not known whether MAT 13762B cells have such receptors. Opioid peptides and morphine, as mentioned, release hypophyseal hormones, including prolactin and ACTH (Morley, 1983), which might promote tumor progression. For example, some tumor lines carry PRL receptors. In fact, many experimental breast tumors, including the solid form of MAT 13762B (Bogden *et al.*, 1974), progress faster under the influence of elevated levels of PRL. Adrenal corticosteroids are powerful immune suppressants in rodents and could contribute to the enhanced growth or metastasis of tumors following stressors. It has been shown that the MAT 13762B tumor induces a specific immune response (Kreider *et al.*, 1978), and hence may be sensitive to steroid-induced impairment of immune function. It is also possible that other physiological changes caused by opioids (e.g., cardiovascular or thermoregulatory) affect the degree of tumor vascularization or the incidence and pattern of metastases. However, the most likely explanation for the connection between enhanced progression of MAT 13762B by intermittent footshock and morphine is the reduction of NK cell cytotoxicity.

In order to test this hypothesis, we have recently studied the MADB106 mammary adenocarcinoma cell line (Ben-Eliyahu *et al.*, 1989). It was previously shown (Barlozzari *et al.*, 1985) that rats treated with an anti-NK cell antibody (anti-asGM1) have a decreased ability to destroy circulating MADB106 cells, leading to an increased incidence of pulmonary metastases. Treatment with this antibody inhibits NK activity without affecting T-cell-mediated immunity and macrophage cytotoxicity. Adaptive transfer of large granular lymphocytes with high NK activity, but not T cells, restored the ability of NK-suppressed rats to inhibit the development of pulmonary metastases. These results indicate that NK cells are involved in resistance to this tumor strain (Barlozzari *et al.*, 1985).

Based on these lines of evidence, Fischer 344 rats injected with either naltrexone (10 mg/kg) or saline solution were subjected to the intermittent forced swim stress procedure described above or were not stressed. One hour after the end of the stressful procedure, 1×10^5 MADB106 tumor cells were injected intravenously. Twelve days later, surface lung metastases were counted. In a second experiment, rats were sacrificed 1 h after the end of the swim stress, and their spleens were removed and dissociated into a single-cell suspension. These cells were cocultured with chromium-labeled MADB106 target cells, and NK cell cytotoxicity against them was determined by the release of chromium after 16 h. The stressful procedure significantly suppressed the cytotoxic activity of splenic NK cells against the MADB106 cells; it also significantly enhanced the number of MADB106 metastases *in vivo*. A similar effect was observed after exposure to surgical stress (Page *et al.*, 1990). In contrast to our previous findings with intermittent footshock, naltrexone had no effects on either the suppression of NK cell cytotoxicity or the enhanced tumor growth (Ben-Eliyahu *et al.*, 1989).

In a recent study we assessed the role of the autonomic nervous system in mediating the effects of swim stress on tumor growth (Ben-Eliyahu *et al.*, 1990). We found that the increase in metastases number produced by exposure to swim stress could be significantly attenuated by preadministration of the ganglionic blocker chlorisondamine or the β-2 adrenergic receptor antagonist butoxamine. Neither drug affected number of metastases in nonstressed animals. These findings suggest that activation of adrenergic receptors by the sympathetic nervous system is important in mediating the effects of stress on tumor progression.

In a parallel set of experiments (Yirmiya *et al.*, 1990b) the effects of two opiate drugs, morphine and fentanyl, on NK cell activity and tumor growth were studied. Rats were injected with either naltrexone (10 mg/kg) or saline solution 20 min before a second injection of either morphine (50 mg/kg), fentanyl (35 μg/kg), or saline. One hour after the second injection, 1×10^5 MADB106 tumor cells were injected intravenously. Twelve days later, surface lung metastases were counted. In another experiment, rats were sacrificed 1 h after the second injection, and the cytotoxic activity of their NK cells against MADB106 cells was determined as described above. The administration of both morphine and fentanyl produced an increase in the number of MADB106 metastases *in vivo*, and suppressed the cytotoxic activity of NK cells against MADB106 *in vitro*. Naltrexone completely blocked the effects of both drugs on the suppression of NK cell cytotoxicity and the enhancement of tumor growth. In another experiment (Yirmiya *et al.*, 1990b), we found that administration of the glucocorticoid antagonist RU38486 (25 mg/kg, one hour before morphine administration) did not attenuate morphine-induced increase in lung metastases, indicating that the effect of morphine is not mediated by glucocorticoids.

To evaluate farther the hypothesis that opiates increase MADB106 metastases by suppressing NK activity, we studied the effects of morphine in NK depleted rats. Rats were divided into two groups injected with either normal rabbit serum (NRS) or anti-asGM1 (a monoclonal antibody directed at NK cells). Two days later, rats within each group were further divided into two subgroups and injected either with saline or morphine. One hour later all animals were injected with MADB106 tumor cells. Morphine administration produced a marked increase in the number of metastases in NRS-treated rats, but had no effect in anti-asialoGM1 treated rats. This finding strongly supports a causal relationship between the immune suppressive and tumor enhancing effects of opiates.

Alcohol has been shown to act as stressor to activate the brain–pituitary–adrenal axis (Redei *et al.*, 1986, 1988). Several lines of evidence suggest that alcohol consumption also increases risk for cancer. One possible explanation for this association is that ethanol is immunosuppressive (Seitz and Simanowski, 1988). Therefore, we have studied the effects of both chronic and acute ethanol administration on NK cell activity *in vivo* and *in vitro*, and on tumor metastases (Yirmiya *et al.*, 1989a,c).

In a series of chronic experiments, Fischer 344 rats were fed either a liquid diet containing ethanol (5% w/v) or a control diet. After 3 weeks, animals were injected intravenously with MADB106 tumor cells. Two weeks later, the animals were sacrificed and their lungs were examined for surface metastases. In a second experiment, animals were sacrificed after 3 weeks on the diet and their splenic NK cell cytotoxic activity against MADB106 cells was assayed. In acute experiments, rats were injected with either saline or ethanol (1.5–3.5 g/kg). One hour later, animals were injected with MADB106 tumor cells, sacrificed 12 days later, and metastases on the lung surface were counted. Another group thus treated was sacrificed, and the cytotoxic activity of their splenic NK cells was assessed. Because many of the effects of ethanol are known to be mediated by opioid mechanisms (Trachtenberg and Blum, 1987; Yirmiya and Taylor, 1989), animals were pretreated with naltrexone in order to determine whether it influences the effects of an acute injection of ethanol on tumor growth. Finally, the direct effect of ethanol on NK cell cytotoxic activity *in vitro* was studied by incubating splenic and MADB106 cells together in solutions containing various concentrations of ethanol.

Ethanol treatment significantly increased the number of metastases in both the chronic and the acute experiments. This effect was not influenced by prior naltrexone administration, nor was it correlated with plasma concentrations of corticosterone. However, in these experiments ethanol did not affect NK cell cytotoxicity in a standard assay. In contrast, direct incubation of effector and target cells in physiologically relevant concentrations of ethanol significantly suppressed NK cell cytotoxicity. These results indicate that ethanol increases tumor growth and that this effect is not mediated by opioids. It is possible that at least some of this ethanol-induced tumor growth results from a direct effect of ethanol on the interaction between NK and tumor cells.

In order to test the generality of these findings we also studied the effects of ethanol on progression of CRNK-16 leukemia. This leukemia occurs spontaneously and is a major cause of death in aged Fischer rats. Although a relationship between NK cells and CRNK-16 leukemia is not fully established, tumor cells can be destroyed by interleukin-2 activated NK (LAK) cells. We found that chronic ethanol treatment had no significant effect on mortality of rats injected with CRNK-16 leukemia cells after two weeks on the ethanol-containing diet. However, acute administration of ethanol (at doses equal to or greater than 1.5 mg/kg) one hour before tumor inoculation significantly reduced survival time (Yirmiya *et al.*, 1990a).

IV. Conclusions

A summary of our results is presented in Table I. The data indicate that some stressful procedures can suppress immune function in rats and decrease their resistance to tumor challenge. Opioid peptides seem to mediate the effects of some stressors (e.g., intermittent footshock), and these effects are mimicked by high doses of morphine given systemically or by minute amounts intracerebroventricularly. Furthermore, the suppression of NK cell cytotoxicity by centrally administered morphine may be mediated by opiate receptors in the brain. In other forms of stressful procedures, such as swim stress, nonopioid mechanisms seem to be involved in mediating the effects on NK cells and tumor growth. The nature of these mechanisms can at this time only be a subject of speculation, but involvement of one or several of the neuropeptides described in this chapter can be suggested. Our data suggest that the final common path that mediates the effects of at least some stressors on NK activity and tumor development involves activation of the autonomic nervous system.

Although our knowledge of the precise manner by which components

Table I
Summary of Results

Experimental manipulation	Target cell	Effect on NK cytotoxicity	Tumor cell	Effect on tumor growth	Attenuated by naltrexone
Opioid form of footshock stress (4 days)	YAC-1	Suppressed	MAT 13762B	Reduced survival	Yes
Nonopioid form of footshock stress (4 days)	YAC-1	No effect	MAT 13762B	No effect	No
Opioid form of footshock stress (1 session)	YAC-1	Suppressed			Yes
Nonopioid form of swimming stress (1 session)	MADB106 YAC-1	Suppressed Suppressed	MADB106	Increased metastasis	No
Morphine injection (30 or 50 mg/kg; 4 days)	YAC-1	Suppressed	MAT 13672B	Reduced survival	Yes
Single morphine injection (50 mg/kg)	MADB106 YAC-1	Suppressed Suppressed	MADB106	Increased metastasis	Yes
Single fentanyl injection (30, 35 µg/kg)	MADB106 YAC-1	Suppressed Suppressed	MADB106	Increased metastasis	Yes
ICV morphine administration (20 or 40 µg)	YAC-1	Suppressed	MADB106	Increased metastasis	Yes
Chronic ethanol consumption (3 or 5 weeks)	MADB106 YAC-1	No effect No effect	MADB106	Increased metastasis	Not tested
Single ethanol injection (1.5–3.5 g/kg)	MADB106 YAC-1	No effect No effect	MADB106	Increased metastasis	No
Incubation with ethanol (at concentration ≥0.1 mg/ml)	MADB106 YAC-1	Suppressed Suppressed			

of the immune system carry out surveillance against tumors is limited, there is evidence to suggest that NK cells play an important role in this process (Herberman and Ortaldo, 1981; Barlozzari et al., 1985). Further evidence in support of the role of NK cells in averting tumor progression and metastases is provided by the studies summarized in this chapter. We found that the effects of intermittent footshock and morphine on NK cytotoxic activity closely parallel their effects on the survival of rats challenged with tumor cells. In fact, in our early work with the MAT 13762B tumor every manipulation that caused an opioid-mediated suppression of NK cytotoxicity in rats also decreased their resistance to tumor challenge. More recently we have shown that swim stress and opiate drugs increase the development of pulmonary metastases of MADB106 cells *in vivo* and suppress NK cell activity against them *in vitro,* thus providing evidence of a possible causal relationship between stress, suppression of NK cell cytotoxicity, and increases in tumor metastases.

These studies also make it clear that Selye's concept of stress (Selye, 1956) is no longer tenable (Weiner, 1988). The experiments reported here show that stress is not a unitary phenomenon. Seemingly minor differences in stress parameters (e.g., the same total amount of footshock applied intermittently versus continuously) determine whether or not a stressor will suppress NK cell activity and enhance tumor growth, while also producing different forms of analgesia. Moreover, different stressful procedures that suppress NK cell activity and enhance tumor metastases may be mediated by different neurochemical systems (e.g., intermittent footshock stress is mediated by opioid peptides whereas swim stress is not).

Our findings also support the view that stressors, by altering brain and plasma levels of certain neuropeptides and hormones, play a role in regulating NK cell activity and tumor surveillance in animals. They add further substance to the data and concepts of behavioral neuroimmunology (Ader, 1981) and reinforce the need for continuing efforts to clarify the neural and neurohumoral mechanisms by which a stressful environment can alter the organism's immune system and susceptibility to and progression of disease.

Acknowledgments

R. Yirmiya and S. Ben Eliyahu were supported by the William S. Bettingen Endowment Fund for Psychoneuroimmunology. Y. Shavit was supported by the John D. and Catherine T. MacArthur Foundation. This research was supported by NIH grant NS07628 and an Unrestricted Pain Research Grant from the Bristol-Myers Company (J. C. Liebeskind), VA Medical Research Service and grant AA06744 (A. N. Taylor), and a grant from the Israel Institute for Psychobiology (R. Yirmiya).

References

Aarstad, H. J., Gaudernack, G., and Seljelid, R. (1983). Stress causes reduced natural killer activity in mice. *Scand. J. Immunol.* **18**, 461–464.

Ader, R., ed. (1981). "Psychoneuroimmunology" Academic Press, New York.

Anisman, H., Pizzino, A., and Sklar, L. S. (1980). Coping with stress, norepinephrine depletion and escape performance. *Brain Res.* **191**, 583–588.

Aravich, P. F., Silverman, W. F., Sladek, C. D., Felten, S. Y., Felten, D. L., and Sladek, J. R., Jr. (1987). Aging and water deprivation alter vasopressin content in lymphoid tissue and gut. *Soc. Neurosci. Abstr.* **13**, 1369.

Arrenbrecht, S. (1974). Specific binding of growth hormone to thymocytes. *Nature (London)* **252**, 255–257.

Axelrod, J., and Reisine, T. D. (1984). Stress hormones: Their interaction and regulation. *Science* **224**, 452–459.

Barlozzari, T., Leonhardt, J., Wiltrout, R. H., Herberman, R. B., and Reynolds, C. W. (1985). Direct evidence for the role of LGL in the inhibition of experimental tumor metastases. *J. Immunol.* **134**, 2783–2789.

Beilin, B., Martin, F. C., Shavit, Y., and Liebeskind, J. C. (1989). Suppression of natural killer (NK) cell activity in rats by various narcotic agents. *Brain, Behav., Immun.* **3**, 129–137.

Bellussi, G., Muccioli, G., Ghe, C., and Di Carlo, R. (1987). Prolactin binding sites in human erythrocytes and lymphocytes. *Life Sci.* **41**, 951–959.

Ben-Eliyahu, S., Yirmiya, R., Gale, R. P. G., and Liebeskind, J. C. (1989). Evidence for a causal relationship between the suppressive effect of stress on natural killer cell activity and enhanced metastatic tumor growth in rats. *Soc. Neurosci. Abstr.*

Ben Eliyahu, S., Yirmiya, R., Page, G., Boun, S. A., Taylor, A. N., Gale, R. P., Weiner, H., and Liebeskind, J. C. (1990). Sympathetic involvement in the stress-induced increase of metastatic spread: Studies of a natural killer-sensitive tumor. *Soc. Neurosci. Abs.*

Ben-Eliyahu, S., Yirmiya, R., Shavit, Y., and Liebeskind, J. C. (1990). Stress-induced suppression of natural killer cell cytotoxicity in the rat: A naltrexone-insensitive paradigm. *Behav. Neurosci.* **104**, 235–238.

Berczi, I., and Nagy, E. (1982). A possible role of prolactin in adjuvant arthritis. *Arthritis Rheum.* **25**, 591–594.

Berczi, I., Nagy, E., Asa, S. L., and Kovacs, K. (1983). Pituitary hormones and contact sensitivity in rats. *Allergy* **38**, 325–330.

Bernton, E., Meltzer, S., and Holaday, J. (1988). Suppression of macrophage activation and T-lymphocyte function in hypoprolactinemic mice. *Science* **239**, 401–404.

Blalock, J. E., Bost, K. L., and Smith, E. M. (1985). Neuroendocrine peptide hormones and their receptors in the immune system. *J. Neuroimmunol.* **10**, 31–40.

Bodnar, R. J., Zimmerman, E. A., Nilaver, G., Mansour, A., Thomas, L. W., Kelly, D. D., and Glusman, M. (1980). Dissociation of cold-water swim and morphine analgesia in Brattleboro rats with diabetes insipidus. *Life Sci.* **26**, 1581–1590.

Bogden, A. E., Taylor, D. J., Kuo, E. Y. H., Mason, M. M., and Speropoulos, A. (1974). The effect of perphenazine-induced serum prolactin response on estrogen primed mammary tumor-host systems, 13762 and R-35 mammary adeno-carcinomas. *Cancer Res.* **34**, 3018–3025.

Brown, G. M., and Martin, J. B. (1974). Corticosterone, prolactin, growth hormone response to handling and new environment in the rat. *Psychosom. Med.* **36**, 241–247.

Brown, G. M., Schalch, D. S., and Reichlin, S. (1971). Patterns of growth hormone and cortisol responses to psychological stress in the squirrel monkey. *Endocrinology (Baltimore)* **88**, 956–963.

Brown, M. R., and Fisher, L. A. (1989). Role of CRF in regulating autonomic nervous system responses to stress. *In* "Frontiers of Stress Research: Neuronal Control of Bodily Function: Basic and Clinical Aspects" (H. Weiner, D. Hellhammer, I. Florin, and R. C. Murison, eds.), pp. 233–239. Hans Huber, Toronto.

Chatterton, R. T., Jr., Murray, C. L., and Hellman, L. (1973). Endocrine effects on leukocytopoiesis in the rat. I. Evidence for growth hormone secretion as the leukopoietic stimulus following acute cortisol-induced lymphopenia, *Endocrinology (Baltimore)* **92**, 775–787.

Comsa, J., and Leonhardt, H. (1975). Influence of the thymus-corticotropin-growth hormone interaction on the rejection of skin allografts in the rat. *Ann. N.Y. Acad. Sci.* **249**, 387–401.

Comsa, J., Schwarz, J. A., and Neu, H. (1974). Interaction between thymic hormone and hypophysial growth hormone on production of precipitating antibodies in the rat. *Immunol. Commun.* **3**, 11–18.

Davila, D. R., Brief, S., Simon, J., Hammer, R. E., Brinster, R. L., and Kelly, K. W. (1987). Role of growth hormone in regulating T-dependent immune events in aged, nude, and transgenic rodents. *J. Neurosci. Res.* **18**, 108–116.

Dougherty, T. F. (1952). Effects of hormones on lymphatic tissue. *Physiol. Rev.* **32**, 379–401.

Faith, R. E., Liang, H. J., Murgo, A. J., and Plotnikoff, N. P. (1984). Neuroimmunomodulation with enkephalins: Enhancement of human natural killer (NK) cell activity in vitro. *Clin. Immunol. Immunopathol.* **31**, 412–418.

Fauci, A. S. (1978). Mechanisms of the immunosuppressive and anti-inflammatory effects of glucocorticoids. *J. Immunopharmacol.* **1**, 1–25.

Felten, D. L., Felten, S. Y., Carlson, S. L., Olschowka, J. A., and Livnat, S. (1985). Noradrenergic and peptidergic innervation of lymphoid tissue. *J. Immunol.* **135**, 755s–765s.

Fischer, E. G. (1988). Opioid peptides modulate immune functions. A review. *Immunopharmacol. Immunotoxicol.* **10**, 265–326.

Gibbs, D. M. (1986). Vasopressin and oxytocin: Hypothalamic modulators of the stress response: A review. *Psychoneuroendocrinology* **11**, 131–140.

Gillies, G. E., Linton, E. A., and Lowry, P. J. (1982). Corticotropin releasing activity of the new CRF is potentiated several times by vasopressin. *Nature (London)* **299**, 4355–4357.

Gisler, R., and Schenkel-Hulliger, L. (1971). Hormonal regulation of the immune response. II. Influence of pituitary and adrenal activity on immune responsiveness *in vitro*. *Cell. Immunol.* **2**, 646–657.

Glaser, R., Rice, J., Stout, J. C., Speicher, C. E., and Kiecolt-Glaser, J. K. (1986). Stress depresses interferon production by leukocytes concomitant with a decrease in natural killer cell activity. *Behav. Neurosci.* **100**, 675–678.

Guillemin, R., Vargo, T., Rossier, J., Minick, S., Ling, N., Rivier, C., Vale, W., and Bloom, F. E. (1977). Beta-endorphin and adrenocorticotropin are secreted concomitantly by the pituitary gland. *Science* **197**, 1367–1369.

Hartmann, D. P., Holaday, J. W., and Bernton, E. W. (1989). Inhibition of lymphocyte proliferation by antibodies to prolactin. *FASEB J.*, **3**, 2194–2202.

Hayashida, T., and Li, C. H. (1957). Influence of adrenocorticotropic and growth hormone on antibody formation. *J. Exp. Med.* **105**, 93–98.

Herberman, R. B., and Ortaldo, J. R. (1981). Natural killer cells: Their role in defenses against disease. *Science* **214**, 24–30.

Hochman, P. S., and Cudkowicz, G. (1978). Suppression of natural cytotoxicity by spleen cells of hydrocortisone-treated mice. *J. Immunol.* **123**, 968–976.

Ijaz, M. K., Dent, D., and Babiuk, L. A. (1990). Neuroimmunomodulation of in vivo anti-rotavirus humoral immune response. *J. Neuroimmunol.*, **26**, 159–171.

Irwin, M. R., Vale, W., and Britton, K. T. (1987). Central corticotropin-releasing factor suppresses natural killer cytotoxicity. *Brain, Behav., Immun.* 1, 81–87.

Irwin, M. R., Hauger, R. L., Brown, M. R., and Britton, K. T. (1988). CRF activates autonomic nervous system and reduces natural killer cytotoxicity. *Am. J. Physiol.* 255, R744–R747.

Irwin, M. R., Vale W., and Rivier C. (in press). Central corticotropin releasing factor mediates the suppressive effect of stress on natural killer cytotoxicity. *Endocrinology.*

Jobin, M., Feland, L., Cote, J., and Labrie, R. (1975). Effect of exposure to cold on hypothalamic TRH and plasma levels of TSH and prolactin in the rat. *Neuroendocrinology* 18, 204–212.

Johnson, H. M., Farrar, W. L., and Torres, B., A. (1982a). Vasopressin replacement of interleukin 2 requirement in gamma interferon production: Lymphokine activity of a neuroendocrine hormone. *J. Immunol.* 129, 983–986.

Johnson, H. M., Smith, E. M., Torres, B. A., and Blalock, J. E. (1982b). Regulation of the *in vitro* antibody response by neuroendocrine hormones. *Proc. Natl. Acad. Sci. U.S.A.* 79, 4171–4174.

Johnson, H. M., Torres, B. A., Smith, E. M., Dion, L. D., and Blalock, J. E. (1984). Regulation of lymphokine (gamma-interferon) production by corticotropin. *J. Immunol.* 132, 246–250.

Kant, G. J., Leu, J. R., Anderson, S. M., and Mougey, E. H. (1987). Effect of chronic stress on plasma corticosterone, ACTH and prolactin. *Physiol. Behav.* 40, 775–779.

Kastin, N. W. (1986). Characteristics of body temperature, vasopressin, and oxytocin responses to endotoxin in the rat. *Can. J. Physiol. Pharmacol.* 64, 1575–1578.

Kelly, K. W., Brief, S., Westly, H. J., Novakofski, J., Bechtel, P. J., Simon, J., and Walker, E. B. (1986). GH3 pituitary adenoma cells can reverse thymic aging in rats. *Proc. Natl. Acad. Sci. U.S.A.* 83, 5663–5667.

Kiess, W., Holtmann, H., Butenandt, O., and Eife, R. (1983). Modulation of lymphoproliferation by human growth hormone. *Eur. J. Pediatr.* 140, 47–50.

Kiess, W., Doerr, H., Butenandt, O., and Belohradsky, B. H. (1986). Lymphocyte subsets and natural-killer activity in growth hormone deficiency. *N. Engl. J. Med.* 314, 321.

Kreider, J. W., Bartllet, G. L., Purnell D. M., and Webb, S. (1978). Immunotherapy of an established rat mammary adenocarcinoma (13762A) with intratumor injection of *Corynebacterium parvum. Cancer Res.* 38, 689–692.

Lenox, F. H., Kant, G. J., Sessions, G. R., Pennington, L. L., Mougey, E. H., and Meyerhoff, J. L. (1980). Specific hormonal and neurochemical responses to different stressors. *Neuroendocrinology* 21, 300–308.

Levins, R., and Lewontin, R. (1985). "The Dialectical Biologist." Harvard Univ. Press, Cambridge, Massachusetts.

Lewis, J. W., Cannon, J. T., and Liebeskind, J. C. (1980). Opioid and nonopioid mechanisms of stress analgesia. *Science* 208, 623–625.

Lewis, J. W., Shavit, Y., Terman, G. W., Gale, R. P., and Liebeskind J. C. (1983a). Stress and morphine affect survival of rats challenged with a mammary ascites tumor (MAT 13762B). *Nat. Immun. Cell Growth Regul.* 3, 43–50.

Lewis, J. W., Shavit, Y., Terman, G. W., Nelson, L. R., Gale, R. P., and Liebeskind, J. C. (1983b). Apparent involvement of opioid peptides in stress-induced enhancement of tumor growth. *Peptides (N.Y.)* 4, 635–638.

Locher, R., Vetter, W., and Block, L. H. (1983). Interactions between 8-L-arginine vasopressin and prostaglandin-E2 in human mononuclear phagocytes. *J. Clin. Invest.* 71, 884.

Maier, S. F., Sherman, J. E., Lewis, J. W., Terman, G. W., and Liebeskind, J. C. (1983). The opioid-nonopioid nature of stress-induced analgesia and learned helplessness, *J. Exp. Psychol., Anim. Behav. Processes* 9, 80–90.

Mandler, R. N., Biddison, W. E., Mandler, R., and Serrate, S. A. (1986). β-endorphin augments the cytolytic activity and interferon production of natural killer cells. *J. Immunol.* **136**, 934–939.

Markwick, A. J., Lolait, S. J., and Funder, J. W. (1986). Immunoreactive arginine vasopressin in the rat thymus. *Endocrinology (Baltimore)* **119**, 1690–1696.

Martin, F. C., Shavit, Y., Terman, G. W., Pechnick, R. N., Oh, C., and Liebeskind, J. C. (1985). Stereospecificity of opiate immunosuppression in rats. *Soc. Neurosci. Abstr.* **11**, 86.

Mathews, P. M., Froelich, C. J., Sibbit, W. L., Jr., and Bankhurst, A. D. (1983). Enhancement of natural cytotoxicity by β-endorphin. *J. Immunol.* **130**, 1658–1662.

McCann, S. M., Antunes-Rodrigues, J., Nallar, R., and Valtin, H. (1966). Pituitary-adrenal function in the absence of vasopressin. *Endocrinology (Baltimore)* **79**, 1058–1064.

Medawar, P. B., and Sparrow, E. M. (1956). Effect of adrenocortical hormones, adrenocorticotropic hormone and pregnancy on skin transplantation. *J. Endocrinol.* **14**, 240–256.

Meeker, M. L., Meeker, R. B., and Hayward, J. N. (1987). Accumulation of circulating endogenous and exogenous immunoglobulins by hypothalamic magnocellular neurons. *Brain Res.* **423**, 45–55.

Mercola, K. E., Cline, M. J., and Golde, D. W. (1981). Growth hormone stimulation of normal and leukemic human T-lymphocyte proliferation *in vitro*. *Blood* **58**, 337–340.

Millan, M. J., Millan, M. H., Colpaert, F. C., and Herz, A. (1985). Chronic arthritis in the rat: differential changes in discrete brain pools of vasopressin as compared to oxytocin. *Neurosci. Lett.* **54**, 33–37.

Mirsky, I. A., Stein, M., and Paulisch, G. (1954). The secretion of an antidiuretic substance into the circulation of rats exposed to noxious stimuli. *Endocrinology (Baltimore)* **54**, 491–505.

Miyabo, S., Asato, T., and Mizushima, N. (1979). Psychological correlates of stress-induced cortisol and growth hormone release in neurotic patients. *Psychosom. Med.* **41**, 515–523.

Monjan, A. A. (1981). Stress and immunologic competence: Studies in animals. *In* "Psychoneuroimmunology" (R. Ader, ed.), pp. 185–228. Academic Press, New York.

Morley, J. E. (1983). Neuroendocrine effects of endogenous opioid peptides in human subjects: A review. *Psychoneuroendocrinology* **8**, 361–379.

Nagy, E., Berczi, I., and Friesen, H. G. (1983a). Regulation of immunity in rats by lactogenic and growth hormones. *Acta Endocrinol. (Copenhagen)* **102**, 351–357.

Nagy, E., Berczi, I., Wren, G. E., Asa, S. L., and Kovacs, K. (1983b). Immuno-modulation by bromocriptine. *Immunopharmacology* **6**, 231–243.

Okimura, T., Ogawa, M., and Yamauchi, T. (1986). Stress and immune response. III. Effect of restraint stress on delayed type hypersensitivity (DTH) response, natural killer (NK) activity and phagocytosis in mice. *Jpn. J. Pharmacol.* **41**, 229–235.

Osgood, C. K., and Favour, C. B. (1951). Effect of adrenocorticotropic hormone on inflammation due to tuberculin hypersensitivity and turpentine and on circulating antibody levels. *J. Exp. Med.* **94**, 415–430.

Owens, P. C., Chan, E. C., Lovelock, M., Falconer, J., and Smith, R. (1988). Immunoreactive methionine-enkephalin in cerebrospinal fluid and blood plasma during acute stress in conscious sheep. *Endocrinology (Baltimore)* **122**, 311–317.

Page, G. G., Ben ELiyahu, S., Yirmiya, R., and Liebeskind, J. C. (1990). Surgical stress increases the number of breast cancer metastases in rats. *Soc. Neurosci. Abs.*

Rappaport, R., Oleske, J., Ahdieh, H., Solomon, S., Delfaus, C., and Denny, T. (1986). Suppression of immune function in growth hormone-deficient children during treatment with human growth hormone. *J. Pediatr.* **109**, 434–439.

Redei, E., Branch, B. J., and Taylor, A. N. (1986). Direct effect of ethanol on adrenocorticotropin (ACTH) release *in vitro. J. Pharmacol. Exp. Ther.* 237, 59–64.

Redei, E., Gholami, F., Lin, E. Y. R., and Taylor, A. N. (1988). Effects of ethanol on CRF
release *in vitro. Endocrinology (Baltimore)* 123, 27–36.

Riegel, G. D., and Meites, J. (1976). The effects of stress on serum prolactin in the female rat.
Proc. Soc. Exp. Biol. Med. 152, 441–447.

Riley, V. (1981). Psychoneuroendocrine influences on immunocompetence and neoplasia. *Science* 212, 1100–1109.

Ritter, S., and Pelzer, N. L. (1978). Magnitude of stress-induced norepinephrine depletion
varies with age. *Brain Res.* 152, 170–175.

Rivier, C., and Vale, W. (1985). Involvement of corticotropin-releasing factor and somatostatin in stress-induced inhibition of growth hormone secretion in the rat. *Endocrinology (Baltimore)* 117, 2478–2482.

Rivier, C., Rivier, J., and Vale, W. (1982). Inhibition of adrenocorticotropic hormone secretion
in the rat by immunoneutralization of corticotropin-releasing factor. *Science* 218, 377–
379.

Rivier C., Rivier, J., and Vale, W. (1986). Stress-induced inhibition of reproductive functions:
Role of endogenous corticotropin-releasing factor. *Science* 231, 607–609.

Rossier, J., French, E., Rivier, C., Shibasaki, T., Guillemin, R., and Bloom, F. E. (1980). Stress-
induced release of prolactin: Blockade by dexamethasone and naloxone may indicate
beta-endorphin mediation. *Proc. Natl. Acad. Sci. U.S.A.* 77, 666–669.

Saxena, Q. B., Saxena, R. K., and Adler, W. H. (1980). Regulation of natural killer cell activity
in vivo. I. Loss of natural killer cell activity during stravation. *Indian J. Exp. Biol.* 18,
1383–1386.

Saxena, Q. B., Saxena, R. K., and Adler, W. H. (1982). Regulation of natural killer cell activity
in vivo. III. Effect of hypophysectomy and growth hormone treatment on the natural
killer activity of the mouse spleen cell population, *Int. Arch. Allergy Appl. Immunol.*
67, 169–174.

Seitz, H. K., and Simanowski, U. A. (1988). Alcohol and carcinogenesis. *Annu. Rev. Nutr.* 8,
99–119.

Selye, H. (1936). A syndrome produced by diverse nocuous agents. *Nature (London)* 148, 84–
85.

Selye, H. (1956). "The Stress of Life." McGraw-Hill, New York.

Selye, H. (1970). The evolution of the stress concept. *Am. Sci.* 61, 692–699.

Shavit, Y., Lewis, J. W., Terman, G. W., Gale, R. P., and Liebeskind, J. C. (1984). Opioid
peptides mediate the suppressive effect of stress on natural killer cell cytotoxicity. *Science* 223, 188–190.

Shavit, Y., Depaulis, A., Martin, F. C., Terman, G. W., Pechnick, R. N., Zane, C. J., Gale, R.
P., and Liebeskind, J. C. (1986a). Involvement of brain receptors in the immune-
suppressive effect of morphine. *Proc. Natl. Acad. Sci. U.S.A.* 83, 7114–7117.

Shavit, Y., Terman, G. W., Lewis, J. W., Zane, C. J., Gale, R. P., and Liebeskind, J. C. (1986b).
Effects of footshock stress and morphine on natural killer lymphocytes in rats: Studies
of tolerance and cross-tolerance. *Brain Res.* 372, 382–385.

Shavit, Y., Martin, F. C., Yirmiya, R., Ben-Eliyahu, S., Terman, G. W., Weiner, H., Gale,
R. P., and Liebeskind, J. C. (1987). Effects of a single administration of morphine or
foot-shock stress on natural killer cell cytotoxicity. *Brain, Behav., Immun.* 1, 318–
328.

Shin, S. H. (1979). Prolactin secretion in acute stress is controlled by prolactin releasing factor.
Life Sci. 25, 1829–1835.

Sibinga, N. E. S., and Goldstein, A. (1988). Opioid peptides and opioid receptors in cells of
the immune system. *Annu. Rev. Immunol.* 6, 219–249.

Simon, R. H., Arbo, T. E., and Lundy, J. (1984). β-Endorphin injected into the nucleus of the raphe magnus facilitates metastatic tumor growth. *Brain Res. Bull.* **12,** 487–491.

Sklar, L. S., and Anisman, H. (1981). Stress and cancer. *Psychol. Bull.* **89,** 369–406.

Sohn, J. H., Shavit, Y., Morgan, M. M., Martin, F. C., Melendez, A. R. J., Gale, R. P., and Liebeskind, J. C. (1986). Brain μ-opioid receptors are involved in morphine-induced suppression of immune function. *Soc. Neurosci. Abstr.* **12,** 339.

Solomon, G. F., and Amkraut, A. A. (1981). Psychoneuroendocrinological effects on the immune response. *Annu. Rev. Microbiol.* **35,** 155–184.

Spangelo, B. L., Hall, N. R., NcGillis, J. P., and Goldstein, A. L. (1984). Evidence for an interaction between prolactin and the primary immune response. *Fed. Proc., Fed. Am. Soc. Exp. Biol.* **43,** 1610.

Terman, G. W., Shavit, Y., Lewis, J. W., Cannon, J. T., and Liebeskind, J. C. (1984). Intrinsic mechanisms of pain inhibition: Activation by stress. *Science* **226,** 1270–1277.

Thoa, N. B., Tizabi, Y., and Yacobowitz, D. M. (1977). The effect of isolation on chatacolamine concentration and turnover in discrete areas of the rat brain. *Brain Res.* **131,** 259–269.

Tobach, E., and Bloch, H. (1958). Effect of stress by crowding prior to and following tuberculous infection, *Am. J. Physiol.* **187,** 399–402.

Torres, B. A., and Johnson, H. M. (1988). Arginine vasopressin (AVP) replacement of helper cell requirement in IFN-gamma production: Evidence for a novel AVP receptor on mouse lymphocytes. *J. Immunol.* **140,** 2179–2183.

Trachtenberg, M. C., and Blum, K. (1987). Alcohol and opioid peptides: Neuropharmacological rationale for physical craving of alcohol. *Am. J. Alcohol Abuse* **13,** 365–372.

Vale, W., Spiess, J., Rivier, C., and Rivier, J. (1981). Characterization of a 41 residue ovine hypothalamic peptide that stimulates the secretion of corticotropin and β-endorphin. *Science* **213,** 1394–1397.

Webster, E. L., and De Souza, E. (1988). Corticotropin-releasing factor receptors in mouse spleen: Identification, autoradiographic localization, and regulation by divalent cations and guanine nucleotides. *Endocrinology,* **122,** 609–617.

Weigent, D. A., and Blalock, J. E. (1987). Interactions between the neuroendocrine and immune systems: Common hormones and receptors. *Immunol. Rev.* **100,** 79–108.

Weiner, H. (1988). The concept of stress in the light of studies on distress, unemployment and loss: A critical analysis. *In* "Stress in Health and Disease" (R. Zales, ed.), pp. 24–94. Brunner/Mazel, New York.

Weiner, H., Stephens, R. L., Garick, T., and Tache, Y. (1989). Gastric erosion formation by stress: Brain stem mechanisms. *In* "Molecular Biology of Stress" (S. Breznitz and O. Zinder, eds.), pp. 241–249. Alan R. Liss, New York.

Weiss, J. M. (1971). Effect of coping behavior in different warning signal conditions on stress pathology in rats. *J. Comp. Physiol. Psychol.* **77,** 23–30.

Wideman, C. H., and Murphy, H. M. (1985). Effects of vasopressin deficiency, age, and stress on stomach ulcer induction in rats. *Peptides (N.Y.)* **6** Suppl., 63–67.

Wimer, R. E., Norman, R., and Elefthériou, B. E. (1974). Serotonin levels in the hippocampus: Striking variations associated with mouse strain and treatment. *Brain Res.* **63,** 397–401.

Yahya, M. D., and Watson, R. R. (1987). Immunomodulation by morphine and marijuana. *Life Sci.* **41,** 2503–2510.

Yirmiya, R., and Taylor, A. N. (1989). Genetic differences in brain opiate receptor concentration and sensitivity to ethanol's effects. *Pharmacol., Biochem. Behav.* **33,** 793–796.

Yirmiya, R., Ben-Eliyahu, S., Gale, R. P., Shavit, Y., Weiner, H., Liebeskind, J. C., and Taylor, A. N. (1989a). Effects of ethanol on tumor growth and NK cell cytotoxicity. *Soc. Neurosci. Abstr.* **15,** 720.

Yirmiya, R., Ben-Eliyahu, S., Gale, R. P., Liebeskind, J. C., and Taylor, A. N. (1990a). Acute ethanol administration reduces survival of leukemic rats. *Alcoholism: Clin. Exp. Res.,* **14,** 354.

Yirmiya R., Ben-Eliyahu, S., Shavit, Y., Gale, R. P., Taylor, A. N., Weiner, H., Page, G., Lee, N., and Liebeskind, J. C. (1990b). Opiate-induced increase in tumor metastases is caused by suppression of NK activity and is not mediated by glucocorticoids. *Soc. Neurosci. Abs.*

Yirmiya, R., Shavit, Y., Ben-Eliyahu, S., Martin, F. C., Weiner, H., and Liebeskind, J. C. (1989b). Natural killer cell activity in vasopressin-deficient rats (Brattleboro strain). *Brain Res.* **479,** 16–22.

Yirmiya, R., Taylor, A. N., Gale, R. P., Ben-Eliyahu, S., Shavit, Y., and Liebeskind, J. C. (1989c). Ethanol increases tumor growth, *Alcohol.: Clin. Exp. Res.* **13,** 330.

Zagon, I. S., and McLaughlin, P. J. (1986). Endogenous opioid systems, stress and cancer. *In* "Enkephalins and Endorphins: Stress and the Immune System" (N. P. Plotnikoff, R. E. Faith, A. J. Murgo, and R. A. Good, eds.), pp. 81–100. Plenum, New York.

14

Stress Responses and the Pathogenesis of Arthritis

E. M. Sternberg

Clinical Neurosciences Branch, National
Institute of Mental Health, and
Arthritis and Rheumatism Branch, NIAMS
Bethesda, Maryland 20892

R. L. Wilder

Arthritis and Rheumatism Branch, NIAMS
Bethesda, Maryland 20892

G. P. Chrousos

Developmental Endocrinology Branch
NICHD
Bethesda, Maryland 20892

P. W. Gold

Clinical Neuroendocrinology Branch
National Institute of Mental Health
Bethesda, Maryland 20892

I. Introduction

Although psychological stress and depression have long been thought to be associated with the initial onset and exacerbations of inflammatory and autoimmune diseases, such as rheumatoid arthritis (RA), strong scientific proof of this thesis has remained elusive. In part, the lack of an apparent biological basis for such a relationship has made testing of the hypothesis difficult. Recent developments in the field of neuroendocrine immunology, however, now provide a biochemical and molecular framework for hypothesizing that a relationship between depression and rheumatoid arthritis may be rooted in a common neuroendocrine defect. Both inflammatory and behavioral stresses, through stimulation of the corticotropin-releasing hormone (CRH) neuron, activate a final common neuroendocrine pathway: the hypothalamic–pituitary–adrenal axis. The association between psychological stress and development of inflammatory disease may therefore be related to alterations of this common pathway, or to defects in the intricate feedback loops that exist between the immune system and the central nervous system. This chapter will review the evidence for an association between stress, depression, and rheumatoid arthritis, as well as current concepts of the immune system–central nervous system feedback loop, with emphasis on the hypothalamic–pituitary–adrenal axis. We will review our recent findings that relate interruptions of this loop to susceptibility to arthritis, as well as our recent findings of the relationship of interruptions of this loop to depressive disorders.

II. Depression and Arthritis

Most studies addressing the association between depression and arthritis have been epidemiological studies, designed to determine whether an association does exist, and if so whether the depression is associated with severity of disease. The latter question addresses the important but more difficult issue of whether depression is secondary to the disease process, or rather is an independent but coexistent problem. A number of factors inherent in both RA and depression, as well as factors related to the techniques used to identify, define, and quantitate depression in these studies, contribute to the difficulty in answering these questions (Bishop, 1988). Depression is a symptom complex, with heterogeneous causes and clinical presentations. Depressive symptomatology could result from a coexistent major affective disorder, or could result from the effects of chronic disease on mood. It is not surprising therefore that no clear-cut association has been found between RA and this mixed symptom complex, and that results of studies addressing this issue are conflicting. That many of the symptoms of RA are also symptoms of depression (e.g., hypersomnia, lack of energy, fatigue), the fact that chronic pain affects mood, and the variation over time of the potentially mood-altering symptomatology of rheumatoid arthritis, make the relationship between RA and depression almost impossible to dissect with a single psychological instrument, at a single point in time. Further complicating the issue is the fact that many of the psychiatric instruments used to define and quantitate mood have not been normed in chronically ill populations (Bishop, 1988), and some instruments, (such as MMPI) may respond to features of rheumatoid arthritis, rather than to mood, resulting in "criterion contamination" (Pincus *et al.*, 1986; Smythe, 1984). Finally, it is difficult to compare studies in which different instruments have been used, since each instrument is designed to test a different aspect of affective disorder.

Two recent prospective studies (McFarlane and Brooks, 1988; Hawley and Wolfe, 1988) have attempted to control for these variables. McFarlane and Brooks (1988), using the Middlesex Hospital Questionnaire (MHQ), Illness Behavior Questionnaire (IBQ), and Beck Depression Inventory, found that the psychological state of the RA patients and their degree of physical impairment were relatively independent variables. There was no correlation between depressive and anxiety symptoms, and RA disease activity. Hawley and Wolfe (1988), utilizing the Arthritis Impact Measurement Scales (AIMS) test, found that while 25% of the variance in the initial depression and anxiety scores could be explained by the clinical variables in the study, most of the anxiety and depression observed were not explained by these variables. Depression appeared to be associated with socioeconomic, not clinical, features, and neither worsening nor improvement of clinical scores correlated with alteration in depression and anxiety scores. Furthermore, RA patients' scores were similar to those of other rheumatic disease patients. Other previous studies (Cassileth *et al.*, 1984; Mason *et al.*, 1983), using the same or similar instruments, also found no difference in anxiety and depression scores in RA compared to other rheumatic diseases, nor any association with severity of the rheumatic disorder. The AIMS instrument, however, was not developed to sensitively discriminate between different forms or causes of depression, and therefore data derived from this instrument must be interpreted cautiously.

In summary, the lack of a clear-cut answer in these studies is related to the lack of a clear-cut question, or viable pathophysiological hypothesis, on which to base the analytic approach. However, recent advances in our understanding of the interactions of the immune system and the central nervous system (CNS) and the central role of corticotropin-releasing hormone (CRH) in the stress response provide the context for a hypothesis that posits that vulnerability to rheumatoid arthritis and major depression constitute different manifestations of the same pathogenetic change in the CNS.

III. The Hypothalamic–Pituitary–Adrenal Axis: The Final Common Pathway of Stress

The hypothalamic–pituitary–adrenal (HPA) axis is one of the principal final common pathways of the stress response to a variety of stressful stimuli from the external environment. Corticotropin-releasing hormone, synthesized by CRH neurons in the paraventricular nucleus (PVN) of the hypothalamus, is secreted into the portal blood, and stimulates corticotropin (ACTH) release from the anterior pituitary. ACTH in turn stimulates synthesis and release of corticosteroids from the adrenal cortex. While centrally directed CRH sets into motion a variety of behavioral and physiological alterations adaptive during stressful situations, peripherally directed CRH, through transport via the hypophyseal portal system to the anterior pituitary, promotes pituitary–adrenal activation. Although the functions of glucocorticoid secretion during threatening situations have not been definitively elucidated, it has been suggested that a principal role is to counterregulate or restrain the stress response to prevent its excessive or prolonged activation.

CRH synthesis and release in the PVN of the hypothalamus are under the close control of a variety of regulatory substances and neurotransmitter pathways. Data available from *in vitro* hypothalamic organ culture suggest that noradrenergic, serotonergic, and cholinergic (Calogero *et al.*, 1988a) inputs stimulate CRH release, while gamma-aminobutyric acid (GABA) and opiate (Calogero *et al.*, 1988c) pathways are inhibitory. Glucocorticoids, ACTH, and CRH (Calogero *et al.*, 1988b) itself exert negative feedback effects upon PVN CRH neurons as well. Recent studies have shown that immune mediators are also important regulators of the CRH neuron, and molecules such as interleukin-1 (IL-1) and interleukin-2 (IL-2) provide another means of stimulating the HPA axis via the CRH neuron (Sternberg, 1988).

IV. Corticotropin-Releasing Hormone in the Major Depressive Syndromes: Potential Relevance to the Depression Associated with Rheumatoid Arthritis

The sequencing and subsequent synthesis of corticotropin-releasing hormone in 1981 by Vale and colleagues have been of great interest to neurobiologists concerned with the problem of major depression. Indeed, the best documented finding of a biological abnormality in psychiatry is that patients with major melancholic depression show evidence of a pathological activation of the hypothalamic–pituitary–adrenal axis, potentially attributable to a defect in CRH regulation (Gold *et al.*, 1988a). In addition, CRH is the principal signal for the cleavage and release of ACTH and beta-endorphin from neurons containing pro-opiomelancortin (POMC) in the arcuate nucleus of the hypothalamus, which is the principal central source for both of these behaviorally active neuropeptides (Gold *et al.*, 1988b).

CRH is of great potential interest to neurobiologists for reasons other than its role in modulating peripheral pituitary–adrenal function and the production of ACTH and beta-endorphin in the CNS. CRH is synthesized not only in the PVN for axonal transport to the median eminence or to POMC-containing neurons in the arcuate nucleus, but also in the floor of the third ventricle for secretion into the CSF. Moreover, extrahypothalamic CRH cell bodies and terminal fields are located in disparate regions of the neuroaxis, especially in close association with the central autonomic system, the locus ceruleus (LC), and in many periventricular locations. This distribution of CRH within and beyond the boundaries of the hypothalamus provides an anatomical context for the observation that CRH can simultaneously activate and coordinate a series of metabolic, cardiovascular, and behavioral responses that are adaptive during threatening or stressful situations. Hence, in the rat, the intracerebroventricular administration of CRH leads not only to activation of the pituitary–adrenal axis, but also to activation of the sympathetic nervous system (Rock *et al.*, 1984; Brown *et al.*, 1982; Sutton *et al.*, 1982) and to several behavioral changes characteristic of the stress response. These include decreased exploration in familiar surroundings (Swerdlow *et al.*, 1986), enhanced vigilance (Swerdlow *et al.*, 1986), decreased feeding (Britton *et al.*, 1982), and inhibition of central programs subserving growth and reproduction (Sirinathsinghji *et al.*, 1983; Rivier and Yale, 1984). In larger doses, CRH produces behavioral effects that can be construed as anxiogenic, ranging from hyperresponsiveness to acoustic startle, enhancement of the acquisition of conditioned-fear responses and ultimately assumption of a freeze posture or disruption of apparently purposeful behavior (Sutton *et al.*, 1982).

In addition to direct receptor-mediated effects at target neurons, CRH may also promote arousal by interacting with the other principal arousal producing system in brain, namely, the locus ceruleus–norepinephrine (LC-NE) system found in the region of the mid pons. Several lines of data indicate that these two systems may mutually reinforce each other's functional activity. For example, Valentino (see Valentino *et al.*, 1983) has shown that the direct application of CRH onto locus ceruleus neurons in awake free-ranging rats markedly increases the locus ceruleus firing rate, while we have shown that the intracerebroventricular (icv) administration of CRH significantly enhances glucose utilization in the LC in a dose- and time-dependent fashion (G. Perini, unpublished observations). Conversely, our group has shown that NE is a potent stimulus to the *in vitro* release of CRH (Calogero *et al.*, 1988c), while propranolol has been shown to attenuate the arousal-producing effects of centrally administered CRH.

V. Differential Function of the CRH Neuron in Subtypes of Depression

A. Melancholia

Melancholic depression represents a consistent cluster of symptoms that indicate that depression need not reflect a state of emotional and cognitive inactivation (Gold *et al.*, 1988a). Indeed, the principal psychological components of the syndrome of melancholic depression include indices of pathologic arousal such as an obsessional preoccupation with personal inadequacy and the inevitability of loss. The physiological concomitants of melancholic depression also suggest a state of pathologic arousal and include not only physiologic evidence of arousal such as hypercortisolism and sympathetic activation, but also inhibiton of vegetative pathways subserving feeding and sexual function. Accordingly, among the cardinal manifestions of melancholic depression are anorexia, hypothalamic hypogonadism, and decreased libido.

Our group has advanced several lines of data suggesting that the hypercortisolism of major melancholic depression reflects a defect at or above the hypothalamus resulting in the hypersecretion of endogenous CRH (Gold *et al.*, 1988a). First, plasma ACTH responses to synthetic ovine CRH are attenuated in major depression and negatively correlated with basal plasma cortisol levels, indicating that the pituitary corticotroph cell is appropriately restrained by the negative feedback of glucocorticoids (Gold *et al.*, 1984, 1986). Second, normal controls given a continuous infusion of CRH have the pattern and magnitude of hypercortisolism seen in major depression (Schulte *et al.*, 1985). Third, CRH in the cerebrospinal fluid (CSF) correlates positively with indices of pituitary–adrenal activation (Roy *et al.*, 1987). These data, indicative of an activation of the CRH neuron in melancholic depression, are of interest in light of the fact that many of the cardinal clinical and biochemical manifestations of melancholic depression can be accounted for on the basis of the concerted behavioral and physiological effects attributable to the activation of the CRH system.

B. Atypical Depression

The pathologic hyperarousal of melancholic depression, which we attribute to the concomitant activation of the CRH and LC-NE systems, represents the classic and best described major depressive syndrome. In contrast to this state of intense arousal, however, is the pathologic inactivation that defines the other major depressive syndrome, commonly referred to as atypical depression. In many respects, this syndrome seems the antithesis of melancholic depression. On the one hand, melancholic depression represents preferential activation of arousal-producing pathways subserving vigilence, anxiety, and aggression, coupled with inhibition of pathways mediating vegetative functions such as feeding and sleep; in contrast, atypical depression seems associated with inhibition of pathways mediating arousal, and preferential activation of those subserving vegetative and reparative functions (Gold *et al.*, 1988a). Hence, the cardinal melancholic symptoms of anorexia and early morning awakening in melacholic depression stand in marked contrast to the hyperphagia and hypersomnia that define atypical depression (Gold *et al.*, 1988a,b). Moreover, in contrast to the intense anxiety about self and the ruminative preoccupation with the inevitability of loss characteristic of melancholia, patients with atypical depression seem passive, anergic, and apathetic.

The marked differences in the clinical manifestations of the melancholic and atypical depressive syndromes are associated with clear differences in biochemical features. As an example, while hypercortisolism is the cardinal neuroendocrine manifestation of melancholic depression, this finding is generally absent in patients with atypical depression. Parenthetically, this absence of frank hypercortisolism in atypical depression has been interpreted to suggest normal hypothalamic–pituitary–adrenal function. It should be noted, however, that it can be difficult or impossible to demonstrate a decrease in the functional activity of the CRH system with commonly used clinical tests assessing the functional integrity of the hypothalamic–pituitary–adrenal axis (Gold *et al.*, 1988b). In this regard, given the fact that CRH biases the CNS in the direction of arousal by activating pathways subserving fight-or-flight responses and inhibiting pathways subserving vegetative functions, the possibility of a pathologic inactivation of the CRH and/or NE-LC systems in atypical depression should be considered (Gold *et al.*, 1988b). To support this notion, we have shown that the atypical depression that almost invariably accompanies Cushing's disease is associated with a marked decrease in the levels of CSF CRH (Kling *et al.*, 1990). Moreover, we found that most patients with Cushing's disease whom we studied after transphenoidal adenectomy (at a time when basal ACTH levels were uniformly undetectable), had small but detectable ACTH responses to exogenous ovine CRH. We surmise that the postoperative adrenal insufficiency in these patients partly reflected the hypofunction of neurons secreting CRH: neurons that had been physiologically suppressed by exposure to the negative feedback of longstanding hypercortisolism. These findings, indicative of a central CRH deficiency in Cushing's disease associated with signs of atypical depression, are compatible with our data that the hypercortisolism of this disorder represents a peripheral rather than a centrally mediated defect, and are supported by our recent *in vitro* data indicating that PVN CRH-containing cells are eminently glucocorticoid-suppressible.

In summary, our clinical data suggest that the pathological hyperarousal of melancholic depression is associated with an activation of the CRH neuron, while the pathological inactivation of atypical depression is associated with a hypofunctioning of the CRH system. In the following sections, we shall review the role of the CRH neuron as a regulator of the immune response and as a factor conferring susceptibility to the development of arthritis. Our data suggest that a defect in the regulation of biosynthesis and secretion of CRH is associated with susceptibility to arthritis; we speculate that this defect may also be relevant to the depressive syndrome frequently associated with rheumatoid arthritis.

VI. HPA Axis–Immune System Interactions

In addition to the behavioral effects of CRH, and the concomitant pathophysiological implications of imbalances of CRH on the pathogenesis of depression, CRH's role as the central stimulator of the HPA axis has profound implications in relation to regulation of the immune system. Through stimulation of corticosteroid secretion, CRH plays a central role in counterregulation of the immune response, and CRH imbalances therefore also have important implications for the pathogenesis of susceptibility or resistance to inflammatory disease.

A. The Immune Activation Cascade

Exposure of cells of the immune system, such as lymphocytes and macrophages, to an immune stimulus, such as an antigen, initiates a cascade of cell–cell and cell–mediator interactions during which lymphocytes and macrophages become activated, differentiate, and act together to affect various aspects of the immune response (Sternberg and Parker, 1988). During lymphocyte activation, T lymphocytes proliferate and differentiate into effector T-cell subtypes, such as suppressor, helper, or cytotoxic T lymphocytes. These subtypes act in concert to produce the cellular immune response. The B lymphocytes differentiate to plasma cells, which secrete antibodies, the final effector molecules in the humoral immune response. During activation, macrophages differentiate to become antigen-presenting cells, capable of "presenting" antigens to lymphocytes. Such macrophages express class II antigen (major histocompatibility antigens, i.e., HLA-DR) on their surface. They process antigens, that is, they ingest and degrade large antigenic proteins to small peptide fragments, which are reexpressed on the macrophage surface together with class II antigen. Antigen expressed in this form is recognized by the T-lymphocyte receptor for antigen, thus beginning the cascade of T-lymphocyte activation and differentiation.

During the course of an immune response, activated macrophages and lymphocytes produce interleukins. These proteins, initially defined by the immune system cell that produced them, as well as the target cell upon which they were found to act, are now known to affect a much broader range of targets than originally defined. Up to eight interleukins have now been identified. During immune or inflammatory stimulation, activated lymphocytes produce lymphokines, such as interferon gamma, that stimulate macrophages to produce monokines such as interleukin-1 (IL-1) and tumor necrosis factor (TNF). IL-1 stimulates T lymphocytes to express interleukin-2 (IL-2) receptors and to produce IL-2, which in turn further stimulates T lymphocytes to proliferate and differentiate to one of the effector subtypes. Thus, a plethora of inflammatory mediators and interleukins is released during the immune response, and through the multiple amplification loops the cascade of an immune/inflammatory response is perpetuated.

Although lymphokines and monokines were initially defined as interleukins because they were considered molecules important in interactions between immune cells, or leukocytes, the current definition now comprises a class of molecules that are synthesized by and have effects on a large variety of cells in addition to monocytes and lymphocytes. These include not only nonimmune cells such as fibroblasts and endothelial cells, but also cells of the central nervous system. A variety of cytokines, including IL-1 alpha and IL-1 beta, TNF, and IL-2, have now been shown to stimulate the HPA axis. A recent series of elegant studies has shown that IL-1 stimulates hypothalamic CRH secretion as well as pituitary ACTH secretion (Sternberg, 1988, 1989; Sternberg et al., 1989b; Berkenbosch et al., 1987; Bernardini et al., 1988; Bernton et al., 1987; Besedovsky et al., 1986; Brown et al., 1987; Lumpkin, 1987; Sapolsky et al., 1987; Uehara et al., 1987.) IL-1 injected in vivo intracerebroventricularly, or added to hypothalamic explant tissue in vitro, stimulates CRH secretion. IL-1 injected in vivo intraperitoneally increases plasma ACTH and corticosterone in rats and mice. The precise mechanism through which IL-1 injected peripherally stimulates the HPA axis is not known, since there is no direct evidence that it can cross the blood–brain barrier. It may stimulate the hypothalamus directly, at sites contiguous with the circumventricular organs, or it may stimulate indirectly via a second messenger such as prostaglandin E_1 (PGE_1). In addition to this neuroendocrine HPA axis-stimulating effect of IL-1, IL-1 neuronal pathways have also been described in the central nervous system. These CNS

IL-1 pathways probably serve a physiologic role in the central component of the acute-phase response (Breder *et al.*, 1988), distinct from peripheral, circulating IL-1 effects on the HPA axis. It is not known whether peripheral IL-1 interacts with central IL-1 pathways in coordinating these two aspects of the stress response.

B. Corticosteroid Effects on the Immune Response

In the interaction of the immune system with the HPA axis, corticosteroids are the effector end point in an important physiologic negative feedback loop between the immune system and the central nervous system. Inflammatory and immune mediators can stimulate the axis both at the level of the hypothalamus and at the level of the pituitary gland. Direct stimulation of the adrenal glands by these immune system hormones has not been shown.

The overall effect of corticosteroids on the immune/inflammatory response is suppressive, completing the critical negative feedback loop which acts to keep the immune system under control. Corticosteroids inhibit the immune cascade at virtually every level, from the level of antigen presentation to the level of mature effector cell function, and essentially induce a state of temporary immune tolerance (Sternberg and Parker, 1988; Sternberg *et al.*, 1989c). Corticosteroids inhibit class II antigen expression on the surface of macrophages, IL-1 and IL-2 secretion, IL-2 receptor expression, lymphocyte proliferation, generation of helper and cytotoxic lymphocytes, and helper and cytotoxic cell function. Since the body is constantly exposed to a barrage of inflammatory stimuli from the environment that have the potential to induce inflammatory reactions, the suppressive effects of corticosteroids, released within hours of exposure to inflammatory stimuli, serve a critical physiologic function: to prevent inflammation from going on unchecked. The HPA axis thus acts as a sensitive thermostat that maintains the inflammatory/immune system under constant control.

VII. HPA Axis and Susceptibility to Arthritis

We have recently found that an important component of susceptibility to development of arthritis in the streptococcal cell wall (SCW) induced arthritis model in the Lewis (LEW/N) rat is a defect in the effector arm of the HPA axis response to inflammatory and other stress mediators (Sternberg *et al.*, 1989a,b). After a single intraperitoneal injection of SCW, LEW/N rats develop a symmetrical inflammatory and erosive polyarthritis that mimics many of the features of human rheumatoid arthritis. In the course of the inflammation induced by SCW, various inflammatory and immune mediators are released, including IL-1. We have found that LEW/N rats have a profound defect in corticosterone and ACTH responses to these inflammatory mediators, which is secondary to a defect in regulation of corticotropin-releasing hormone biosynthesis and secretion in the paraventricular nucleus of the hypothalamus. The lack of suppression of inflammation, resulting from deficient corticosterone release in response to inflammatory stimuli, leads to unchecked and chronic inflammation in LEW/N rats. Conversely, arthritis-resistant histocompatible Fischer (F344/N) rats have intact, robust corticosterone and ACTH responses to inflammatory mediators, resulting in suppression of inflammation once it begins, and protection from chronic inflammatory disease. Interruption of the HPA axis at its final effector end point, with the glucocorticoid receptor antagonist RU 486, results in development of severe inflammatory disease, and arthritis in response to SCW in otherwise inflammation-resistant F344/N rats. Thus, interruption of the HPA axis responses to inflammatory mediators on a genetic basis, as in LEW/N rats, or on a pharmacologic basis, as in F344/N rats treated with RU 486, is associated with development of susceptibility to inflammatory disease.

LEW/N rats are susceptible not only to streptococcal cell wall induced arthritis, but also to a large variety of experimentally induced inflammatory diseases, including experimental allergic encephalomyelitis (EAE), uveitis, nephritis, and orchitis (Allen and Wilder, 1987; Beraud et al., 1986; Caspi et al., 1986; Davis et al., 1982; Griffiths and DeWitt, 1984; Hill and Yu, 1987; Kohashi et al., 1986; Lehman et al., 1984). The specific pattern of inflammatory disease that develops is related to the specific antigenic or proinflammatory agent to which they are exposed. Thus, in response to myelin basic protein, LEW/N rats develop EAE; in response to retinal protein, they develop uveitis; in response to collagen they develop collagen arthritis; in response to adjuvant, they develop adjuvant arthritis. This suggests that the pattern of inflammatory disease that develops in LEW/N rats is determined by the nature of the environmental trigger, while their susceptibility to development of inflammatory disease, and the course and severity of inflammation that develops in response to that trigger, is at least partially related to the HPA axis defect we have described.

VIII. Summary

The central role played by the CRH neuron in this model of susceptibility to arthritis, together with its central role in the pathogenesis of depression, suggests a mechanism that could potentially link both depressive symptomatology and susceptibility to arthritis to a common defect in CRH responses. Within this framework, therefore, approaches to dissecting the associations between depression, susceptibility to inflammatory disease, and neuroendocrine abnormalities may be developed and tested in human diseases, such as rheumatoid arthritis and depression.

References

Allen, J. B., and Wilder, R. L. (1987). Variable severity and Ia antigen expression in streptococcal-cell-wall-induced hepatic granulomas in rats. *Infect. Immun.* 55, 674–679.

Beraud, E., Reshef, T., Vanderbark, A. A., Offner, H., Fritz, R., Chou, C. H. J., Bernard, D., and Cohen, I. R. (1986). Experimental autoimmune encephalomyelitis mediated by T lymphocyte lines: Genotype of antigen-presenting cells influences immunodominant epitope of basic protein. *J. Immunol.* 136, 511–515.

Berkenbosch, F., Oers, J. V., Del Ray, A., Tilders, F., and Besedovsky, H. (1987). Corticotropin-releasing factor-producing neurons in the rat activated by interleukin-1. *Science* 238, 524.

Bernardini, R., Calogero, A. E., Gold, P. W., Luger, A., Chiarenza, A., Legakis, J., and Chrousos, G. P. (1988). Cytokine stimulation of corticotropin releasing hormone (CRH) secretion in vitro In "New Trends in Brain and Female Reproductive Function" (A. R. Genazzani, U. Montemagno, C. Nappi, and F. Petraglia, eds.), pp. 35–99. CIC Edizioni Internazionali, Rome.

Bernton, E. W., Beach, J. E., Holaday, J. W., Smallridge, R. C., and Fein, H. G. (1987). Release of multiple hormones by a direct action of interleukin-1 on pituitary cells. *Science* 238, 519.

Besedovsky, H., Del Ray, A., Sorkin, E., and Dinarello, C. A. (1986). Immunoregulatory feedback bewteen interleukin-1 and glucocorticoid hormones. *Science* 233, 652.

Bishop, D. S. (1988). Depression and rheumatoid arthritis. *J. Rheumatol.* 15, 888-889.

Breder, C. D., Dinarello, C. A., and Saper, C. B. (1988). Interleukin-1 immunoreactive innervation of the human hypothalamus. *Science* 120, 2492

Britton, D. R., Koob, G. F., Rivier, J., and Vale, W. (1982). Intraventricular corticotropin-releasing factor enhances behavioral effects of novelty. *Life Sci.* 31, 363–367.

Brown, M. R., Fisher, L. A., Spiess, J., Rivier, C., Rivier, J., and Vale, W. (1982). Corticotropin-releasing factor: Actions on the sympathetic nervous system and metabolism. *Endocrinology (Baltimore)* 111, 928–931.

Brown, S. L., Smith, L. R., and Blalock, J. E. (1987). Interleukin-1 and interleukin-2 enhance proopiomelanocortin gene expression in pituitary cells. *J. Immunol.* 139, 3181.

Calogero, A. E., Gallucci, W. T., Chrousos, G. P., and Gold, P. W. (1988a). Interaction between GABAergic neurotransmission and rat hypothalamic corticotropin-releasing hormone secretion in vitro: Theorectical and clinical implications. *Brain Res.* 463, 28–36.

Calogero, A. E., Gallucci, W. T., Gold, P. W., and Chrousos, G. P. (1988b). Multiple feedback regulatory loops upon rat hypothalamic corticotropin-releasing hormone secretion. *J. Clin. Invest.* 82, 767–814.

Calogero, A. E., Gallucci, W. T., Chrousos, G. P., and Gold, P. W. (1988c). Catecholamine effects upon rate hypothalamic corticotropin-releasing hormone secretion. Clinical implications. *J. Clin. Invest.* 82, 839–846.

Caspi, R. R., Roberge, F. G., McCallister, M., El-Sared, M., Kuwabara, T., Gery, I., Hanna,

E., and Nussenblatt, R. B. (1986). T cell lines mediating experimental autoimmune uveoretinitis (EAU) in the rat. *J. Immunol.* **136**, 928–933.

Cassileth, B. R., Lusk, E. J., Strouse, T. B., Miller, D. S., Brown, L. L., Cross, P. A., and Tenaglia, A. N. (1984). Psychological status in chronic illness. A comparative analysis of six diagnostic groups. *N. Engl. J. Med.* **311**, 506–511.

Davis, J. K., Throp, R. B., Maddox, P. A., Brown, M. B., and Cassell, G. H. (1982). Murine respiratory mycoplasmosis in F344 and LEW rats: Evolution of lesions and lung lymphoid cell populations. *Infect. Immun.* **36**, 720–729.

Gold, P. W., Chrousos, G. P., Kellner, C., Post, R., Roy, A., Augerinos, P., Schulte, H., Oldfield, E., and Loriaux, D. L. (1984). Psychiatric implications of basic and clinical studies with corticotropin-releasing factor. *Am. J. Psychiatry* **141**, 619–627.

Gold, P. W., Loriaux, D. L., Roy, A., Kling, M. A., Calabrese, J. R., Kellner, C. H., Nieman, L. K., Post, R. M., Pickar, D., Gallucci, W., Avgerinos, P., Paul, S., Oldfield, E. H., Cutler, G. B., and Chrousos, G. P. (1986). Responses to corticotropin-releasing hormone in the hypercortisolism of depression and Cushing's disease: pathophysiologic and diagnostic implications. *N. Engl. J. Med.* **314**, 1329–1335.

Gold, P. W., Goodwin, F. K., and Chrousos, G. P. (1988a). Clinical and biochemical manifestations of depression. Part 1. *N. Engl. J. Med.* **319**, 348–353.

Gold, P. W., Goodwin, F. K., and Chrousos, G. P. (1988b). Clinical and biochemical manifestations of depression. Part 2. *N. Engl. J. Med.* **319**, 413–420.

Griffiths, M. M., and DeWitt, C. W. (1984). Genetic control of collagen-induced arthritis in rats: The immune response to type II collagen among susceptible and resistant strains and evidence for multiple gene control. *J. Immunol.* **132**, 2830–2836.

Hawley, D. J., and Wolfe, F. (1988). Anxiety and depression in patients with rheumatoid arthritis: A prospective study of 400 patients. *J. Rheumatol.* **15**, 932–941.

Hill, J. L., and Yu, D. T. Y. (1987). Development of an experimental animal model for reactive arthritis induced by *Yersinia enterocolitica* infection. *Infect. Immun.* **55**, 721–726.

Kling, M. A., Perini, G. I., Demitrack, M. A., Geracioti, T. A., Linnoila, M., Chrousos, G. P., and Gold, P. W. (1990). Stress-responsive neurohormonal systems and the symptom complex of affective illness. *Psychopharmacol. Bull.* **25**, 312–318.

Kohashi, O., Kohashi, Y., Takahashi, T., Ozawa, A., and Shigematsu, N. (1986). Suppressive effect of *Escherichia coli* on adjuvant-induced arthritis in germ-free rats. *Arthritis Rheum.* **29**, 547–553.

Lehman, T. J. A., Allen, J. B., Plotz, P. H., and Wilder, R. (1984). *Lactobacillus Casei* cell wall-induced arthritis in rats: Cell wall fragment distribution and persistence in chronic arthritis-susceptible LEW/N and resistant F344/N rats. *Arthritis Rheum.* **27**, 939–942.

Lumpkin, M. D. (1987). The regulation of ACTH secretion by IL-1. *Science* **238**, 452.

Mason, J. H., Weener, J. L., Gertman, P. M., and Meenan, R. F. (1983). Health status in chronic disease: A comparative study of rheumatoid arthritis. *J. Rheumatol.* **10**, 763–768.

McFarlane, A. C., and Brooks, P. M. (1988) An Analysis of the relationship between psychological morbidity and disease activity in rheumatoid arthritis. *J. Rheumatol.* **15**, 926–931.

Mendelson, W. B., Slater, S., Gold, P. W., and Gillian, J. C. (1980). The effect of growth hormone administration on human sleep: A dose-response study. *Biol. Psychiatry* **15**, 613–618.

Pincus, T., Callahan, L. F., Bradley, L. A., Vaughn, W. K., and Wolfe, F. (1986). Elevated MMPI scores for hypochondriasis, depression and hysteria in patients with rheumatoid arthritis reflect disease rather than psychological status. *Arthritis Rheum.* **29**, 1456–1466.

Rivier C., and Vale, W. (1984). Influence of corticotropin-releasing factor on reproductive functions in the rat. *Enocrinology (Baltimore)* **114**, 914–121.

Rock, J. P., Oldfield, E. H., Schulte, H. M., Gold, P. W., Kornblith, P. L., Loriaux, L., and Chrousos, G. P. (1984). Corticotropin releasing factor administered into the ventricular CSF stimulates the pituitary-adrenal axis. *Brain Res.* **323**, 365–368.

Roy, A., Pickar, D., Paul, S., Doran, A., Chrousos, G. P., and Gold, P. W. (1987). CSF corticotropin-releasing hormone in depressed patients and normal control subjects. *Am. J. Psychiatry* **144**, 641–645.

Sapolsky, R., Rivier, C., Yamamoto, G., Plotsky, P., and Vale, W. (1987). Interleukin-1 stimulates the secretion of hypothalamic corticotropin releasing factor. *Science* **238**, 522.

Schulte, H. M., Chrousos, G. P., Gold, P. W., Booth, J. D., Oldfield, E. H., Cutler, G. B., Jr., and Loriaux, D. L. (1985). Continuous administration of synthetic ovine corticotropin-releasing factor in man: Physiological and pathophysiological implications. *J. Clin. Invest.* **75**, 1781–1785.

Sirinathsinghji, D. J. S., Rees, L. H., Rivier, J., and Vale, W. (1983). Corticotropin-releasing factor is a potent inhibitor of sexual receptivity in the female rate. *Nature (London)* **305**, 232–235.

Smythe, H. A. (1984). Problems with the MMPI (editorial). *J. Rheumatol.* **11**, 417–418.

Sternberg, E. M. (1988). Monokines, lymphokines and the brain. *In* "The Year in Immunology" (J. M. Cruse and H. J. Wedner, eds.), Vol. 5, pp. 205–217. Karger, Basel.

Sternberg, E. M., and Parker, C. W. (1988). Immunopharmacologic aspects of lymphocyte regulation. *In* "Lymphocyte Structure and Function" J. J. Marchalonis, (ed.), pp. 1–53. Dekker, New York.

Sternberg, E. M., Hill, J. M., Chrousos, G. P., Kamilaris, T., Listwak, S. J., Gold, P. W., and Wilder, R. L. (1989a). Inflammatory mediator-induced hypothalamic-pituitary-adrenal axis activation is defective in streptococcal cell wall arthritis susceptible Lewis rats. *Proc. Natl. Acad. Sci. U.S.A.* **86**, 2374–2378.

Sternberg, E. M., Young, W. S., III, Bernardini, R., Calogero, A. E., Chrousos, G. P., Gold, P. W., and Wilder, R. L. (1989b). A central nervous system defect in biosynthesis of corticotropin-releasing hormone is associated with susceptibility to steptococcal cell wall athritis in Lewis rats. *Proc. Natl. Acad. Sci. U.S.A.* **86**, 4771–4775.

Sternberg, E. M., Wilder, R. L., Gold, P. W., and Chrousos, G. P. (1989c). The central nervous system–immune system feedback loop and arthritis susceptibility. *Prog. NeuroEndocrinImmunol.* **2**, 102–108.

Sutton, R. E., Koob, G. F., LeMoal, M., Rivier, J., and Vale, W. (1982). Corticotropin releasing factor produces behavioural activiation in rats. *Nature (London)* **297**, 331–333.

Swerdlow, N. R., Geyer, M. A., Vale, W. W., and Koob, G. F. (1986). Corticotropin-releasing factor potentiates acoustic startle in rats: Blockade by chlordiazepoxide. *Psychopharmacology (Berlin)* **88**, 147–152.

Uehara, A., Gillis, S., and Arimura, A. (1987). Effect of interleukin-1 on hormone release from normal rat pituitary cells in primary culture. *Neuroendocrinology* **45**, 343.

Vale, W., Spiess, J., Rivier, C., and Rivier, J. (1981). Characterization of a 41-residue ovine hypothalamic peptide that stimulates secretion of corticotropin and β-endorphin. *Science* **213**, 1394–1397.

Valentino, R. J., Foote, S. L., and Aston-Jones, G. (1983). Corticotropin-releasing hormone activates noradrenergic neurons of the locus coeruleus. *Brain Res.* **270**, 363–367.

Zis, A. P., Grof, P., and Goodwin, F. K. (1979). The natural course of affective disorders: implications for lithium prophylaxis. *In* "Lithium: Controversies and Unresolved Issues" (T. B. Cooper, S. Gershon, N. S. Kline, and M. Schou, eds.), pp. 381–391. Excerpta Medica, Amsterdam.

IV
Gastrointestinal Function

15

Brain Peptides and Gastrointestinal Transit

Thomas F. Burks
Department of Pharmacology
College of Medicine
University of Arizona
Tucson, Arizona 85724

I. Introduction

Acquisition and assimilation of nutrients are fundamental necessities for survival of any organism. Existence of a species is often determined by its nutritional success. Typically, the more important a particular function is to survival, the more elaborate are the regulatory processes that control the critical function. Because well-regulated gastrointestinal motility is a requirement for survival of mammals, it is predictable that motility functions of the gastrointestinal tract are subject to multiple levels of control. Regulatory peptides, including neurotransmitters, hormones, and immunomodulators, act at chemosensitive sites in the brain, spinal cord, endocrine system, peripheral ganglia, and in the enteric nervous system to influence the time and place that contractions of gastrointestinal smooth muscle will occur. The regulatory power of the brain over gastrointestinal motility is presently understood to be of great physiological, pathophysiological, and pharmacological importance. The most direct pathway by which the brain influences gastrointestinal motility is by interactions with the enteric nervous system.

A. Regulation of Motility

Motility of the gastrointestinal tract is regulated primarily by nerves of the enteric nervous system, now recognized as a distinct division of the autonomic nervous system, that control the excitability of the gastrointestinal smooth muscle. The enteric nervous system is comprised of two major neural plexuses, the myenteric plexus that lies between the outer longitudinal muscle coat and the inner circular muscle coat, and the submucosal plexus that lies between the circular muscle and the mucosa. These plexuses consist of nerve cell bodies organized in distinct ganglia, axons, interneurons, and fascicals that provide nerve pathways extending over long distances. The myenteric plexus is responsible mainly for motor control of the longitudinal and circular smooth muscle; the submucosal plexus is responsible for integration of sensory information and regulates, via motor pathways, mucosal transport of fluid, electrolytes, and nutrients. Both efferent and afferent neural pathways are represented in the nerve plexuses of the enteric nervous system. The well-coordinated interplay of nerve activity assures great precision in regulation of motility events.

In addition to the enteric nervous system control, gastrointestinal smooth muscle contractions are influenced also by the central nervous system, the endocrine system, and the immune system (Figure 1). Sensory information from the gastrointestinal tract is relayed to the central nervous system over parasympathetic (primarily vagal and pelvic nerve) pathways and over sympathetic pathways. The wall of the intestine is thought to contain mechanoreceptors, chemoreceptors, osmoreceptors, thermoreceptors, and nociceptors that serve primary afferent neurons with cell bodies in the nodose ganglion of the vagus or the dorsal root ganglia of the spinal cord. The information concerning muscle tension, chemical composition, and osmolarity of luminal content, temperature, and pain stimuli is integrated in the spinal cord and brain to generate appropriate regulatory output. Efferent nerves from the brain or spinal cord terminate on intrinsic ganglia of the enteric nervous system. The parasympathetic and sympathetic nerves modulate, facilitate, or inhibit neurotransmission within the enteric nervous

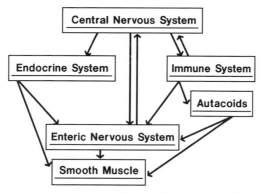

Figure 1 Schematic representation of regulation of gastrointestinal smooth muscle by the enteric nervous system, central nervous system, endocrine system, and immune system. The enteric nervous system is the primary controller of smooth muscle contractions. Regulatory modulation of the enteric nervous system is provided by the central nervous system, the endocrine system, and the immune system, plus effects of local hormones or autacoids.

system. Thus, the central nervous system can, for example, select a fed or fasting motility pattern.

B. Patterns of Motility

The fed pattern of motility consists of irregular phasic contractions that serve to mix intestinal contents and move them slowly in an aborad direction, although short (5–10 cm) propulsive contractions may also occur (Figure 2). The rate at which phasic contractions occur is determined by the excitability of the smooth muscle cells and by the local frequency of myogenic slow waves. Excitability of the smooth muscle is regulated primarily by neurotransmitter substances released from nerves of the enteric nervous system. Enteric neurotransmitters include acetylcholine, substance P, 5-hydroxytryptamine, cholecystokinin, vasoactive intestinal peptide, enkephalins, neurotensin, and neuropeptide Y (Lundgren et al., 1989). The myogenic slow waves are very regular changes in membrane potential of muscle cells at rates of approximately 3 per minute in distal stomach, 17 per minute in upper small intestine, and 12 per minute in distal small intestine in humans. Because of the proximal to distal gradient of slow wave frequencies in the small intestine, there tends also to be a gradient of frequencies of phasic contractions with more contractions in the duodenum than in the ileum. As suggested by the relationship in contractile frequency, phasic contractions in the stomach and small intestine occur in conjunction with slow waves. If smooth muscle cells are rendered excitable by neurotransmitters,

Segmenting Contractions   **Propulsive Contractions**

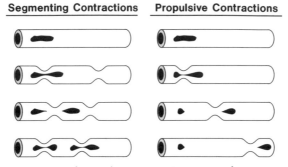

Figure 2 Both segmenting and propulsive contraction can produce net movement (propulsion) of intestinal content (depicted by shaded area) in the aborad direction.

contraction will occur during the depolarization phase of slow waves. Depending on the degree of excitation of smooth muscle cells, an individual slow wave may or may not generate a contraction. Neural influences determine whether an area of intestine with a slow wave frequency of 12 develops 1, 6, or 12 phasic contractions per minute.

The fasting pattern of motility is a fascinating demonstration of brain–gut coordination. Some 1–4 h after eating, bands of phasic contractions develop in the stomach or proximal small intestine and slowly travel aborally to the terminal ileum (Szurszewski, 1987). The bands of intense phasic contractions represent the gastrointestinal migrating motor complex (MMC). MMCs require approximately 90–120 min to progress from the duodenum to the terminal ileum, and they cycle continuously, day and night, until the next meal is consumed. The MMC waves in the stomach may be perceived as "hunger pangs." When a meal is eaten, MMC activity at all levels of the intestine abruptly ceases and the fed pattern of motility is immediately initiated.

The central nervous system has the ability to determine whether the enteric nervous system will direct a fed or fasting pattern of motility, the general incidence and intensity of contractions, and local activity in each portion of the gastrointestinal tract.

The endocrine and immune system can also influence gastrointestinal motility by actions of hormones and cytokines on nerves of the enteric nervous system, by direct effects on smooth muscle, or by actions mediated through the central nervous system. The gastrointestinal mucosa is itself an endocrine organ and is responsible for release of such hormones as gastrin, secretin, cholecystokinin, motilin, gastric inhibitory peptide, neurotensin, and gastrin-releasing peptide (Solcia et al., 1987). Release of motilin may be associated with initiation of MMC activity during interdigestive periods. Hormones of the pituitary, adrenal medulla and cortex, pancreas, and gonads also can affect gastrointestinal motility. Less is known about cytokine actions, but interleukin-1α has recently been shown to influence motility (Vander Hamm *et al.*, 1989). Finally, the autocoid substances released locally in the stomach or intestine, such as histamine, 5-hydroxytryptamine, and prostanoids, can influence both neural and muscle elements and can thereby affect motility.

Propulsion or transit of gastrointestinal content depends on pressure gradients favoring aboral flow. Under normal conditions the pressure gradients are generated by contractions of circular smooth muscle, although in pathological hypersecretory conditions, hydrostatic pressure is sufficient to provide gradients sufficient for brisk flow. Normal postprandial transit, except in the esophagus, proceeds slowly as a result of phasic mixing contractions. Propulsion of swallowed boluses of food or drink in the esophagus is accomplished by aborad propulsive contractions. Gastric emptying is regulated by both the frequency and amplitude of contractions in the antrum and pyloric canal as well as by the contractile state of the proximal duodenum. Contractions of the duodenum can elevate intraluminal pressure and abolish the antral–duodenal pressure gradient essential for flow of gastric content into the duodenum. Transit through the small intestine and colon is determined by local patterns of phasic contractions, although propulsive "mass movements" occur from time to time in the colon to move contents from the right to the left colon.

C. Relationship to Stress

A connection between emotional states, such as fear or anxiety, and gastrointestinal propulsion is well established in popular scatology but has not been extensively studied in scientific investigations. Walter Cannon (1902) noted that exposure of cats to a growling dog resulted in altered transit of intestinal contents in the subject cats. Psychological stress was found over 30 years ago to change colonic motility in a human volunteer (Almy, 1951). The decreases in motility and transit associated with fear of physical harm are explained adequately by centrally directed mass sympathoadrenal discharge, resulting in catecholamine-mediated inhibition of excitatory neural pathways in the enteric nervous system. The complex changes in motility and transit associated with more psychological stress (often a combination of psychic and physical stress) are more difficult to explain. Studies of animals and humans indicate that different stressors produce somewhat different patterns of specific changes in transit and motility, but some common themes can be detected. Psychological stress in humans generally does not significantly alter the rate of gastric emptying, can increase or decrease transit through the small intestine, and nearly always results in increased colonic motility (Wingate and Kumar, 1988). In animals, stressors such as partial restraint decrease small intestinal transit, increase colonic transit, and increase fecal excretion (Williams *et al.*, 1988). The profound effects of psychic stress on gastrointestinal transit in animals and humans provide evidence for central nervous system-directed changes in gastrointestinal function of both laboratory and clinical importance. Irritable bowel syndrome (IBS) is an example of a prevalent functional disorder of motility and transit that is a result of stress or is at least exacerbated by stress (Narducci *et al.*, 1985; Valori *et al.*, 1986).

II. Opioids

Opium and opiates, such as morphine, have been known since antiquity to inhibit gastrointestinal transit, and opium was used for centuries in the treatment of diarrhea. It is now recognized that opioids can affect gastrointestinal transit by actions in the central nervous system (Burks, 1978). The first direct demonstration of centrally mediated opioid effects on gastrointestinal motility came from a study of intestinal myoelectric activity in cats given small doses of morphine directly into the cerebral ventricles by means of cannulas implanted through the skull (Stewart *et al.*, 1977). Morphine caused an increase in myoelectric spikes recorded from the intestine, indicative of increased contractions of circular muscle, the typical intestinal response to morphine in cats (Pruitt *et al.*, 1974).

Parolaro *et al.* (1977) and Stewart *et al.* (1978) went on to find that morphine administered intracerebroventricularly (icv) in rats produced inhibition of intestinal transit measured by propulsion of an orally given charcoal meal or by distribution of radioactivity in the intestinal lumen after intraduodenal instillation of radiochromium. Subsequent investigations revealed that morphine was much more potent as an antitransit drug when given icv than when given peripherally (Galligan and Burks, 1983). However, when morphine is administered systemically, it exerts antitransit effects by actions at both peripheral and central sites (Tavani *et al.*, 1979; Manara *et al.*, 1986; Burleigh *et al.*, 1981; Shook *et al.*, 1987c). The peripheral site of morphine action is thought to be primarily the myenteric plexus of the enteric nervous system (Manara *et al.*, 1986).

Another advance in understanding the central regulation of gastrointestinal transit was the discovery that intrathecally (i.t.) administered morphine also inhibited gastrointestinal transit (Porreca *et al.*, 1983a; Porreca and Burks, 1983b). This finding suggested that both the brain and the spinal cord contain chemosensitive sites at which drugs can act to affect gastrointestinal transit. It has now become important to establish the gastrointestinal actions of substances at brain, spinal, and peripheral sites.

A. Opioid Peptides

The discovery that endogenous opioid peptides occur in the central nervous-system (Hughes, 1975; Hughes *et al.*, 1975) raised the possibility of functional significance of central opioid systems in regulation of gastrointestinal motility and transit (Burks and Galligan, 1982). Several studies, summarized in Table I, were conducted to characterize the effects of natural opioid peptides on gastrointestinal transit after icv or i.t. injection. In rats, several opioid peptides, including β-endorphin-(1–31), were found to inhibit intestinal transit after icv but not after intraperitoneal (ip) administration even in much higher doses (Galligan and Burks, 1982). The modified natural opioid peptide DAMEA (Tyr-D-Ala-Gly-Phe-Met-NH$_2$) produced inhibition of transit in rats when given icv in doses of 25 μg or greater, but failed to inhibit transit when given ip in doses up to 1000 μg. A systematic series of studies in mice, featuring both icv and i.t. injections, revealed significant differences among relatively closely related peptides (Table I). Peptide E-(1–25), derived from proenkephalin, produced inhibition of transit when given either icv or i.t. in small doses. BAM 22P, which corresponds to peptide E-(1–22), did not significantly inhibit transit in mice at doses up to 100 μg when given icv, but did inhibit transit when given i.t. in a dose of 60 μg. These data are curious because peptide E-(1–25) contains [Met^5]enkephalin

Table I

Effects of Natural Opioid Peptides on Gastrointestinal Transit in Mice

Peptide	icv Dose	icv Geometric center[a]	i.t. Dose	i.t. Geometric center[a]
β-Endorphin-(1–31)	5 μg	2.2 ± 0.2[b]	5 μg	1.2 ± 0.1[b]
Dynorphin-(1–13)	100 μg	5.9 ± 0.4	100 μg	5.1 ± 0.5
Peptide E	10 μg	2.7 ± 0.3[b]	10 μg	1.9 ± 0.5[b]
BAM 22P	10 μg	3.2 ± 0.5[b]	10 μg	2.3 ± 0.5[b]
BAM 12P	100 μg	4.1 ± 0.9	60 μg	1.8 ± 0.2[b]
Peptide F	40 μg	3.6 ± 0.9	40 μg	2.4 ± 0.4[b]
MEAGL	200 μg	4.7 ± 0.4	200 μg	3.1 ± 0.5[b]
MEAP	100 μg	3.7 ± 0.4	100 μg	2.4 ± 0.2[b]
Saline	5 μl	5.7 ± 0.4	5 μl	5.4 ± 0.2

[a]Geometric center is an expression of transit derived from the distribution of radioactivity within the lumen of the intestine after intragastric administration of ^{51}Cr. A geometric center of 1.0 indicates no transit and a value of 10.0 indicates complete transit through the small intestine.

[b]Significantly different from saline control, $p < 0.05$. Data from Davis *et al.*, (1985); Porreca and Burks (1983b), Porreca *et al.* (1983b), and Shook *et al.* (1988). Sequences of the peptides are given in Burks *et al.* (1987).

(Tyr-Gly-Gly-Phe-Met) at the N-terminus, and BAM 22P and BAM 12P can be viewed simply as C-terminal extended analogs of [Met^5]enkephalin. Peptide F is a proenkephalin-derived 34-amino-acid residue peptide with [Met^5]enkephalin sequences at both the N and C terminals. Peptide F inhibited transit when given i.t. but not when given icv in a dose of 40 μg, whereas peptide E, which has a [Met^5]enkephalin sequence at the N-terminus but a [Leu^5]enkephalin sequence at the C terminus, was active icv in a dose of 10 μg. MEAGL ([Met^5]enkephalin-Arg-Gly-Leu) and MEAP ([Met^5]enkephalin-Arg-Phe) were also relatively inactive when given icv, but were effective in inhibiting transit when given i.t. Natural [Met^5]enkephalin inhibited transit when given icv in a dose of 400 μg. These data indicate that C-terminal extended enkephalins, such as BAM 12P, peptide F, MEAGL, and MEAP, are more active as antitransit agents in the spinal cord than in the brain, suggesting that the spinal cord contains a population of opioid receptors linked to gastrointestinal regulation not found in the brain. Peptide E and BAM 22P were able to act potently in the brain to inhibit transit, indicating that these peptides act at a different population of supraspinal receptors linked to gastrointestinal regulation.

β-Endorphin-(1–31), derived from pro-opiomelanocortin, produced antitransit effects when given icv in rats (Galligan and Burks, 1982) and in mice (Shook *et al.*, 1988). A major peptide derived from the third major opioid gene product, prodynorphin, was examined in detail. Dynorphin-(1–13) and dynorphin-(1–9) failed to inhibit transit when given icv in rats (Galligan and Burks, 1982) or when given icv or i.t. in mice (Porreca *et al.*, 1983b). The dynorphin peptides, however, induced analgesia when given i.t. (Porreca *et al.*, 1983b).

These studies with natural opioid peptides revealed three distinct patterns of antitransit actions: peptides that inhibited transit by actions both in the brain and spinal cord, those that were active only in the spinal cord, and those that failed to alter transit after either brain or spinal administration. These patterns, of course, suggested effects at multiple types of opioid receptors.

B. Receptor-Selective Opioids

Based on the insight of Martin *et al.* (1976) and Lord *et al.* (1977), it is now recognized that there are at least three types (mu, delta, and kappa) of opioid receptors of importance in mammals (Dougall, 1988). As selective agonists for each type of opioid receptor became available, it was possible to determine which brain, spinal cord, and peripheral receptors were responsible for opioid antitransit effects. The selective agonists used in our studies were DAMGO (Tyr-D-Ala-Gly-N-methyl-Phe-Gly-ol) (Handa *et al.*, 1981) and PL017 (Tyr-Pro-Phe-Pro-NH$_2$) (Chang *et al.*, 1983) for mu receptors, DPDPE (cyclic Tyr-D-Pen-Gly-Phe-D-Pen) (Mosberg *et al.*, 1983) for delta receptors, and U-50488 (*trans-(d,l)*-3,4-dichloro-N-methyl-N -[2-(-pyrrolidinyl) cyclohexyl]-benzeneacetamide methane sulfonate) (von Voigtlander *et al.*, 1983) for kappa receptors. Interestingly, these selective agonists reproduced the pattern of antitransit effects noted before with natural opioid peptides: those that acted both in brain and spinal cord, those that acted only in the spinal cord, and those that acted at neither brain nor spinal cord.

In rats, DAMGO, the selective mu agonist, and morphine, the classical mu agonist, produced dose-related inhibition of intestinal transit when administered icv (Galligan *et al.*, 1984). In contrast, the selective delta agonist DPDPE and the selective kappa agonist U-50,488 had little or no effect on transit when given icv (data summarized in Table II). All of the agonists produced analgesia, indicating that the doses administered icv were sufficient to induce opioid effects. These findings indicated that mu, but not delta or kappa, receptors in the brain are linked to gastrointestinal transit effects.

Both brain and spinal effects of receptor selective opioids were assessed in mice (Porreca *et al.*, 1984); the results are summarized in Table III. As in rats, icv administration of the mu agonists, DAMGO and morphine, caused dose-related inhibition of gastrointestinal transit in mice, while the delta agonist, DPDPE, and the kappa agonist, U-50,488, had little or no effects. However, all three types of opioid agonists, mu, delta, and kappa, produced analgesia when given icv.

Table II

Effects of Receptor-Selective Opioid Agonists on
Intestinal Transit and Hot-Plate Latency in Rats[a]

| Agonist | D$_{50}$ values (nmol/rat) | |
	Antitransit	Analgesia
DAMGO	0.56	0.14
Morphine	5.75	2.02
DPDPE	~1000	35.5
U-50,488	~1000	120.8

[a]All agents were administered icv. Approximate antitransit D$_{50}$ values for DPDPE and U-50,488 were estimated by extrapolation from very slight effects at the highest doses tested. Data from Galligan *et al.* (1984).

Table III

Effects of Receptor-Selective Opioid Agonists on Intestinal Transit and Hot-Plate Latency
in Mice[a]

| Agonist | D_{50} values (nmol/rat) | | | |
| | Antitransit | | Analgesia | |
	icv	i.t.	icv	i.t.
DAMGO	0.051	0.051	0.0095	0.56
Morphine	1.69	2.60	0.40	0.37
DPDPE	Inactive	3.10	10.14	1.52
U-50,488	Inactive	215.0	32.5	107.7

[a]The approximate antitransit D_{50} value for U-50,488 after i.t. injection was estimated by extrapolation from slight effects produced by the highest dose administered. Data from Porreca et al. (1984).

When the selective opioid agonists were administered i.t., a different pattern of effects became evident. Both mu and delta agonists produced dose-related antitransit effects after spinal injection, whereas the kappa agonist was nearly inactive. DAMGO, morphine, and DPDPE also produced analgesia when given i.t., whereas U-50,488 was only weakly active in the hot plate test of antinociception after i.t. administration.

The receptor-selective opioid agonists produced distinct patterns of antitransit effects related to the particular type of receptor at which they act: mu receptors in both brain and spinal cord are associated with antitransit effects, delta receptors in the spinal cord but not in the brain are linked to antitransit mechanisms, and central nervous system kappa receptors seem not to produce significant antitransit effects.

When administered peripherally by subcutaneous (sc) injection in mice, mu agonists (morphine and PLO17) produced dose-related inhibition of gastrointestinal transit, whereas delta (DPDPE) and kappa agonists (U-50,488) had essentially no effect (Shook et al., 1987c). The antitransit effects of sc mu agonists were blocked by naloxone and CTP, a highly selective mu antagonist (Shook et al., 1987a,b). Peripherally administered mu agonists produced their antitransit effects mainly by actions at peripheral sites (Shook et al., 1987c).

The effects of receptor selective opioid agonists on small intestinal transit are summarized in Table IV. The patterns of action of these ligands suggest that the patterns of antitransit effects produced by the natural opioid peptides can be explained by their profiles of receptor actions. β-Endorphin, peptide E, and BAM 22P exert pronounced agonist effects at mu opioid receptors (Shook et al., 1987c; Wuster et al., 1979; Lewis et al., 1979). Relatively shorter C-terminus extended enkephalins BAM 12P, MEAGL,

Table IV

Effects of Neuropeptides and Peptide Mimetics on Small Intestinal
Transit in Rats and Mice after icv, i.t., or Peripheral Administration[a]

Agonists	icv	i.t.	iv, sc, ip
DAMGO, PL017	↓	↓	↓
Morphine	↓	↓	↓
DPDPE	0	↓	↓
U-50,488	0	0	0
Bombesin	↓	↓	↓
CRF	↓	NT	↓

[a] ↓, Decrease in transit; 0, little or no effect on transit; NT, not tested.

and MEAP, as well as the enkephalins themselves and peptide F, possess
relatively less preference for mu receptors and greater preference for delta
receptors (Leslie, 1987; Höllt, 1986). Dynorphin is relatively selective for
kappa opioid receptors (Corbett *et al.*, 1982; Yoshimura *et al.*, 1982). Thus,
there is great consistency in the effects of both natural and synthetic opioids
in terms of their antitransit effects when receptor selectivity and sites of
action are taken into account.

C. Intestinal Motility

The relationship between gastrointestinal motility (contractions) and transit
(propulsion) is complicated because contractions of circular muscle of the
intestine both provide normal pressure gradients that direct luminal flow
aborally and increase resistance to luminal flow. In many mammalian species, mu opioids induce contractions of the circular muscle that retard transit by increasing resistance to flow (Burks, 1976; Hirning *et al.*, 1985). On
the other hand, intestinal transit can be enhanced by administration of
drugs, such as neostigmine, that induce coordinated propulsive contractions
(Galligan and Burks, 1986).

Intestinal intraluminal pressure was measured in unanesthetized rats
by means of chronically implanted catheters. Contractions were measured
in the upper half of the small intestine, duodenum and jejunum, because
radiochromium was placed in the duodenum for measurement of its distribution in the small intestine in studies of transit. Administration of morphine icv or sc produced inhibition of contractions in the small intestine
(Galligan and Burks, 1983). The time sequence of the response and dose
requirements by the different routes of administration showed great correspondence between inhibition of contractions and inhibition of transit. Opi-

oid peptides with mu receptor agonist actions were also found to inhibit intestinal contractions in rats after icv administration (Burks and Galligan, 1982). Morphine was approximately 25-fold more potent both in inhibiting transit and in decreasing contractions when administered icv than when administered sc (Galligan and Burks, 1983).

III. Bombesin

Bombesin is a 14-amino-acid residue peptide, isolated originally from the skin of frogs, that shares considerable sequence homology and essentially identical pharmacological properties with mammalian gastrin-releasing peptide (GRP). Bombesin/GRP occurs in the rat brain, spinal cord, and gastrointestinal tract (Brown et al., 1978). Peripherally administered bombesin produces contractions of the pylorus in rats and delays gastric emptying in rats and humans (Bertaccini and Impicciatore, 1975; Scarpignato and Bertaccini, 1981; Scarpignato et al., 1982). In addition to effects observed after peripheral administration, bombesin has been found to produce profound changes in gastrointestinal transit by actions in the central nervous system (Porreca et al., 1988).

Administration of small doses of bombesin icv in rats resulted in dose-related inhibition of gastric emptying and inhibition of small intestinal transit (Porreca and Burks, 1983a). The bombesin-induced inhibition of gastric emptying was attenuated by subdiaphragmatic vagotomy, indicating that icv bombesin altered gastroduodenal flow via vagal pathways. Bombesin administered icv in rats produced transient stimulation of colonic transit. Gmerek et al. (1983) found that bombesin given i.t. in rats also inhibits gastric emptying and intestinal transit.

In mice, bombesin was found to inhibit gastrointestinal transit after icv, i.t., or ip injection (Koslo et al., 1986a). Bombesin given icv was approximately 13–14 times more potent in inhibiting transit than when given i.t. and over 3000 times more potent icv than ip. Colonic propulsion was assessed in mice by expulsion of small glass beads inserted 2 cm into the rectum. Colonic bead expulsion was inhibited by bombesin given icv and i.t., whereas bombesin was completely inactive when given ip even in doses up to 3000-fold higher than the icv D_{50}.

Data obtained in rats and mice suggested the great potency and possible importance of bombesin central actions as related to gastrointestinal regulation. The consistently greater potency of bombesin when given icv than when given i.t. raised the question of whether bombesin acts independently at brain and spinal sites to bring about changes in gastrointestinal transit or whether interaction between the brain and spinal cord are necessary for expression of bombesin action. Bombesin was administered icv and i.t. to normal mice and to mice with spinal transections at the level of the second thoracic vertebra that eliminated both neural and cerebrospinal fluid communication between the brain and spinal cord below the thoracic level. Bombesin was completely effective in inhibiting gastrointestinal transit and colonic bead expulsion after icv injection in both intact and spinal transected mice. Bombesin given i.t. was effective in intact mice, but not in spinally transected mice (Koslo *et al.*, 1986a). In contrast to results with bombesin, morphine was shown in the same study to inhibit colonic bead expulsion when given i.t. below the level of transection in spinally transected mice as well as when given icv.

These data indicate that gastrointestinal antipropulsive effects of spinally administered bombesin require intact connections between the cord and the brain. Intrathecal bombesin may activate supraspinal centers to initiate antitransit effects, whereas those centers can be activated directly by icv injections of bombesin. Bombesin given i.t. therefore may act at chemosensitive sites in ascending cord pathways to influence gastrointestinal propulsion. As vagotomy blocks at least some of the antitransit effects of bombesin, part of the supraspinal action of bombesin may be to alter vagal outflow to the gastrointestinal tract. However, other mechanisms may also be involved in bombesin's effects. For example, Gmerek and Cowan (1984) found that ablation of either the pituitary or adrenals prevented the antitransit effects of icv bombesin in rats. Similarly, Koslo *et al.* (1986b) established that an intact pituitary–adrenal axis is required for spinally mediated antitransit effects of bombesin.

Central gastrointestinal effects of bombesin seem to involve multiple effector mechanisms, including the pathways classically associated with responses to stress. Bombesin inhibition of gastric emptying appears to be mediated at least in part by vagal mechanisms, because subdiaphragmatic vagotomy diminishes ability of centrally administered bombesin to delay gastric emptying. The centrally directed effects of bombesin on intestinal propulsion, on the other hand, depend on pituitary and adrenal mechanisms. It is probably significant that spinally administered bombesin requires intact spinal cord–brain connections and seems to share identical effector mechanisms with icv administered bombesin.

A. Intestinal Motility

The intestinal antitransit effects of icv administered mu opioids, including morphine and β-endorphin, are associated with decreases in intestinal motility. To determine whether the antitransit effects of icv bombesin are also explained by decreased intestinal motility, intestinal intraluminal pressure

Table V

Effects of Mu Opioids and Bombesin on Intestinal Motility and
Transit in Rats[a]

Agonist	Contractions	Transit
Morphine	↓	↓
β-Endorphin-(1–31)	↓	↓
Bombesin	↑	↓

[a]Data from Burks and Galligan (1982); Galligan and Burks (1983), and
Porreca *et al.* (1985).

was measured in unanesthetized rats (Porreca *et al.*, 1985). Patterns of contractions after icv bombesin were strikingly different from those that occur after icv morphine. Bombesin produced dose-related increases in the frequency and amplitude of intestinal contractions within 30 min after icv injection. These stimulatory effects persisted for at least 1 h. No effect was observed when bombesin was given ip, even in doses 200 times greater than those used icv. These data indicate that bombesin given icv, but not peripherally, produces an increase in intestinal contractions and a decrease in intestinal transit. Morphine and related mu opioids, on the other hand, decrease contractions and decrease transit. Obviously, the specific pattern of motility initiated by centrally acting neuropeptides determines whether transit will be affected (Table V).

IV. Corticotropin-Releasing Factor

Corticotropin-releasing factor (CRF) is a 41-amino-acid residue peptide first identified in extracts of ovine hypothalamus (Vale *et al.*, 1981). CRF is a critical mediator of stress responses and is released from the hypothalamus to stimulate production of adrenocorticotropin (ACTH) and β-endorphin by the pituitary (Rivier *et al.*, 1982). In addition to its pituitary actions, CRF also exerts a number of extrapituitary effects on the cardiovascular and reproductive systems (Fisher *et al.*, 1982; Sirinathsinghji *et al.*, 1983). Because of its widespread distribution within the central nervous system and its multiple actions, often associated with stress, CRF has been proposed as a "master transmitter" that is capable of eliciting coordinated endocrine and autonomic events characteristic of the stress response.

Within the brain, CRF immunoreactivity is associated with regions that regulate both endocrine and autonomic functions (Swanson *et al.*, 1983). CRF is also present in the stomach and small intestine in many species (Nieuwenhuyzen-Kruseman *et al.*, 1982; Petrusz *et al.*, 1985). Several studies had examined effects of exogenously administered CRF on gastrointestinal functions. CRF given icv was found to inhibit gastric acid secretion and to delay gastric emptying (Taché *et al.*, 1983; Konturek *et al.*, 1985; Bueno and Fioramonti, 1986). Administration icv of CRF in dogs suppressed gastric, but not jejunal, migrating motor complexes (MMCs), but was inactive when administered iv (Bueno *et al.*, 1986). The presence of CRF-like immunoreactivity in central structures relevant to gastrointestinal control demonstrated effects of CRF on aspects of gastrointestinal function, and recently recognized effects of stress on intestinal propulsion (Williams *et al.*, 1988; Williams and Burks, 1989) predicted that CRF could possess unique effects on gastrointestinal transit.

Administration of CRF icv in doses of 0.3–10 μg in unanesthetized rats resulted in dose-related inhibition of gastric emptying, inhibition of small intestinal transit, and stimulation of colonic transit (Williams *et al.*, 1987). The stimulation of colonic transit was associated with increased fecal output and, at the highest doses tested, diarrhea. CRF administered iv and CRF administered icv were essentially equieffective. The functional consequences of CRF (0.3 μg icv) and stress induced by partial wrap restraint were strikingly similar (Table VI). Both CRF and stress induced inhibition of small intestinal transit and stimulation of colonic transit and fecal output. In addition, both CRF and stress produced increases in plasma levels of ACTH (Williams *et al.*, 1987). The possible mediator role of CRF in gastrointestinal responses to stress was greatly strengthened by the finding that a CRF antagonist, α-helical CRF-(9–41) (Rivier *et al.*, 1985), inhibited the stimulation of colonic transit induced by CRF or stress (Williams *et al.*, 1987).

Further studies have provided additional evidence for a critical role of

Table VI

Effects of icv Corticotropin-Releasing Factor (CRF) and Stress
in Unanesthetized Rats[a]

Parameter	CRF (0.3 μg icv)	Stress
Gastric emptying	0	0
Small intestinal transit	↓	↓
Colonic transit	↑	↑
Fecal output	↑	↑
ACTH release	↑	↑

[a]0, Little or no change; ↓, decrease; ↑, increase. Data from Williams *et al.* (1987).

CRF in gastrointestinal responses to stress. Lenz *et al.* (1988a) confirmed that icv administration of CRF in rats resulted in decreased gastric emptying and small intestinal transit and stimulation of colonic transit. The CRF antagonist, α-helical CRF-(9–41), was found to block stress-induced changes in small intestinal transit, colonic transit, and gastric acid secretion (Lenz *et al.*, 1988b). Acoustic stress and cold stress in mice that had been fed a meal containing fat were found to increase gastric emptying (Bueno and Gué, 1988). The stressors evidently reversed fat-induced inhibition of gastric emptying in these animals. Importantly, the ip administration of CRF antiserum blocked the effects of the stressors on gastric emptying, again suggesting a role of CRF in mediation of gastrointestinal responses to stress. It is important to note that ip injections of CRF antiserum also blocked the effects of icv CRF on gastric emptying, indicating that immunoneutralization of circulating CRF may effectively eliminate responses to icv CRF as well as to stress. Along this line, Williams *et al.* (1987) found that α-helical CRF-(9–41) given either icv or iv prevented stress-induced stimulation of colonic transit. It is therefore not clear whether brain or peripheral sites of action are responsible for CRF-induced changes in gastrointestinal transit.

Clearly, present evidence implicates CRF in mediation of gastrointestinal responses to stress. Because hypophysectomy and adrenalectomy did not block responses to stress (Williams *et al.*, 1988), the effects of CRF are thought to involve extrapituitary actions. Precise definition of the mechanism of CRF effects will require further experimentation.

V. Other Peptides

In addition to opioids, bombesin/GRP, and CRF, several other peptides have been shown to act in the central nervous system to alter gastrointestinal motility. These include thyrotropin-releasing hormone (TRH), cholecystokinin (CCK), somatostatin, calcitonin, calcitonin gene-related peptide (CGRP), neurotensin, and interleukin-1α (IL-1α). In several cases, the consequences of motility changes on transit have not been established.

A. Thyrotropin-Releasing Hormone

Thyrotropin-releasing hormone is a tripeptide that produces a variety of effects after central administration (Horita *et al.*, 1986). TRH given icv was found in anesthetized rabbits to increase contractions of the small intestine, cecum, and colon (La Hann and Horita, 1982). These effects apparently are mediated by central vagal mechanisms, as they were blocked by atropine, hexamethonium, and bilateral vagotomy. Subsequent studies revealed that icv administered TRH increased transit in the proximal colon of anesthetized rabbits, resulting in diarrhea when given in sufficiently high doses (Horita and Carino, 1982). Interestingly, the effects of TRH on colonic transit and diarrhea were not sensitive to blockade by atropine, but were inhibited by hexamethonium, vagotomy, cyproheptadine, and cinanserin. These results suggest that the stimulation of colonic transit induced by icv TRH is vagally mediated, but results from release of 5-hydroxytryptamine rather than acetylcholine. An opioid link in the TRH centrally directed increase in colonic transit is indicated by the finding that systemic administration of opioid antagonists, naloxone and naltrexone, blocked the transit effect and diarrhea (Horita *et al.*, 1985). These results are anomalous because endogenous opioid peptides, at least in the brain, generally exert antitransit and antidiarrheal effects (Burks and Galligan, 1982; Shook *et al.*, 1987c). However, it is possible that peripheral, naloxone-sensitive opioid mechanisms participate in a presently unrecognized manner in fluid secretion in the colon.

In rats, TRH administered intracisternally (ic) increases contractions of the stomach and increases gastric emptying (Garrick *et al.*, 1987; Maeda-Hagiwara and Taché, 1987). The stimulating effect of centrally administered TRH on the stomach was blocked by vagotomy and partially inhibited by atropine, indicating mediation by vagal mechanisms. The gastric motility effects of ic TRH did not occur when the peptide was given iv.

Data obtained in studies of rabbits and rats therefore suggest that TRH can act in the brain, but not peripherally, to increase motility at all levels of the gastrointestinal tract. The motility changes result in stimulation of gastric emptying and colonic transit (Table VII). The central effects of TRH are vagally mediated, and possible effector mechanisms involve acetylcholine, 5-hydroxytryptamine, and possibly opioids.

Table VII

Effects of Selected Neuropeptides on Gastrointestinal Motility[a]

Peptides	Effect (icv)	Sites
TRH	↑ Contractions, transit	Stomach, small intestine, colon
CCK	↓ MMC frequency	Small intestine
Somatostatin	↑ MMC frequency	Small intestine
Calcitonin	↑ MMC induction	Small intestine
Neurotensin	↑ MMC induction	Small intestine
Substance P	↓ Fed pattern duration	Small intestine
IL-1α	↑ Transit	Small intestine

[a]MMC, migrating motor complex. Data from references in Section V.

B. Cholecystokinin

Given peripherally, CCK increases contractions of the small intestine and gall bladder and increases small intestinal transit in humans (Walsh, 1987). When administered icv in rats, CCK-8 decreased the frequency of migrating motor complexes (MMCs) in fasted rats (Bueno and Ferre, 1982). The effects of centrally administered CCK on intestinal transit have not been evaluated.

C. Somatostatin

The effects of centrally administered somatostatin have been examined in only one study. Bueno and Ferre (1982) found that icv somatostatin in fasted rats increased the frequency of occurrence of MMC cycles in the duodenum and jejunum (Table VII).

D. Calcitonin, Neurotensin, and Substance P

Bueno *et al.* (1983) studied the effects of calcitonin, neurotensin, and substance P on myoelectric activity in fed or fasted rats (Table VII). Both calcitonin and neurotensin restored fasted MMC patterns in the small intestine when administered icv to rats displaying fed patterns of motility. That is, the irregular contractions that occurred after feeding were converted by the peptides to regular MMC cycles. Substance P given icv reduced the duration of the postprandial fed motility pattern, but did not immediately convert it to the fasting MMC pattern.

    The ability of icv calcitonin to induce cyclic MMC activity in fed rats was found to be blocked by indomethacin, indicative of a possible role of prostaglandins in the calcitonin effect (Fargeas *et al.*, 1984). Prostaglandin E_2 administered icv produced motility effects identical to those induced by icv calcitonin. The ability of prostaglandin E_2 to induce MMCs was not blocked by indomethacin.

E. Interleukin-1α

Interleukin-1α was recently discovered to stimulate transit in the small intestine of mice after icv administration (Vander Hamm *et al.*, 1989). The effects of icv IL-1α on transit were not prevented by hypophysectomy, indicating that pituitary effects were not responsible for the stimulation of transit. A pituitary role was examined because of the reported ability of IL-1 to release pituitary hormones (Bernton *et al.*, 1987). The effects of IL-1α on transit are nevertheless of interest because it is one of the few centrally acting peptides found to increase propulsion in the small intestine.

VI. Conclusion

Peptide neuroregulators can act at multiple chemosensitive sites in the mammalian brain, spinal cord, and periphery to modify gastrointestinal motility and transit. The peripheral sites of action often involve receptors in the enteric nervous system. Actions of directly administered peptides in the brain or spinal cord result in altered efferent signals from the central nervous system to the enteric nervous system, either over neural pathways or by means of endocrine influences.

Some peptide families, such as opioids, have been demonstrated to act at multiple types of receptors to bring about their regulatory changes. Each type of receptor, mu, delta, or kappa, is associated with a distinct functional pattern depending on the site of drug administration in the brain, spinal cord, or periphery. Actions of a receptor-selective opioid at multiple sites, a nonselective opioid at a single site, or a nonselective opioid at multiple sites can generate a complex pattern of effects representing the summation of many different individual effects. It is therefore often impossible to generalize the motility effects of a class of peptides to a single statement.

It is also evident that individual parts of the gastrointestinal tract are regulated differently by centrally acting peptides. The stomach, small intestine, cecum, and colon are subject to independent regulatory influences. Specific peptides may increase, decrease, or not change motility and propulsion in each of these organs.

Finally, it must be recognized that motility and transit in the gastrointestinal tract are related in complex ways. Effective transit or propulsion depends on the particular pattern of contractions in each part of the digestive tube. A specific pattern of motility may or may not result in effective propulsion, independently of whether the incidence of contractions is increased or decreased.

All of these factors complicate definition of the possible roles of individual neuropeptides in stress responses. The strongest evidence implicating neuropeptides as mediators in gastrointestinal responses to stress is found with CRF and TRH, but further research will probably expand the list to include other peptides.

Acknowledgments

The author is grateful to Rita Sainz for preparation of this manuscript. Work from the author's laboratory described in this manuscript was supported by U.S. Public Health Service grants DA02163, DK36289, and DK33547.

References

Almy, T. P. (1951). Experimental studies on irritable colon. *Am. J. Med.* **10**, 60–67.

Bernton, E. W., Beach, J. E., Holaday, J. W., Smallridge, R. C., and Fein, H. G. (1987). Release of multiple hormones by a direct action of interleukin-1 on pituitary cells. *Science* **238**, 519–521.

Bertaccini, G., and Impicciatore, M. (1975). Action of bombesin on the motility of the stomach. *Naunyn-Schmiedeberg's Arch. Pharmacol.* **289**, 149–156.

Brown, M., Allen, R., Villarreal, J., Rivier, J., and Vale, W. (1978). Bombesin-like activity: Radioimmunologic assessment in biological tissues. *Life Sci.* **23**, 2721–2728.

Bueno, L., and Ferre, J.-P. (1982). Central regulation of intestinal motility by somatostatin and cholecystokinin octapeptide. *Science* **216**, 1427–1429.

Bueno, L., and Fioramonti, J. (1986). Effects of CRF, corticotropin, and cortisol on gastrointestinal motility in dogs. *Peptides (N.Y.)* **7**, 73–77.

Bueno, L., and Gué, M. (1988). Evidence for the involvement of cotricotropin-releasing factor in the gastrointestinal disturbances induced by acoustic and cold stress in mice. *Brain Res.* **441**, 1–4.

Bueno, L., Ferre, J. P., Fioramonti, J., and Honde, C. (1983). Effects of intracerebroventricular administration of neurotensin, substance P and calcitonin on gastrointestinal motility in normal and vagotomized rats. *Regul. Pept.* **6**, 197–205.

Bueno, L., Fargeas, M. J., Gué, M., Peeters, T. L., Bormans, V., and Fioramonti, J. (1986). Effects of corticotropin-releasing factor on plasma motilin and somatostatin levels and gastrointestinal motility in dogs. *Gastroenterology* **91**, 884–889.

Burks, T. F. (1976). Gastrointestinal pharmacology. *Annu. Rev. Pharmacol. Toxicol.* **16**, 15–31.

Burks, T. F. (1978). Central sites of action of gastrointestinal drugs. *Gastroenterology* **74**, 322–324.

Burks, T. F., and Galligan, J. J. (1982). Central regulation of intestinal transit: Possible role of endogenous opiates. *In* "Motility of the Digestive Tract" (M. Wienbeck, ed.), pp. 73–78. Raven Press, New York.

Burks, T. F., Galligan, J. J., Hirning, L. D., and Porreca, F. (1987). Brain, spinal cord and peripheral sites of action of enkephalins and other endogenous opioids on gastrointestinal motility. *Gastroenterol. Clin. Biol.* **11**, 44B–51B.

Burleigh, D. E., Galligan, J. J., and Burks, T. F. (1981). Subcutaneous morphine reduces intestinal propulsion in rats partly by a central action. *Eur. J. Pharmacol.* **75**, 283–287.

Cannon, W. B. (1902). The movement of the intestines studied by means of the Roentgen rays. *Am. J. Physiol.* **6**, 251–277.

Chang, K.-J., Wei, E. T., Killian, A., and Chang, J.-K. (1983). Potent morphiceptin analogs: Structure activity relationships and morphine-like activities. *J. Pharmacol. Exp. Ther.* **227**, 403–408.

Corbett, A. D., Paterson, S. J., McKnight, A. T., Magnan, J., and Kosterlitz, H. W. (1982). Dynorphin-(1–8) and dynorphin-(1–9) are ligands for the κ-subtype of opiate receptor. *Nature (London)* **299**, 79–81.

Davis, T. P., Porreca, F., Burks, T. F., and Dray, A. (1985). The proenkephalin A fragment, peptide E: Central processing and CNS activity *in vivo*. *Eur. J. Pharmacol.* **111**, 177–184.

Dougall, I. G. (1988). A critical review of the classification of opioid receptors. *Biotechnol. Appl. Biochem.* **10**, 488–499.

Fargeas, M. J., Fioramonti, J., and Bueno, L. (1984). Prostaglandin E_2: A neuromodulator in the central control of gastrointestinal motility and feeding behavior by calcitonin. *Science* 225, 1050–1052.

Fisher, L. A., Rivier, J., Rivier, C., Spiess, J., Vale, W., and Brown, M. R. (1982). Corticotropin-releasing factor (CRF): Central effects on mean arterial pressure and heart rate in rats. *Endocrinology (Baltimore)* 110, 2222–2224.

Galligan, J. J., and Burks, T. F. (1982). Opioid peptides inhibit intestinal transit in the rat by a central mechanism. *Eur. J. Pharmacol.* 85, 61–68.

Galligan, J. J., and Burks, T. F. (1983). Centrally mediated inhibition of small intestinal transit and motility by morphine in the rat. *J. Pharmacol. Exp. Ther.* 226, 356–361.

Galligan, J. J., and Burks, T. F. (1986). Cholinergic neurons mediate intestinal propulsion in the rat. *J. Pharmacol. Exp. Ther.* 238, 594–598.

Galligan, J. J., Mosberg, H. I., Hurst, R., Hruby, V. J., and Burks, T. F. (1984). Cerebral delta opioid receptors mediate analgesia but not the intestinal motility effects of intracerebroventricularly administered opioids. *J. Pharmacol. Exp. Ther.* 229, 641–648.

Garrick, T., Buack, S., Veiseh, A., and Taché, Y. (1987). Thyrotropin-releasing hormone (TRH) acts centrally to stimulate gastric contractility in rats. *Life Sci.* 40, 649–657.

Gmerek, D. E., Cowan, A., and Vaught, J. L. (1983). Intrathecal bombesin in rats: Effects on behavior and gastrointestinal transit. *Eur. J. Pharmacol.* 94, 141–143.

Gmerek, D. E., and Cowan, A. (1984). Pituitary-adrenal mediation of bombesin-induced inhibition of gastrointestinal transit in rats. *Regul. Pept.* 9, 299–304.

Handa, B. K., Lane, A. C., Lord, J. A. H., Morgan, B. A., Rance, M. J., and Smith, C. F. C. (1981). Analogues of beta-LPH$_{61-64}$ possessing selective agonist activity at mu-opiate receptors. *Eur. J. Pharmacol.* 70, 531–540.

Hirning, L. D., Porreca, F., and Burks, T. F. (1985). Mu, but not kappa, opioid agonists induce contractions of the canine small intestine, ex vivo. *Eur. J. Pharmacol.* 109, 49–54.

Höllt, V. (1986). Opioid peptide processing and receptor selectivity. *Annu. Rev. Pharmacol. Toxicol.* 26, 59–77.

Horita, A., and Carino, M. A. (1982). Centrally administered thyrotropin-releasing hormone (TRH) stimulates colonic transit and diarrhea production by a vagally mediated serotonergic mechanism in the rabbit. *J. Pharmacol. Exp. Ther.* 222, 367–371.

Horita, A., Carino, M. A., and Pae, Y.-S. (1985). Blockade by naloxone and naltrexone of the TRH-induced stimulation of colonic transit in the rabbit. *Eur. J. Pharmacol.* 108, 289–293.

Horita, A., Carino, M. A., and Lai, H. (1986). Pharmacology of thyrotropin-releasing hormone. *Annu. Rev. Pharmacol. Toxicol.* 26, 311–322.

Hughes, J. (1975). Isolation of an endogenous compound from the brain with pharmacological properties similar to morphine. *Brain Res.* 88, 295–306.

Hughes, J., Smith, T. W., Kosterlitz, H. W., Fothergill, L. H., Morgan, B. A., and Morris, H. (1975). Identification of two related pentapeptides from the brain with potent opiate agonist activity. *Nature (London)* 255, 577–579.

Konturek, S. J., Bilski, J., Pawlik, W., Thor, P., Czarnobilski, K., Szoke, B., and Schally, A. V. (1985). Gastrointestinal secretory, motor, and circulatory effects of corticotropin-releasing factor (CRF). *Life Sci.* 37, 1231–1240.

Koslo, R. J., Burks, T. F., and Porreca, F. (1986a). Centrally administered bombesin affects gastrointestinal transit and colonic bead expulsion through supraspinal mechanisms. *J. Pharmacol. Exp. Ther.* 238, 62–67.

Koslo, R. J., Gmerek, D. W., Cowan, A., and Porreca, F. (1986b). Intrathecal bombesin-induced inhibition of gastrointestinal transit: Requirement for an intact pituitary adrenal axis. *Regul. Pept.* 14, 237–242.

La Hann, T. R., and Horita, A. (1982). Thyrotropin releasing hormone: Centrally mediated effects on gastrointestinal motor activity. *J. Pharmacol. Exp. Ther.* 222, 66–70.

Lenz, H. J., Burlage, M., Raedler, A., and Greten, H. (1988a). Central nervous system effects of corticotropin-releasing factor on gastrointestinal transit in the rat. *Gastroenterology* **94,** 598–602.

Lenz, H. J., Raedler, A., Greten, H., Vale, W. W., and Rivier, J. E. (1988b). Stress-induced gastrointestinal secretory and motor responses in rats are mediated by endogenous corticotropin-releasing factor. *Gastroenterology* **95,** 1510–1517.

Leslie, F. M. (1987). Methods used for the study of opioid receptors. *Pharmacol. Rev.* **39,** 197–249.

Lewis, R. V., Stern, A. S., Rossier, J., Stein, S., and Undenfriend, S. (1979). Putative enkephalin precursors in bovine adrenal medulla. *Biochem. Biophys. Res. Commun.* **89,** 822–829.

Lord, J. A. H., Waterfield, A. A., Hughes, J., and Kosterlitz, H. W. (1977). Endogenous opioid peptides: Multiple agonists and receptors. *Nature (London)* **267,** 495–499.

Lundgren, O., Svanvik, J., and Jivegåard, L. (1989). Enteric nervous system. I. Physiology and pathophysiology of the intestinal tract. *Dig. Dis. Sci.* **34,** 264–283.

Maeda-Hagiwara, M., and Taché, Y. (1987). Central nervous action of TRH to stimulate gastric emptying in rats. *Regul. Pept.* **17,** 199–207.

Manara, L., Bianchi, G., Ferretti, P., and Tavani, A. (1986). Inhibition of gastrointestinal transit in the rat results primarily from direct drug action on gut opioid sites. *J. Pharmacol. Exp. Ther.* **237,** 945–949.

Martin, W. R., Eades, C. G., Thompson, J. A., Huppler, R. E., and Gilbert, P. E. (1976). The effect of morphine- and nalorphine-like drugs in the non-dependent and morphine-dependent chronic spinal dog. *J. Pharmacol. Exp. Ther.* **197,** 517–523.

Mosberg, H. I., Hurst, R., Hruby, V. J., Gee, K., Yamamura, H. I., Galligan, J. J., and Burks, T. F. (1983). Bis-penicillamine enkephalins possess highly improved specificity toward δ-opioid receptors. *Proc. Natl. Acad. Sci. U.S.A.* **80,** 5871–5874.

Narducci, F., Snape, W. J., Battle, W. M., London, R. L., and Cohen, S. (1985). Increased colonic motility during exposure to a stressful situation. *Dig. Dis. Sci.* **30,** 40–44.

Nieuwenhuyzen-Kruseman, A. C., Linton, E. A., Lowry, P. J., Rees, L. H., and Besser, G. M. (1982). CRF-like immunoreactivity in the human gastrointestinal tract. *Lancet* **2,** 1245–1246.

Parolaro, D. L., Sala, M., and Gori, E. (1977). Effect of intracerebroventricular administration of morphine upon intestinal motility in rat and its antagonism with naloxone. *Eur. J. Pharmacol.* **46,** 329–338.

Petrusz, P., Merchenthaler, I., Maderdrut, J. L., and Heitz, P. U. (1985). Central and peripheral distribution of corticotropin-releasing factor. *Fed. Proc., Fed. Am. Soc. Exp. Biol.* **44,** 229–235.

Porreca, F., and Burks, T. F. (1983a). Centrally administered bombesin affects gastric emptying and small and large bowel transit in the rat. *Gastroenterology* **85,** 313–317.

Porreca, F., and Burks, T. F. (1983b). The spinal cord as a site of opioid effects on gastrointestinal transit in the mouse. *J. Pharmacol. Exp. Ther.* **227,** 22–27.

Porreca, F., Filla, A., and Burks, T. F. (1983a). Spinal cord-mediated opiate effects on gastrointestinal transit in mice. *Eur. J. Pharmacol.* **86,** 135–136.

Porreca, F., Filla, A., and Burks, T. F. (1983b). Studies in vivo with dynorphin-(1-9): Analgesia but not gastrointestinal effects following intrathecal administration to mice. *Eur. J. Pharmacol.* **91,** 291–294.

Porreca, F., Mosberg, H. I., Hurst, R., Hruby, V. J., and Burks, T. F. (1984). Roles of mu, delta and kappa opioid receptors in spinal and supraspinal mediation of gastrointestinal effects and hot-plate analgesia in the mouse. *J. Pharmacol. Exp. Ther.* **230,** 341–348.

Porreca, F., Fulginiti, J. T., and Burks, T. F. (1985). Bombesin stimulates small intestinal motility after intracerebroventricular administration to rats. *Eur. J. Pharmacol.* **114,** 167–173.

Porreca, F., Burks, T. F., and Sheldon, R. J. (1988). Central and peripheral visceral effects of bombesin. *Ann. N.Y. Acad. Sci.* **547**, 194–203.

Pruitt, D. B., Grubb, M. N., Jacquette, D. L., and Burks, T. F. (1974). Intestinal effects of 5-hydroxytryptamine and morphine in guinea pigs, dogs, cats and monkeys. *Eur. J. Pharmacol.* **26**, 298–305.

Rivier, C., Brownstein, M., Spiess, J., Rivier, J., and Vale, W. (1982). In vivo corticotropin-releasing factor-induced secretion of adrenocorticotropin, β-endorphin, and corticosterone. *Endocrinology (Baltimore)* **110**, 272–278.

Rivier, J., Rivier, C., and Vale, W. (1985). Synthetic competitive antagonists of corticotropin-releasing factor-induced ACTH secretion in the rat. *Science* **224**, 889–891.

Scarpignato, C., and Bertaccini, G. (1981). Bombesin delays gastric emptying in the rat. *Digestion* **21**, 104–106.

Scarpignato, C., Micali, B., Vitulo, F., Zimbaro, G., and Bertaccini, G. (1982). Inhibition of gastric emptying by bombesin in man. *Digestion* **23**, 128–131.

Shook, J. E., Pelton, J. T., Wire, W. S., Hirning, L. D., Hruby, V. J., and Burks, T. F. (1987a). Pharmacological evaluation of a cyclic somatostatin analog with antagonist activity at mu-opioid receptors in vitro. *J. Pharmacol. Exp. Ther.* **240**, 772–777.

Shook, J. E., Pelton, J. T., Lemcke, P. K., Porreca, F., Hruby, V. J., and Burks, T. F. (1987b). Mu opioid antagonist properties of a cyclic somatostatin octapeptide in vivo: Identification of mu receptor-related function. *J. Pharmacol. Exp. Ther.* **242**, 1–7.

Shook, J. E., Pelton, J. T., Hruby, V. J., and Burks, T. F. (1987c). Peptide opioid antagonist separates peripheral and cental opioid antitransit effects. *J. Pharmacol. Exp. Ther.* **243**, 392–500.

Shook, J. E., Kazmierski, W., Wire, W. S., Lemcke, P. K., Hruby, V. J., and Burks, T. F. (1988). Opioid receptor selectivity of B-endorphin in vitro and in vivo: Mu, delta and epsilon receptors. *J. Pharmacol. Exp. Ther.* **246**, 1018–1025.

Sirinathsinghji, D. J. S., Rees, L. H., Rivier, J., and Vale, W. (1983). CRF is a potent inhibitor of sexual activity in the female rat. *Nature (London)* **305**, 230–235.

Smith, J. R., La Hann, T. R., Chesnut, R. M., Carino, M. A., and Horita, A. (1977). Thyrotropin-releasing hormone: Stimulation of colonic activity following intracerebroventricular administration. *Science* **196**, 660–661.

Solcia, E., Capella, C., Buffa, R., Usellini, L., Fiocca, R., and Sessa, F. (1987). Endocrine cells of the digestive system. *In* "Physiology of the Digestive Tract" (L. R. Johnson, ed.), 2nd ed., pp. 111–130. Raven Press, New York.

Stewart, J. J., Weisbrodt, N. W., and Burks, T. F. (1977). Centrally mediated intestinal stimulation by morphine. *J. Pharmacol. Exp. Ther.* **202**, 174–181.

Stewart, J. J., Weisbrodt, N. W., and Burks, T. F. (1978). Central and peripheral actions of morphine on intestinal transit. *J. Pharmacol. Exp. Ther.* **205**, 547–555.

Swanson, L. W., Sawchenko, P. E., Rivier, J., and Vale, W. W. (1983). Organization of ovine CRF immunoreactive cells and fibers in the rat brain: An immunohistochemical study. *Neuroendocrinology* **136**, 165–186.

Szurszewski, J. H. (1987). Electrical basis for gastrointestinal motility. *In* "Physiology of the Digestive Tract" (L. R. Johnson, ed.), 2nd ed., pp. 383–422. Raven Press, New York.

Taché, Y., Goto, Y., Gunion, M. W., Vale, W., Rivier, J., and Brown, M. (1983). Inhibition of gastric acid secretion in rats by intraventricular injection of CRF. *Science* **222**, 935–937.

Tavani, A., Bianchi, G., and Manara, L. (1979). Morphine no longer blocks gastrointestinal transit but retains antinociceptive action in diallylnormorphine-pretreated rats. *Eur. J. Pharmacol.* **59**, 151–154.

Vale, W., Spiess, J., Rivier, C., and Rivier, J. (1981). Characterization of a 41-residue ovine hypothalamic factor that stimulates secretion of corticotropin and β-endorphin. *Science* **213**, 1394–1397.

Valori, R. M., Kumar, D., and Wingate, D. L. (1986). Effects of different types of stress and of "prokinetic" drugs on the control of the fasting motor complex in humans. *Gastroenterology* **90**, 1890–1900.

Vander Hamm, D. G., Ayers, E. A., Lemcke, P. K., and Burks, T. F. (1989). Interleukin-1 stimulates small intestinal transit by factors other than the hypothalamic pituitary axis. *Pharmacologist* **31**, 168.

von Voigtlander, P. F., Lahti, R. A., and Ludens, J. H. (1983). U-50, 488H: A selective and structurally novel non-mu (kappa) opioid agonist. *J. Pharmacol. Exp. Ther.* **224**, 7–12.

Walsh, J. H. (1987). Gastrointestinal hormones. *In* "Physiology of the Gastrointestinal Tract" (L. R. Johnson, ed.), 2nd ed., pp. 181–253. Raven Press, New York.

Williams, C. L., and Burks, T. F. (1989). Stress, opioids, and gastrointestinal transit. *In* "Neuropeptides and Stress" (Y. Taché, J. E. Morley, and M. R. Brown, eds.), pp. 175–187. Springer-Verlag, Berlin and New York.

Williams, C. L., Peterson, J. M., Villar, R. G., and Burks, T. F. (1987). Corticotropin-releasing factor directly mediates colonic responses to stress. *Am. J. Physiol.* **253**, G582-G586.

Williams, C. L., Villar, R. G., Peterson, J. M., and Burks, T. F. (1988). Stress-induced changes in intestinal transit in the rat: A model for irritable bowel syndrome. *Gastroenterology* **94**, 611–621.

Wingate, D. L., and Kumar, D. (1988). Stress and gastrointestinal motility. *In* "An Illustrated Guide to Gastrointestinal Motility" (D. Kumar and S. Gustavsson, eds.), pp. 255–264. Wiley, Chichester.

Wuster, M., Schulz, R., and Herz, A. (1979). Specificity of opioids towards the μ-, δ- and ε-opiate receptors. *Neurosci. Lett.* **15**, 193–198.

Yoshimura, K., Huidobro-Toro, J. P., Lee, N. M., Loh, H. H., and Way, E. L. (1982). Kappa opioid properties of dynorphin and its peptide fragments on the guinea pig ileum. *J. Pharmacol. Exp. Ther.* **222**, 71–79.

16

Stress, Peptides, and Regulation of Ingestive Behavior

Allen S. Levine
Neuroendocrine Research Laboratory
Veterans Administration Medical Center
Minneapolis, Minnesota 55417
and Departments of Food Science and
Nutrition, Medicine, Psychiatry, and
Surgery
University of Minnesota
Minneapolis/St. Paul, Minnesota 55455

Charles J. Billington
Neuroendocrine Research Laboratory
Veterans Administration Medical Center
Minneapolis, Minnesota 55417
and Department of Medicine
University of Minnesota
Minneapolis, Minnesota 55455

I. Introduction

The concept of stress is both powerful and nonspecific. The stress concept has informed and framed a rich field of scientific investigation. At the same time, stress remains a generalized neural and physiological response to any unpleasant stimulus. In this review we have narrowed the field to consideration of the effects of stress on one activity, eating. The impact of stress even on this single behavior is variable; stress can be shown to increase and decrease eating. In an attempt to grapple with the mechanistic basis for these stress effects, we first review developing information about alterations in feeding behavior produced by administration of various stress-related neurotransmitters to sites within the brain. We then review what is known about stress effects on the overall behavior of feeding.

II. Corticotropin-Releasing Factor and Consummatory Behaviors

Every since Hans Selye (1979) discussed a mythical factor that releases cortisol from the adrenal during stressful events, individuals have searched for such a substance. Early in this decade such a factor was identified, isolated, and found to contain 41 amino acids (Spiess *et al.*, 1981; Vale *et al.*, 1981). This peptide, corticotropin-releasing factor (CRF), is released following stress and stimulates the secretion of adrenocorticotropin (ACTH) as well as other peptides processed from pro-opiomelanocortin (POMC) (Brown *et al.*, 1982). CRF alters endocrine, gastrointestinal, cardiovascular, and immune function (Lenz, 1987). It also alters locomotion (Britton *et al.*, 1982), sexual activity (Sirinathsinghji *et al.*, 1983), feeding (Britton *et al.*, 1982; Morley and Levine, 1982), grooming (Morley and Levine, 1982), and other behaviors. Following intracerebroventricular (icv) injection of CRF rats groom more, move and rear less in the open field, and move about more when in a familiar environment (Britton *et al.*, 1982; Morley and Levine, 1982; Suton *et al.*, 1983). Such behaviors resemble those seen following exposure to "stressors." Centrally administered CRF decreases food intake in spontaneously-feeding, starved, muscimol-, norepinephrine-, dynorphin-, or insulin-treated rats (Levine *et al.*, 1983). This action of CRF is independent of the pituitary and adrenals, indicating that CRF does not decrease eating due to release of ACTH and cortisol, which are usually thought to participate in the stress response (Gosnell *et al.*, 1983; Morley and Levine, 1982). We injected CRF into five regions of the brain—the striatum, globus pallidus, ventromedial hypothalamus, lateral hypothalamus, and paraventricular hypothalamic nucleus (PVN)—and measured food intake following 24 h of food deprivation (Krahn *et al.*, 1988). After injection of CRF into the PVN, deprived rats ingested about 63% less food than the control rats. However, CRF had no effects on feeding following injection into the other four brain regions. This is somewhat puzzling since CRF not only is found in the PVN but also is found in the other four brain regions we studied. In addition to the effects on feeding, PVN administration of CRF resulted in increased grooming and increased locomotion. These events were independent of the length of food deprivation, suggesting that CRF does not alter grooming simply as part of the normal satiety sequence.

Brown *et al.* (1982) demonstrated that a somatostatin agonist was capable of decreasing the rise in plasma epinephrine and glucose due to CRF administration. Shibasaki *et al.* (1988) recently reported that somatostatin pretreatment can also reverse the suppression of food intake induced by intraventricular administration of CRF. At doses of 0.11 nmol and 0.21 nmol CRF (0.5 and 1.0 µg) CRF decreased deprivation-induced food intake by 33.3 and 14.1% of control. Intraventricular administration of somatostatin 14 or 28 partially attenuated the effect of CRF on feeding. Somatostatin 14 had no effect on feeding when administered by itself; however, somatostatin 28 decreased feeding slightly. Shibasaki *et al.* (1988) suggest that CRF may have some importance in anorexia nervosa, since these patients have elevated concentrations of CRF but decreased concentrations of somatostatin in the CSF.

In a series of studies using an antagonist of CRF, Krahn *et al.* (1986) demonstrated that CRF may be involved in stress related decreases in feeding. First they demonstrated that the CRF antagonist alpha-helical CRF-(9–41) decreased the CRF-induced suppression of feeding in deprived rats. Next it was reported that food deprived rats which were placed into restraint cages for one hour ate less food when returned to their home cage. However, if these rats were pretreated with alpha-helical CRF-(9–41), restraint did not result in decreased food intake. The CRF antagonist failed to alter feeding in nonrestrained animals at a variety of doses. Such data suggest that CRF plays an important role in stress-induced decreases in consummatory behaviors.

Further evidence that CRF may play an endogenous role in stress responses is demonstrated by the study of Lenz *et al.* (1988). Gastrointestinal secretion, a response related to feeding, also can be affected by administration of CRF. Both CRF administration and partial body restraint decrease gastric acid secretion, gastric emptying, and small bowel transit time while increasing large bowel transit time (see Lenz *et al.*, 1988). Lenz *et al.* (1988) found that pretreatment of animals with alpha-helical CRF-(9–41) reversed all of the gastrointestinal responses due to CRF and partial body restraint.

III. Opioid-Induced Changes in Eating Behavior

Opioids are thought to be important mediators of the stress response. Blockade of the opioid receptor decreases the release of various stress hormones, such as prolactin and growth hormone (Morley, 1983). Also, following stressful events levels of β-endorphin increase as a result of CRF-induced release of POMC (Akil *et al.*, 1984). Administration of β-endorphin decreases ACTH and cortisol levels in humans (Taylor *et al.*, 1983). Associated with the increased opioid activity that occurs during stress in animals and humans is an elevation of the pain threshold (Cohen *et al.*, 1982).

Pinching the tail of a rat results in eating behavior that is not observed when the rat's tail is not being pinched. This so-called stress-induced eating appears to be regulated by a variety of neuroregulatory substances. We suggested that opioid peptides represent one group of regulators of such stress-induced feeding (Morley and Levine, 1980). Naloxone decreased food intake observed during a tail-pinch session, and chronic tail pinching resulted in withdrawal symptoms that resembled withdrawal from exogenous opioids. Like morphine, tail pinching suppressed "wet-dog" shakes in rats (Ornstein, 1981). Naloxone's effect on tail pinch-induced feeding also occurs in mice and even slugs (Kavaliers and Hirst, 1986). Levels of dynorphin were altered following tail pinching for 10 min (Morley et al., 1982). Tail pinching might also alter pain threshold by altering opioid levels. Antelman and Caggiula (1977) found that tail pinching induced indifference to pin pricks. Also, tail-pinch-induced consummatory behaviors were blocked by injection of xylocaine into the tail of rat (Levine and Morley, 1982). Diabetic animals that are less sensitive to pain as measured by tail-flick latency demonstrate prolonged latency to the induction of tail-pinch behavior (Levine et al., 1982). Such an interaction between pain, feeding, and stress may be of importance in protecting an animal from pain during the hunt for food.

There is a large body of literature related to the effect of opioids on feeding (Baile et al., 1986; Cooper et al., 1988; Levine et al., 1985; Reid, 1985). In general, opioid peptides, when injected centrally, increase food intake for about 4 h after injection. Administration of opioid antagonists tends to decrease short-term food intake induced by a variety of means. Long-term administration of opiates, such as morphine, has been shown to decrease food intake and body weight in rats when given centrally or peripherally. Based on such data, it appears that opioids could be involved in stress-related decreases or increases in feeding. Patients with anorexia nervosa have increased opioid concentrations in their cerebrospinal fluid (Kaye et al., 1982). Elevated levels of opioids in the CSF could potentially alter not only food consumption, but might also change metabolic rate (Mandenoff et al., 1982). The increased levels of CRF found in anorectic patients should result in an increase in β-endorphin levels, since this opioid peptide is derived from POMC, which is released following peaks of CRF activity. Although central administration of β-endorphin and other opioid peptides increases feeding (Levine et al., 1985), peripheral administration of β-endorphin results in a decrease in food intake in rats (Morley and Levine, 1982).

The "stress" of exercise has also been associated with changes in feeding behavior as well as changes in opioid levels. Running, bicycling, and swimming have been shown to alter blood and tissue levels of opioids (Farrell et al., 1982; Langenfeld et al., 1985; Pyle et al., 1986; Wardlow and Frantz, 1980). Addiction to endogenous opioid has been reported, and neurospeculation has led to the idea that the runners' high is associated with autoaddiction to opioids. Several reports have suggested that running leads to a decrease in feeding (Harri and Kuusela, 1986; Mayer et al., 1954; Thomas and Miller, 1958). Unfortunately this effect is generally quantitated hours to days after the exercise. Vaswani and colleagues (1988) have reported that acute swim stress results in elevated feeding that is naloxone reversible. Also, these rats chose high-fat diets, a diet known to be preferred by rats injected with opioids. Fishman and Carr (1983) found that naloxone inhibited exercise-stimulated drinking; however, this effect was not specific to exercised rats. In preliminary experiments we found that cold-water swim stress actually decreased feeding (Waggoner et al., 1985). More recently Vaswani et al. (1988) found that cold-swim stress caused a 42% decrease in pituitary β-endorphin, but increased the level of this peptide in the hypothalamus by 36% and in the plasma by 337%. Dynorphin levels decreased by 62% in the hypothalamus, but did not change in the pituitary. Enkephalin levels decreased in the adrenal gland, but were not altered in the brain. Thus the literature is not clear as to the role of opioids in exercise-related changes in feeding behavior.

IV. Other Regulators of Stress-Induced Eating

The monoamine serotonin is another neuroregulator that participates in both the regulation of food intake and stress. Stressed animals display altered serotonin levels in the central nervous system (CNS), in particular, increased levels with chronic stress (Donohoe, 1984; Campbell et al., 1981). Manipulations that destroy serotonin receptors increase feeding, whereas stimulation of serotonin receptors or enhancing synaptic levels of serotonin decreases feeding (Blundell, 1977). It has been suggested that serotonin or its precursor tryptophan decreases carbohydrate ingestion, a pattern observed in patients with anorexia nervosa (Wurtman, 1982). The serotonin antagonist cyproheptadine has been demonstrated to increase food intake in such patients (Halmi et al., 1983). Perhaps serotonin may be important in protecting the organism against some of the effects of stress. A diet that is deficient in tryptophan, which lowers the serum tryptophan levels and presumably then decreases serotonin levels in the brain, results in an exacerbation of gastric ulcers in rats that were immobilized (Natelson et al., 1981).

Aside from opioids, other factors seem to be involved in the tail-pinch model of stress-induced eating. Tail-pinch induced eating is blocked by bilateral injections of 6-hydroxydopamine in the substantia nigra or by administration of dopamine antagonists (Marshall et al., 1974). This type of stress-induced eating is also blocked by injection of serotonin agonists and by a variety of neuropeptides, such as cholecystokinin, bombesin, thyrotropin-releasing hormone, calcitonin, somatostatin, and substance P (Antelman *et al.*, 1979; Blundell, 1977; Campbell *et al.*, 1981; Donohoe, 1984; Halmi *et al.*, 1983; Marshall *et al.*, 1974; Morley *et al.*, 1983; Natelson *et al.*, 1981; Rowland *et al.*, 1982; Vaswani *et al.*, 1988; Wurtman, 1982). We should emphasize, however, that many of these substances also decrease feeding induced by other means than tail pinch, indicating that they are not specific regulators of stress-induced eating.

β-Phenylethylamine, an analog of amphetamine that is found in the blood, brain, urine, and various tissues such as the adrenal medulla, stimulates motor activity in rats and mice, reinforces self-administration of drugs, and releases catecholamines into the central nervous system (Snoddy *et al.*, 1985). This amphetamine-like compound also decreases food intake in rats and has been implicated as an important regulator of appetite control. Of interest is the fact that the cardiovascular, neurochemical, and behavioral changes observed upon exposure to environmental stressors are similar to those observed after administration of amphetamines. Following stressful situations, normal humans have marked increases in the urinary excretion of β-phenylethylamine (Paulos and Tessel, 1982). Snoddy *et al.* (1985) reported that cold restraint in the rat produces an elevation of endogenous β-phenylethylamine excreted in the urine. Such a change could not be attributed to altered urinary pH, glomerular filtration rate, or food consumption. Thus, this amphetamine-like compound could play a role in stress-induced decreases in food intake.

The benzodiazepines represent a group of drugs that are used to treat a variety of stress-related ailments including anxiety and muscle tension. One of the earliest benzodiazepines to be used was chlordiazepoxide, a drug that was reported to increase food intake in animals, ranging from laboratory rats to baboons (Randall *et al.*, 1960). Several investigators have attributed such feeding to the anxiolytic properties of these drugs. For example, there are anecdotal tales of diazepam stimulating feeding in captive animals that generally refuse to eat new foods when brought into captivity. T. Kreeger *et al.* (unpublished observation) recently found that diazepam will also stimulate food intake in captive wolves that have adapted to dog food and a kennel environment. This supports the view of others that indicate that the benzodiazepines stimulate feeding in a manner that appears to be unrelated to the anxiolytic properties of these drugs. Cooper (1990) has suggested that the role of benzodiazepines in food intake can be separated from their role as anxiolytics. For example, zolpidem binds with high affinity to the benzodiazepine receptor and acts as an anxiolytic agent, resulting in sedative and hypnotic effects (Yerbury and Cooper, 1990). However, it fails to increase consumption of a palatable food in rats. Another exmple is that of the pyrazoloquinolines, drugs that resemble diazepam but in fact act as antagonists of benzodiazepine-induced hyperphagia (Cooper and Yerbury, 1986). The roles that these drugs play in stress effects on food intake are not clear, since an endogenous ligand and an antagonist of this ligand have not been identified unequivocally.

V. Effect of Stress on Consummatory Behavior in Humans

Stressful events in life are known to alter ingestive behaviors and associated physiological events such as gastric acid secretion and gastrointestinal motility. Tense family situations that result in child abuse, parental neglect, and family separation have been reported to result in pica, a compulsive ingestion of nonfood substances including clay, soil, grass, leaves, paint chips, and paper (Sayetta, 1986; Singhi and Singhi, 1983). Reports of incidences of poisoning are more common in children exposed to stress (Bithoney *et al.*, 1985). Disorders of feeding behavior are also linked with stressful situations. Women in prisons often gain weight due to hyperphagia (Shaw *et al.*, 1985). In one study, 30 of 34 patients linked a traumatic life event with the onset of bulimia (Pyle *et al.*, 1981). Women that binged followed by vomiting reported problems in interpersonal relationships (56%), social interactions (54%), work/school activities (52%), family relationships (37%), recreation activities (33%), and financial status (24%) (Pyle *et al.*, 1986). Binge eating rarely resulted in a feeling of relaxation in these women (6/34). Abnormalities in chewing behavior also occur during or following stress. Anxious, stressed children are reported to more frequently grind their teeth (Lefer, 1971). The compulsive biting of the tongue, lips, and fingers which occurs in children with Lesch–Nyan syndrome is exacerbated during periods of stress (Seegmiller, 1980).

Everyone seems to have encountered individuals who either eat less or more during a stressful life event. Willenbring *et al.* (1986) attempted to quantify this observation in 80 subjects through a series of questions. The results showed that 48% ate less, 44% ate more, and 8% did not change their food consumption when stressed. Stressed eaters said they preferred crunchy foods with a low water content that were calorically dense. Forty-six percent preferred sweet foods, 29% salty foods, and the remainder did not demonstrate a preference. Forty-six percent stated that boredom resulted in an increase of food. The stress eaters who answered these questions were not stressed nor overweight at the time they filled out the questionnaire. Leon and Chamberlain (1973) found that subjects that lost weight and regained their weight ate due to "feelings of emotional arousal." Those that lost weight and maintained their weight loss ate due to boredom. Normal weight subjects seemed to eat only when they were hungry.

Obese subjects often complain that they gain weight due to stress-induced hyperphagia. For example, obese girls complained of stress-induced eating during periods of examinations at school. The "night eating syndrome" was characterized by Stunkard *et al.* (1955) in the 1950s. These people were found to eat more than 25% of their total calories after supper. They slept poorly and felt guilty at breakfast, choosing not to eat much food at this meal. Life stress seemed to exacerbate this condition. One patient spent some time at the hospital due to phlebitis. Even though she was ill, the hospital setting seemed tranquil and she stopped eating late at night, slept well, and ate a normal breakfast.

Various studies evaluating the effects of stress in the obese patient have been conducted. For example, lean executives placed in high-stress environments lose weight, whereas body weight does not correlate with stress level in obese executives (Beller, 1977). One of the difficulties with studies of this sort is how to define stress. Types of stress have ranged from unpredicted mild shock to false heart-rate monitoring causing anxiety in the subject. Schachter *et al.* (1968) found that electric shock reduced the number of crackers eaten in sated subjects, whereas in the obese, electric shock failed to alter intake. Obese subjects also failed to alter eating after being told that they would have social problems and that they would not have successful marriages (Abramson and Wunderlick, 1972). In a cleverly designed study, Slochower (1976) created anxiety by allowing individuals to listen to what they assumed was their own heart rate, although what they heard was a recording of a rapid (88 beats/min) or normal heart rate (70 beats/min). One group, the labeled subjects, were told that rapid heart rate was due to the acoustics in the room, whereas the unlabeled subjects were given no specific details about the cause of the heart rate. After listening to "their" heart rate they were told to complete a 3-min thinking task, during which time a tin of cashew nuts was placed on the table. Normal subjects ingested only a few nuts during the high-stress state, whereas the obese subjects ingested markedly more cashews during this period. In a second experiment Slochower and Kaplan (1980) used the same paradigm but added a group whose members were told that they could control their heart rate by breathing slowly. This knowledge decreased the intake of nuts in the obese group; however, it did not alter food intake in the normal subjects. Eating in the nonobese subjects was positively correlated with hunger and negatively correlated with degree of anxiety. Obese subjects also increase food intake during exposure to noise, flickering lights, or insoluble puzzles. Intense illumination of a food also increased feeding in the obese (Ross, 1974).

VI. Stress-Induced Consummatory Behavors in Animals

Studies in wild and laboratory animals have helped define the role of stress in feeding and have led to investigations concerning regulators of feeding behavior. When an animal is exposed to danger it often begins to groom and preen itself—events defined as displacement-type behavior. Male jungle birds peck at the ground during fights, a behavior more characteristic of the winners than the losers (Kruijt, 1964). Between bouts of aggression, cichlids (a type of fish) bite at the substratum, throwing the rocks and sand about (Immelman, 1980). Electroshock treatment of sticklebacks leads to a frantic feeding behavior resembling starvation-induced eating (Tugendhat, 1960).

Laboratory animals also display consummatory behaviors when exposed to stress ranging from noise to pain. Rats, rabbits, and guinea pigs will search for food, chew, and ultimately eat due to loud sounds, such as rapid water jets or a buzzer sounding (Drew, 1937; Kupferman, 1964). Isolation, confinement, and electroshock treatment enhance oral behaviors in laboratory animals (Denton and Nelson, 1980; Morgan, 1973; Morley et al., 1986). For example, immobilization of mice for 15 min resulted in an increase in drinking of a salt solution, but not water (Kuta et al., 1984). Rats that were immobilized or isolated for 14 days in an unpredictable manner ingested alcohol in preference to saccharin solutions, an unusual finding in the nonstress animal (Nash and Maickel, 1985). Tail pinching in cats, rats, mice, Limax maximus (a giant slug), and Aplysia sp. (a mollusk) leads to increased consummatory behaviors (Kavaliers and Hirst, 1986; Kupferman and Weiss, 1981; Sprague et al., 1963). Attack of a smaller mouse by a larger mouse leads to increased eating in the smaller creature after the defeat. Certain types of stress, such as restraint or cold-water swimming, can decrease feeding in the rat (Krahn et al., 1986; Waggoner et al., 1986). Thus, as is true in humans, rats may respond to stress by either eating more or less.

VII. Conclusion

Despite many years of diligent work by many scientists, we still cannot formulate an overall explanation of stress effects on feeding behavior. The complexity of the physiologic response of stress is certainly one barrier to understanding, as is the apparent individual variability of the response. It may be also that the wide variety of "stressors" and experimental designs employed have not been conducive to understanding. In future, it may be necessary to categorize the type of stress as well as the observed response, as in this case of feeding, during intensive study.

Acknowledgments

This work was supported by the Veterans Administration Medical Center.

References

Abramson, E. E., and Wunderlick, R. A. (1972). Anxiety, fear and eating: A test of the psycho-somatic concept of obesity. *J. Abnorm. Psychol.* **79**, 317–321.

Akil, H., Watson, S. J., Young, E., *et al.* (1984). Endogenous opioids: Biology and function. *Annu. Rev. Neurosci.* **7**, 223–225.

Antelman, S. M., and Caggiula, A. R. (1977). Tails of stress-related behavior: A neuropharma-cological model. *In* "Animal Models in Psychiatry and Neurology" (I. Hanin and E. Usdin, eds.), p. 277. Pergamon, New York.

Antelman, S. M., Caggiula, A. R., Eichler, A. J., *et al.* (1979). The importance of stress in assessing the effects of anorectic drugs. *Curr. Med. Res. Opin.* **6**, 73–82.

Baile, C. A., McLaughlin, C. L., and Della-Fera, M. A. (1986). Role of cholecystokinin and opioid peptides in control of food intake. *Physiol. Rev.* **66**, 172–234.

Beller, A. S. (1977). "Fat and Thin: A Natural History of Obesity." McGraw-Hill, New York.

Bithoney, W. G., Snyder, J., Michalek, J., *et al.* (1985). Childhood ingestions as symptoms of family distress. *Am. J. Dis. Child.* **139**, 456–459.

Blundell, J. E. (1977). Hyperphagia and obesity following serotonin depletion by intraventricu-lar *p*-chlorophenylalanine. *Int. J. Obes.* **1**, 15–42.

Britton, D R., Koob, G. F., Rivier, J., and Vale, W. (1982). Intraventricular corticotropin-releasing factor enhances behavioral effects of novelty. *Life Sci.* **31**, 363–367.

Brown, M. R., Fisher, L. A., Rivier, J., *et al.* (1982). Corticotropin-releasing factor: Effects on the sympathetic nervous system and oxygen consumption. *Life Sci.* **30**, 207–210.

Campbell, I., Cohen, R. M., Murphy, D. L., *et al.* (1981). *In* "Metabolic Disorders of the Nervous System" (F. C. Rose, ed.), pp. 446–460. Pitman, London.

Cohen, M. R., Pickar, D., Dubois, M., *et al.* (1982). Stress-induced plasma beta-endorphin immunoreactivity may predict postoperative morphine usage. *Psychiatry Res.* **6**, 7–12.

Cooper, S. A., Jackson, A., Kirkham, T. C., and Turkish, S. (1988). Endorphins, opiates and food intake. *In* "Endorphin, Opiates and Behavioral Processes" (R. J. Rodgers and S. J. Cooper, eds.), pp. 143–186. Wiley, New York.

Cooper, S. J. (1990). Benzodiazepine receptor-mediated enhancement and inhibition of taste reactivity, food choice and intake. *Ann. N.Y. Acad. Sci.* **575**, 321–337.

Cooper, S. J., and Yerbury, R. E. (1986). Benzodiazepine-induced hyperphagia: Stereospecific-ity and antagonism by pyrazoloquinolines, CGS 9895 and CGS 9896. *Psychopharma-cology (Berlin)* **89**, 462–466.

Denton, D. A., and Nelson, J. F. (1980). The influence of reproductive processes on salt appe-tite. *In* "Biological and Behavioral Aspects of Salt Intake" (M. R. Kare, M.D. Fregley, and R. A. Bernard, eds.), pp. 229–246. Academic Press, New York.

Donohoe, T. P. (1984). Stress-induced anorexia: Implications for anorexia nervosa. *Life Sci.* **34**, 203–218.

Drew, G. C. (1937). Recurrence of eating in rats after apparent satiation. *Proc. Zool. Soc. London* **107**, 95–106.

Farrell, P. A., Gates, W. K., Maksud, M. G., and Morgan, W. P. (1982). Increases in plasma beta-endorphin/beta-lipotropin immunoreactivity after treadmill running in humans. *J. Appl. Physiol.* **52**, 1245–1249.

Fishman, S. M., and Carr, D. B. (1983). Naloxone blocks exercise-stimulated water intake in the rat. *Life Sci.* **32** 2523–2527.

Gosnell, B. A., Morley, J. E., and Levine, A. S. (1983). Adrenal modulation of the inhibitory effect of corticotropin-releasing factor on feeding. *Peptides (N.Y.)* **4**, 807–812.

Halmi, K. A., Eckert, E. D., and Falk, J. R. (1983). Cyproheptadine: An antidepressant and weight-inducing drug for anorexia nervosa. *Psychopharmacol. Bull.* **19**, 103–105.

Harri, M., and Kuusela, P. (1986). Is swimming exercise or cold exposure for rats? *Acta Physiol. Scand.* **126**, 189–197.

Immelman, K. (1980). "Introduction to Ethology." Plenum, New York.

Kavaliers, M., and Hirst, M. (1986). Naloxone-reversible stress-induced feeding and analgesia in the slug limax maximus. *Life Sci.* **38**, 203–209.

Kaye, W. H., Pickar, D., Naber, D., *et al.* (1982). Cerebrospinal fluid opioid activity in anorexia nervosa. *Am. J. Psychiatry* **139**, 643–645.

Krahn, D. D., Gosnell, B. A., Grace, M., *et al.* (1986). CRF antagonist partially reverses CRF- and stress-induced effects on feeding. *Brain Res. Bull.* **17**, 285–289.

Krahn, D. D., Gosnell, B. A., Levine, A. S., and Morley, J. E. (1988). Behavioral effects of corticotropin-releasing factor: Localization and characterization of central effects. *Brain Res.* **443**, 63–69.

Kruijt, J. P. (1964). Ontogeny of social behaviour in Burmese Red jungle fowl *(Gallus gallus spadiceus)* Bonnaterre. *Behaviour, Suppl.* **12**, 1–201.

Kupferman, I. (1964). Eating behavior induced by sounds. *Nature London* **201**, 324.

Kupferman, I., and Weiss, K. R. (1981). Tail pinch and handling facilitate feeding behavior in *Aplysia. Behav. Neural Biol.* **32**, 126–132.

Kuta, C. C., Bryant, H. U., Zabik, J. E., *et al.* (1984). Stress, endogenous opioids and salt intake. *Appetite* **5**, 53–60.

Langenfeld, M. E., Hart, L. S., and Cao, P. C. (1985). Effects of plasma beta-endorphin of one hour bicycling and running exercise at 60% VO2MAX. *Med. Sci. Sports Exercise* **17**, 235.

Lefer, L. (1971). Psychic stress and the oral cavity. *Postgrad. Med.* **49**, 171–175.

Lenz, H. J. (1987). Extrapituitary effects of corticotropin-releasing factor. *Horm. Metab. Res.* **16**, 17–23.

Lenz, H. J., Raedler, A., Greten, H., Vale, W. W., and Rivier, J. E. (1988). Stress-induced gastrointestinal secretory and motor responses in rats are mediated by endogenous corticotropin-releasing factor. *Gastroenterology* **95**, 1510–1517.

Leon, G. R., and Chamberlain, K. (1973). Emotional arousal, eating patterns, and body image as differential factors associated with varying success in maintaining a weight loss. *J. Consult. Clin. Psychol.* **40**, 474–477.

Levine, A. S., and Morley, J. E. (1982). Gnawing is the preferred consummatory behavior initially induced by tail pinch. *Appetite* **3**, 135–138.

Levine, A. S., Morley, J. E., Wilcox, G., *et al.* (1982). Tail pinch behavior and analgesia in diabetic mice. *Physiol. Behav.* **28**, 39–43.

Levine, A. S., Rogers, B., Kneip, J., *et al.* (1983). Effect of centrally administered corticotropin-releasing factor (CRF) on multiple feeding paradigms. *Neuropharmacology* **22**, 337–339.

Levine, A. S., Morley, J. E., Gosnell, B. A., Billington, C. J., and Bartness, T. J. (1985). Opioids and consummatory behavior. *Brain Res. Bull.* **14**, 663–672.

Mandenoff, A., Fumeson, F., Apfelbaum, M., *et al.* (1982). Endogenous opiates and energy balance. *Science* **215**, 1536–1538.

Marshall, J. F., Richardson, J. S., and Teitelbaum, P. (1974). Nigrostriatal bundle damage and the lateral hypothalamic syndrome. *J. Comp. Physiol. Psychol.* **87**, 808–830.

Mayer, J., Marshall, N. B., Vitale, J. J., Christensen, J. H., Mashayekhi, M. B., and Stare, F. J. (1954). Exercise, food intake and body weight in normal rats and genetically obese adult mice. *Am. J. Physiol.* 177, 544–548.

Morgan, M. J. (1973). Effects of post-weaning environment on learning in the rat. *Anim, Behav.* 21, 429–442.

Morley, J. E. (1983). Neuroendocrine effects of endogenous opioid peptides in human subjects: A review. *Psychoneuroendocrinology* 8, 361–379.

Morley, J. E., and Levine, A. S. (1980). Stress-induced eating is mediated through endogenous opiates. *Science* 209, 1259–1261.

Morley, J. E., and Levine, A. S. (1982). Corticotropin-releasing factor, grooming and ingestive behavior. *Life Sci.* 31, 1459–1467.

Morley, J. E., Elson, M. K., Levine, A. S., *et al.* (1982). The effects of stress on central nervous system concentrations of the opioid peptide, dynorphin. *Peptides (N.Y.)* 3, 901–906.

Morley, J. E., Levine, A. S., and Rowland, N. E. (1983). Minireview: Stress induced eating. *Life Sci.* 32, 2169–2182.

Morley, J. E., Levine, A. S., and Willenbring, M. L. (1986). Stress-induced feeding disorders. *In* "Pharmacology of Eating Disorders: Theoretical and Clinical Developments" (M. O. Carruba and J. E. Blundell, eds.), pp. 71–99. Raven Press, New York.

Nash, J. F., Jr., and Maickel, R. P. (1985). Stress-induced consumption of ethanol by rats. *Life Sci.* 37, 757–765.

Natelson, B. H., Janocko, L., and Jacoby, J. H. (1981). An interaction between dietary tryptophan and stress in exacerbating gastric disease. *Physiol. Behav.* 26, 197–200.

Ornstein, K. (1981). Suppression of wet-dog shakes by tail and scruff-pinch. *Physiol. Behav.* 27, 13–17.

Paulos, M. A., and Tessel, R. E. (1982). Excretion of beta-phenylethylamine is elevated in humans after profound stress. *Science* 215, 1127–1129.

Pyle, R. L., Mitchell, J. E., and Eckert, E. D. (1981). Bulimia: A report of 34 cases. *J. Clin. Psychiatry* 42, 60–64.

Pyle, R. L., Halvorson, P. A., Neuman, P. A., *et al.* (1986). The increasing prevalence of bulimia in freshman college students. *Int. J. Eat. Disord.* 5, 631–647.

Randall, L. W., Schallek, W., Heise, G. A., Keith, E. F., and Bagdon, R. E. (1960). The psychosedative properties of methaminodiazepoxide. *J. Pharmacol. Exp. Ther.* 129, 163–171.

Reid, L. D. (1985). Endogenous opioid peptides and regulation of drinking and feeding. *Am. J. Clin. Nutr.* 42, 1099–1132.

Ross, L. (1974). Effects of manipulating salience of food upon consumption by obese and normal eaters. *In* "Obese Humans and Rats" (S. Schacter and J. Rodin, eds.), pp. 43–51. Erlbaum Associates, Potomac, Maryland.

Rowland, N., Antelman, S. M., and Kocan, D. (1982). Differences among 'serotonergic' anorectics in a cross-tolerance paradigm: Do they all act on serotonin systems? *Eur. J. Pharmacol.* 81, 57–66.

Sayetta, R. B. (1986). Pica: An overview. *Am. Fam. Physician* 33, 181–185.

Schachter, S., Goldman, R., and Gordon, A. (1968). Effects of fear, food deprivation and obesity on eating. *J. Pers. Soc. Psychol.* 10, 91–97.

Seegmiller, J. E. (1980). Diseases of purine and pyrimidine metabolism. *In* "Metabolic Control and Disease" (P. K. Bondy and L. E. Rosenberg, eds.), pp. 777–937. Saunders, Philadelphia, Pennsylvania.

Selye, H. (1979). "The Stress of My Life: A Scientist's Memoirs," 2nd ed. Van Nostrand/Reinhold, New York.

Shaw, N. S., Rutherdale, M., and Kenny, J. (1985). Eating more and enjoying it less. U.S. prison diets for women. *Women Health* 10, 39–57.

Shibasaki, T., Kim, Y. S., Yamauchi, N., Masuda, A., Imaki, T., Hotta, M., Demura, H., Wakabayashi, I., Ling, N., and Shizume, K. (1988). Antagonistic effect of somatostatin on corticotropin-releasing factor-induced anorexia in the rat. *Life Sci.* **42**, 329–334.

Singhi, P., and Singhi, S. (1983). Nutritional status and psycho-social stress in children with pica. *Indian Pediatr.* **20**, 345–349.

Sirinathsinghji, D. T. S., Rees, L. H., Rivier, J., and Vale, W. (1983). Corticotropin-releasing factor is a potent inhibitor of sexual receptivity in the female rat. *Nature (London)* **305**, 232–235.

Slochower, J. (1976). Emotional labeling and overeating in obese and normal weight individuals. *Psychosom. Med.* **38**, 131–139.

Slochower, J., and Kaplan, S. P. (1980). Anxiety, perceived control, and eating in obese and normal weight persons. *Appetite* **1**, 75–79.

Snoddy, A. M., Heckathorn, D., and Tessel, R. E. (1985). Cold-restraint stress and urinary endogenous beta-phenylethylamine excretion in rats. *Pharmacol., Biochem. Behav.* **22**, 497–500.

Spiess, J., Rivier, J., Rivier, C., *et al.* (1981). Primary structure of corticotropin-releasing factor from ovine hypothalamus. *Proc. Natl. Acad. Sci. U.S.A.* **78**, 6517–6521.

Sprague, J. M., Levitt, M., Robson, K., *et al.* (1963). A neuroanatomical and behavioral analysis of the syndromes resulting from midbrain lemniscal and reticular lesions in the cat. *Arch. Ital. Biol.* **101**, 225–295.

Stunkard, A. J., Grace, W. J., and Wolff, H. G. (1955). The night-eating syndrome: A pattern of food intake among certain obese patients. *Am. J. Med.* **19**, 78–86.

Sutton, R. E., Koob, G. F., LeMoal, M., Rivier, J., and Vale, W. (1983). Corticotropin-releasing factor produces behavioral activation in rats. *Nature (London)* **297**, 165–186.

Taylor, T., Dluhy, R. G., and Williams, G. H. (1983). Beta-endorphin suppresses adrenocorticotropin and cortisol levels in normal human subjects. *J. Clin. Endocrinol. Metab.* **57**, 592–596.

Thomas, B. M., and Miller, A. T., Jr. (1958). Adaptation to forced exercise in the rat. *Am. J. Physiol.* **193**, 350–354.

Tugendhat, B. (1960). Feeding in conflict situations and following thwarting. *Science* **132**, 896–897.

Vale, W., Spiess, J., Rivier, C., *et al.* (1981). Characterization of a 41-residue ovine hypothalamic peptide that stimulates secretion of corticotropin and beta-endorphin. *Science* **213**, 1394–1397.

Vaswani, K. K., Richard, C. W., and Tejwani, G. A. (1988). Cold swim stress-induced changes in the levels of opioid peptides in the rat CNS and peripheral tissues. *Pharmacol., Biochem. Behav.* **29**, 163–168.

Waggoner, D., Wager-Srdar, S. A., Levine, A. S., and Morley, J. E. (1985). A model of stress-induced anorexia. *Fed. Proc., Fed. Am. Soc. Exp. Biol.* **44**, 1281.

Waggoner, D., Krahn, D. D., Grace, M., and Levine, A. S. (1986). Corticotropin releasing factor (CRF) suppresses tail pinch induced feeding. *Fed. Proc., Fed. Am. Soc. Exp. Biol.* **45**, 795.

Wardlaw, S. L., and Frantz, A. G. (1980). Effect of swimming stress on brain beta-endorphin and ACTH. *Clin. Res.* **28**, A482.

Willenbring, M. L., Levine, A. S., and Morley, J. E. (1986). Stress induced eating and food preference in humans: A pilot study. *Int. J. Eat. Disord.* **5**, 855–864.

Wurtman, R. J. (1982). Nutrients that modify brain function. *Sci. Am.* **246**, 50–59.

Yerbury, R. E., and Cooper, S. J. (1989). Novel benzodiazepine receptor ligands: Palatable food consumption following administration of zolpidem, CGS 17867A or Ro23-0364, in the rat. *Pharmacol. Biochem. Behav.* **33**, 303–307.

V
Cardiovascular Regulation

17

Peptides Derived From ACTH and the N-Terminal Region of Pro-Opiomelanocortin in the Regulation of Central Autonomic Drive

Kenneth A. Gruber *
Department of Medicine
Wake Forest University Medical Center
Winston-Salem, North Carolina 27103

Michael F. Callahan
Department of Medicine
Wake Forest University Medical Center
Winston-Salem, North Carolina 27103

I. Introduction

Our initial interest in the cardiovascular effects of peptides derived from pro-opiomelanocortin (POMC) was a result of our hypothesis that some of the hypertensive and natriuretic effects of chronic ACTH treatment (Scoggins *et al.*, 1984) were due to direct effects of the hormone or its metabolites. We first became interested in these possibilities after reading the reports of Lohmeier and Carroll (1982) on their inability to produce the cardiovascular effects of chronic ACTH treatment in dogs by substituting infusions of mineralocorticoids and/or glucocorticoids. The possibility of an unknown factor responsible for the cardiovascular effects of ACTH was hypothesized. A review of the literature revealed that while there is a high incidence (>75%) of hypertension associated with Cushing's disease (Plotz

*Current Address: Department of Physiology, University of Puerto Rico, San Juan, Puerto Rico 00936

343

et al., 1952), the occurrence of the disease in steroid-treated patients is 5–16% (Maunsell *et al.*, 1968; Savage *et al.*, 1962)). These data suggested that a factor(s) other than mineralocorticoids or glucocorticoids played a role in the etiology of the disease.

One potential explanation for these data was that the ACTH molecule itself was having direct effects on vascular smooth muscle to produce hypertension and/or increased vascular reactivity. In support of this possibility, Zeiler *et al.* (1982) showed that the ability of ACTH to potentiate the contractile effects of norepinephrine in atrial muscle was associated with specific binding of ACTH to the tissue.

Another hypothesis was derived from the evidence that administration of ACTH results in the production of circulating fragments of the molecule (Hudson and McMartin, 1980). It appeared conceivable to us that these fragments might possess direct natriuretic and cardiovascular effects. Experiments exploring this latter possibility formed the basis for the work reported in this chapter.

II. Hypertensive and Natriuretic Activities of ACTH(4–10)

Our initial approach to examine the possibility that fragments of ACTH had direct hypertensive or natriuretic activity was to compare ACTH to other peptides known to have natriuretic or pressor activity to look for amino acid sequence homologies. We quickly appreciated the fact that alpha and beta melanocyte-stimulating hormone (MSH), peptides known to possess a significant degree of natriuretic activity (Orias and McCann, 1972), had a 7-amino-acid residue sequence in common with ACTH; ACTH(4–10)/alpha MSH(4–10)/beta MSH(7–13) (Figure 1).

When the ACTH(4–10) sequence was tested in a rat bioassay, we found it had significant natriuretic activity, with a molar potency equivalent to alpha or beta MSH (Figure 2) (Gruber *et al.*, 1984). Further, the unique pattern of the natriuretic activity of the MSH peptides, a delayed response that peaked 30–60 min after intravenous (iv) administration, was also seen with ACTH(4–10). These data suggested that the natriuretic activity of these peptides was contained within this 7-amino-acid residue sequence.

During the course of our natriuresis studies, we also examined the effect of ACTH(4–10) administration on mean arterial pressure (MAP) and heart rate (HR) in chronically instrumented rats. We were able to demonstrate significant pressor and cardioaccelerator effects of the peptide after iv administration (Gruber *et al.*, 1984) (Figure 3). These actions appeared to be catecholamine dependent, since alpha-adrenergic receptor blockade (with phentolamine) attenuated the pressor effect, while beta-adrenergic receptor blockade (with metoprolol) prevented the cardioaccelerator effect.

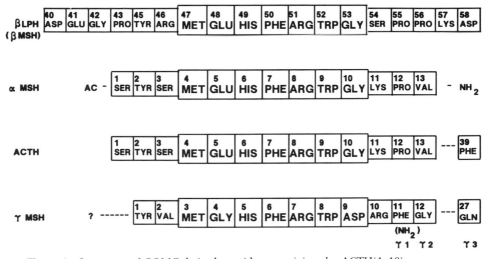

Figure 1 Structures of POMC-derived peptides containing the ACTH(4–10) or gamma MSH(3–9) sequences. In gamma MSH, residues 1–12 are the structure of gamma-2 MSH. Gamma-1 MSH is the des-Gly-12, C-terminal amide product of further posttranslational processing of the C-terminus of gamma-2 MSH. Gamma-3 MSH is a 15-amino-acid residue extension of gamma-2 MSH. The question mark at the N-terminus of gamma MSH indicates the possibility (discussed in the text) that N-terminal extensions of gamma-1 and 2 MSH have been reported to be the predominant naturally occurring forms of these peptides. [Reprinted from Gruber, *Hypertension* **10** *Suppl.* **I,** I-48-I-51 (1987), by permission of the American Heart Association.]

Initial studies in our laboratory with rats treated with mecamylamine (a ganglionic blocker) did not show a reduction in the pressor response to iv ACTH(4–10). This indicated an effect of the peptide on the postganglionic limb of the sympathetic nervous system, or its target tissues. These data were consistent with the work of Zeiler *et al.* (1982) and Bassett *et al.* (1978), in that these groups reported ACTH-mediated potentiation of the contractile effects of catecholamines on atrial tissue. Since these effects appeared to be due to specific binding of the ACTH molecule to atrial tissue, our data could be interpreted as suggesting a similar effect of ACTH(4–10), that is, an interaction with ACTH binding sites. However, subsequent work with more active analogs of ACTH(4–10) and with more efficient ganglionic blockers has shown our initial hypotheses to be incorrect (see below).

The doses of ACTH(4–10) required to produce cardiovascular and natriuretic effects were above the range for physiological effects. However, we felt that our pharmacological data suggested that the cardiovascular effects of the peptide were specific, implying the existence of a more potent naturally occurring agonist.

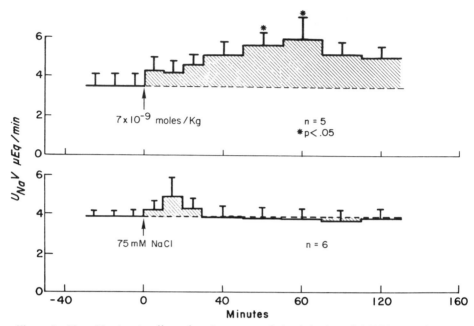

Figure 2 Top: Natriuretic effect of an intravenous bolus injection of ACTH(4–10) in an anesthetized rat bioassay. Urine was collected over 10-min sampling periods prior to peptide administration, and for 10- or 20-min periods postinjection. Data are expressed as mean ± standard error. Bottom: Natriuretic effects of a saline vehicle.

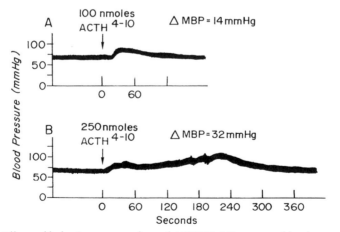

Figure 3 Effects of bolus intravenous does of ACTH(4–10) on mean blood pressure (MBP) in an anesthetized rat bioassay preparation.

An approach to demonstrating the specificity of a biological action is to show that the effects are receptor mediated. The presence of receptors mediating a biological action has been used to imply the existence of a naturally occurring ligand for the receptor. Since receptors are binding sites that recognize specific topochemical and conformational properties of a ligand, this implies that changing the chemical properties and/or secondary structure of a ligand could change its biological activity. We therefore used these principles in studies of ACTH(4–10).

III. Conformation–Activity Relationships of ACTH(4–10)

Evidence suggests that the biological effects of humoral factors, particularly peptides, are mediated by an interaction with specific binding sites on target cell membranes (i.e., receptors). Receptors are membrane-bound protein complexes, which have a region of their structure accessible to interaction with extracellular substances (i.e. ligands). It is now well established that receptor–ligand interaction or "binding" requires specific steric and topological properties to be present in the ligand that are complementary to the binding site of the receptor (Hruby, 1981, 1982; Sawyer *et al.*, 1982). If the cardiovascular effects of ACTH(4–10) were due to structural similarities to a naturally occurring analog, then these actions should be due to recognition at a receptor. Biological activity would therefore be critically dependent on a specific stereochemical configuration of the molecule.

Established approaches to demonstrating a specific receptive site are via changing the primary structure of the ligand, and by the synthesis of conformationally restricted analogs. The information that could be gained from such experiments is twofold. Demonstrating that a specific amino acid sequence is required for a biological response clearly implies a certain degree of specificity for the effect. Further, the design and synthesis of ACTH(4–10) analogs with enhanced biological activity would suggest the secondary structure requirements for receptor binding.

We first tested the effects of peptides composed of some of the amino acids found in ACTH(4–10), but in a totally different sequence ("nonsense" peptides). The nonsense peptides that were tested included Glu-Arg-Trp-His and Arg-Glu-Trp-His, administered in iv doses of 1–1000 nmol/kg. These peptide sequences produced no significant increases in MAP or HR above that produced by normal saline injections (Gruber *et al.*, 1984).

We then used an approach to predict the secondary structure of ACTH(4–10) by analyzing the tendency of each amino acid residue to contribute to the formation of an alpha-helix or beta-sheet conformation. This method, first described by Chou and Fasman (1974), is based on empirical rules for predicting the initiation and termination of helical and beta sheet or turn regions. In the method, data from statistical analyses of proteins of known conformation and amino acid sequence are used to assign numerical values, which predict the alpha-helix or beta-sheet forming potential ($P\alpha$ or $P\beta$) of specific amino acid residues.

Assignment of these predictive values (Fasman coordinates) to each residue in ACTH(4–10) predicted an alpha-helix as the preferred conformation of the peptide (Klein *et al.*, 1985) (Table I). While these data raised

Table I

Empirical Analysis of the Secondary Structure of ACTH(4–10)-Like Peptides in Terms of Alpha-Helical Potential (P_α) and Beta-Sheet Potential (P_β)

	Fasman coordinates	
	P_α	P_β
ACTH(4–10)[a]		
Met	1.20	1.67
Glu	1.53	0.26
His	1.24	0.71
Phe	1.12	1.28
Arg	0.79	0.90
Trp	1.14	1.19
Gly	—	—
Mean[c]	1.17	1.00
Gamma MSH(3–9)[b]		
Met	1.20	1.67
Gly	0.53	0.81
His	1.24	0.71
Phe	1.12	1.28
Arg	0.79	0.90
Trp	1.14	1.19
Asp	—	—
Mean[d]	[1.00]	[1.10]

[a]Potential in terms of 4–9.
[b]Potential in terms of 3–8.
[c]If for six consecutive residues $[P\alpha] > [P\beta]$ and $[P\alpha] \geqslant 1.03$, then an alpha-helix can be postulated. These as well as other conditions (see Chou and Fasman, 1974) are met by ACTH(4–10).
[d]If for six consecutive residues $[P_\beta] > [P_\alpha]$ and $[P_\beta] \geqslant 1.09$, then a beta-sheet can be postulated. These as well as other conditions (Chou and Fasman, 1974) are met by gamma MSH(3–9). Thus, two peptides with similar biological activities (see Figures 4 and 5) have different secondary conformation tendencies. Since no definitive conclusions could be drawn from these analyses, we approached this problem through the use of sterically hindered analogs (see text).

the possibility that an alpha-helix was the peptide conformation that was required for biological activity, examination of a naturally occurring and analogous peptide sequence with similar biological activities raised questions about this conclusion. Gamma MSH(3–9) is a peptide sequence found in pro-opiomelanocortin (POMC), the precursor to the adrenocorticotrophic and melanotrophic hormones. The amino-terminus of this protein contains a region that has structural similarities to alpha melanocyte-stimulating hormone. In the core sequence of the gamma MSH region, five of seven amino acid residues are identical to ACTH(4–10) (Nakanishi *et al.*, 1979). The differences lie in the second and seventh amino acid residues: glutamyl and glycine residues in ACTH(4–10), versus glycyl and aspartic acid residues in gamma MSH(3–9) (Figure 1). Based on the Fasman coordinates of these amino acid residues, there was clearly a significantly reduced tendency of gamma MSH(3–9) to assume an alpha-helix conformation, with sufficient evidence to predict a beta-sheet (Table I). However, the cardiovascular activity of gamma MSH(3–9) was virtually identical to that of ACTH(4–10) (Figures 4 and 5) (Klein *et al.*, 1985).

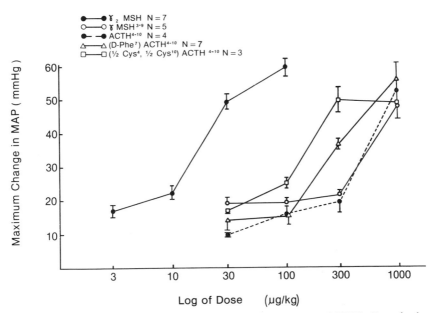

Figure 4 Blood-pressure-elevating effects of ACTH(4–10), gamma MSH(3–9), and related peptides in conscious rats. The maximum increment in MAP following bolus iv administration of the peptides is shown. The bars represent the standard error for each mean response. Note that all peptides produce a significant and dose-dependent response, but gamma-2 MSH was greater than an order of magnitude more potent than any other peptide. [Reprinted from Klein *et al.* (1985) by permission of Pergamon Press.]

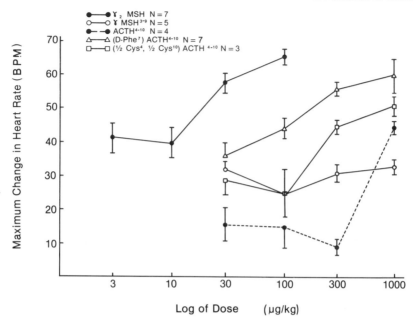

Figure 5 Cardioaccelerator effects of ACTH(4–10), gamma MSH(3–9), and related peptides in conscious rats. The maximum beat per minute (BPM) increment in heart rate is depicted. The bars represent the standard error for each mean response. While all peptides produced significant cardioacceleration, their effects were dose independent. However, gamma-2 MSH was at least one order of magnitude more potent than any other peptide. [Reprinted from Klein *et al.* (1985) by permission of Pergamon Press.]

These data highlight a potential problem in peptide structural analysis approaches based on crystallographic or other physical determinations of molecular structure. This is the rarely confirmed assumption that the minimum energy conformation, the conformer produced and analyzed in these methods, is in fact the receptor-bound structure. There are numerous examples in biological systems of conformational changes being produced when two molecules interact. For example, allosteric effects in enzymes clearly demonstrate the ability of a small molecule to change the three-dimensional conformation of a large protein. It is entirely logical to assume the reverse situation can also occur. Since small peptides are relatively flexible molecules, the least energy conformation in a symmetrical solution is not necessarily the conformer assumed when it is subjected to the asymmetrical force field associated with a "binding" protein, that is, a receptor (for a review of the above concepts, see Marshall *et al.*, 1979).

Based on the ACTH(4–10) /gamma MSH(3–9) cardiovascular activity comparison, we then investigated the possibility that a beta-turn was the molecular conformation preferred for these effects. Our approaches to this problem were derived from the work of Victor Hruby and associates on the conformation of alpha MSH preferred for receptor binding. Through the use of sterically restricted analogs, Sawyer *et al.* (1982) had shown that a beta-turn was the most likely candidate for the conformation assumed when biological effects are produced. Several of the alpha MSH agonists synthesized involved amino acid substitutions in the region of the molecule containing the ACTH(4–10) (i.e., alpha MSH 4–10) sequence, and/or involved derivatizations that would produce secondary structure changes within this sequence.

Using the work of Hruby (1981, 1982) and Sawyer *et al.* (1982) as a model, we utilized D-amino acid substitution, or isosteric substitution combined with side-chain-to-side-chain cyclization, to produce sterically restricted analogs of ACTH(4–10). Both of these analogs had significantly enhanced pressor and cardioaccelerator activity (Figures 4 and 5).

The implications for these conformational changes producing enhanced biological activity are as follows. Substitution of a D-amino acid into a peptide composed of L-amino acid residues acts as a strong alpha-helix breaker, and beta-turn former. The basis for these effects is the work of Ramachandran and associates (Ramachandran and Sasiskharan, 1968; Chandrasekaran *et al.*, 1973) on the inability of racemic peptides to assume an alpha-helix conformation, and the stabilizing effect of D-amino acid residues on beta-turns in L-amino acid residue peptides. Thus, a "D" for "L" Phe substitution in ACTH(4–10) significantly increased an empirical prediction of a beta-turn for the molecular configuration assumed to initiate a cardiovascular effect.

Final evidence for a reverse or beta-turn as the three-dimensional configuration assumed by ACTH(4–10) when a cardiovascular effect was produced resulted from a dicysteine-substituted analog. The replacement of cysteine residues for the Met-4 and Gly-10 residues of ACTH(4–10) produces an "isosteric" derivative—that is, there is a structural and steric similarity between the side-chain groups of cysteine and the methionyl and glycine residues of ACTH(4–10). The intermediate free disulfhydryl analog was oxidized to its intramolecularly disulfide-bridged derivative, forming a cyclic analog of ACTH(4–10). The steric restriction induced in this derivative is compatible with a beta-turn conformation. The superagonist activity present in this peptide provided further evidence in favor of a beta-turn as the receptor-bound conformation of ACTH(4–10), which produces cardiovascular effects.

Similar results were seen when we examined the natriuretic activity of the synthetic analog (D-Phe-7) ACTH(4–10). This peptide had approximately 1000-fold more natriuretic activity than ACTH(4–10) (Gruber *et al.*, 1985b).

Thus, our studies on ACTH(4–10) analogs indicated that the cardiovascular activity could be enhanced in a sterically restricted structure that did not appear to be the predicted minimal energy conformer of the naturally occurring sequence. This provided indirect evidence for a receptor that induces and then "recognizes" a specific conformation of the molecule.

IV. Naturally Occurring Analogs of ACTH(4–10): Gamma MSH

Our pharmacological data suggesting the existence of stereospecific effects for ACTH(4–10)-like peptides encouraged us to test naturally occurring peptides containing the ACTH(4–10) sequence, to ascertain their relative cardiovascular and natriuretic activities. While alpha or beta MSH has natriuretic activity similiar to ACTH(4–10), these peptides were devoid of pressor and cardioaccelerator activity (Klein *et al.*, 1985). However, the elucidation of the entire primary structure of POMC revealed the existence of another family of peptides with an ACTH(4–10)-like sequence, the gamma MSHs.

Gamma MSH peptides contain a core 7-amino-acid residue sequence that is very similar to ACTH(4–10). Initially three gamma MSH peptides were hypothesized to occur naturally. These were gamma-1 MSH, with 11 amino acid residues; gamma-2 MSH, a C-terminus Gly extension of gamma-1 MSH; and gamma-3 MSH, a 15-amino-acid residue C-terminus extension of gamma-2 MSH (Ling *et al.*, 1979). While the biological studies reported in this chapter were performed with the 11- or 12-amino-acid residue forms of gamma MSH, recent work has revealed that the predominant naturally occurring forms of these peptides may be of a considerably higher molecular weight (Bjartell *et al.*, 1987; Fenger, 1988; Fenger and Johnson, 1988). The high-molecular-weight forms of these peptides are due to an N-terminal extension of their originally hypothesized structure, plus glycosylation, producing a molecular size >5000 daltons. This may have significant implications for the biological activities of these peptides (see below).

Initial attempts to isolate gamma-1 or gamma-2 MSH from rat pituitary failed to detect these peptides, and could only find gamma-3 MSH (Browne *et al.*, 1981). This appeared to be consistent with the fact that the Arg-Arg sequence that appears at the C-terminus of the gamma MSH region in the POMC molecule of most species was replaced by a Pro-Arg sequence in rodents (Uhler and Herbert, 1983). It was assumed that this amino acid substitution prevented enzymatic processing of POMC to form lower-molecular-weight gamma MSH peptides. However, these data did not reconcile the fact that the molar quantities of gamma-3 MSH in rat neurointermediate lobe only accounted for the processing of 50% of the total quantity of POMC found in the tissue (Browne *et al.*, 1981).

Lin *et al.* (1987) have detected circulating gamma MSH immunoreactivity in rat plasma and pituitary, using an antibody made against synthetic gamma-2 MSH. Chromatographic examination of the immunoreactive substances revealed the presence of five peaks, with molecular masses between 2 and 23 kDa. These molecular weights are considerably larger than that of synthetic gamma-2 MSH, and could account for the failure of Browne *et al.* (1981) to detect low-molecular-weight forms of gamma MSH. The evidence, presented subsequent to the reports of Brown *et al.* and Uhler and Herbert, that a Pro-Arg sequence can be a signal for posttranslational enzymatic cleavage (Oikawa *et al.*, 1984; Reeve *et al.*, 1983) as well as the evidence for high-molecular- weight forms of gamma-1 and gamma-2 MSH, provides additional support for the hypothesis that the rat may indeed possess gamma-1 and gamma-2 MSH-like peptides.

Certain gamma MSH peptides were found to be superagonists of ACTH(4–10) or gamma MSH(3–9). When the cardiovascular effects of iv gamma-2 MSH were evaluated in conscious rats, we noted a >10-fold enhancement of pressor and cardioaccelerator activities compared to ACTH(4–10) or gamma MSH(3–9) (Klein *et al.*, 1985). Gamma-1 MSH was slightly, though significantly, less potent than gamma-2 MSH on these parameters (Gruber *et al.*, 1985a). Gamma-3 MSH had little, if any, pressor or cardioaccelerator activity (Klein *et al.*, 1985), with its biological activities apparently confined to actions as a potentiator of the steroidogenic effects of ACTH, as well as an adrenocorticotrophic hormone in its own right (Pedersen *et al.*, 1980; Al-Dujaili *et al.*, 1981). The natriuretic effect of gamma-2 MSH was approximately 1000-fold greater than ACTH(4–10), with an efficacy similiar to the sterically restricted analog (D-Phe-7) ACTH(4–10) (Lymangrover *et al.*, 1984).

To ensure that the basis of the enhanced pressor and cardioaccelerator effects of gamma-1 or gamma-2 MSH was dependent on the same mechanisms as those of ACTH(4–10), we performed a series of adrenergic receptor blockade studies. Using the alpha-1-adrenoreceptor antagonist prazosin, we were able to attenuate >80% of the pressor response of iv gamma-2 MSH (Callahan *et al.*, 1985). As with ACTH(4–10), prevention of sympathetic chronotropic effects, by beta-adrenoreceptor blockade with metoprolol, did not reveal the presence of baroreceptor mediated bradycardia.

To further explore the possibility that the pressor response to gamma-2 MSH was accompanied by inhibition of the cardiac baroreceptor reflex, we tested the effects of the peptide in rats treated with methylatropine. If parasympathetic drive to the heart was limiting the cardiovascular effects of the peptide by minimizing cardioacceleration, then blocking cholinergic receptors should enhance the pressor and cardioaccelerator effects of gamma MSH. This did not occur, though the dose of methylatropine we used was sufficient to prevent phenylephrine-induced bradycardia (Callahan *et al.*, 1985). It therefore appears that the appropriate physiological response to the degree of blood pressure elevation produced by gamma MSH (+ 60 mmHg)—that is, an increase in parasympathetic drive to the heart—was lacking.

Our work with ACTH(4–10) in rats treated with mecamylamine (a ganglionic blocker) suggested that the effects of this peptide were directed against the postganglionic limb of the sympathetic nervous system or its target tissues. To confirm these effects with gamma MSH, a more potent agonist, we tested this peptide in rats treated with chlorisondamine. The latter is a ganglionic blocking agent with approximately 10-fold more potency than mecamylamine (Aviado, 1971). This treatment reduced the pressor effect of gamma-2 MSH by almost 90% (Callahan *et al.*, 1985). Thus, the effects of iv gamma-2 MSH appeared to be directed toward the preganglionic limb of the sympathetic nervous system, or structures proximal to it. These data were interpreted as evidence that our previous studies of ACTH(4–10) in mecamylamine-treated rats were carried out under conditions of, for the stimulus used, incomplete blockade. The ability of potent central sympathoexcitatory stimuli to overcome ganglionic blockade has previously been reported (Aviado, 1971).

While our pharmacological data on the basis of the cardiovascular response of ACTH(4–10)/gamma MSH peptides suggested a crucial role for the sympathetic nervous system, it did not differentiate between adrenal medullary catecholamine release and that of sympathetic terminals. Our data with ACTH(4–10) in bilaterally adrenalectomized rats (Gruber *et al.*, 1984) provided one line of evidence for a predominant role of sympathetic terminal catecholamine release in the cardiovascular effects of these peptides.

Another approach to this problem would be to use drugs that specifically block sympathetic terminal or adrenal medullary catecholamine release, permitting an immediate evaluation of the effects of these peptides. One such drug is bretylium, which prevents sympathetic terminal catecholamine release, while leaving the activity of the sympatho–medullary system intact (McCarty and Kopin, 1979). Bretylium-treated rats showed a dramatic decrease in their pressor and cardioaccelerator responses to gamma MSH, suggesting that sympathetic terminal catecholamine release is the major component to these cardiovascular effects (Callahan *et al.*, 1988c).

The evidence for a preganglionic site of action of gamma MSH suggested that the circulating peptide might have direct effects on the central nervous system. A fortuitous collaborative experiment with Dr. Lee Mitchell (University of Iowa) provided insight into the problem of anatomical substrates for the central actions of circulating gamma MSH.

Administration of gamma MSH into the internal carotid artery (via a cannulated external carotid artery) produced an increase in the firing rate of vasopressinergic neurons in the supraoptic nucleus, which preceded the pressor effects of the peptide (Mitchell *et al.*, 1989). In addition, the pressor effects of the peptide were present at doses that were significantly below those required to produce the effect upon iv administration. These experiments raised the possibility that circulating gamma MSH acted in the forebrain to activate vasopressinergic neurons. A subsequent series of experiments investigated this concept.

A comparison of intracarotid versus intrajugular pressor dose-response curves in rats showed that the former route produced a fivefold increase in sensitivity (i.e., a shift to the right in the dose-response curve) (Callahan *et al.*, 1988b). This strongly implied that the forebrain was the site of action for the acute cardiovascular effects of the circulating peptide. A logical anatomical substrate for the action of the circulating peptide was the forebrain circumventricular organs (CVOs).

The CVOs are periventricular structures that lack a blood–brain barrier, and are known to act as receptive sites for humoral substances. In particular, forebrain CVOs are known to detect circulating levels of angiotensin II (AII) or osmolality (Bealer, 1983; Brody and Johnson, 1980; Haywood *et al.*, 1980) and are crucial to the production of the appropriate physiological response. Electrolytic lesions of forebrain CVOs prevent the central actions of hyperosmolality or circulating AII (Bealer, 1983; Brody and Johnson, 1980). To assess the role of these structures in the cardiovascular response to gamma MSH, we tested the peptide in rats with lesions of forebrain periventricular tissue. There was a significant decrease in the pressor response to iv gamma MSH in lesioned rats compared to a group with sham lesions (Callahan *et al.*, 1988a). The specificity of the effect in the lesioned group was demonstrated by equivalent pressor responses to phenylephrine in lesioned and sham-lesioned rats. Taken with the previous series of experiments, these results suggest that the pressor effects of circulating gamma MSH are due to an interaction with forebrain CVOs.

It is well established that efferent projections from forebrain CVOs are important stimulatory influences upon vasopressinergic neurons (Brody and Johnson, 1980). However, the role of the sympathetic nervous system in the cardiovascular effects of gamma MSH appeared to be inconsistent with a circulating vasopressin component in these effects. To further investigate the importance of circulating vasopressin in the cardiovascular response to iv gamma MSH, we tested the peptide in rats treated with a vascular vasopressin receptor antagonist. While this treatment prevented >80% of the pressor effect of exogenous iv vasopressin, it had no effect upon the gamma MSH response (Gruber and Eskridge, 1986).

Since these experiments appeared to rule out a role for hypophyseal vasopressin in the cardiovascular response to gamma MSH, we decided to evaluate the contribution of the central vasopressin system. In addition to magnocellular vasopressinergic projections to the pituitary, parvocellular vasopressinergic neurons appear to innervate hindbrain vasomotor centers (Sofroniew, 1980). The potential role of this central vasopressin system in cardiovascular regulation has been investigated using intraventricular, intrathecal, and microinjection procedures (Berecek *et al.*, 1984; Matsuguchi *et al.*, 1982; Pittman *et al.*, 1982; Riphagen and Pittman, 1985). The results of these experiments have consistently shown that central administration of vasopressin produces a sympathetically mediated pressor and cardioaccelerator effect. These actions are similar to the effects of iv gamma MSH, and were therefore consistent with the possibility that the central vasopressin system was a mediator of the central actions of circulating gamma MSH. To investigate this hypothesis, we employed both pharmacological and genetic model approaches.

The sympathoexcitatory effects of central vasopressin appear to be mediated by a receptor that has some similarity to the vascular or V-1 vasopressin receptor, since central administration of V-1 antagonists prevents the sympathoexcitatory effect of centrally administered vasopressin (Berecek *et al.*, 1984). We therefore tested the pressor effect of iv gamma MSH before and after central administration of a V-1 vasopressin antagonist. Central vasopressin receptor blockade attenuated >80% of the gamma MSH pressor response (Gruber and Eskridge, 1986).

While these data suggested that the central vasopressin system was one of the anatomical pathways mediating the central sympathoexcitatory effect of circulating gamma MSH, it is possible to critique the specificity of these pharmacological blockade studies, since the V-1 antagonist has not yet been shown to be totally specific for central nervous system vasopressin receptors. We therefore performed a parallel series of experiments in Brattleboro rats.

Rats of the Brattleboro strain have a genetic defect in vasopressin synthesis that renders them deficient in both central and hypophyseal vasopressin. When gamma MSH was administered to Brattleboro rats there was >80% reduction in their pressor response compared to Long-Evans rats (their genetic controls) (Gruber and Eskridge, 1986). Since several lines of evidence showed no role for circulating vasopressin in the cardiovascular effects of iv gamma MSH, the Brattleboro rat data was consistent with a role for the central vasopressin system. In addition, these data provide further evidence that the majority of the cardiovascular effects produced by iv gamma-1 or gamma-2 MSH administration are mediated via central nervous system mechanisms.

V. Physiological Significance of Circulating Gamma MSH

Circulating gamma MSH is a product of POMC peptide secretion by the corticotrophs of the anterior pituitary lobe and the melanotrophs of the neurointermediate lobe. Many other POMC-derived peptides are cosecreted with the gamma MSHs. Indeed, it was the roughly parallel secretory rates of these other peptides (e.g., ACTH, beta lipotrophin, alpha MSH, beta endorphin, etc.) that provided the first hints that all of these peptides were derived from a common precursor (for a review, see Eipper and Mains, 1980). Evidence is accumulating that gamma-1 and gamma-2 MSH are co-synthesized with gamma-3 MSH in both the anterior and neurointermediate lobes of the pituitary (Bjartell *et al.*, 1987; Fenger, 1988; Fenger and Johnson, 1988). This indicates that POMC molecules undergo differential post-translational processing, since the production of the sympathoexcitatory forms (gamma-1 or gamma-2 MSH) versus steroidogenic forms (gamma-3 MSH) of this hormone are mutually exclusive.

Since the gamma MSH family was the last group of POMC peptides to be structurally defined, there are still relatively few reports of their measurement in experimental or pathophysiologial states. Contributing to this problem is the recently presented evidence on potential problems in the quantitative extraction of gamma-1 or gamma-2 MSH from biological samples (Bjartell *et al.*, 1987). Therefore, it may be useful to describe conditions known to increase the secretion of POMC peptides from the pituitary, and review the physiology of these states in light of the autonomic effects of these peptides.

One of the first physiological states in which high levels of a POMC-derived peptide could be measured was experimental stress. Sandman *et al.* (1973) reported that rats subjected to footshock had elevated circulating levels of alpha MSH and ACTH. In retrospect, these data indicated stress-induced secretion of POMC peptides from both the anterior and neurointermediate lobe. More recently, Pedersen *et al.* (1982) have measured increased circulating levels of N-terminal POMC-derived peptides in rats subjected to an intraperitoneal injection. A well-established hallmark of many forms of stress is an increase in central sympathetic drive, and increased circulating levels of N-terminal POMC peptides with sympathoexcitatory activity could contribute to the autonomic effects of stress.

Circulatory shock, which includes the models of endotoxemia, hypovolemia (i.e. hemorrhage), anaphylaxis, and spinal trauma, is associated with elevated levels of ACTH, as well as other POMC-derived peptides (e.g., beta endorphin). Holaday and co-workers (Holaday, 1983; Bernton *et al.*, 1985) have investigated the role of endogenous opioids in shock, since the actions these peptides produce (cardiodepression and hypotension) are similar to the effects of circulatory shock. Naloxone treatment increased the survival rate of animals subjected to various forms of circulatory shock, suggesting that the cardiodepressant effects of opioids may be active in these models. Since large quantities of pituitary-derived beta endorphin circulate in shock, Holaday and co-workers hypothesized that hypophysectomy would reduce the circulating levels of these cardiodepressant peptides and thus improve survival. However, studies with acute hemorrhagic or endo-toxic shock in hypophysectomized rats demonstrated a sensitization to the hypotensive effects of these experimental states. While these investigators suggested that the lack of ACTH-mediated glucocorticoid secretion was re-sponsible for this effect, the removal of sympathoexcitatory or cardiotonic pituitary-derived POMC peptides may have played a role in the detrimental effects of hypophysectomy in shock.

In support of the latter concept, Bertolini et al. (1986) have shown that several POMC peptide fragments containing the ACTH (4–10) se-quence, including ACTH(4–10) itself, can increase the survival rate of rats subjected to acute hemorrhage. The protective effects of these peptides ap-peared to be related to their ability to acutely increase arterial pressure in hemorrhaged rats, as well as controls. The cardiovascular actions of these peptides are similar to those reported by us for gamma MSH, which is the naturally occurring analog of ACTH(4–10) as regards its natriuretic and cardiovascular effects. When combined with the work of Holaday (1983), these studies suggest that part of the sensitivity of hypophysectomized rats to hemorrhage may be the lack of POMC-derived peptides with sympa-thoexcitatory activity.

Chan et al. (1983) have provided evidence that N-terminal POMC peptides are cosecreted with ACTH in several disease states, including Cushing's or Addison's disease, Nelson's syndrome, and chronic renal fail-ure. In these situations the magnitude of increase in N-terminal derived pep-tides far exceeded that of ACTH. This may reflect the enhanced resistance to enzymatic degradation that has been reported for these peptides (Lu et al., 1983), possibly a reflection of the fact that they are glycosylated. This is a posttranslational derivitization step that protects peptides from enzyma-tic attack, prolonging their circulating half-life (Loh and Gainer, 1979). The N-terminal peptides secreted in the above disease states do not include gamma-3 MSH, since direct measurements of this peptide have produced circulating levels below that of ACTH. Another clinical state in which high circulating levels of N-terminal derived POMC peptides have been found is cardiac arrest (Wortsman et al., 1985).

Large quantities of gamma-1 MSH immunoreactivity have been de-tected in all POMC-containing cells of the human pituitary (Ali-Rachedi et *al.*, 1983), and high-molecular-weight gamma-1 MSH has been isolated from human pituitary (Fenger and Johnson, 1988). It is therefore not unreasonable to suggest that appropriate plasma extraction techniques might detect elevated circulating levels of gamma-1 MSH peptides in certain disease states.

VI. Conclusions

The iv cardiovascular and natriuretic activities of ACTH(4–10) appear to be due to the structural similarity of this peptide to a naturally occurring family of hypophyseal hormones, the gamma MSHs. Evidence that gamma MSH peptides produce their cardiovascular actions via effects on sympathetic drive were initially based on the ability of adrenergic receptor or ganglionic blockade to attenuate the pressor and cardioaccelerator effects of iv gamma MSH. Further work has shown that central nervous system lesions or the lack of a central vasopressin system will also prevent the full pressor effect of iv gamma MSH. In contrast, circulating vasopressin plays no role in the cardiovascular effects of gamma MSH.

The evidence that hypophyseal POMC-derived peptides, including gamma MSH, are released in various states of stress, shock, or cardiovascular distress suggests potential roles for these peptides in the changes in autonomic drive known to occur in these conditions. The recent evidence that gamma MSH peptides may occur as high-molecular-weight molecules, as well as improvements in the extraction techniques for these peptides (Bjartell *et al.*, 1987; Fenger, 1988), may now facilitate the precise assay of these hormones in blood.

Acknowledgments

The work in this review was supported by the following groups: William Randolph Hearst Foundation, R. J. Reynolds Industries, North Carolina Affiliate of the American Heart Association, and National Institutes Of Health Grants 1R01 HL 33506 and 1R01 HL 35112. K. A. Gruber held Research Career Development Award 1K04 HL 00804 during the course of most of these studies.

References

Al-Dujaili, E. A. S., Hope, J., Estivariz, F. E., Lowry, P. J., and Edwards, C. R. W. (1981). Circulating human pituitary pro-gamma-melanotropin enhances the adrenal response to ACTH. *Nature (London)* **291**, 156–159.

Ali-Rachedi, A., Ferri, G.-L., Varndell, I. M., Van Noorden, S., Schot, L. P. C., Ling, N., Bloom, S. R., and Polak, J. M. (1983). Immunohistochemical evidence for the presence of gamma-1-MSH-like immunoreactivity in pituitary corticotrophs and ACTH-producing tumors. *Neuroendocrinology* 37, 427–433.

Aviado, D. M. (1971). Ganglionic stimulant and blocking drugs. *In* "Drill's Pharmacology in Medicine" (J. R. De Palma, ed.), 4th ed., Chapter 35, pp. 708–731. McGraw-Hill, New York.

Bassett, J. R., Strand, F. L., and Cairncross, K. D. (1978). Glucocorticoids, adrenocorticotropic hormone and related polypeptides on myocardial sensitivity to noradrenalin. *Eur. J. Pharmacol.* 49, 243–249.

Bealer, S. L. (1983). Hemodynamic mechanisms in CNS-induced natriuresis in the conscious rat. *Am. J. Physiol.* 244 (Renal, Fluid, Electrolyte Physiol. 13), F376-F382.

Berecek, K. H., Olpe, H. R., Jones, R. S. G., and Hofbauer, K. G. (1984). Microinjection of vasopressin into the locus coeruleus of conscious rats. *Am. J. Physiol.* 247 (Heart Circ. Physiol. 16), H675-H681.

Bernton, E. W., Long, J. B., and Holaday, J. W. (1985). Opioids and neuropeptides: Mechanisms in circulatory shock. *Fed. Proc., Fed. Am. Soc. Exp. Biol.* 44, 290–299.

Bertolini, A., Guarini, S., Rompianesi, E., and Ferrari, W. (1986). Gamma-MSH and other ACTH fragments improve cardiovascular function and survival in experimental hemorrhagic shock. *Eur. J. Pharmacol.* 130, 19–26.

Bjartell, A., Ekman, R., and Sundler, F. (1987). Gamma-MSH-like immunoreactivity in porcine pituitary and adrenal medulla. An immunochemical and immunohistochemical study. *Regul. Pept.* 19, 291–306.

Brody, M. J., and Johnson, A. K. (1980). Role of the anteroventral third ventricle (AV3V) region in fluid and electrolyte balance, arterial pressure regulation, and hypertension. *In* "Frontiers in Neuroendocrinology" (L. Martini and W. F. Ganong, eds.), Vol. 6, pp. 249–291. Raven Press, New York.

Browne, C. A., Bennett, H. P. J., and Solomon, S. (1981). The isolation and characterization of gamma-3-melanotropin from the neurointermediate lobe of the rat. *Biochem. Biophys. Res. Commun.* 100, 336–343.

Callahan, M. F., Kirby, R. F., Wolff, D. W., Strandhoy, J. W., Lymangrover, J. R., Johnson A. K., and Gruber, K. A. (1985). Sympathetic nervous system mediation of acute cardiovascular actions of gamma-2-melanocyte stimulating hormone. *Hypertension* 7, Suppl. I, I-145–I-150.

Callahan, M. F., Cunningham, J. T., Kirby, R. F., Johnson, A. K., and Gruber, K. A. (1988a). Role of the anteroventral third ventricle (AV3V) region of the rat brain in the pressor response to gamma-2-melanocyte-stimulating hormone (gamma MSH). *Brain Res.* 444, 177–180.

Callahan, M. F., Gruber, K. A., and Eskridge-Sloop, S. L. (1988b). Peripherally administered gamma-MSH can have a central site of action for its cardiovascular effects. *Soc. Neurosci. Abst.* 505.

Callahan, M. F., Kirby, R. F., Johnson, A. K., and Gruber, K. A. (1988c). Sympathetic terminal mediation of the acute cardiovascular response of gamma-2-MSH. *J. Auton. Nerv. Syst.* 24, 179–182.

Chan, J. S. D., Seidah, N. G., and Chrétien, M. (1983). Measurement of N-terminal (1-76) of human proopiomelanocortin in human plasma: Correlation with adrenocorticotropin. *J. Clin. Endocrinol. Metab.* 56(4), 791–796.

Chandrasekaran, R., Lakshminarayanan, U. V., Pandya, U. V., and Ramachandran, G. N. (1973). Conformation of the LL and LD hairpin beds with internal hydrogen bonds in proteins and peptides. *Biochim. Biophys. Acta* 303, 14–27.

Chou, P. Y., and Fasman, G. D. (1974). Prediction of protein conformation. *Biochemistry* **13**, 222–245.

Eipper, B. A., and Mains, R. E. (1980). Structure and biosynthesis of proadrenocorticotropin/endorphin and related peptides. *Endocr. Rev.* **1**, 1–27.

Fenger, M. (1988). Pro-opiomelanocortin-derived peptides in the pig pituitary: Alpha and gamma-1-melanocyte-stimulating hormones and their glycine extended forms. *Regul. Pept.* **20**, 345–357.

Fenger, M., and Johnson, A. H. (1988). Alpha-amidated peptides derived from pro-opiomelanocortin in normal human pituitary. *Biochem. J.* **250**, 781–788.

Gruber, K. A. (1987). Natriuretic response to hydromineral imbalance. *Hypertension* **10**, I48–I151.

Gruber, K. A., and Eskridge, S. L. (1986). Central vasopressin system mediation of acute pressor effect of gamma MSH. *Am. J. Physiol.* (Endocrinol. Metab. 14), E134–E137.

Gruber, K. A., Klein, M. C., Hutchins, P. M. Buckalew, V. M., Jr., and Lymangrover, J. R. (1984). Natriuretic and hypertensive activities reside in a fragment of ACTH. *Hypertension* **6**, 468–474.

Gruber, K. A., Callahan, M. F., Kirby, R. F., Johnson, A. K., and Lymangrover, J. R. (1985a). Natriuretic and hypertensionogenic pro-opiomelanocortin derived peptides. *Regul. Pept.* Suppl 4, 118–123.

Gruber, K. A., Klein, M. C., and Lymangrover J. R. (1985b). Natriuretic peptides derived from pro-opiocortin. *In* "Endocoids" (H. Lal, F. LaBella, and J. Lane, eds.), pp. 213–220. Alan R. Liss, New York.

Haywood, J. R., Fink, G. D., Buggy, J., Phillips, M. I., and Brody, M. J. (1980). The area postrema plays no role in the pressor action of angiotensin in the rat. *Am. J. Physiol.* **239** (Heart, Circ. Physiol. 8), H108–H113.

Holaday, J. W. (1983). Cardiovascular effects of endogenous opiate systems. *Annu. Rev. Pharmacol. Toxicol.* **23**, 541–594.

Hruby, V. J. (1981). Structure and conformation related to the activity of peptide hormones. *In* "Perspectives in Peptide Chemistry," pp. 207–220. Karger, Basel.

Hruby, V. J. (1982). Conformational restriction of biologically active petides via amino acid side chain groups. *Life Sci.* **31**, 189–199.

Hudson, A. M., and McMartin, C. (1980). Mechanisms of catabolism of corticotrophin-(1–24)-tetracosapeptide in the rat *in vivo. J. Endocrinol.* **85**, 93–103.

Klein, M. C., Hutchins, P. M., Lymangrover, J. R., and Gruber, K. A. (1985). Pressor and cardioaccelerator effects of gamma MSH and related peptides. *Life Sci.* **36**, 769–775.

Lin, S. Y., Chaves, C., Wiedemann, E., and Humphreys, M. H. (1987). A γ melanocyte stimulating hormone-like peptide causes reflex natriuresis after acute unilateral nephrectomy. *Hypertension* **10**, 619–627.

Ling, N., Ying, S., Minick, S., and Guillemin, R. (1979). Synthesis and biological activity of four gamma-melanotropin peptides derived from the cryptic region of adrenocorticotropin/B lipotropin precursor. *Life Sci.* **25**, 1773–1180.

Loh, Y. P., and Gainer, H. (1979). The role of the carbohydrate in the stabilization, processing and packaging of the glycosylated adrenocorticotropin-endorphin common precursor in toad pituitaries. *Endocrinology (Baltimore)* **105**, 474–487.

Lohmeier T. E., and Carroll, R. G. (1982). Chronic potentiation of vasoconstrictor hypertension by adrenocorticotropic hormone. *Hypertension, Suppl.* **II**, II-138–II-148.

Lu, C-L., Chan, J. S. D., DeLean, A., Chen, A., Seidah, N. G., and Chretien, M. (1983). Metabolic clearance rate and half-time disappearance rate of human N-terminal and adrenocorticotropin of pro-opiomelanocortin in the rat: a comparative study. *Life Sci.* **33**, 2599–2608.

Lymangrover, J. R., Buckalew, V. M., Jr., Harris, J., Klein, M. C., and Gruber, K. A. (1984). Gamma-2-MSH is natriuretic in the rat. *Endocrinology (Baltimore)* **116,** 1227–1229.

Marshall, G. R., Barry, C. D., Bassard, H. E., Dammkoehler, R. A., and Dunn, D. A. (1979). The conformational parameter in drug design: The active analog approach. *Am. Chem. Soc. Symp. Ser.* **112,** 205–226.

Matsuguchi, H., Sharabi, F. M., Gordon, F. J., Johnson, A. K., and Schmid, P. G. (1982). Blood pressure and heart rate responses to microinjection of vasopressin into the nucleus tractus solitarius region of the rat. *Neuropharmacology* **21,** 687–693.

Maunsell, K., Pearson, R. S. B., and Livingstone, J. C. (1968). Long-term corticosteroid treatment of asthma. *Br. Med. J.* **1,** 661–665.

McCarty, R., and Kopin, I. J. (1979). Stress and alterations in plasma catecholamines and behavior in rats: Effect of chlorisondamine and bretylium. *Behav. Biol.* **27,** 249–265.

Mitchell, L. D., Callhan, M. F., Wilkin, L. D., Gruber K. A., and Johnson, A. K. (1989). Activation of supraoptic magnocellular neurons by gamma-2-melanocyte stimulating hormone (gamma-2-MSH). *Brain Res.* **480,** 388–392.

Nakanishi, S., Inoue, A., Kita, T., Nakamura, M., Chang, A. C. Y., Cohen, S. N., and Numa, S. (1979). Nucleotide sequence of cloned cDNA for bovine corticotropin-B lipotropin precursor. *Nature (London)* **278,** 423–427.

Oikawa, S., Imai, M., Ueno, A., Tanaka, S., Noguchi, T., Nakazato, H., Kangawa, K., Funda, A., and Matsuo, H. (1984). Clonning and sequence analysis of DNA encoding a precursor for human atrial natriuretic polypeptide. *Nature (London)* **309,** 724–726.

Orias, R., and McCann, S. M. (1972). Natriuresis induced by alpha and beta MSH in rats. *Endocrinology (Baltimore)* **90,** 700–706.

Pedersen, R. C., Brownie, A. C., and Ling, N. (1980). Proadrenocorticotropin/endorphin-derived peptides: Coordinate action on adrenal steroidogenesis. *Science* **208,** 1044.

Pedersen, R. C., Ling, N., and Brownie, A. C. (1982). Immunoreactive gamma-melanotropin in rat pituitary and plasma: A partial characterization. *Endocrinology (Baltimore)* **110,** 825–834.

Pittman, O. T., Lawrence, T. D., and McKean, L. (1982). Central effects of arginine vasopressin on blood pressure in rats. *Endocrinology (Baltimore)* **110,** 1058–1060.

Plotz, C. M., Knowlton, A. I., and Ragan, C. (1952). Natural history of Cushing's disease. *Am. J. Med.* **13,** 597–614.

Ramachandran, G. N., and Sasiskharan, V. (1968). Conformation of polypeptides and proteins. *Adv. Protein Chem.* **23,** 284–437.

Reeve, J. R., Jr., Walsh, H. H., Chew, P., Clark, B., Hawke, D., and Shively, J. E. (1983). Amino acid sequences of bombesin-like peptides from canine intestine extracts. *J. Biol. Chem.* **258,** 5582–5588.

Riphagen, G. L., and Pittman, O. J. (1985). Cardiovascular responses to intrathecal administration of arginine vasopressin in rats. *Regul. Pept.* **10,** 293–298.

Sandman, C. A., Kastin, A. J., Schally, A. V., Kendall, J. W., and Miller L. H., (1973). Neuroendocrine responses to physical and psychological stress. *J. Comp. Physiol. Psychol.* **84,** 386–390.

Savage, O., Copeman, W. S. C., Chapman, L., Wells, M. V., and Treadwell, B. L. J. (1962). Pituitary and adrenal hormones in rheumatoid arthritis. *Lancet* **1,** 232–235.

Sawyer, T. K., Hruby, V. J., Darman, P. S., and Hadley, M. E. (1982). [Half-cys[4], half-cys[10]] α melanocyte-stimulating hormone: A cyclic α-melanotropin exhibiting superagonist biological activity. *Proc. Natl. Acad. Sci. U.S.A.* **79,** 1751–1755.

Scoggins, B. A., Denton, D. A., Whitworth, J. A., and Coghlan, J. P. (1984). ACTH dependent hypertension. *Clin. Exp. Hypertens., Part A* **A6,** 599–646.

Sofroniew, M. V. (1980). Projection from vasopressin, oxytocin, and neurophysin neurons to neural targets in the rat and human. *J. Histochem. Cytochem.* **28**, 475–478.

Uhler, M., and Herbert, E. (1983). Complete amino acid sequence of mouse pro-opiomelanocortin derived from the nucleotide sequence of pro-opiomelanocortin cDNA. *J. Biol. Chem.* **258**, 257–261.

Wortsman, J., Frank, S., Wehrenberg, W. B., Petra, P. H., and Murphy, J. E. (1985). Gamma-3-melanocyte-stimulating hormone immunoreactivity is a component of the neuroendocrine response to maximal stress (cardiac arrest). *J. Clin. Endocrinol. Metab.* **61**(2), 355–360.

Zeiler, R. H., Strand, F. L., and El-Sherif, M. (1982). Electrophysiological and contractile responses of canine atrial tissue to adrenocorticotropin. *Peptides (N.Y.* **3**, 815–822.

18

Atrial Natriuretic Factor Systems and Experimental Hypertension

Robert E. Stewart
Department of Psychology and Graduate
Program in Neuroscience
University of Virginia
Charlottesville, Virginia 22903

Richard McCarty
Department of Psychology
University of Virginia
Charlottesville, Virginia 22903

I. Introduction

A. Atrial Natriuretic Factor and Hypertension

A recently discovered family of peptides, collectively known as atrial natriuretic factor, exerts powerful effects on physiological systems involved in the regulation of body fluid homeostasis and blood pressure. Because of the diversity and robust nature of these effects, many investigators have suggested that atrial natriuretic factor plays important causative roles in the development and maintenance of hypertension. In this chapter, we will con-

Stress, Neuropeptides, and Systemic Disease

Table I

Summary of Several Models of Hypertension in Laboratory Rats

Model	Stock of origin	Year started	Developed by	Reference
Dahl salt-sensitive (DS)	Sprague-Dawley	1961	Dahl	Rapp (1982, 1984)
Dahl salt-resistant (DR)	Sprague-Dawley	1961	Dahl	Rapp (1982, 1984)
Inbred Dahl hypertension-sensitive (S/JR)	Dahl salt-sensitive	1975	Rapp	Rapp (1982, 1984)
Inbred Dahl hypertension-resistant (R/JR)	Dahl salt-resistant	1975	Rapp	Rapp (1982, 1984)
Spontaneously hypertensive (SHR)	Wistar–Kyoto	1959	Okamoto and Aoki	Yamori (1984)
Wistar–Kyoto normotensive (WKY)	Wistar–Kyoto	1959	Okamoto and Aoki	Yamori (1984)
Stroke-prone SHR (SHRSP)	SHR	1970	Yamori and Okamoto	Yamori (1984)

sider the portion of the atrial natriuretic factor literature that addresses such roles for these peptides in two models of genetic experimental hypertension, the inbred Dahl hypertensive rat and the spontaneously hypertensive rat. Table I highlights the contrasts between these models of genetic hypertension.

In this first section, the widely varied actions that provide support for the idea that atrial natriuretic factor is involved in hypertension are briefly considered. This discussion of the actions of ANF is included also to foster an appreciation for the varied and potent effects of this peptide on fluid and electrolyte homeostasis and cardiovascular regulation. Following this brief review, separate sections evaluating the potential involvement of atrial natriuretic factor in the development of hypertension in Dahl rats and spontaneously hypertensive rats are presented.

B. Biological Effects of Atrial Natriuretic Factor

Atrial natriuretic factor (ANF) is synthesized, stored, and secreted by mammalian atrial myocytes (deBold *et al.*, 1981). The primary circulating form of ANF in rats and humans is a 28-residue peptide [ANF-(99–126)], formed by cleavage from the storage form of ANF, ANF-(1–126) (Bloch *et al.*,

1985; Eskay *et al.*, 1986; Lang *et al.*, 1985; Thibault *et al.*, 1986). It is currently thought that secretion of ANF from specific atrial granules is influenced by several factors relating to cardiac function and coronary hemodynamics, including heart rate, intraatrial pressure, and atrial stretch (Lang *et al.*, 1985; Naruse *et al.*, 1987; Edwards *et al.*, 1988). These peptides possess powerful natriuretic and diuretic properties, as first noted by deBold *et al.*, (1981), and have since been shown to exert a wide range of physiological effects in a variety of peripheral and central target tissues.

Abundant evidence indicates that ANF plays a major role in the maintenance of body fluid and electrolyte homeostasis, as well as in cardiovascular regulation. For example, systemic intravenous bolus injections or infusions of ANF are attended by a prompt and intense, though short-lived, natriuresis and diuresis and a transient decrease in arterial blood pressure (deBold *et al.*, 1981; Cantin and Genest, 1985). Chronic infusions of ANF at low doses reduce arterial blood pressure to normotensive values in spontaneously hypertensive and Goldblatt two-kidney, one-clip hypertensive rats (Garcia *et al.*, 1985a,b) and inhibit the onset of hypertension induced by chronic infusions of norepinephrine (Yasujima *et al.*, 1985). ANF also potently inhibits renin secretion from kidney, particularly in states of exaggerated basal or stimulated secretion of renin (Atlas and Laragh, 1986; Atlas *et al.*, 1986; Burnett *et al.*, 1984), and supresses aldosterone (ALDO) synthesis in the adrenal zona glomerulosa (Kudo and Baird, 1984; Goodfriend *et al.*, 1984). In addition, ANF possesses potent, though regionally selective, vasorelaxant properties, most notably in blood vessels precontracted with angiotensin II (AII) (Atlas and Laragh, 1986; Winquist, 1987). Finally, ANF exerts several cardioinhibitory effects, including decreased cardiac output, lowered stroke volume, and decreased cardiac contractility (Lappe *et al.*, 1985a; Sasaki *et al.*, 1985; Seymour *et al.*, 1987).

It is certain that circulating ANF exerts its actions at target tissues via specific receptors, and binding sites for ANF have been localized and characterized in a wide variety of tissues in several species, including rat, rabbit, guinea pig, and human. Such binding sites are found in kidney (Figure 1), vasculature, adrenal zona glomerulosa (Figure 2), lung, spleen, and thymus (see Stewart *et al.*, 1988a, for a review). These findings, along with others, suggest strongly that ANF in the periphery serves as an important humoral factor involved in cardiovascular and body fluid regulation.

Recent evidence also points to the existence of a parallel, functional ANF system in the central nervous system (CNS). In laboratory rats, ANF-like immunoreactivity has been detected in neuronal cell bodies and fibers in a variety of discrete brain areas (Figure 3). High concentrations of ANF-like immunoreactivity are found in several hypothalamic nuclei, including periventricular, median preoptic, and paraventricular nuclei, as well as in

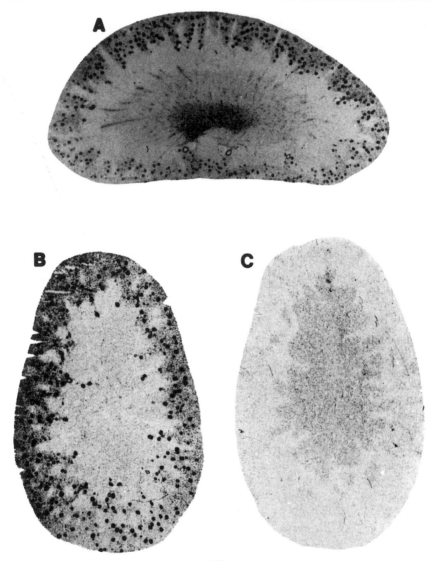

Figure 1 Autoradiographic localization of ^{125}I-ANF binding sites in 16-μm sections of rat kidney. Sections were incubated in 100 pM ^{125}I-ANF for 60 min, washed, dried, and later opposed to ^{3}H-sensitive Ultrofilm for 48 h. (A) Longitudinal section at the midline. (B) Horizontal section. (C) Horizontal section incubated in the presence of 10^{-6} M unlabeled ANF. Note the high density of ANF binding sites within the glomeruli and the papilla. Adapted from Swithers *et al.* (1987).

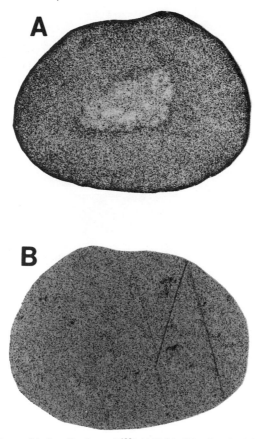

Figure 2 Autoradiographic localization of ^{125}I-ANF binding sites in 16-μm sections of rat adrenal. Sections were incubated as described in Figure 1 and opposed to ^{3}H-sensitive Ultrofilm for 36 h. (A) Cross section. (B) Cross section incubated with 10^{-6} M unlabeled ANF. Note the high density of ANF binding sites within the zona glomerulosa. Adapted from Swithers *et al.* (1987).

the organum vasculosum of the lamina terminalis (Zamir *et al.*, 1985; Kawata *et al.*, 1985; Standaert *et al.*, 1986). These areas may be important in central regulation of cardiovascular function and fluid and electrolyte homeostasis (Brody and Johnson, 1980; Johnson, 1985). Other brain regions, including neocortical, amygdalar, and hippocampal structures, contain lower amounts of ANF-like immunoreactivity. Primary transcripts of ANF mRNA in brain have been isolated and appear to be generally homologous, if not identical, to ANF mRNA isolated from heart (in Quirion,

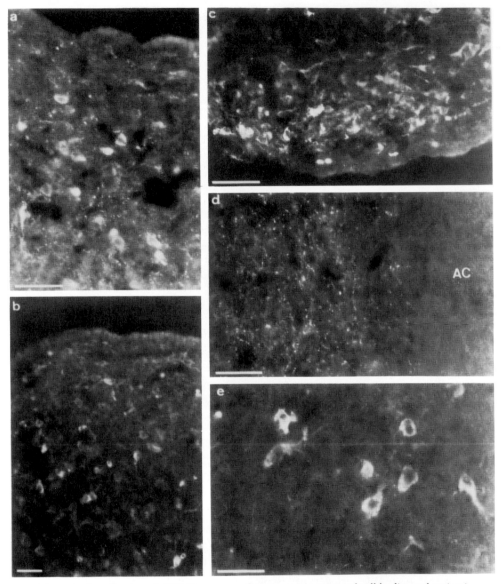

Figure 3 Localization of ANF-like immunofluorescence in neuronal cell bodies and varicosities within selected areas of colchicine-treated rat brain. (a) Paraventricular nucleus. (b) Arcuate nucleus. (c) Periventricular preoptic nucleus. (d) Ventral part of the bed nucleus of the stria terminalis; AC, anterior commissure. (e) Dorsolateral tegmental nucleus. Scale bars are 50 μm. Adapted from Jacobowitz *et al.* (1985).

1988). The primary forms of ANF in brain, however, correspond to 25- and 24-amino acid peptides, ANF-(101–126) and ANF-(102–126), respectively (Shiono *et al.*, 1986).

Like ANF in the periphery, ANF in brain appears to exert a variety of actions directed at regulation of cardiovascular function and body fluid and electrolyte balance. For instance, intracerebroventricular (icv) administration of ANF in laboratory rats greatly attenuates spontaneous or AII-induced drinking (Masotto and Negro-Vilar, 1985) and blunts salt appetite (Fitts *et al.*, 1985), potentially via direct effects on the subfornical organ (Buranarugsa and Hubbard, 1988), an area enriched with binding sites for ANF (Quirion *et al.*, 1984, 1986; Bianchi *et al.*, 1986). ANF delivered icv also enhances renal water and sodium excretion (Fitts *et al.*, 1985; Israel and Barbella, 1986; Lee *et al.*, 1987; Shimizu *et al.*, 1986) and suppresses the pressor response to centrally administered AII (Shimizu *et al.*, 1986; Casto *et al.*, 1987a). This latter effect could be mediated, in part, by the potent inhibitory effect of icv ANF on vasopressin secretion (Casto *et al.*, 1987b; Poole *et al.*, 1987), perhaps via direct inhibition of hypothalamic vasopressinergic neurons (Standaert *et al.*, 1987). Binding sites for ANF are localized in several discrete brain areas that correlate well with the actions of ANF in brain following icv administration (see Figure 4). These sites include the subfornical organ (SFO), nucleus of the solitary tract, the anteroventral third ventricle region of hypothalamus, and the area postrema, all areas considered to play important roles in cardiovascular regulation and body fluid and electrolyte homeostasis (Brody and Johnson, 1980; Johnson, 1985). Notably, the SFO, area postrema, and other circumventricular organs are accessible to circulating ANF, as shown by *in vivo* ultrastructural autoradiography (Bianchi *et al.*, 1986).

In addition to the presence of ANF in brain, Sudoh and colleagues (1988) have described the existence of a brain natriuretic peptide (BNP) originally isolated from porcine brain tissue. More recently, BNP has been isolated from porcine atria, heart perfusate, and plasma in much higher quantity than in porcine brain (Saito *et al.*, 1989). BNP has also been localized within canine (Itoh *et al.*, 1989) and rat (Holmes *et al.*, 1988) brain. In addition, BNP has been shown to exert effects similar to those of ANF in both the CNS and the periphery (see Itoh *et al.*, 1988; Shirakami *et al.*, 1988; Tang *et al.*, 1989; Higuchi *et al.*, 1989). Most strikingly, BNP apparently acts via the ANF receptor (Higuchi *et al.*, 1989; Oehlenschlager *et al.*, 1989). Although this peptide shares considerable homology with the primary structure of ANF, *ANF and BNP appear to be derived from separate and distinct genes* (Sudoh *et al.*, 1988). While it is beyond the scope of this chapter to include a detailed review of this exciting, novel area of research,

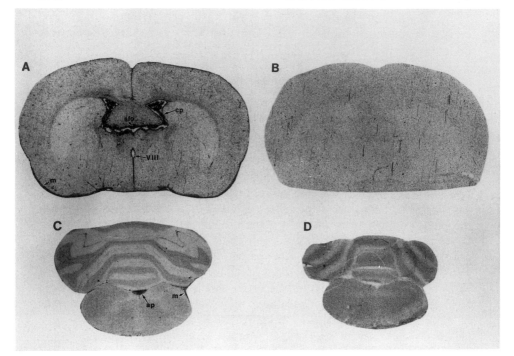

Figure 4 Autoradiographic localization of ^{125}I-ANF binding sites in 16-μm coronal sections of rat brain. Sections were incubated in 40 pM ^{125}I-ANF for 60 min, washed, dried, and later opposed to ^{3}H-sensitive Ultrofilm for 72–96 h. (A) Forebrain section at the level of the subfornical organ. (B) Forebrain section as in (A) but incubated with 10^{-6} M unlabeled ANF. (C) Brainstem section at the level of the area postrema, incubated as in (A). (D) Brainstem section as in (C) but incubated in the presence of 10^{-6} M unlabeled ANF. Note the high density of ANF binding sites in the subfornical organ (sfo), choroid plexs (cp), area postrema (ap), the meninges (m), and the ependyma lining the third ventricle (VIII). Adapted from Stewart *et al.* (1988a).

it is important to emphasize that BNP, in addition to ANF, may play an important role in the regulation of body fluid homeostasis and blood pressure.

These findings, among others, demonstrate clearly the considerable involvement of ANF in body fluid and electrolyte homeostasis and regulation of blood pressure. As indicated above, and as shown in Figure 5, the biological effects of ANF are noted in a vast array of tissues. To date, a substantial body of literature has accumulated that addresses the role of peripheral and central ANF systems in Dahl and SHR rats. As will be seen in the following sections, this literature is frought with many problems. Our consideration of this literature indicates that the inconsistency of available

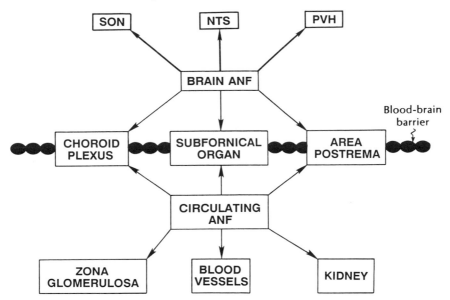

Figure 5   A summary of the major sites of action of ANF in central and peripheral tissues. *Abbreviations:* SON, supraoptic nucleus of the hypothalamus; NTS, nucleus of the solitary tract; PVH, paraventricular nucleus of the hypothalamus.

data and the lack of important research leave the role of ANF in hypertension uncertain.

II. Dahl Salt-Susceptible and Salt-Resistant Rats

In the early 1960s, Lewis Dahl initiated a program of selective breeding at Brookhaven National Laboratories that separated from a normal Sprague-Dawley breeding colony animals that exhibited differential blood pressure responses following maintenance on a high salt diet (8% NaCl). Those animals that demonstrated substantial increases in arterial blood pressure when fed this high salt diet were termed salt-susceptible (DS), and those that showed no significant change in arterial blood pressure were termed salt-resistant (DR) (Rapp, 1982, 1984). Today, when placed on a high-NaCl diet, DS rats reliably develop pronounced hypertension and exhibit increased mortality rates, whereas DR rats show little or no increment in blood pressure when maintained on a high-salt diet. DS rats maintained on normal or low-salt diets do not develop hypertension. The development of these rat lines, often referred to as the Brookhaven strains, has provided a useful and interesting model of the environmentally labile expression of a hypertensive phenotype. However, Dahl and co-workers avoided inbreeding of these rats, except in the first several generations of the selective breeding program. Therefore, DS and DR rats are not fully inbred and do not represent genotypically homozygous populations (Rapp, 1982, 1984).

In the 1970s, John Rapp initiated a rigorous program of inbreeding DS and DR rat lines. Today, after more than 35 generations of brother–sister mating, Rapp and his colleagues have produced the inbred Dahl hypertension-sensitive (S/JR) and Dahl hypertension-resistant (R/JR) rat strains, sometimes referred to as the Toledo strains. Interestingly, S/JR rats spontaneously and rapidly develop fulminant hypertension (systolic blood pressures above 180 mmHg) between 7 and 12 weeks of age (Rapp, 1982; Stewart *et al.*, 1988b). A diet high in salt content is not necessary for the expression of hypertension but will greatly accelerate the development of

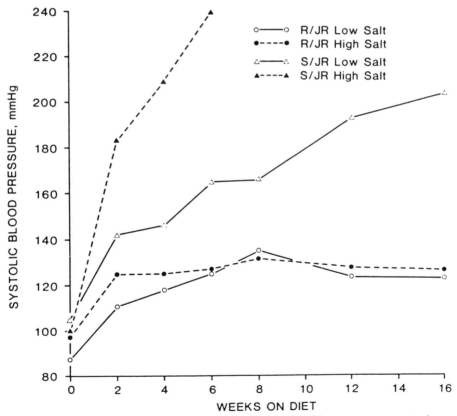

Figure 6 Development of arterial blood pressure in inbred Dahl rat strains maintained on normal or high salt diet. S/JR, inbred Dahl hypertension-sensitive rats. R/JR, inbred Dahl hypertension resistant rats. Adapted with permission from Rapp (1984).

elevated arterial blood pressure and significantly enhance morbidity in the S/JR rat strain (see Figure 6) (Rapp, 1982, 1984). In contrast, rats of the R/JR strain maintain sytolic blood pressures typically between 100 and 110 mmHg throughout adulthood (Stewart *et al.*, 1988b). The reader is asked to bear in mind the distinction between the Dahl rat lines (Brookhaven rats) and the inbred Dahl rat strains (Toledo rats). In the following section, these subsets within the Dahl model of experimental hypertension will be treated separately.

III. ANF Systems in Dahl Rats

A. Tissue and Plasma Levels of ANF in Dahl Rats

One hypothesis regarding the role of ANF systems in the development and maintenance of hypertension in Dahl rats proposes that ANF synthesis and/ or release are pathologically compromised in these models of hypertension. To this extent, the great majority of research regarding ANF systems in Dahl rats has been focused upon atrial content and circulating plasma levels of the peptide. These studies have attempted to discover abnormalities in ANF synthesis and secretion mechanisms in DS and S/JR rats. These studies have provided somewhat inconsistent results and, for simplicity, are summarized in Tables II and III.

Table II

Atrial Content of ANF in Dahl Rats[a]

Line/strain	Age	Method	Diet	Relative atrial content	Reference
DS and DR	Adult	Bioassay	4.0% NaCl	DS > DR	Hirata *et al.*(1984)
			0.11 NaCl	DS > DR	
DS and DR	Adult	RIA	8.0% NaCl	DS = DR	Tanaka and
			0.4% NaCl	DS = DR	Inagami (1986)
DS, DR, and WKY	10 weeks	RIA	8.0% NaCl	DS = DR = WKY	Gutkowska *et al.* (1986)
S/JR and R/JR	4, 8, 28 weeks	RIA	8.0% NaCl	S/JR > R/JR	Snajdar and Rapp
			0.3% NaCl	S/JR > R/JR	(1985)
S/JR and R/JR	2 weeks	RIA	1.0% NaCl	S/JR = R/JR	Snajdar *et al.* (1987)
	4 weeks	RIA	1.0% NaCl	S/JR > R/JR	
	8 weeks	RIA	1.0% NaCl	S/JR > R/JR	
	4, 6, 8 weeks	RIA	NaCl deficient	S/JR > R/JR	
	4, 6, 8 weeks	RIA	8.0% NaCl	S/JR > R/JR	
S/JR and R/JR	8 and 14 weeks	RIA	0.9% NaCl	S/JR = R/JR	Sterzel *et al.* (1987)
			8.0% NaCl	S/JR = R/JR	

[a]DS, Dahl salt-susceptible rat; DR, Dahl salt-resistant rat; S/JR, inbred Dahl hypertension-sensitive rat; R/JR, inbred Dahl hypertension-resistant rat; WKY, Wistar–Kyoto rat; RIA, radioimmunoassay.

Table III

Plasma ANF Levels in Dahl Rats[a]

Line/strain	Age	Sampling condition	Diet	Method	Relative plasma ANF levels	References
DS and DR	Adult	Pentobarbital anesthesia	8.0% NaCl 0.4% NaCl	RIA RIA	DS >> DR DS = DR	Tanaka and Inagami (1986)
DS, DR, and WKY	10 weeks	Pentobarbital anesthesia	8.0% NaCl	RIA	DS >> DR = WKY	Gutkowska et al. (1986)
S/JR and R/JR	8 weeks	Pentobarbital anesthesia	1.0% NaCl 8.0% NaCl	RIA RIA	S/JR = R/JR S/JR > R/JR	Snajdar and Rapp (1986)
	20–24 weeks		1.0% NaCl	RIA	S/JR > R/JR	
S/JR and R/JR	8 and 14 weeks	Decapitation	0.9% NaCl 8.0% NaCl	RIA RIA	S/JR = R/JR S/JR = R/JR	Sterzel et al. (1987)

[a]DS, Dahl salt-susceptible rat; DR, Dahl salt-resistant rat; S/JR, inbred Dahl hypertension-sensitive rat; R/JR, inbred Dahl hypertension-resistant rat; WKY, Wistar–Kyoto rat; RIA, radioimmunoassay.

1. Dahl Rat Lines

Hirata *et al.* (1984) first described line- and diet-related alterations in atrial content of ANF in Dahl rat lines. Utilizing natriuresis in normal Sprague-Dawley bioassay rats as a marker for ANF activity, these workers observed that infusions of atrial extracts from DS rats induced a significantly greater diuresis and natriuresis than extracts of atria from DR rats. In addition, 5-day maintenance of DS and DR rats on a high-salt (4% NaCl) diet resulted in enhanced atrial ANF content in DR rats only, as determined by bioassay. This effect was reversible, as atrial extracts from DR rats given a low-salt (0.11% NaCl) diet following 5 days of high salt induced a natriuresis similar to values for control, low-salt-diet DR rats. These investigators also showed that intravenous infusions of pooled atrial extracts from the hearts of normal Sprague-Dawley rats into 9-week-old normotensive DS and DR rats induced greater renal sodium excretion in DR rats as compared to DS rats. While this result implies impaired renal responses to ANF in DS rats, others have been unable to detect any differences between DS and DR rats in renal responsiveness to synthetic ANF infusions (Sonnenberg *et al.*, 1987). Other work has demonstrated that synthesis of ALDO is inhibited by ANF equally in suspensions of adrenal zona glomerulosa cells from salt-loaded hypertensive DS and normotensive DR rats (Racz *et al.*, 1986).

In a subsequent experiment featuring radioimmunoassay for ANF, Tanaka and Inagami (1986) detected no differences in atrial ANF content between DS and DR rats, regardless of dietary salt content (0.4% or 8.0% NaCl), although high-salt diets were associated with a slight, nonsignificant decrease in DS rat atrial ANF concentrations. In striking contrast, these authors observed that DS rats made hypertensive by maintenance on 8% NaCl feed exhibited twofold higher levels of circulating plasma ANF as opposed to normotensive DR rats on a matched diet, or normotensive DS and DR rats fed a 0.4% NaCl diet. These findings were replicated later by Gutkowska et al. (1986a), who also showed by radioimmunoassay that atrial ANF content was similar among DS, DR, and Wistar rats maintained on 8% NaCl chow from weaning to about 10 weeks of age. In further agreement with Tanaka and Inagami (1986), these investigators detected greatly elevated (two- to threefold) levels of circulating plasma ANF in hypertensive DS rats (see Tables II and III). Both groups concluded that elevated plasma ANF was most probably a consequence and not a cause of increased arterial blood pressure in this model of hypertension. Such increases in circulating ANF could also be related to increased fluid volume or atrial pressure (considered a major stimulus for ANF release) (Lang et al., 1985).

Discrepancies in the results described above may be due to the use of bioassay with atrial extracts. Methods used to extract atria require boiling, which could degrade or denature ANF differentially between these rat lines, thus altering apparent biological activity and masking true ANF activity and tissue content. Divergent results in studies of renal responsiveness of Dahl rat lines to ANF could stem from different bioassay procedures, and particularly from the use of different anesthetic agents and of atrial extracts versus synthetic ANF. Until these issues can be clarified more completely, the role of ANF in the pathogenesis of salt-induced hypertension remains unresolved. The information gained so far, however, tends to support the notion that observed changes in ANF secretion during states of hypertension are not a precipitating factor in the development of hypertension.

2. Dahl Rat Strains

Increasing plasma levels of ANF in parallel with increasing arterial blood pressure have been described in studies examining ANF systems in inbred S/JR and R/JR rat strains. Using natriuresis in Long-Evans bioassay rats as an indicator, Snajdar and Rapp (1985) reported that extracts of atria from prehypertensive S/JR rats contained significantly more ANF than did atria from age-matched R/JR controls at 1 and 2 months of age, when systolic blood pressures were similar between strains. This strain-related difference in atrial ANF content was still noted in animals at 7 months of age when S/JR rats exhibited pronounced hypertension. Interestingly, these authors found that at all ages 8% dietary NaCl resulted in decreases in atrial ANF content to comparable extents in both S/JR and R/JR rats.

In the same study, pooled atrial extracts from normal Sprague-Dawley rats were infused intravenously into S/JR and R/JR rats fed normal (~1% NaCl) feed at 1, 2, and 7 months of age to assess renal responsiveness to ANF in these strains. These experiments revealed that young (1 month old) S/JR had a decreased natriuretic response to such infusions compared to R/JR, while at 2 months of age, S/JR rats had similar renal responses to such infusions versus R/JR rats. Most strikingly, at 7 months of age, after the establishment of hypertension, S/JR rats responded with a significantly more robust natriuresis than did R/JR normotensive controls following infusion of atrial extracts.

Later reports by this same group indicated that for any given cardiac preload, isolated heart–lung preparations from inbred S/JR rats released more ANF into perfusate compared to preparations from age-matched R/JR control (Onwochei et al., 1987). Additionally, a significant positive correlation between left or right atrial pressure and ANF release was found in both strains. The age of the animals employed in this experiment was not mentioned, but these findings may support the observation by Snajdar and Rapp (1986) that plasma immunoreactive ANF is elevated in 2-month-old S/JR rats made rapidly hypertensive with 8% dietary NaCl and also in 6-month-old hypertensive S/JR rats maintained on normal feed as compared to age-matched normotensive S/JR (2 months old) and R/JR rats. A later study (Snajdar et al., 1987) demonstrated that such enhanced atrial content and secretion of ANF in the S/JR strain is probably due to factors regulating the transcription and/or translation of ANF and not to strain-related differences in the structure of the ANF gene. In this study, atrial ANF content was similar between strains at 15 days of age, while at 30 and 60 days of age, ANF levels were higher in atria of S/JR rats.

Another group has presented data that are in sharp contrast to those of the Toledo group. Sterzel et al. (1987) measured atrial and plasma immunoreactive ANF in 8-week-old normotensive S/JR and R/JR rats maintained on normal diet, and in 14-week-old hypertensive S/JR and normotensive R/JR rats maintained either on normal or high NaCl (8%) diets. No strain-, age-, blood pressure-, or diet-related differences in plasma or atrial immunoreactive ANF levels could be detected. Regardless of age, dietary salt, or blood pressure, infusions of synthetic ANF were attended by similar increases in diuresis and natriuresis, renal blood flow, and glomerular filtration rate in both strains. Also, similar, transient decreases in blood pressure (both age groups) were noted in both strains, regardless of dietary salt content or baseline blood pressure.

It is difficult to surmise what might account for such divergent results; however, it should be noted that differences in protocol, including the use of different aged rats, different anesthetics, different radioimmunoassays, and widely variable dietary salt levels could be contributing factors. For instance, Sterzel *et al.* (1987) maintained that the anesthetic Inactin, unlike ether, did not elevate plasma ANF levels as compared to levels in plasma obtained from awake rats following decapitation. However, grasping the rat for decapitation could cause a rapid redistribution of blood volume and result in increases in plasma ANF, which, in a comparison, could mask the effects of anesthetic agents, including Inactin. Ideally, blood should be collected from conscious, undisturbed, freely behaving rats via methods such as chronic cannulation of an artery or vein. While it is difficult to reconcile the differences in the results presented for plasma and atrial ANF levels in inbred Dahl rats, it may be useful to compare them with results from studies in Dahl rat lines. In this case, reports of consistently increased circulating plasma ANF in S/JR rats after the establishment of hypertension may be tentatively (and cautiously) accepted as valid. Again, the results described above tend to reject the idea that abnormalities in the synthesis and release of ANF predate or contribute to the expression of hypertension in Dahl rat lines and strains.

B. ANF Binding and Bioactivity in Dahl Rats

Others have examined the possibility that pathological alterations in the bioactivity or utilization of ANF in target tissues of S/JR rats contribute to the development of hypertension in this strain. Such alterations could include reductions in target ANF binding site number or affinity or defective transduction of the ANF signal. Several biochemical and biophysical studies have been performed to examine these issues.

1. Kidney

The notion that plasma ANF may be elevated in hypertensive S/JR rats fits well with findings regarding ANF binding sites and cyclic guanosine monophosphate (cGMP, the presumed second messenger for ANF) accumulation in kidneys of inbred Dahl rats. Using quantitative film autoradiography, Stewart *et al.* (1987) reported significantly elevated maximum binding site capacity (B_{max}) for ANF in renal glomeruli of 7-week-old prehypertensive S/JR rats as compared to age-matched R/JR controls. Consistent with the finding that plamsa ANF is elevated in hypertensive S/JR, 10-week-old hypertensive S/JR rats exhibited a downregulation in the number of ANF binding sites in glomeruli such that strain-related differences in B_{max} were no longer noted. This type of receptor downregulation by high ambient levels of ANF is well documented in vascular smooth muscle cell cultures (Hirata *et al.*, 1987; Neuser and Bellemann, 1987; Roubert *et al.*, 1987). Conceivably, elevations in B_{max} for ANF in kidneys of S/JR rats at 7 weeks of age could account for roughly equivalent renal responses to infusions of atrial extracts in S/JR and R/JR rats at this age, as observed by Snajdar and Rapp (1985). Similarly, elevated plasma ANF in hypertensive S/JR rats, in conjunction with glomerular receptor densities roughly equivalent to those seen in R/JR rats at 10 weeks of age, could account for the enhanced natriuresis noted in 7-month-old hypertensive S/JR rats (Snajdar and Rapp, 1985).

Hinko *et al.* (1987) obtained similar results in studies of ANF binding to renal membranes from 9-week-old S/JR and R/JR rats. These researchers detected no strain-related differences in either B_{max} or dissociation constant (K_d) for ANF binding in these tissues. In the same study, ANF-induced accumulation of cGMP in renal membrane preparations was found to be similar for both S/JR and R/JR rats, although others (Appel and Dunn, 1987) have shown that cGMP accumulation is slightly, though significantly, enhanced in isolated papillary collecting tubules from 13-week-old R/JR as compared to age-matched, hypertensive S/JR rats. This reduction in ANF-induced cGMP accumulation in hypertensive S/JR rats, again, could be related to downregulation of renal ANF receptors (see Hirata *et al.*, 1987) by high ambient ANF levels in these rats.

2. Other Peripheral Tissues

ANF binding in other tissues of inbred Dahl rats has also been characterized. In the adrenal zona glomerulosa, the B_{max} for ANF binding was similar in S/JR and R/JR rats at 7 weeks of age, while blood pressures between strains were not significantly different (Stewart *et al.*, 1987). At 10 weeks of age, after the sharp increase in arterial blood pressure characteristic of the S/JR strain, B_{max} for ANF in zona glomerulosa was increased some 20% in S/JR rats versus normotensive R/JR controls. At no age were strain-related changes in K_d for ANF in adrenal zona glomerulosa observed. These changes may reflect compensatory responses to elevated blood pressure in the S/JR strain. Such alterations could serve to decrease net sodium and fluid retention in these rats by inhibition of the renin–angiotensin–aldosterone system.

3. Central Nervous System

In the CNS, 7-week-old prehypertensive S/JR rats showed enhanced B_{max} for ANF in SFO compared with values for age-matched R/JR rats (Stewart *et al.*, 1988b). Again, such an elevation in the number of ANF binding sites may serve as a compensatory mechanism in the CNS to antagonize the activity of the central AII system. The net effect of such antagonistic actions could be a reduction of fluid and salt intake, or perhaps suppression of vasopressin secretion. At present, virtually no research has explored the actions of ANF in the CNS of Dahl rats. Until studies are carried out that characterize the central actions of ANF in this model of genetic hypertension, the possible function implications of alterations in ANF binding sites in SFO of S/JR rats will remain unknown.

The involvement of ANF systems in the pathogenesis of hypertension in the Dahl rat models of hypertension is far from established. It would appear, however, that alterations in circulating levels of ANF in plasma of Dahl rat lines and strains are a consequence rather than a cause of hypertension. Further work is required to establish more reliably the true renal responsiveness of Dahl rats to ANF. Additionally, the relevance of alterations in binding sites for ANF in peripheral and central tissues of inbred Dahl rats awaits further work examining the biological potency of these alterations, particularly in the CNS. It would appear, at least in kidney, that age-related downregulation of ANF binding site density in S/JR is a consequence of elevated plasma ANF in this strain, rather than a pathological precursor to the development of hypertension.

IV. Spontaneously Hypertensive Rats

The spontaneously hypertensive rat (SHR) was developed initially by Okamoto and Aoki at Kyoto University beginning in the late 1950s. These workers selectively bred Wistar–Kyoto rats that exhibited elevated blood pressure for at least 1 month prior to mating. In turn, offspring that exhibited the spontaneous development of hypertension were mated. Through their efforts, Okamoto and Aoki were able to establish (as described in 1963) a colony of animals that uniformly and reliably developed hypertension spontaneously (Yamori, 1984). By 1969, this line of rats had been fully inbred by Yamori (1984).

SHR rats slowly develop elevated arterial blood pressures typically between 7 and 15 weeks of age, when systolic pressures tend to plateau at about 200 mmHg. By comparison, Wistar–Kyoto (WKY) normotensive control rats maintain systolic pressures of about 130 mmHg throughout adulthood. A closely related substrain, the stroke-prone SHR (SHRSP), shows a similar, though somewhat accelerated, time course in arterial blood pressure increases. Additionally, SHRSP rats attain systolic blood pressure values near 250 mmHg; cerebral vascular accident is the greatest cause of morbidity in this substrain, affecting greater than 80% of the population (Yamori, 1984). Figure 7 provides a summary of the development of elevated arterial blood pressures in SHR and SHRSP rats strains.

Together, these rat strains, and in particular the SHR strain, comprise the most widely employed and studied animal model of human essential

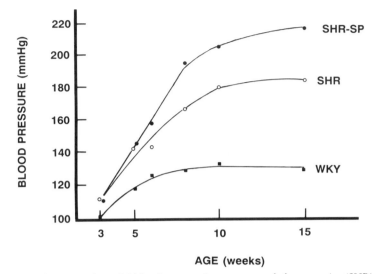

Figure 7 Development of arterial blood pressure in spontaneously hypertensive (SHR), spontaneously hypertensive stroke-prone (SHRSP), and Wistar-Kyoto (WKY) normotensive rats. Adapted from Nagaoki and Lovenberg (1976).

hypertension. To date, a great deal of research has been directed at identifying the factors that contribute to the pathogenesis and maintenance of hypertension in the SHR rat strain. Such factors include a wide variety of genetically determined and environmentally aggravated pathologies such as structural changes in vasculature, increased sympathetic nerve discharge, and altered central regulation of cardiovascular function (Yamori, 1984). More recently, the role of central and peripheral ANF systems in the onset of hypertension in SHR has been investigated. In the next section, the considerable literature detailing the activity of ANF systems in SHR and SHRSP will be considered together.

V. ANF Systems in Spontaneously Hypertensive Rats

A. Tissue and Plasma Levels of ANF in SHR

In contrast to the paucity of literature that describes ANF systems in Dahl rats, a substantial body of work exists regarding ANF systems in SHR. Similar to work done on Dahl rats, however, a large volume of research has examined plasma and atrial levels of ANF in SHR in an attempt to discover possible decreases in ANF synthesis and/or secretion that could contribute to the development of hypertension. Like studies of tissue and plasma levels of ANF in Dahl rats, these studies have generated widely divergent results.

Table IV

Atrial Content of ANF in SHR (and Related Strains)[a]

Age	Method	Diet	Relative atrial content	Reference
16–17 weeks	Bioassay	Normal	WKY > SHR	Sonnenberg et al. (1983)
12, 15 weeks	RIA	Normal	Left: WKY > SHR Right: WKY = SHR	Imada et al. (1985)
5, 10, 20 weeks	RIA	Normal	SHRSP, SHR > WKY	Kato et al. (1987)
8 weeks	RIA	Normal	WKY > SHR	Ruskoaho and Leppaluoto (1988)
24 weeks	RIA	Normal	WKY = SHR	Ruskoaho and Leppaluoto (1988)
52 weeks	RIA	Normal	WKY > SHR	Ruskoaho and Leppaluoto (1988)
4 weeks	RIA	Normal	Left: WKY − SHR Right: SHR > WKY	Haass et al. (1987)
14 weeks	RIA	Normal	WKY = SHR	Haass et al. (1987)
9 weeks	RIA	1.0% NaCl 8.0% NaCl	WKY = SHR-SS WKY = SHR-SS	Jin et al. (1988)

[a]SHR, spontaneously hypertensive rat; SHRSP, stroke-prone SHR; SHR-SS, salt-sensitive SHR; WKY, Wistar–Kyoto normotensive rat; RIA, radioimmunoassay.

Summaries of these studies and their assay conditions are provided in Tables IV and V.

An early report by Sonnenberg and colleagues (1983), which featured a bioassay to assess atrial ANF content, indicated that atria from 16- to 17-week-old SHR contained less ANF than age-matched WKY. These workers suggested that reduced cardiac ANF in SHR was due to enhanced chronic secretion of ANF from atrial stores. This view was later supported by the findings of Imada et al. (1985), who showed by radioimmunoassay that circulating ANF in plasma of anesthetized SHR was elevated versus age-matched normotensive WKY rats at 8, 12, and 15 weeks of age, after arterial blood pressure in SHR was significantly increased compared with WKY controls. In addition, left atrial ANF content in SHR was significantly reduced versus WKY at 12 and 15 weeks of age. These findings are supported by the observation that ANF mRNA levels in left atria of SHR were significantly elevated, while immunoreactive ANF in left atria was decreased relative to WKY normotensive controls (Arai et al., 1987), implying increased synthesis and secretion of ANF from this tissue in SHR. Similarly, Gutkowska et al. (1986b) observed that plasma ANF levels in anesthetized SHR, compared with levels for WKY, increased with the progression of hypertension in this strain.

Table V

Plasma Levels of ANF in SHR (and Related Strains)[a]

Age	Sampling condition	Diet	Method	Relative plasma ANF levels	Reference
3 weeks	Pentobarbital anesthesia	Normal	RIA	SHR = WKY	Imada et al. (1985)
8, 12, 15 weeks	Pentobarbital anesthesia	Normal	RIA	SHR > WKY	Imada et al. (1985)
16 weeks	Conscious, undisturbed	Normal	RIA	SHR = WKY	Haass et al. (1986)
5 weeks	Decapitation	Normal	RIA	WKY, SHRSP > SHR	Kato et al. (1987)
10, 20 weeks	Decapitation	Normal	RIA	SHR, SHRSP > WKY	Kato et al. (1987)
4, 16 weeks	Conscious, undisturbed	Normal	RIA	SHR = WKY	Haass et al. (1987)
8, 24 weeks	Conscious, undisturbed	Normal	RIA	SHR = WKY	Ruskoaho and Leppaluoto (1988)
52 weeks	Conscious, undisturbed	Normal	RIA	SHR > WKY	Ruskoaho and Leppaluoto (1988)
20 weeks	Decapitation	Normal 1% NaCl H_2O	RIA	SHR > WKY SHR >> WKY	Kohno et al. (1986)
9 weeks	Conscious, undisturbed	1.0% NaCl 8.0% NaCl	RIA	SHR-SS = WKY SHR-SS = WKY	Jin et al. (1988)

[a]SHR, spontaneously hypertensive rat; SHRSP, stroke-prone SHR; SHR-SS, salt-sensitive SHR; WKY, Wistar–Kyoto normotensive rat; RIA, radioimmunoassay.

Others (Kato et al., 1987) confirmed these results, reporting increased concentrations of ANF in plasma of SHR compared with WKY at 10 and 20 weeks of age, but not at 5 weeks of age, when, in fact, plasma ANF in SHR was markedly lower than in WKY. In addition, these researchers demonstrated that SHRSP rats, which exhibit more rapid increases in arterial pressure, had higher plasma levels of ANF at 5 weeks of age versus age-matched SHR and at 5, 10, and 20 weeks of age versus WKY rats. In contrast to previous findings, however, Kato et al. (1987) found that atrial ANF content was elevated in SHR and SHRSP versus WKY in a manner that reflected the progression of hypertension in these strains. A later study performed by this group (Kato et al., 1988) again pointed to increased levels of immunoreactive ANF in extracted plasma of SHR versus WKY, and further described the presence of ANF immunoreactivity bound to a high-molecu-lar-weight protein in unextracted plasma, possibly a carrier protein for ANF. Ratios of "free" ANF to "bound" ANF were higher in plasma of SHR and SHRSP compared with WKY. The importance of the bound form of ANF, particularly in this model of hypertension, is currently unknown. The studies described so far employed anesthetized animal preparations or involved decapitation for collection of blood samples.

Other laboratories have measured plasma ANF levels in blood of SHR and WKY collected from undisturbed, freely behaving rats and have derived results in sharp contrast to those presented above. An early report (Haass *et al.*, 1986) indicated that both basal and stimulated levels of plasma ANF were similar between 16-week-old SHR and WKY, despite pronounced differences in arterial blood pressure between the strains at this age. These workers later reported that basal plasma ANF concentrations were similar in 1-month-old SHR and WKY, although when challenged with an acute volume expansion, SHR responded with an attenuated release of ANF into plasma as compared with WKY controls (Haass *et al.*, 1987). Similar results were obtained by Morris and co-workers (1987), who measured plasma ANF and vasopressin in conscious SHR, SHRSP, and WKY following both acute volume load with 5% dextrose and hemorrhage (1.5 ml/100 g body weight). In this study, SHR, SHRSP, and WKY at 15–18 weeks of age all exhibited similar baseline and stimulated levels of ANF and vasopressin in plasma, as determined by radioimmunoassay. A more recent study revealed that at 2 and 6 months of age, basal or volume-stimulated plasma ANF levels were similar for SHR and WKY (Ruskoaho and Leppaluoto, 1988). This relationship changed, however, when rats were 12 months old; at this age, baseline values of plasma ANF in SHR were markedly increased as compared to age-matched WKY controls. Still others have obtained nearly identical results in measurements of plasma ANF from conscious SHR and WKY (Petersson *et al.*, 1986; Jin *et al.*, 1988).

Several laboratories have demonstrated that certain antihypertensive treatments can alter circulating levels of ANF in SHR. For instance, chronic treatment of SHR with the angiotensin I converting-enzyme inhibitors captopril or enalapril significantly reduced systolic blood pressure (but not to normotensive values) compared with untreated SHR, and resulted in significant reductions in plasma ANF, again as compared with untreated SHR (Kohno *et al.*, 1987a). Some investigators (Stasch *et al.*, 1987) have shown that chronic administration of the calcium antagonist nisoldipine lowered blood pressure and immunoreactive plasma ANF in 70-week-old SHR to values similar to those in age-matched normotensive WKY controls. In contrast, untreated SHR had greatly increased values of blood pressure and plasma ANF. Another group (Oda *et al.*, 1988) has shown that antihypertensive treatment with CS622, a novel angiotensin-converting-enzyme inhibitor, and hydralazine, a vasodilator, had differential effects on plasma ANF in SHR. Specifically, while chronic treatment with either drug reduced blood pressure to similar degrees in SHR, only CS622 was associated with a concomitant decline in circulating ANF. These findings imply an interaction between ANF and AII in the maintenance of hypertension in this strain.

Others have less directly examined possible interactions between the renin–angiotensin–aldosterone and ANF systems in SHR. Kohno and co-workers (1986) described a significant increase in plasma immunoreactive ANF in 18-week-old SHR maintained for 2 weeks on a high sodium (1% NaCl in tap water) diet as compared with diet-control and pure control SHR and WKY rats. This diet induced a slight, though significant, increase in systolic blood pressure in SHR rats. Another study (Jin et al., 1988) employed 9-week-old SHR sodium-sensitive rats (SHR-SS), which exhibit a pronounced exacerbation of hypertension when placed on a high-sodium (8% NaCl in feed) diet as compared with normal SHR. Rats of this substrain demonstrated no change in plasma levels of ANF regardless of dietary sodium. On the other hand, WKY rats receiving high dietary sodium showed enhanced levels of circulating ANF. These results suggest an impaired capacity of SHR-SS to respond to chronic and acute sodium loads. Additionally, no strain-related differences were noted between SHR-SS and WKY rats maintained on normal feed. Unfortunately, these workers did not include normal SHR as controls in addition to WKY normotensive rats. Their study did, however, benefit from the use of conscious, undisturbed, freely behaving rats during blood collection. Together, these findings may reflect either a relative hyperactivity of the renin–angiotensin–aldosterone system or an impaired ability of ANF systems to antagonize the renin–angiotensin–aldosterone system in SHR.

It seems clear that methods of blood collection, particularly methods that include the use of anesthesia or decapitation, strongly influence determinations of plasma immunoreactive ANF. Studies employing anesthesia or decapitation for collection of blood samples from SHR have consistently reported baseline values of plasma ANF two- to threefold higher than accepted baseline values of circulating ANF in normal, conscious rats (i.e., less than 100 pg/ml) (Horky et al., 1985; Lang et al., 1985; Eskay et al., 1986). Additionally, it has been demonstrated that certain anesthetic agents can strongly influence plasma levels of ANF in rats (Horky et al., 1985; Lang et al., 1985). In contrast, values of circulating ANF derived from plasma of conscious SHR are within the accepted range for plasma ANF in normal rats. For these reasons, reports of increased circulating ANF in SHR should be viewed with caution. Results from preparations employing conscious animals, therefore, probably provide the most accurate indication of baseline ANF secretion in these strains. These results, particularly the findings of elevated plasma ANF in older (12 month) SHR, fit nicely with the findings of increasing heart failure at this age in SHR (in Ruskoaho and Leppaluoto, 1988) and increased concentrations of ANF in plasma of rats with induced chronic heart failure (Tsunoda et al., 1986). In addition, they call attention to the possibility that release of cardiac ventricular ANF may contribute to circulating ANF in these strains.

Takayanagi et al. (1987) described the presence of ANF mRNA in rat ventricles, and further showed that ventricles from 15-week-old SHR rats contained a threefold higher content of immunoreactive ANF as compared to ventricles from age-matched WKY controls. Levels of ANF in ventricles from both strains were several orders of magnitude lower than levels measured in atrial tissue. In agreement with these results, Arai et al. (1988) observed that both ventricular immunoreactive ANF and ANF mRNA were increased in 27-week-old SHR and SHRSP, as compared to age-matched WKY. These increases were not noted in 6-week-old SHR, and only slight elevations in ANF and ANF mRNA were noted in 6-week-old SHRSP, possibly reflecting the effects of increased blood pressure and/or ventricular hypertrophy in these strains. Ruskoaho and Leppaluoto (1988), on the other hand, described decreased ventricular immunoreactive ANF in SHR at 12 months of age, but suggested this was due to enhanced release of ANF from this tissue to compensate for, or inhibit, the development of cardiac hypertrophy in this strain. Furthermore, a recent ultrastructural examination of immunoreactive ANF in heart tissues from SHR and WKY (Gu and Gonzalez-Lavin, 1988) indicated that ventricular (particularly left ventricle) ANF levels increased with the progression of hypertension from 6 to 18 weeks of age in SHR compared with age-matched WKY normotensive controls. These authors suggest, based upon the increased number and size of specific granules containing ANF, that SHR ventricles could contribute significantly to the circulating pool of ANF in SHR. In agreement with some previous results, these workers found atrial levels of the peptide decreased with the development of hypertension in SHR. Notably, the high levels of ANF in ventricles of SHR are similar to levels of the peptide in ventricles of fetal and newborn rats (Cantin et al.,1987). In ventricles of adult normotensive rats, the presence of ANF and secretory granules is practically undetectable. The pathophysiological implications of these unique and curious alterations in the locus of ANF synthesis and secretion in SHR and SHRSP are not well understood, but could prove to be of great significance in understanding the role of ANF in this model of genetic hypertension. A more detailed and complete determination of the dynamics of ANF synthesis and release in relation to the ontogeny of hypertension in SHR should provide more information regarding possible pathophysiological roles for ANF in the development of hypertension in this strain.

B. Physiological Responses to Peripheral Administration of Exogenous ANF in SHR

Many researchers have sought to describe pathological impairment in ANF bioactivity and/or target tissue responsiveness in SHR. To this extent, the effects of peripheral administration of ANF to SHR have met with similar variability in results, probably because of widely divergent ANF dose and administration protocols. These results are summarized in Table VI.

Infusion via miniosmotic pumps of low doses of ANF (100 ng/h) over a 7-day period gradually reduced systolic blood pressure in conscious 14- to 15-week-old SHR to normotensive values, while age-matched normotensive WKY showed no significant change in systolic pressure after this infusion regimen (Garcia *et al.*, 1985b). This reduction of blood pressure in SHR

TABLE VI

Relative Effects of Peripheral Administration of Exogenous ANF on Blood Pressure and Renal Function in Adult SHR and WKY[a]

Delivery	Approximate dose	Delivery time	Lowered BP?	Natriuresis?	Diuresis?	Reference
Infusion	35 pmol/h	7 days	SHR only	No	No	Garcia *et al.* (1985b)
Bolus	350 pmol	Acute	SHR > WKY	SHR > WKY	SHR > WKY	Pang *et al.* (1985)
Infusion	720–3000 pmol/hr	20 min	SHR > WKY	SHR = WKY	SHR = WKY	Marsh *et al.* (1985)
Infusion	5700–11,400 pmol/h	20 min	SHR > WKY	WKY > SHR	WKY > SHR	Marsh *et al.* (1985)
Infusion	160 pmol + 310 pmol/h	90 min	SHR > WKY	SHR only	SHR only	Gellai *et al.* (1986)
Infusion	1600 pmol + 3100 pmol/h	90 min	SHR > WKY	SHR = WKY	SHR = WKY	Gellai *et al.* (1986)
Bolus	16, 160, 1600, 16,000 pmol	Acute	SHR only	N/D	N/D	Gellai *et al.* (1986)
Bolus	1600–160,000 pmol	Acute	SHR only	N/D	N/D	De Mey *et al.* (1987)
Infusion	160 pmol/h	7 days	SHR only	No	No	De Mey *et al.* (1987)
Infusion	1600 pmol/h	7 days	SHR only	No	SHR = WKY	De Mey *et al.* (1987)

[a]SHR, spontaneously hypertensive rat; WKY, Wistar–Kyoto normotensive rat; N/D, not determined.

occurred without any apparent changes in renal water or sodium excretion. A lack of natriuresis or diuresis due to chronic ANF infusion was similarly noted in WKY. In contrast, this same group (Pang *et al.*, 1985) demonstrated later that acute bolus injections of very high doses of ANF (~4 µg/kg) in anesthetized SHR and WKY induced significant, transient declines in arterial pressure and increases in diuresis and natriuresis and urinary cGMP excretion in both strains. While urinary cGMP was elevated to a similar extent in both strains following ANF injection, the blood pressure lowering and natriuretic and diuretic effects were markedly greater in SHR compared with WKY. These early findings immediately indicated differential physiological responses relating to dose and duration of ANF administration.

Roughly similar findings were reported by Marsh and associates (1985), who showed that 20-min infusions of ANF at high doses ranging from 12 to 190 pmol/min decreased arterial blood pressure in both conscious hypertensive SHR and normotensive WKY, although to a significantly greater extent in SHR. At lower loses (12–50 pmol/min) of ANF, renal responsiveness was similar for SHR and WKY. However, at higher doses (95–190 pmol/min), SHR responded with blunted natriuresis and diuresis as compared with WKY. In sharp contrast to the results of Pang *et al.* (1985), these workers described practically no effect of ANF infusion on cGMP excretion in SHR, except a slight increase in urinary cGMP at the highest infusion dose (190 pmol/min). WKY rats responded in a dose-related fashion to all doses of ANF with significantly enhanced cGMP excretion. It is important to note that baseline values of urinary cGMP in SHR were nearly threefold lower than in WKY, according to Marsh *et al.* (1985), while Pang *et al.* (1985) reported similar values of resting urinary cGMP between strains.

Gellai *et al.* (1986) clarified these results somewhat by assessing the differential effects of infusions and bolus injections of low and high doses (bolus: 0.1, 1.0, 10, 100 ng/kg; infusions: 1 µg/kg + 2 µg/h and 10 µg/kg + 20 µg/kg/h) of ANF in conscious, unrestrained SHR and WKY. These researchers observed gradual, dose-dependent reductions in blood pressure in both strains following 90-min infusions of ANF, although SHR showed a significantly greater hypotensive response than WKY. Significant changes in renal sodium and water excretion were noted only in SHR at the high dose infusion. Infusions at the highest dose were also attended by slight, but significant, decreases in heart rate in SHR. Bolus injections of ANF were associated with dose-dependent, transient and rapid decreases in arterial pressure only in SHR without changes in heart rate.

Others (De Mey *et al.*, 1987) have reported that low-dose (4.0 nmol/kg/) infusions of ANF over a 7-day period resulted in pronounced decreases in arterial pressure in SHR, but not in normotensive Sprague-Dawley rats.

Slight increases in renal water excretion were noted in both strains on day 6 of chronic infusion, long after the maximal lowering effect of ANF on blood pressure. Similarly, acute intravenous bolus injection of ANF in low doses (4–400 nmol/kg) reduced blood pressure transiently only in SHR. This study indicated similar rates of ANF biodegradation in renal tissues of both SHR and Sprague-Dawley rats, precluding the possibility that increased duration of ANF activity in SHR could account for the observed strain-related differences in blood pressure responses following ANF administration. ANF was also shown to relax isolated, precontracted aortic strips and mesenteric and coronary microarteries from SHR and Sprague-Dawley rats to similar degrees. It is important to note that infusion doses of ANF in this study were approximately three- to 30-fold higher than the dose utilized by Garcia and colleagues (1985b).

Renal and blood pressure responses to peripheral administration of ANF in SHR and WKY also appear to be labile in response to changes in dietary sodium content. Chronic administration of a relatively low dose of ANF (100 ng/h, 7 days) to conscious, sodium-replete SHR and WKY was found to induce enhanced chronic urinary sodium excretion in SHR only. In a sodium-depleted state induced by low-sodium feed, urinary sodium excretion remained similar between strains (Kondo *et al.*, 1986). In striking contrast to results noted above, these workers observed decrements in blood pressure of similar magnitude following 7 days of ANF infusion, regardless of diet or strain. On the other hand, Gradin and Persson (1987) found that increasing dietary sodium (1.5% NaCl in tap water) for 3 weeks was associated with an attenuated natriuretic response to acute bolus injections of considerably higher amounts of ANF (8 or 16 nmol/kg) in SHR versus diet-WKY and pure-control SHR and WKY rats. These researchers also detected transient reductions in blood pressure of equal magnitude regardless of strain or diet.

Critical differences in these studies clearly include the great variability in doses and in rate and duration of ANF infusions and injections. These factors, among other differences in protocols, necessarily limit assessment of ANF-induced effects to distinct time windows during the physiological response to administration of ANF. A more extensive comparison of the dynamic and equilibrium responses to administered ANF could provide greater, more meaningful insight regarding the physiological responsiveness of SHR to ANF administration. An important consideration in future studies exploring the effects of exogenous ANF in SHR will be the use of doses of ANF that do not represent grossly pharmacological amounts of the peptide.

Despite the variability in the results above, it seems clear that the hypotensive effect of exogenously administered ANF, particularly the enhanced hypotensive response in SHR, is an effect independent of renal responses to ANF. This is reflected in the consistent finding of reductions in blood pressure in SHR often with little or no change in sodium or water excretion. Also, those studies that report changes in renal function concurrent with decreases in blood pressure typically utilized rather high doses of ANF in the form of bolus injections or short-term (hours versus days) infusions (see Table VI). Other support for this notion comes from the work of Garcia et al. (1987), who showed that 5-day continuous infusion of ANF in conscious SHR at 100 ng/h induced no significant changes in plasma, extracellular, blood, or interstitial fluid volumes, but significantly reduced systolic blood pressure to near normotensive levels. Similarly, these parameters were unaffected in conscious WKY normotensive controls, which exhibited no change in systolic blood pressure following chronic ANF infusion. Therefore, large, acute increases in plasma ANF due to high dose, bolus ANF administration or to extreme "natural" stimuli (e.g., hypertonic or volume-expanding stimuli) could recruit renal responses to reinstate immediately a homeostatic balance. It appears likely, however, that chronic, slight increases in plasma ANF observed after chronic ANF administration in several studies (De Mey et al., 1987; Garcia et al., 1987) do not affect renal function appreciably, while they exert pronounced effects on blood pressure.

C. ANF Binding and Bioactivity in Peripheral Tissues of SHR

1. Vasculature

The mechanisms mediating the exaggerated ANF-induced hypotension in SHR remain uncertain, as does the role of ANF in the development and maintenance of hypertension in this strain. In addition to work listed above, research has been focused upon ANF binding and biological activity in several specific tissues. To this extent, one possible explanation for the apparently enhanced hypotensive effect of exogenous ANF administration in SHR could be an increased sensitivity of SHR vasculature to the vasodilatory actions of ANF. In support of this concept, radioreceptor assay of radiolabeled ANF binding to cultured SHR vascular smooth muscle cells from carotid artery revealed significantly elevated numbers of binding sites versus normotensive WKY and American Wistar control cultures (Khalil et al., 1987). However, binding sites in SHR cell cultures had lower affinity for the ligand as compared to WKY and American Wistar. A persistently reduced affinity for ANF at these binding sites could account, in part, for the observation that isolated aorta from 12- and 16-week old SHR are less responsive to ANF than WKY aorta following precontraction with a variety of agents (Sauro and Fitzpatrick, 1987; de Leon et al., 1987). Sauro et al.

(1988) later showed that ANF-induced cGMP production in isolated aortic rings of 8- or 9-week-old SHR was significantly attenuated as compared to tissue from age-matched normotensive WKY. Cauvin et al. (1987) also described a reduced vasodilation response to ANF in isolated, norepinephrine-contracted mesenteric resistance vessels from adult SHR as compared to vessels from WKY. Likewise, Mulvany (1987) found similar relaxant effects of ANF in 20-week-old SHR and WKY isolated renal arcuate arteries, although these tissues from SHR at 5 weeks of age were actually hypersensitive to the application of ANF. ANF binding sites of moderate density have been detected over renal arcuate arteries (Healy and Fanestil, 1986). Taken together, these findings do not support the notion that enhanced vasodilation in SHR after ANF administration results from hyperresponsiveness of vasculature to the peptide.

2. Kidney

The findings of Mulvany (1987) may be reflected in the results of several studies that have addressed the binding of ANF in kidneys of SHR and WKY. Utilizing a radioreceptor assay, Saito et al. (1986) demonstrated in an early study that renal basolateral membranes from 14-week-old SHR and SHRSP had significantly reduced affinity and numbers of binding sites for ANF. However, at 5 weeks of age, prior to the establishment of pronounced hypertension, ANF binding parameters were similar among these strains. In slight contrast, another group (Ogura et al., 1987) was unable to detect by radioreceptor assay any significant differences in values of K_d between SHR and WKY rats, but demonstrated that 12-week-old SHR have greatly reduced values of B_{max} for ANF binding in renal membrane preparations as compared with normotensive WKY controls. Using quantitative autoradiography of whole kidney sections, another laboratory described marked reductions in B_{max} and K_d for ANF binding in renal glomeruli of SHR as compared to WKY at 14 weeks of age (Swithers et al., 1987).

It is attractive to speculate that these apparent age-related alterations in ANF binding in kidney precede the age-related changes in renal arcuate artery responsiveness. Such alterations could be due to elevations in circulating ANF levels. Accordingly, it has been shown that renal ANF binding sites are seemingly sensitive to moderate changes in blood pressure and/or circulating levels of ANF. Treatment of 12-week-old SHR with the antihypertensive agent indapamide was associated with a significant reduction in B_{max} and elevation in affinity for ANF binding in kidney membranes versus untreated control SHR (Ogura et al., 1986). The mechanism of this curious alteration in renal ANF binding site properties may be related to a direct effect of the drug on the receptor protein or to indirect effects of blood pressure lowering. In contrast, Oda et al. (1988) have recently shown that following a 21-week treatment with CS622, a potent angiotensin I converting-enzyme inhibitor, 41-week-old SHR exhibited significantly reduced arterial blood pressure and plasma ANF levels compared with untreated SHR. In addition, CS622-treated SHR exhibited significantly increased values for B_{max} in ANF binding in kidney membranes as compared to untreated SHR. Based upon their findings, these workers suggested that alterations in ANF binding-site profiles in kidneys of SHR noted in earlier studies were due to increases in circulating plasma ANF. However, they failed to examine ANF binding characteristics in kidney membranes of SHR chronically treated with hydralazine from their own study, an intervention that reduced blood pressure but did not reduce plasma levels of ANF. Therefore, while high ambient plasma ANF could account for downregulation of renal ANF binding sites in SHR, such a relationship remains to be established directly.

3. Adrenal Gland

In the adrenal zona glomerulosa, another prominent target tissue for ANF, differences in the biological activity of the peptide between SHR and WKY have not been detected. Data from several studies support this idea nicely. Swithers and her colleagues (1987) were unable to demonstrate strain-related differences in ANF binding to adrenal zona glomerulosa in 14-week-old SHR and normotensive WKY controls. In agreement with these results, Racz *et al.* (1986) and Uchida *et al.* (1987) were unable to reveal any differences in the ability of ANF to inhibit differentially basal or stimulated aldosterone synthesis in adrenal zona glomerulosa cells from SHR and WKY at 12 (Racz *et al.*, 1986) or 14 weeks of age (Uchida *et al.*, 1987). These results suggest that if ANF systems in SHR are defective in their ability to antagonize the effects of the renin–angiotensin–aldosterone system, the site for such a defect probably does not include the adrenal zona glomerulosa. Other peripheral tissues, however, show marked differences in ANF binding that may be related to altered bioactivity of ANF in SHR.

4. Other Peripheral Tissues

Using quantitative autoradiographic techniques, Kurihara *et al.* (1987) examined ANF binding kinetics in spleen cells and thymocytes in SHR and WKY at 4 and 14 weeks of age. Their results indicated that numbers of ANF binding sites in cells from thymic medulla and spleen white pulp were significantly reduced in 4- and 14-week-old SHR as compared to age-matched WKY. Despite the pronounced differences in ANF binding to these tissues, these investigators noted that ANF-stimulated cGMP formation was similar between SHR and WKY. Such discrepant results in binding profiles and biological activity may reflect the existence of so-called "ANF-C," or clearance, receptors, which reportedly possess no biological activity (Maack *et al.*, 1987).

A recent investigation has revealed the presence of immunoreactive ANF and ANF binding sites in sympathetic ganglia. Kuchel and associates (1988) described significant age-related changes in the content of immunoreactive ANF in celiac ganglion of SHR. SHR and WKY at 4 weeks of age showed similar levels of ANF in celiac ganglion, while at 12 weeks of age, after the establishment of hypertension, SHR rats exhibited significantly elevated levels of ANF in this sympathetic ganglion. This alteration was unique to the celiac ganglion, as no strain- or age-related differences in immunoreactive ANF were noted in superior cervical ganglion. Interestingly, Gutkind and colleagues (1987) have detected significant age- and strain-related alteration in ANF binding to superior cervical and stellate ganglia in SHR and WKY. Specifically, SHR at 4 and 14 weeks of age had a profoundly reduced number of binding sites for ANF in these sympathetic ganglia. In contrast, ANF stimulated cGMP production to a similar extent in tissues from both strains. A more thorough examination of ANF binding and biological activity in other sympathetic ganglia, including celiac ganglion, could be quite informative in regard to ANF and sympathetic activity. While the meaning of these alterations is unclear, increased celiac ANF could be related to increased splanchnic nerve outflow in states of hypertension in SHR. Moreover, others (Tsuda *et al.* 1987) have demonstrated that exogenous administration of ANF inhibits electrically stimulated sympathetic nerve norepinephrine outflow to a lesser degree in SHR than in WKY. These results fit well with early reports (Lappe *et al.*, 1985b) that regional vasoconstriction in response to ANF infusion in conscious SHR was related to reflex increases in sympathetic tone. Further experiments examining the role of ANF in the modulation of sympathetic tone and outflow could be of crucial importance and could reveal the mechanisms of the hypotensive activity of ANF.

D. ANF Binding and Bioactivity in Central Tissues of SHR

In the CNS, highly consistent results have been obtained from studies of immunoreactive ANF and ANF binding in brain regions of SHR WKY rats. Several investigators have described significantly increased levels of brain immunoreactive ANF in several hypothalamic and pontine regions of SHR brain (Imada *et al.*, 1985; Ruskoaho and Leppaluoto, 1988; Jin *et al.*, 1988), particularly in the anterior hypothalamus, a region implicated in central regulation of cardiovascular function (Jin *et al.*, 1988). In addition, the absolute hypothalamic content of immunoreactive ANF appears to be reduced in SHR following chronic treatment with the hypotensive agent minoxidil (Ruskoaho and Leppaluoto, 1988). These blood pressure-related changes in brain ANF content in SHR may reflect compensatory responses to increased arterial pressure in this strain.

Quantitative autoradiographic examination of ANF binding characteristics in discrete brain areas of SHR and WKY revealed that 4- and 14-week old SHR rats possessed significantly lower numbers of binding sites for ANF in SFO and choroid plexus versus age-matched normotensive WKY controls (Figure 8) (McCarty and Plunkett, 1986). Moreover, at 14 weeks of age SHR rats exhibited increased affinity for ANF binding in choroid plexus. Roughly similar findings were reported by another group in two separate communications (Saavedra, 1986; Saavedra *et al.*, 1986a), although these investigators failed to detect any strain-related differences in K_d in 19-week-old SHR brain areas (Saavedra *et al.*, 1986a) or indicated a higher K_d in SFO of SHR versus WKY at 14 weeks of age. These studies also addressed binding of ANF to area postrema (AP) but detected no strain-related differences in ANF binding kinetics in this brain area.

A striking overlap of ANF and AII binding sites occurs in several dis-

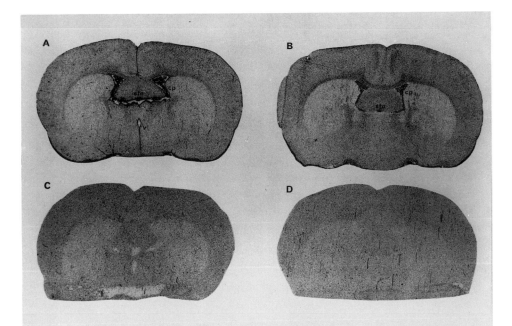

Figure 8 Autoradiographic localization ^{125}I-ANF binding sites in 16-μm coronal sections of representative 4-week-old male SHR and WKY forebrains at the level of the subfornical organ. Sections were incubated in 40 pM ^{125}I-ANF and later opposed to the same sheet of ^{3}H-sensitive ultrofilm for 96 h. (A) 4-Week-old WKY. (B) 4-Week-old SHR. (C,D) Sections from 4-week-old WKY and SHR, respectively, incubated in the presence of 10^{-6} M unlabelled ANF. Note the high density of ANF binding sites in subfornical organ (sfo), choroid plexus (cp), meninges, and the ependymal cells lining the third ventricle (v). Adapted from McCarty and Plunkett (1986).

crete areas of rat brain. Like the distribution of binding sites for ANF in rat brain, high densities of high-affinity binding sites for AII have been demonstrated in SFO and AP, with other areas of overlap including the nucleus of the solitary tract and the organum vasculosum of the lamina terminalis of the hypothalamus (Mendelsohn et al., 1984). Interestingly, binding of ANF and AII to the SFO is inversely related in SHR and WKY rats. SHR rats exhibit augmented AII binding in conjunction with reduced ANF binding in SFO as compared with WKY rats (Saavedra et al., 1986b). The reciprocal alterations in the binding of these important cardiovascular and body fluid regulatory peptides in brain of SHR may indicate a pathological imbalance in their central activities in rats of this strain.

To identify a possible pathological relationship of central ANF and AII systems in SHR, several laboratories have undertaken studies to characterize the effects of ANF and AII administered centrally in SHR. Intracerebroventricular infusions of ANF were shown to attenuate AII-induced drinking to a similar extent in both SHR and WKY (Itoh et al., 1987). However, in SHR a lower dose of ANF was required to suppress deprivation-induced drinking, and the magnitude of this reduction was significantly greater in SHR versus WKY rats. Similarly, chronic icv infusions of ANF were shown to reduce salt appetite significantly in SHR but not in WKY rats. These effects may be related to an enhanced effect of central ANF on the activity of the central renin–angiotensin system in SHR. This apparent hypersensitivity of the central ANF system in SHR is in contrast with data regarding brain ANF binding in this strain. However, as seen in the periphery, such alterations in binding may be related to the existence of biologically silent ANF receptor types. This notion could be reflected by data that demonstrate that ANF-induced cGMP accumulation is significantly enhanced in brain slices from SHR as compared to WKY (Takayanagi et al., 1986). While the authors note that the greatest effect of ANF on cGMP formation was seen in slices that contained areas known to possess dense populations of ANF binding sites, these results must be viewed with extreme caution due to the lack of anatomical resolution afforded by their methods.

While some workers have focused their efforts on the role of central ANF systems in regulating fluid and sodium intake, others have explored the role of central ANF in blood pressure control. As noted earlier, in addition to the pronounced effects of central ANF on fluid and sodium intake, icv ANF attenuates the pressor response to central AII (Shimizu et al., 1986; Casto et al., 1987a). While some have been unable to detect any effect of icv ANF on blood pressure in SHR (Nakamaru et al., 1986), others (Levin et al., 1988) have demonstrated that fourth ventricular infusions of ANF in rather high doses significantly reduced resting arterial pressure to similar extents in both SHR and WKY. Additionally, these workers found that administration of adrenergic agonists or pretreatment with 6-hydroxydopamine abolished the depressor response to icv injections of ANF, implying a relationship between central ANF and α_2-adrenergic mechanisms. However, how such an interaction might be altered or pathological in SHR is unknown. Again, results from these studies have provided divergent results. It is therefore still unclear whether the activity of ANF in brain of SHR is compromised in such a way as to contribute to the pathogenesis of hypertension in this strain. However, continued research into the emerging concept of interactions between brain ANF systems and the sympathetic nervous system and the possible participation of ANF in the regulation of blood pressure could provide information of crucial importance.

VI. Summary and Conclusions

In this chapter, we have summarized the findings of numerous studies regarding ANF systems in two experimental models of genetic hypertension, Dahl and spontaneously hypertensive rats. We have sought to describe the possible involvement of ANF systems in the development and maintenance of hypertension in these widely used models of hypertension. In this regard, we have considered possible pathologies in ANF synthesis and secretion, in tissue responsiveness to exogenous ANF, and in bioactivity and binding properties of ANF in central and peripheral target tissues in both Dahl and spontaneously hypertensive rats.

In Dahl rat lines and inbred rat strains, it appears that ANF systems respond to changes in the homeostatic state of the organism that parallel the increasing severity of hypertension. Based upon available data, it seems that plasma levels of ANF increase in parallel with increasing arterial blood pressure in both DS and S/JR rats. In the S/JR rat strain, examination of ANF binding in several target tissues suggests that age- and strain-related alterations in ANF receptor kinetics occur with the progression of hypertension. Specifically, the number of ANF binding sites is increased in kidney glomeruli of prehypertensive S/JR rats compared with R/JR controls. Later, after the establishment of hypertension in S/JR rats, the numbers of binding sites in kidney glomeruli are similar between strains. In addition, the biological responsiveness to ANF (as determined by cGMP accumulation) in renal tissues of S/JR rats appears to be impaired. In brain, prehypertensive S/JR rats exhibit an elevation in the number of binding sites for ANF in the subfornical organ, a structure important in the regulation of fluid and electrolyte intake and vasopressin secretion. However, a virtual absence of studies describing the effects of ANF in the CNS of Dahl rats, and the widely inconsistent results describing the biological activity of ANF in the periphery of Dahl rats, make an accurate assessment of the role of ANF systems in the development of hypertension in these models of experimental hypertension tenuous at best. Based upon current knowledge, however, it is likely that ANF systems do not contribute significantly to the development of hypertension but are sensitive to homeostatic changes concomitant with the development of hypertension in Dahl rats.

In the SHR and related substrains, a different relationship between the onset of hypertension and ANF systems function exists. In contrast to the Dahl rat models, SHR rats do not exhibit increases in plasma ANF levels that parallel the increasing severity of hypertension. This finding may reveal an important lack in ANF system responsiveness to alterations in homeostatic balance in the SHR, which could serve to aggravate or maintain hypertension in rats of this strain. In this context, it has been shown that the hypotensive actions of exogenously administered ANF tend to be more pronounced in SHR than in WKY, perhaps indicating an increased potential for the utilization of available ANF in SHR. This concept lacks empirical support, as a number of researchers have consistently described decreases in ANF bioactivity and binding in several peripheral tissues of SHR, including kidney and vasculature. It may be, instead, that the hypotensive effects of ANF in SHR are mediated primarily by actions of ANF on sympathetic outflow. This novel issue will be an important area of scientific inquiry in the future, and may provide new views on the role of ANF systems in the development of hypertension in SHR. Taken together, evidence presented in this chapter suggests that peripheral ANF systems do not contribute to the development of hypertension in SHR rats.

The possible involvement of central ANF systems in the pathogenesis of hypertension in SHR rats is unknown. The actions of centrally administered ANF tend to be somewhat more pronounced in SHR than in WKY, but, again, results are inconsistent and inconclusive. Intracerebroventricular injections of ANF into SHR antagonize both spontaneous and AII-induced intake to a greater extent than in WKY. Some have shown that central ANF infusions also exert some effect on blood pressure only in SHR and not in WKY. These results are in apparent contrast with the highly consistent finding of persistent reductions in the numbers of ANF binding sites in several discrete brain areas of SHR. The functional significance of the disparity between central ANF binding and bioactivity is completely unclear, and deserves additional experimental attention. As in the Dahl rat models of hypertension, the central activity of ANF as it pertains to blood pressure regulation and hypertension in SHR is a neglected, though extremely important, issue. Current information can neither support nor refute a role for central ANF systems in the development of hypertension in SHR rat strains.

Generally, the actions of ANF are directed toward the regulation of extracellular volume, renal function, blood pressure, and electrolyte balance. Consistent with the major actions of ANF, specific binding sites for the peptide have been localized in a wide variety of target tissues, including kidney, adrenal gland, and vasculature. Also, several discrete regions of brain thought to be involved in the central regulation of blood pressure and fluid and electrolyte balance have been shown to possess high densities of binding sites for ANF. These areas include the circumventricular organs, nucleus of the solitary tract, and the paraventricular nucleus of the hypothalamus. It has been demonstrated in both the periphery and the brain that ANF serves to antagonize the actions of AII and of the angiotensin–renin–aldosterone system in general. Together, peripheral and central ANF systems constitute an interacting neuroendocrine complex that influences the actions of central and peripheral AII systems to provide sensitive and dynamic mechanisms for the regulation of body fluid, electrolytes, and blood pressure. Because of the pronounced effects of ANF on these parameters, the possible involvement of ANF in hypertension is strongly suspected. The considerable body of information that has accumulated regarding the role of ANF systems in hypertension reflects this notion.

After deBold's first description of the considerable hypotensive effects of ANF in 1981 (deBold et al., 1981), many laboratories quickly sought to evaluate the role of ANF in the maintenance of hypertension in humans and the therapeutic potential for exogenous ANF in hypertensive subjects. Closely resembling results from studies in animal models of hypertension, clinical studies of plasma ANF in several hypertensive types have yielded variable results. Several groups (Sagnella et al., 1986; Kohno et al., 1987b; Iimura et al., 1987) have reported increases in circulating ANF in patients with mild, essential or malignant hypertension, as well as in those with chronic renal failure and primary aldosteronism, presumably a response secondary to increased arterial blood pressure. Other researchers have detected no such differences in circulating levels of plasma ANF in hypertensive patients (Genest et al., 1988). These findings imply that while ANF may be involved in the maintenance of hypertension or may serve to compensate for the homeostatic insults concurrent with hypertension, the peptide does not appear to assume an active role in the disease's onset.

As a treatment for hypertension, ANF does not appear to hold the promise initially anticipated, as currently available means for administration of the peptide in humans permit only acute reductions in blood pressure. In patients with a variety of hypertensive etiologies ANF exerts actions consistent with those noted in animal studies at near-physiological concentrations, but current methods for administration do not support long-term reductions in blood pressure (Volpe et al., 1987; Mantero et al., 1987;

Cody *et al.*, 1987). Until some means for convenient, sustained administration (e.g., oral or transdermal) of the peptide is devised, it is unlikely that ANF will be used widely in the treatment of hypertension.

The results summarized in this chapter tend to support the hypothesis that ANF systems in Dahl and SHR rats do not contribute to the pathogenesis of hypertension in these genetic models of the disease. However, this conclusion is necessarily based upon results that are largely inconsistent and, especially in the case of the central activity of ANF systems, often rare. This may be due to the rapid and highly competitive nature of the research that ensued following deBold's now historic communication in 1981, and, most obviously, from the diversity in methods from study to study. As we have stressed, important methodological considerations exist, particularly regarding collection of blood samples and assessment of the dynamic and static physiological effects of exogenous ANF in the whole animal. In addition, the dearth of data characterizing the central effects of ANF as they relate to hypertension constitutes a void in a potentially important and exciting area of hypertension research. The role of ANF systems in brain and the emerging concept of interactions between the autonomic nervous systems and ANF will be critical areas of scientific inquiry in the coming years. As these issues are addressed, it may be possible to propose more informative and more conclusive hypotheses regarding the roles of ANF systems in experimental genetic hypertension.

Acknowledgments

The authors would like to thank David L. Hill and Jeanine Silveira for helpful criticism of an early version of the manuscript, as well as for support and encouragement. The preparation of this chapter was supported in part by U.S. Public Health Service grant HL29906, ADAMHA Research Scientist Development Award MH00529, and NIH training grant HD07323.

References

Appel, R. G., and Dunn, M. J. (1987). Papillary collecting tubule responsiveness to atrial natriuretic factor in Dahl rats. *Hypertension* 10, 107–114.
Arai, H., Nakao, K., Saito, Y., Morii, N., Sugawara, A., Yamada, T., Itoh, H., Shiono, S., Mukoyama, M., Ohkubo, H., Nakanishi, S., and Imura, H. (1987). Simultaneous measurement of atrial natriuretic polypeptide (ANP) messenger mRNA and ANP in rat heart—Evidence for a preferentially increased synthesis and secretion of ANP in left atrium of spontaneously hypertensive rats (SHR). *Biochem. Biophys. Res. Commun.* 148, 239–245.
Arai, H., Nakao, K., Saito, Y., Morii, N., Sugawara, A., Yamada, T., Itoh, H., Shiono, S., Mukoyama, M., Ohkubo, H., Nakanishi, S., and Imura, H. (1988). Augmented expres-

sion of atrial natriuretic polypeptide gene in ventricles of spontaneously hypertensive rats (SHR) and SHR-stroke prone. *Circ. Res.* **62,** 926–930.

Atlas, S. A., and Laragh, J. H. (1986). Atrial natriuretic peptide: A new factor in hormonal control of blood pressure and electrolyte homeostasis. *Annu. Rev. Med.* **37,** 397–414.

Atlas, S. A., Volpe, M., Sosa, R. E., Laragh, J. H., Camargo, M. J. F., and Maack, T. (1986). Effects of atrial natriuretic factor on blood pressure and the renin–angiotensin–aldosterone system. *Fed. Proc., Fed. Am. Soc. Exp. Biol.* **45,** 2115–2121.

Bianchi, C., Gutkowska, J., Ballak, M., Thibault, G., Garcia, R., Genest, J., and Cantin, M. (1986). Radioautographic localization of ^{125}I-atrial natriuretic factor binding sites in the brain. *Neuroendocrinology* **44,** 365–372.

Bloch, K. D., Scott, J. A., Zisfein, J. B., Fallon, J. T., Margolies, M. N., Seidman, C. E., Matsueda, G. R., Homcy, C. J., Graham, R. M., and Seidman, J. G. (1985). Biosynthesis and secretion of proatrial natriuretic factor by cultured rat atriocytes. *Science* **230,** 1168–1171.

Brody, M. J., and Johnson, A. K. (1980). Role of the anteroventral third ventricle (AV3V) region in fluid and electrolyte balance, arterial pressure regulation, and hypertension. *In* "Frontiers in Neuroendocrinology" (L. Martini and W. F. Ganong, eds.), Vol. 6, pp. 249–292. Raven Press, New York.

Buranarugsa, P., and Hubbard, J. I. (1988). Excitatory effects of atrial natriuretic peptide on rat subfornical organ neurons *in vitro*. *Brain Res. Bull.* **20,** 627–631.

Burnett, J. G., Granger, J. P., and Opgenorth, T. S. (1984). Effects of synthetic atrial natriuretic factor on renal function and renin release. *Am. J. Physiol.* **247,** F863–F866.

Cantin, M., and Genest, J. (1985). The heart and the atrial natriuretic factor. *Endocr. Rev.* **6,** 107–127.

Cantin, M., Ding, J., Thibault, G., Gutkowska, J., Salmi, R., Garcia, R., and Genest, J. (1987). Immunoreactive atrial natriuretic factor is present in both atria and ventricles. *Mol. Cell. Endocrinol.* **52,** 105–113.

Casto, R., Hilbig., J., Schroeder., G., and Stock, G. (1987a). Atrial natriuretic factor inhibits central angiotensin II pressor responses. *Hypertension* **9,** 473–477.

Casto, R., Keiler, I., Schroeder, G., and Stock, G. (1987b). Angiotensin II-induced vasopressin release is attenuated by central atrial natriuretic factor. *Clin. Exp. Hypertens., Part A* **A9,** 81–94.

Cauvin, C., Tejerina, M., and van Breemen, C. (1987). Effects of atriopeptin III on isolated mesenteric resistance vessels from SHR and WKY. *Am. J. Physiol.* **253,** H1612–H1617.

Cody, R. J., Atlas, S. A., and Laragh, J. H. (1987). Physiological and pharmacologic studies of atrial natriuretic factor: A natriuretic and vasoactive peptide. *J. Clin. Pharmacol.* **27,** 927–936.

deBold, A. J., Borenstein, H. B., and Veress, A. T. (1981). A rapid and potent natriuretic response to intravenous injection of atrial myocardial extract in rats. *Life Sci.* **28,** 89–94.

de Leon, H., Castaneda-Hernandez, G., and Hong, F. (1987). Decreased ANF atrial content and vascular reactivity to ANF in spontaneous and renal hypertensive rats. *Life Sci.* **41,** 341–348.

De Mey, J. G., Defreyn, G., Lenaers, A., Calderon, P., and Roba, J. (1987). Arterial reactivity, blood pressure and plasma levels of atrial natriuretic peptides in normotensive and hypertensive rats: Effects of acute and chronic administration of atriopeptin III. *J. Cardiovasc. Pharmacol.* **9,** 525–535.

Edwards, B. S., Zimmerman, R. S., Schwab, T. R., Heublein, D. M., and Burnett, J. C., Jr. (1988). Atrial stretch, not pressure is the principal determinant controlling the acute release of atrial natriuretic factor. *Circ. Res.* **62,** 191–195.

Eskay, R., Zukowska-Grojec, Z., Haass, M., and Dave, J. R. (1986). Circulating atrial natri-uretic peptides in conscious rats: Regulation of release by multiple factors. *Science* 232, 636–639.

Fitts, D. A., Thunhorst, R. L., and Simpson, J. B. (1985). Diuresis and reduction of salt appetite by lateral ventricular infusions of atriopeptin II. *Brain Res.* 348, 118–124.

Garcia, R., Thibault, G., Gutkowska, J., Hamet, P., Cantin, M., and Genest, J. (1985a). Effects of chronic infusion of atrial natriuretic factor (ANF 8-33) in conscious two-kidney, one-clip hypertensive rats. *Proc. Soc. Exp. Biol. Med.* 178, 155–159.

Garcia, R., Thibault, G., Gutkowska, J., Horky, K., Hamet, P., Cantin, M., and Genest, J. (1985b). Chronic infusion of low doses of atrial natriuretic factor (ANF Arg101-Tyr126) reduces blood pressure in conscious SHR without apparent changes in sodium excretion. *Proc. Soc. Exp. Biol. Med.* 179, 396–401.

Garcia, R., Cantin, M., Genest, J., Gutkowska, J., and Thibault, G. (1987). Body fluids and plasma atrial peptides after its chronic infusion in hypertensive rats. *Proc. Soc. Exp. Biol. Med.* 185, 352–358.

Gellai, M., DeWolf, R. E., Kinter, L. B., and Beeuwkes III, R. (1986). The effect of atrial natriuretic factor on blood pressure, heart rate, and renal functions in conscious, spon-taneously hypertensive rats. *Circ. Res.* 59, 56–62.

Genest, J., Larochelle, P., Cusson, A. R., Garcia, R., Gutkowska, J., and Cantin, M. (1988). The atrial natriuretic factor in hypertension. *Am. J. Med. Sci.* 295, 299–304.

Goodfriend, T. L., Elliot, M., and Atlas, S. A. (1984). Actions of synthetic atrial natriuretic factor on bovine adrenal zona glomerulosa. *Life Sci.* 35, 1675–1682.

Gradin, K., and Persson, B. (1987). Renal and cardiovascular effects of atrial natriuretic pep-tide in Wistar-Kyoto and spontaneously hypertensive rats during a chronic salt loading. *Acta Physiol. Scand* 131, 273–281.

Gu, J., and Gonzalez-Lavin, L. (1988). Light and electron microscopic localization of atrial natriuretic peptide in the heart of spontaneously hypertensive rat. *J. Histochem. Cyto-chem.* 36, 1239–1249.

Gutkind, J. S., Kurihara, M., Castren, E., and Saavedra, J. M. (1987). Atrial natriuretic peptide receptors in sympathetic ganglia: Biochemical response and alterations in genetically hypertensive rats. *Biochem. Biophys. Res. Commun.* 149, 65–72.

Gutkowska, J., Kuchel, O., Racz, K., Buu, N. T., Cantin, M., and Genest, J. (1986a). Increased plasma immunoreactive atrial natriuretic factor concentrations in salt-sensitive Dahl rats. *Biochem. Biophys. Res. Commun.* 136, 411–416.

Gutkowska, J., Horky, K., Lachance, D., Racz, K., Garcia, R., Thibault, G., Kuchel, O., Gen-est, J., and Cantin, M. (1986b). Atrial natriuretic factor (ANF) in spontaneously hyper-tensive rats. *Hypertension* 8, Suppl. I, I-137–I-140.

Haass, M., Zamir, N., and Zukowska-Grojec, Z. (1986). Plasma levels of atrial natriuretic peptides in conscious adult spontaneously hypertensive rats. *Clin. Exp. Hypertens., Part A* A8, 277–287.

Haass, M., Zamir, N., and Zukowska-Grojec, Z. (1987). Circulating atrial natriuretic peptides in spontaneously hypertensive rats: Altered secretion in early hypertension. *J. Cardi-ovasc. Pharmacol.* 10, Suppl. 5, S28–S33.

Healy, D. P., and Fanestil, D. D. (1986). Localization of atrial natriuretic polypeptide binding sites within the rat kidney. *Am. J. Physiol.* 250, F573–F578.

Higuchi, K., Hashiguchi, T., Ohashi, M., Takayanagi, R., Haji, M., Matsuo, H., and Nawata, H. (1989). Porcine brain natriuretic peptide receptor in bovine adrenal cortex. *Life Sci.* 44, 881–886.

Hinko, A., Thibonnier, M., and Rapp, J. P. (1987). Binding characteristics of atrial factor and the production of cyclic GMP in kidneys of Dahl salt-sensitive and salt-resistant rats. *Biochem. Biophys. Res. Commun.* 144, 1076–1083.

Hirata, Y., Ganguli, M., Tobian, L., and Iwai, J. (1984). Dahl S rats have increased natriuretic factor in atria but are markedly hyporesponsive to it. *Hypertension* **6**, Suppl. I, I-148–I-155.

Hirata, Y., Hirose, S., Takata, S., Takagi, Y., and Matsubara, H. (1987). Down-regulation of atrial natriuertic peptide receptor and cyclic GMP response in cultured rat vascular smooth muscle cells. *Eur. J. Pharmacol.* **135**, 439–442.

Holmes, H. R., Hurley, K. M., and Saper, C. B. (1988). Localization of atrial and brain natriuretic peptides in the rat brain. *Soc. Neurosci. Abstr.* **14**, 354.

Horky, K., Gutkowska, J., Garcia, R., Thibault, G., and Genest, J. (1985). Effect of different anesthetics on immunoreactive atrial natriuretic factor in rat plasma. *Biochem. Biophys. Res. Commun.* **129**, 651–657.

Iimura, O., Shimamoto, K., Ando, T., Ura, N., Ishida, H., Nakagawa, M., Yokoyama, T., Fukuyama, S., Yamaguchi, Y., and Yamaji, I. (1987). Plasma levels of human atrial natriuretic peptide in patients with hypertensive diseases. *Can. J. Physiol. Pharmacol.* **65**, 1701–1705.

Imada, T., Takayanagi, R., and Inagami, T. (1985). Changes in the content of atrial natriuretic factor with the progression of hypertension in spontaneously hypertensive rats. *Biochem. Biophys. Res. Commun.* **133**, 759–765.

Israel, A., and Barbella, Y. (1986). Diuretic and natriuretic action of rat atrial natriuretic peptide (6-33) administered intracerebroventricularly in rats. *Brain Res. Bull.* **17**, 141–144.

Itoh, H., Nakao, K., Morii, N., Sugawara, A., Yamada, T., Shiono, S., Saito, Y., Mukoyama, M., Arai, H., Sakamoto, M., and Imura, H. (1987). Central actions of atrial natriuretic polypeptides in spontaneously hypertensive and normotensive rats. *Jpn. Cir. J.* **51**, 1208–1215.

Itoh, H., Nakao, K., Yamada, T., Shirakami, G., Kangawa, K., Minamino, N., Matsuo, H., and Imura, H. (1988). Antidipsogenic action of a novel peptide, 'brain natriuretic peptide', in rats. *Eur. J. Pharmacol.* **150**, 193–196.

Itoh, H., Nakao, K., Saito, Y., Yamada, T., Shirakami, M., Arai, H., Hosoda, K., Suga, S., Minamino, N., Kangawa, K., Matsuo, H., and Imura, H. (1989). Radioimmunoassay for brain natriuretic peptide (BNP): Detection of BNP in canine brain. *Biochem. Biophys. Res. Commun.* **158**, 120–128.

Jacobowitz, D. M., Skofitsch, G., Keiser, H. R., Eskay, R. L., and Zamir, N. (1985). Evidence for the existence of atrial natriuretic factor-containing neurons in the rat brain. *Neuroendocrinology* **40**, 92–94.

Jin, H., Chen, Y.-F., Yand, R.-H., Meng, Q. C., and Oparil, S. (1988). Impaired release of atrial natriuretic factor in NaCl-loaded spontaneously hypertensive rats. *Hypertension* **11**, 739–744.

Johnson, A. K. (1985). The periventricular anteroventral third ventricle (AV3V): Its relationship with the subfornical organ and neural systems involved in maintaining body fluid homeostasis. *Brain Res. Bull.* **15**, 595–601.

Kato, J., Kida, O., Nakamura, S., Sasaki, A., Kodama, K., and Tanaka, K. (1987). Atrial natriuretic peptide (ANP) in the development of spontaneously hypertensive rats (SHR) and stroke-prone SHR (SHRSP). *Biochem. Biophys. Res. Commun.* **143**, 316–322.

Kato, J., Kida, O., Kita, T., Nakamura, S., Sasaki, A., Kodama, K., and Tanaka, K. (1988). Free and bound forms of atrial natriuretic peptide (ANP) in rat plasma: Preferential increase of free ANP in spontaneously hypertensive rats (SHR) and stroke-prone SHR (SHRSP). *Biochem. Biophys. Res. Commun.* **153**, 1084–1089.

Kawata, M., Nakao, K., Morii, N., Kiso, Y., Yamashita, H., Imura, H., and Sano, Y. (1985). Atrial natriuretic polypeptide: Topographical distribution in the rat brain by radioimmunoassay and immunohistochemistry. *Neuroscience* **16**, 521–546.

Khalil, F., Fine, B., Kuriyama, S., Hatori, N., Nakamura, A., Nakamura, M., and Aviv, A.

(1987). Increased atrial natriuretic factor receptor density in cultured vascular smooth muscle cells of the spontaneously hypertensive rat. *Clin. Exp Hypertens., Part A* **A9**, 741–752.

Kohno, M., Sambhi, M. P., Eggena, P., Clegg, K., Kanayama, Y., Takaori, K., and Takeda, T. (1986). An accelerated increase of circulating atrial natriuretic polypeptide in salt-loaded spontaneously hypertensive rats. *Horm. Metab. Res.* **18**, 147–148.

Kohno, M., Yasunari, K., Matsuura, T., Kanayama, Y., Takaori, K., Murakawa, K., and Takeda, T. (1987a). Effect of chronic treatment with angiotensin I converting enzyme inhibitors on circulating atrial natriuretic polypeptide in spontaneously hypertensive rats. *Clin. Exp. Hypertens., Part A* **A9**, 693–696.

Kohno, M., Yasunari, K., Matsuura, T., Murakawa, K., and Takeda, T. (1987b). Circulating atrial natriuretic polypeptide in essential hypertension. *Am. Heart J.* **113**, 1160–1163.

Kondo, K., Kida, O., Sasaki, A., Kato, J., and Tanaka, K. (1986). Natriuretic effect of chronically administered α human atrial natriuretic polypeptide in sodium depleted or repleted conscious spontaneously hypertensive rats. *Clin. Exp. Pharmacol. Physiol.* **13**, 417–424.

Kuchel, O., Debinski, W., Buu, N. T., Cantin, M., and Genest, J. (1988). Ganglionic immunoreactive atrial natriuretic factor in rat experimental hypertension. *Hypertension* **11**, Suppl. I, I-47–I-51.

Kudo, T., and Baird, A. (1984). Inhibition of aldosterone production in the adrenal zona glomerulosa by atrial natriuretic factor. *Nature (London)* **312**, 756–757.

Kurihara, M., Castren, E., Gutkind, J. S., and Saavedra, J. M. (1987). Lower number of atrial natriuretic peptide receptors in thymocytes and spleen cells of spontaneously hypertensive rats. *Biochem. Biophys. Res. Commun.* **149**, 1132–1140.

Lang, R. E., Tholken, H., Ganten, D., Luft, F. C., Ruskoaho, H., and Unger, T. (1985). Atrial natriuretic factor—A circulating hormone stimulated by volume-loading. *Nature (London)* **314**, 264–266.

Lappe, R. W., Smits, J. F. M., Todt, J. A., Debet, J. J. M., and Wendt, R. L. (1985a). Failure of atriopeptin II to cause arterial vasodilation in the conscious rat. *Circ. Res.* **56**, 606–612.

Lappe, R. W., Todt, J. A., and Wendt, R. L. (1985b). Mechanism of action of vasoconstrictor responses to atriopeptin II in conscious SHR. *Am. J. Physiol.* **249**, R781–R786.

Lee, J., Feng, J. Q., Malvin, R. L., Huang, B.-S., and Grekin, R. J. (1987). Centrally administered atrial natriuretic factor increases renal water excretion. *Am. J. Physiol.* **252**, F1011–F1015.

Levin, E. R., Weber, M. A., and Mills, S. (1988). Atrial natriuretic factor-induced vasodepression occurs through central nervous system. *Am. J. Physiol.* **255**, H616–H622.

Maack, T., Suzuki, M., Almeida, F. A., Nussenveig, D., Scarborough, R. M., McEnroe, G. A., and Lewicki, J. A. (1987). Physiological role of silent receptors of atrial natriuretic factor. *Science* **238**, 675–678.

Mantero, F., Rocco, S., Pertile, F., Carpene, G., Fallo, F., Leone, L., and Boscaro, M. (1987). Effect of alpha-human atrial natriuretic peptide in low renin essential hypertension and primary aldosteronism. *Clin. Exp. Hypertens., Part A* **A9**, 1505–1513.

Marsh, E. A., Seymour, A. A., Haley, A. B., Whinnery, M. A., Napier, M. A., Nutt, R. F., and Blaine, E. H. (1985). Renal and blood pressure responses to synthetic atrial natriuretic factor in spontaneously hypertensive rats. *Hypertension* **7**, 386–391.

Masotto, C., and Negro-Vilar, A. (1985). Inhibition of spontaneous or angiotensin II-stimulated water intake by atrial natriuretic factor. *Brain Res. Bull.* **15**, 523–526.

McCarty, R., and Plunkett, L. M. (1986). Forebrain binding sites for atrial natriuretic factor: Alterations in spontaneously hypertensive (SHR) rats. *Neurochem. Int.* **9**, 177–183.

Mendelsohn. F. A. O., Quirion, R., Saavedra, J. M., Aguilera, G., and Catt, K. J. (1984). Autoradiographic localization of angiotensin II receptors in rat brain. *Proc. Natl. Acad. Sci.* 81, 1575–1579.

Morris, M., Cain, M., and Chalmers, J. (1987). Complementary changes in plasma atrial natriuretic peptide and antidiuretic hormone concentrations in response to volume expansion and haemorrhage: Studies in conscious normotensive and spontaneously hypertensive rats. *Clin. Exp. Pharmacol. Physiol.* 14, 283–289.

Mulvany, M. J. (1987). Enhanced dilatation by atrial natriuretic peptide of renal arcuate arteries from young, but not adult, spontaneously hypertensive rats. *Clin. Exp. Hypertens., Part A* A9, 1789–1801.

Nagaoki, A., and Lovenberg, W. (1976). Plasma norepinephrine and dopamine β-hydroxylase in genetic hypertensive rats. *Life Sci.* 19, 29–34.

Nakamaru, M., Takayanagi, R., and Inagami, T. (1986). Effect of atrial natriuretic factor on central angiotensin II-induced responses in rats. *Peptides (N.Y)* 7, 373–375.

Naruse, M., Higashida, T., Naruse, K., Shibasaki, T., Demura, H., Inagami, T., and Shizume, K. (1987). Coronary hemodynamics and cardiac beating modulate atrial natriuretic factor release from isolated Langendorff-perfused rat hearts. *Life Sci.* 41, 421–427.

Neuser, D., and Bellemann, P. (1987). Receptor binding, cGMP stimulation and receptor desensitization by atrial natriuretic peptides in cultured A10 vascular smooth muscle cells. *FEBS Lett.* 209, 347–351.

Oda, T., Iijima, Y., Sada, T., Nishino, H., Oizumi, K., and Koike, H. (1988). Effects of chronic treatment with a novel angiotensin converting enzyme inhibitor, CS622, and a vasodilator, hydralazine, on atrial natriuretic factor (ANF) in spontaneously hypertensive rats (SHR). *Biochem. Biophys. Res. Commun.* 152, 456–462.

Oehlenschlager, W. F., Baron, D. A., Schomer, H., and Currie, M. G. (1989). Atrial and brain natriuretic peptides share binding sites in the kidney and heart. *Eur. J. Pharmacol.* 161, 159–164.

Ogura, T., Mitsui, T., Yamamoto, I., Katayama, E., Ota, Z., and Ogawa, N. (1986). Effect of indapamide on atrial natriuretic polypeptide receptor in spontaneously hypertensive rat kidney. *Res. Commun. Chem. Pathol. Pharmacol.* 54, 291–298.

Ogura, T., Mitsui, T., Yamamoto, I., Katayama, E., Ota, Z., and Ogawa, N. (1987). Differential changes in atrial natriuretic peptide and vasopressin receptor bindings in kidney of spontaneously hypertensive rat. *Life Sci.* 40, 233–238.

Onwochei, M. O., Snajdar, R. M., and Rapp, J. P. (1987). Release of atrial natriuretic factor from heart-lung preparations of inbred Dahl rats. *Am. J. Physiol.* 253, H1044-H1052.

Pang, S. C., Hoang, M.-C., Trembley, J., Cantin, M., Garcia, R., Genest, J., and Hamet, P. (1985). Effect of natural and synthetic atrial natriuretic factor on arterial blood pressure, natriuresis and cyclic GMP excretion in spontaneously hypertensive rats. *Clin. Sci.* 69, 721–726.

Petersson, A., Rickstein, S. E., Towle, A., Gradin, K., Persson, B., Hedner, J., and Hedner, T. (1986). On the role of atrial natriuretic peptide in cardiovascular regulation in the spontaneously hypertensive rat. *J. Hypertens.* 4, Suppl. 3, S339–S342.

Poole, C. J. M., Carter, D., and Lightman, S. L. (1987). Intracerebroventricular atriopeptin III inhibits vasopressin and oxytocin secretion following haemorrhage in conscious rats. *Neurosci. Lett.* 9, 249–254.

Quirion, R. (1988). Atrial natriuretic factors and the brain: An update. *Trends Neurosci.* 11, 58–62.

Quirion, R., Dalpe, M., De Lean, A., Gutkowska, J., Cantin, M., and Genest, J. (1984). Atrial natriuretic factor (ANF) binding sites in brain and related structures. *Peptides (N.Y.)* 5, 1167–1172.

Quirion, R., Dalpe, M., and Dam, T.-V. (1986). Characterization and distribution of receptors for the atrial natriuretic peptides in mammalian brain. *Proc. Natl. Acad. Sci. U.S.A.* **83,** 174–178.

Racz, K., Kuchel, O., Buu, N. T., Gutkowska, J., Debinski, W., Cantin, M., and Genest, J. (1986). Zona glomerulosa cell responses to atrial natriuretic factor in genetically hypertensive rats. *Am. J. Physiol.* **251,** H689–H692.

Rapp, J. (1982). Dahl salt-susceptible and salt-resistant rats. *Hypertension* **4,** 753–763.

Rapp, J. (1984). Characteristics of Dahl salt-susceptible and salt-resistant rats. *Hand. Hypertens.* **4,** 286–296.

Roubert, P., Lonchampt, M. O., Chabrier, P. E., Plas, P., Goulin, J., and Braquet, P. (1987). Down-regulation of atrial natriuretic factor receptors and correlation with cGMP stimulation in rat cultured vascular smooth muscle cells. *Biochem. Biophys. Res. Commun.* **148,** 61–67.

Ruskoaho, H., and Leppaluoto, J. (1988). Immunoreactive atrial natriuretic peptide in ventricles, atria, hypothalamus and plasma of genetically hypertensive rats. *Cir. Res.* **62,** 384–394.

Saavedra, J. M. (1986). Atrial natriuretic peptide (6-33) binding sites: Decreased number and affinity in the subfornical organ of spontaneously hypertensive rats. *J. Hypertens.* **4,** Suppl. 3, S313–S316.

Saavedra, J. M., Israel, A., Kurihara, M., and Fuchs, E. (1986a). Decreased number and affinity of rat atrial natriuretic peptide (6-33) binding sites in the subfornical organ of spontaneously hypertensive rats. *Circ. Res.* **58,** 389–392.

Saavedra, J. M., Correa, F. M. A., Plunkett, L. M., Israel, A., Kurihara, M., and Shigematsu, K. (1986b). Binding of angiotensin and atrial natriuretic peptide in brain of hypertensive rats. *Nature (London)* **320,** 758–760.

Sagnella, G. A., Shore, A. C., Markandu, N. D., and MacGregor, G. A. (1986). Raised circulating levels of atrial natriuretic peptides in essential hypertension. *Lancet* **1,** 179–181.

Saito, H., Inui, K., Matsukawa, Y., Okano, T., Maegawa, H., Nakao, K., Morii, N., Imura, H., Makino, S., and Hori, R. (1986). Specific binding of atrial natriuretic polypeptide to renal basolateral membranes in spontaneously hypertensive rats (SHR) and stroke-prone SHR. *Biochem. Biophys. Res. Commun.* **137,** 1079–1085.

Saito, Y., Nakao, K., Itoh, H., Yamada, T., Mukoyama, M., Arai, H., Hosoda, K., Shirakami, G., Suga, S., Minamino, N., Kangawa, K., Matsuo, H., and Imura, H. (1989). Brain natriuretic peptide is a novel cardiac hormone. *Biochem. Biophys. Res. Commun.* **158,** 360–368.

Sasaki, A., Kida, O., Kangawa, K., Matsuo, H., and Tanaka, K. (1985). Hemodynamic effects of α-human atrial natriuretic polypeptide (α-hANP) in rats. *Eur. J. Pharmacol.* **109,** 405–408.

Sauro, M. D., and Fitzpatrick, D. F. (1987). Decreased sensitivity of spontaneously hypertensive rat aortic smooth muscle to vasorelaxation by atriopeptin III. *Biochem. Biophys. Res. Commun.* **146,** 80–86.

Sauro, M. D., Fitzpatrick, D. F., and Coffey, R. G. (1988). Defective cyclic GMP accumulation in spontaneously hypertensive rat aorta in response to atrial natriuretic factor. *Biochem. Pharmacol.* **37,** 2109–2112.

Seymour, A. A., Sweet, C. S., Stabilito, I. T., and Emmert, S. E. (1987). Cardiac and hemodynamic responses to synthetic atrial natriuretic factor in rats. *Life Sci.* **40,** 511–519.

Shimizu, T., Katsuura, G., Nakamura, M., Nakao, K., Morii, N., Itoh, Y., Shiono, S., and Imura, H. (1986). Effect of intracerebroventricular atrial natriuretic polypeptide on blood pressure and urine production in rats. *Life Sci.* **39,** 1263–1270.

Shiono, S., Nakao, K., Morii, N., Yamada, T., Itoh, H., Sakamoto, M., Sugawara, A., Saito, Y., Katsuura, G., and Imura, H. (1986). Nature of atrial natriuretic polypeptide in rat brain. *Biochem. Biophys. Res. Commun.* **135**, 728–734.

Shirakami, G., Nakao, K., Yamada, T., Itoh, H., Mori, K., Kangawa, K., Minamino, N., Matsuo, H., and Imura, H. (1988). Inhibitory effect of brain natriuretic peptide on central angiotensin II-stimulated pressor response in conscious rats. *Neurosci. Lett.* **91**, 77–83.

Snajdar, R. M., and Rapp, J. P. (1985). Atrial natriuretic factor in Dahl rats. Atrial content and renal and aortic responses. *Hypertension* **7**, 775–782.

Snajdar, R. M., and Rapp, J. P. (1986). Elevated atrial natriuretic polypeptide in plasma of hypertensive Dahl salt-sensitive rats. *Biochem. Biophys. Res. Commun.* **137**, 876–883.

Snajdar, R. M., Dene, H., and Rapp, J. P. (1987). Partial characterization of atrial natriuretic factor in the hearts of Dahl salt-sensitive and salt-resistant rats. *Endocrinology (Baltimore)* **120**, 2512–2520.

Sonnenberg, H., Milojevic, S., Chong, C. K., and Veress, A. T. (1983). Atrial natriuretic factor: Reduced cardiac content in spontaneously hypertensive rats. *Hypertension* **5**, 672–675.

Sonnenberg, H., Honrath, U., Chong, C. K., Milojevic, S., and Veress, A. T. (1987). Renal responses to saline and atrial natriuretic factor infusions in rats. *Can. J. Physiol. Pharmacol.* **65**, 1680–1683.

Standaert, D. G., Needleman, P., and Saper, C. B. (1986). Organization of atriopeptin-like immunoreactive neurons in the central nervous system of the rat. *J. Comp. Neurol.* **253**, 315–341.

Standaert, D. G., Cechetto, D. F., Needleman, P., and Saper, C. B. (1987). Inhibition of the firing of vasopressin neurons by atriopeptin. *Nature (London)* **329**, 151–153.

Stasch, J.-P., Kazda, S., Hirth, C., and Morich, F. (1987). Role of nisoldipine on blood pressure, cardiac hypertrophy, and atrial natriuretic peptides in spontaneously hypertensive rats. *Hypertension* **10**, 303–307.

Sterzel, R. B., Luft, F. C., Gao, Y., Lang, R. E., Ruskoaho, H., and Ganten, D. (1987). Atrial natriuretic factor in sodium-sensitive and sodium-resistant Dahl rats. *J. Hypertens.* **5**, 17–24.

Stewart, R. E., Swithers, S. E., and McCarty, R. (1987). Alterations in binding sites for atrial natriuretic factor in kidneys and adrenal glands of Dahl hypertension-sensitive rats. *J. Hypertens.* **5**, 481–487.

Stewart, R. E., Swithers, S. E., Plunkett, L. M., and McCarty, R. (1988a). ANF receptors: Distribution and regulation in central and peripheral tissues. *Neurosci. Biobehav. Rev.* **12**, 151–168.

Stewart, R. E., Swithers, S. E., and McCarty, R. (1988b). Brain binding sites for atrial natriuretic factor (ANF): Alterations in prehypertensive Dahl salt-sensitive (S/JR) rats. *Brain Res. Bull.* **20**, 1–8.

Sudoh, T., Kangawa, K., Minamino, N., and Matsuo, H. (1988). A new natriuretic peptide in porcine brain. *Nature (London)* **332**, 78–81.

Swithers, S. E., Stewart, R. E., and McCarty, R. (1987). Binding sites for atrial natriuretic factor (ANF) in kidneys and adrenal glands of spontaneously hypertensive (SHR) rats. *Life Sci.* **40**, 1673–1681.

Takayanagi, R., Grammer, R. T., and Inagami, T. (1986). Regional increase of cyclic GMP by atrial natriuretic factor in rat brain: Markedly elevated response in spontaneously hypertensive rats. *Life Sci.* **39**, 573–580.

Takayanagi, R., Imada, T., and Inagami, T. (1987). Synthesis and presence of atrial natriuretic factor in rat ventricle. *Biochem. Biophys. Res. Commun.* **142**, 483–488.

Tanaka, I., and Inagami, T. (1986). Increased concentration of plasma immunoreactive atrial natriuretic factor in Dahl salt-sensitive rats with sodium chloride-induced hypertension. *J. Hypertens.* **4,** 109–112.

Tang, C. S., Cui, H., Yuan, Q. X., and Tang, J. (1989). Hemodynamic responses to BNP in rats. *Eur. J. Pharmacol.* **159,** 327–328.

Thibault, G., Garcia, R., Gutkowska, J., Lazure, C., Seidah, N. G., Chrétien, M., Genest, J., and Cantin, M. (1986). Identification of the released form of atrial natriuretic factor by the perfused rat heart. *Proc. Soc. Exp. Biol. Med.* **182,** 137–141.

Tsuda, K., Shima, H., Nishio, I., and Masuyama, Y. (1987). Inhibitory action of alpha-human atrial natriuretic polypeptide on vascular adrenergic neurotransmission is attenuated in spontaneously hypertensive rat. *Jpn. Cir. J.* **51,** 589–593.

Tsunoda, K., Hodsman, G. P., Sumithran, E., and Johnston, C. I. (1986). Atrial natriuretic peptide in chronic heart failure in the rat: A correlation with ventricular dysfunction. *Cir. Res.* **59,** 256–261.

Uchida, K., Azukizawa, S., Kamei, M., Yoshida, I., Kigoshi, T., Yamamoto, I., Hosojima, H., and Morimoto, S. (1987). Effect of atrial natriuretic factor on aldosterone and its precursor steroid production in adrenal zona glomerulosa cells from spontaneously hypertensive rats. *Clin. Exp. Hypertens. Part A* **A9,** 2131–2142.

Volpe, M., Mele, A. F., Indolfi, C., De Luca, N., Lembo, G., Focaccio, A., Condorelli, M., and Trimarco, B. (1987). Hemodynamic and hormonal effects of atrial natriuretic factor in patients with essential hypertension. *J. Am. Coll. Cardiol.* **10,** 787–793.

Winquist, R. J. (1987). Modulation of vascular tone by atrial natriuretic factor. *Blood Vessels* **24,** 128–131.

Yamori, Y. (1984). Development of the spontaneously hypertensive rat (SHR) and of various spontaneous rat models, and their implications. *Hand. Hypertens.* **4,**224–239.

Yasujima, M., Abe, K., Kohzuki, M., Tanno, M., Kasai, Y., Sato, M., Omata, K., Kudo, K., Tsunoda, K., Takeuchi, K., Yoshinaga, K., and Inagami, T. (1985). Atrial natriuretic factor inhibits hypertension induced by chronic infusion of norepinephrine in conscious rats. *Circ. Res.* **57,** 470–474.

Zamir, N., Skofitsch, G., Eskay, R. L., and Jacobowitz, D. M. (1985). Distribution of immunoreactive atrial natriuretic peptides in the central nervous system of the rat. *Brain Res.* **365,** 105–111.

19

Stress, Opioid Peptides, and Cardiac Arrhythmias

Richard L. Verrier
Department of Pharmacology
Georgetown University School of Medicine
Washington, D.C. 20007

Daniel B. Carr
Departments of Anesthesia and Medicine
Harvard Medical School
Massachusetts General Hospital
Boston, Massachusetts 02114

   I. Introduction
  II. Endorphins and Receptors in Cardiovascular Control
 III. Opioids and Arrhythmogenesis
  IV. Baroreceptor Modulation and Opioids
   V. Cellular Studies
  VI. Peripheral Opioid Interactions
 VII. Summary and Conclusion
      References

I. Introduction

There are few areas in which the interactions between stress, neuropeptides, and disease carry such potential importance for public health as cardiovascular disease. For some time, physicians have recognized that the brain can exert profound, often deleterious effects upon the heart (Shepherd and Weiss, 1987). In particular, clinical experience and basic studies have clearly shown the importance of neural and psychological factors in arrhythmogenesis and sudden cardiac death (Brodsky *et al.*, 1987; Engel, 1971; Harvey and Levine, 1952; Lown, 1987; Lown and Verrier, 1976; Skinner *et al.*, 1975; Verrier, 1987, 1988, 1990; Verrier *et al.*, 1987; Wolf, 1969). In the past two decades, as the autonomic basis for stress-induced ventricular fibrillation was experimentally probed, identification of endogenous opioids and their receptors has provided unique insights into this often fatal process.

Physiological regulation of heart rate, blood pressure, vascular resistance, and cardiac output depends upon endogenous opioid peptides (Holaday, 1983). Pharmacological stabilization and control of the circulation in cardiac surgical patients routinely begin with the administration of high doses of exogenous opioids (Lowenstein *et al.*, 1969). The rarity of malignant ventricular arrhythmias after opioid administration in cardiac patients during the stress and trauma of major surgery is a remarkable but almost totally ignored daily nonoccurrence.

Although many investigators have described the results of administering opioids or antagonists in various shock models, relatively few have explored the links between behavioral stress, opioid peptides systems, and malignant arrhythmias. Currently, our ability to understand clinical reports of a protective effect from narcotic drugs on stress-induced arrhythmias is now at an early, yet promising, stage. Other contributors to this volume provide authoritative descriptions of the organization of the integrated stress response and functions of opioid and many other peptide subsystems within it. Therefore, we will present evidence of the role of endogenous and exogenous opioids in modulating arrhythmogenesis, describe the autonomic, neuroendocrine, and cellular mechanisms underlying this role, and discuss clinical implications of this work.

II. Endorphins and Receptors in Cardiovascular Control

Many key aspects of cardiovascular status, including myocardial contractility, heart rate, blood pressure, vascular resistance, and cardiac output, are obviously linked, yet may to a degree be independently altered by physiological or pharmacological interventions. This is equally true for opioid receptor activation or blockade, although definition of these effects has not yet coalesced into a simple scheme. A simple picture may, in fact, not be readily assembled, first, because of the variety of endogenous opioid peptides and their detailed processing from their precursor hormones, and the diversity of the types and subtypes of receptors upon which they act. Second, this inherent complexity is due to the wide distribution of endorphins and their receptors throughout the body (Atweh and Kuhar, 1977a,b,c), and there are disparities among the effects of global opiate receptor blockade or activation at varying sites, as is often the case for other neurotransmitters. Third, the compartmental regulation of endorphin content or effects is as a rule diverse, as exemplified by the stress-related reduction in endorphin content in the central nervous system as blood levels rise, and the opposite effects on plasma catecholamine levels that may follow microinjection of opiates at neighboring hypothalamic nuclei (Carr *et al.*, 1985).

Fourth, the effects of both exogenous and endogenous opioids appear to be enhanced during stress and altered from responses during basal states. The contrast between opiates' diminution of stress-induced catecholamines and their stimulation of catecholamine secretion in resting subjects is illustrative. Fifth, opioids are neuromodulators within networks, influencing neural traffic in other circuits and thereby establishing reciprocal, dynamic interactions with other neurochemical systems. Finally, as is true for many hormones, multiple long and short feedback loops exist within endogenous opioid pathways or involve the releasing factors for endorphin secretion and deter attempts to augment or block the actions of opiates (Carr *et al.*, 1982) (Figure 1).

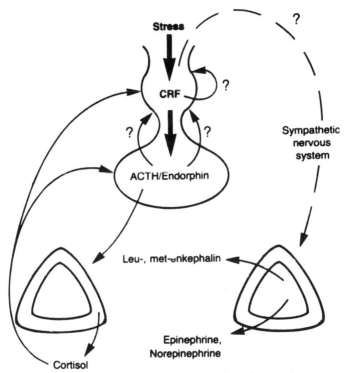

Figure 1   Stress–hormone axis in overview. Stress stimulates the secretion of corticotropin-releasing factor (CRF) from the median eminence of the hypothalamus. CRF is carried down the pituitary stalk and stimulates secretion of ACTH and beta-endorphin into the periphery. Centrally administered CRF produces activation of the sympathetic nervous system, resulting in secretion of epinephrine and norepinephrine from the adrenal medulla. Leu- and met-enkephalin are cosecreted along with epinephrine and norepinephrine from the adrenal medulla into the bloodstream. Inhibitory feedback pathways within this scheme are shown as solid arrows; question marks indicate suspected "short loop" negative feedback (Carr, 1984).

In relation to cardiovascular function, several laboratories have recently described direct, peripheral effects of circulating opioids on myocardial performance. Apparently conflicting effects have been observed depending upon the experimental model used. Whereas in isolated myocytes opioids enhance contractility (Laurent *et al.*, 1985, 1986), in other preparations their effects are chiefly to oppose catecholamine-induced contractility and chronotropy (Ruth and Eiden, 1984; Clo *et al.*, 1985; Caffrey *et al.*, 1985a,b, 1986; Gautret and Schmitt, 1985; Haddad *et al.*, 1986; Liang *et al.*, 1987). This anticatecholamine, modulatory effect is most obvious when probed in conjunction with the beta-adrenergic agonist isoproterenol (Ruth and Eiden, 1984; Clo *et al.*, 1985; Caffrey *et al.*, 1986) and results in a reduction in the normal calcium influx that ordinarily follows beta-agonist binding to the myocardium (Laurent *et al.*, 1986; Ruth and Eiden, 1984). Conversely, peripherally administered opiate receptor antagonists such as naloxone or nalmephene acutely increase myocardial inotropy and chronotropy (Caffrey *et al.*, 1985a,b, 1986; Liang *et al.*, 1987). These effects are particularly enhanced after acute bilateral carotid occlusion (Caffrey *et al.*, 1986) or in chronic cardiac failure produced by tricuspid avulsion and progressive pulmonary artery constriction (Liang *et al.*, 1987), both of which are physiological states in which sympathetic outflow modulates arterial pressure.

The manifestation of opioid effects on the circulation and on vascular resistance is in particular modulated by central and peripheral nervous system interactions with catecholamines (Holaday, 1983; Randich and Maixner, 1984; Feuerstein, 1985; Johnson *et al.*, 1985), as has been demonstrated in naloxone reversal of septic or endotoxic shock. Peripheral vascular effects are determined not only by direct opioid effects on vascular smooth muscle but also by central nervous system activity (Lowenstein *et al.*, 1972) and the intravascular release of histamine (Rosow, 1985). The typical architecture for these examples of neuromodulation mirrors that already recognized at many sites within the central nervous system, in which, for example, opioids inhibit substance P release (in dorsal horn of spinal cord), dopamine release (in hypothalamus or basal ganglia), or norepinephrine release (from locus ceruleus).

III. Opioids and Arrhythmogenesis

The role of opioids in arrhythmogenesis was first studied by the present authors and colleagues a decade ago as part of a larger research effort on the pathophysiology of stress-induced arrhythmias. We were impressed by the wide use of morphine as an analgesic during myocardial infarction when the incidence of ventricular fibrillation is high, notwithstanding the lack of knowledge of its effects on ventricular fibrillation (DeSilva et al., 1978a). Although it had long been recognized that morphine increases vagal tone (Eyster and Meek, 1912), among other autonomic effects, and that electrical stimulation of the vagus nerve decreases ventricular vulnerability (Kent et al., 1974), it remained to be determined whether the vagotonia induced by morphine would influence vulnerability. It was found in chloralose-anesthetized dogs that morphine did indeed result in significant reduction in vulnerability. The drug's influence was then studied in conscious dogs in an aversive stress paradigm (DeSilva et al., 1978b). Within 10 min in the aversive environment, the repetitive extrasystole (RE) threshold decreased 45%, indicating enhanced vulnerability, and heart rate and blood pressure were elevated. Morphine administered during exposure to the aversive environment restored the RE threshold to near-normal values, an effect mediated predominantly by the vagus nerve. A partially protective effect persisted even after muscarinic receptor blockade with atropine, suggesting withdrawal of sympathetic tone, nonspecific alkaloid effects, or direct myocardial effects (Figure 2).

Digitalis intoxication is one model of ventricular arrhythmia that has demonstrated the mixed effects of opioids, but the underlying mechanisms are unclear. Natelson and colleagues have shown that behavioral stress enhances digitalis-induced ventricular arrhythmia (Natelson and Cagin, 1981) and that this is abolished by "low dose" naloxone (4 mg/kg) but not by "high dose" naloxone (20 mg/kg) administration (Natelson et al., 1982). They interpreted these results to mean that endogenous mu blockade was occurring at the lower doses and suggested that in the naloxone-free animal, endogenous mu activation is responsible for the deleterious effects of stress. They also showed that atropine blocked the stress effect, and inferred that during stress, mu activation leads to arrhythmogenic vagal activation (Cagin and Natelson, 1981). This interpretation is questionable since the dose of naloxone that can be considered relatively mu specific is not known, and most investigators would consider 4 mg/kg too high. Furthermore, the arrhythmogenic effect of digitalis depends on autonomic mechanisms and therefore the role of the vagus nerve, which appears to be arrhythmogenic in these studies, must not be generalized to other forms of stress-induced arrhythmia.

In contrast, Rabkin and Roob (1986) have shown that a much lower dose of naloxone (0.1–0.01 mg/kg) increases digitalis-induced arrhythmia and that vagal efferent activity plays a decisive role. These data suggest that endogenous mu activation prevents the arrhythmogenic effects of digitalis, an interpretation exactly opposite that of Natelson's. Rabkin and colleagues (1987) found that i.v. morphine suppressed digitalis-induced arrhythmias in

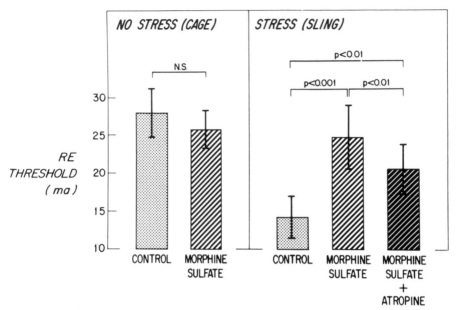

Figure 2 Effect of morphine sulfate (MS) on repetitive extrasystole (RE) threshold in the two environments. Morphine (0.25 mg/kg) significantly elevated RE threshold in the sling environment by 40% (p < 0.001). Administration of atropine sulfate (0.2 mg/kg) following MS partially annulled this effect, but RE threshold still remained significantly above the control level in the sling (p < 0.01). MS was without effect on RE threshold in the cage environment (DeSilva *et al.*, 1978b).

hypokalemic but not normokalemic canines, whereas the mixed mu–delta agonist FK33-824 (intracerebroventricular) enhanced digitalis arrhythmias in guinea pigs. They interpreted these results to suggest that mu activation is protective whereas delta activation is provocative. However, since morphine is not a pure mu agonist, such an inference is open to debate. These studies highlight the pitfalls of work in this area. Many more questions have been raised than answered, and further work will be required before a clear picture of opioid effects in digitalis arrhythmia will be available.

Studies of naloxone's effects on arrhythmias due to coronary ligation and/or ischemia have also been reported. Fagbemi and associates (1982) demonstrated that naloxone diminished ventricular arrhythmias following coronary ligation in anesthetized rats and increased survival rates in conscious rats subject to coronary artery occlusion. They also found that administration of the partial opioid agonist meptazinol led to a reduction in the incidence and severity of arrhythmias following coronary artery occlusion in anesthetized rats (Fagbemi *et al.*, 1983). The apparent contradiction between these and earlier results suggests that different mechanisms were involved in each case. However, another possibility is that a feedback process prevailed over the two opposing pharmacologic interventions.

In contrast, Bergey and Beil (1983) found no protection after naloxone administration in anesthetized pigs and explained these discrepancies on the basis of species differences or of heart size. Zhan and co-workers used an isolated heart preparation to confirm an antiarrhythmic effect of naloxone during myocardial ischemia and reperfusion and showed the same effect in anesthetized dogs (Zhan *et al.*, 1985; Huang *et al.*, 1986). However, our own work (Pinto *et al.*, 1989) using cardiac electrical testing has failed to confirm an antiarrhythmic effect of naloxone during acute coronary artery occlusion in dogs. Although most investigators who have reported an antiarrhythmic effect of naloxone have inferred a role for endogenous opioids in arrhythmogenesis, Frame and Argentieri (1985) showed direct electrophysiologic effects of naloxone *in vitro*, which suggest an alternative explanation. As with the work on digitalis-induced arrhythmias, further studies are required to define better naloxone's putative antiarrhythmic action during acute myocardial ischemia.

IV. Baroreceptor Modulation and Opioids

To define better the structure–activity relationships underlying opioid effects upon cardiac electrical properties, we extended our earlier work on stress-induced ventricular vulnerability using intravenous fentanyl (30 μg/kg) as a probe (Saini *et al.*, 1988). We sought to avoid potentially confusing results, which might be expected from morphine, which is an alkaloid and therefore subject to properties that need not be shared by nonalkaloid (i.e., peptide) narcotic agonists (Sawynok *et al.*, 1979). Furthermore, morphine is active at both delta and mu receptors, while fentanyl is more selective for the mu receptor. Fentanyl increased ventricular fibrillation (VF) threshold in chloralose-anesthetized dogs by 16%. Heart rate and mean arterial pressure declined after fentanyl administration and then remained stable. Hemorrhage effected by means of controlled exsanguination caused a slight decline in VF threshold, but the subsequent administration of fentanyl then elevated the threshold by 33%. Compared to the unstressed model, this amplification of fentanyl's effect was significant. Pretreatment with atropine or the peripherally active derivative atropine methylnitrate did not alter the pattern of elevation of VF threshold after fentanyl administration in hemorrhaged dogs. In contrast, in bilaterally stellectomized dogs, fentanyl's protective effect after hemorrhage was reduced to insignificance, and the heart rate response to hemorrhage was attenuated compared to controls. In vagotomized dogs, hemorrhage caused a slight decline in VF threshold and the subsequent administration of fentanyl was without effect. Thus vagotomy abolished fentanyl's antifibrillatory action (Figure 3).

Fentanyl is recognized as having a central vagotonic and sympatholytic effect (Faden and Holaday, 1979). Since we had found that morphine, an alkaloid with mu and delta agonist properties, acts via vagal activation to decrease vulnerability to VF (DeSilva *et al.*, 1978a,b), we initially surmised that fentanyl's vagal effect would underlie its antifibrillatory action. However, during hemorrhage, muscarinic efferent blockade with atropine did not alter fentanyl's protective effect, whereas stellectomy markedly attenuated it. The facts that an intact vagus nerve is required and that hemorrhage amplifies fentanyl's efficacy suggest that its protective action is mediated through the afferent component of the baroreflex arc.

Substantial experimental literature supports the view that opioids play an important role in modifying baroceptor physiology. Holaday and colleagues (Holaday, 1983; Faden and Holaday, 1979; Vargish *et al.*, 1980) found that naloxone increases heart rate and blood pressure during hemorrhagic shock, implying that endogenous opioid systems buffer the sympathetic response to hypotension. Similar chronotropic and pressor effects of naloxone have been described during nitroprusside-induced hypotension (Petty and Reid, 1981). Montastruc *et al.* (1981) demonstrated that stimu-

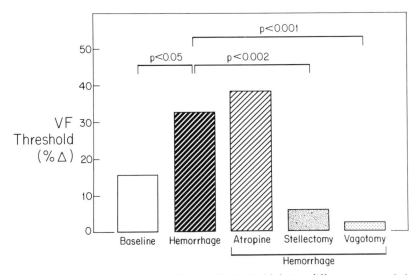

Figure 3 Comparison of fentanyl's effect on VF threshold during different autonomic interventions. Hemorrhage significantly increases fentanyl's antifibrillatory effect. Muscarinic blockade with atropine does not alter the drug's action, whereas stellectomy significantly reduces it. Bilateral cervical vagotomy abolishes fentanyl's effect completely. Values are percent changes in VF threshold after fentanyl (Saini *et al.*, 1988).

lation of vagal afferent fibers produced a pressor response that could be potentiated by naloxone and attenuated by morphine. Weinstock *et al.* (1984) observed in conscious rabbits that naloxone blocked the reflex sympathetic inhibition induced by phenylephrine infusion whereas morphine enhanced the reflex bradycardia of the same pressor stimulus.

There is also evidence that exogenous narcotics enhance depressor responses by increasing the sensitivity of the baroreflex. We found that fentanyl, like morphine, increases baroceptor reflex sensitivity as assessed by phenylephrine infusion (Saini *et al.*, 1988). Laubie *et al.* (1974) reported that fentanyl augments the bradycardia produced by carotid sinus nerve stimulation but not that produced by stimulation of the nucleus tractus solitarius (NTS). This suggests that the drug facilitates transmission of baroreflex traffic at relatively proximal synapses. This action of fentanyl is strongly reminiscent of our earlier experience with clonidine (Rotenberg *et al.*, 1978), which we found to be antifibrillatory in the normal heart. Clonidine, like fentanyl, causes bradycardia and hypotension via a decrease in sympathetic nervous system outflow (Klupp *et al.*, 1970). Clonidine is also known to enhance baroreflex sensitivity to a pressor stimulus, and a major site of action for this effect appears to be the NTS (Walland *et al.*, 1974). Farsang and Kunos (1979) found that naloxone can reverse the hypotensive effect of clonidine in spontaneously hypertensive rats. They further showed *in vitro* that alpha$_2$-adrenoreceptor activation by clonidine appears to release an endogenous opioid (Farsang *et al.*, 1980; Kunos *et al.*, 1984). Clonidine and opioids appear to act upon baroreflex responsiveness through a similar pathway, and their cardiac electrophysiological effects must be added to the list of interactions between central opioid and catecholamine pathways.

The baroreflex may be of particular importance in the cardiovascular adaptation to behavioral stress. Nathan and colleagues (1978; Nathan and Reis, 1977) showed that cats with lesions of the NTS, a major integrating center of the reflex, exhibit a greater hypertensive response to behavioral stress than do controls. Billman and co-workers (1982) found a significantly decreased sensitivity of the baroreflex in a subpopulation of dogs highly susceptible to VF during coronary occlusion. Dworkin and colleagues (1979) and Randich and Maixner (1984) found that a pressor stimulus can induce analgesia, providing further evidence suggesting baroreflex-induced increases in opioid tone. Considering that the sympathoinhibitory action of opioids is often found only in subpopulations, it may be that chronic, recurrent pressor stress can engender long-term alterations in sympathoinhibitory opioid tone and that a variable ability to mount such a response may confer protection or promote risk.

It is important to note that under certain conditions, opioid agents may alter cardiac arrhythmogenesis independently of an influence on the

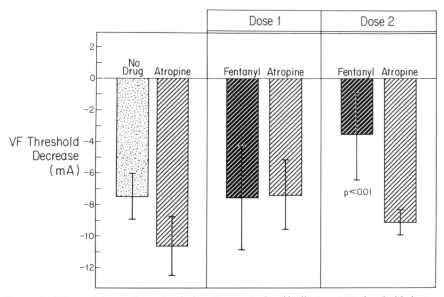

Figure 4 Effect of fentanyl on the decline in ventricular fibrillation (VF) threshold during acute coronary artery occlusion. In the absence of any drug, VF threshold fell by 7.5 mA. After the second dose of fentanyl (30 μg/kg/dose), this decline was significantly reduced to 3.6 mA. Atropine pretreatment increased this decline to 10.6 mA prior to fentanyl administration and prevented the antifibrillatory effect of the second dose of the opioid (Saini *et al.*, 1989).

baroreceptor arc. Specifically, we found during acute myocardial ischemia that mu-receptor activation with fentanyl reduced vulnerability to ventricular fibrillation, an effect that was abolished by blockade of vagal efferent activity with atropine (Figure 4). This is in contrast with its mode of action during hemorrhage, when it enhances vagal afferent inhibition of sympathetic tone, and atropine pretreatment is without effect. In the same study, we found that buprenorphine, a partial mu agonist, had no effect on the ventricular fibrillation threshold, although it caused significant declines in heart rate and arterial blood pressure. Taken collectively, these findings indicate that a full mu agonist increases cardiac electrical stability, but that a partial mu agonist does not. Moreover, the basis for the antifibrillatory action of mu agonism may be specific to the physiological stressor involved (Saini *et al.*, 1989).

V. Cellular Studies

Complementing and strengthening these positive *in vivo* results are a series of advances in the cellular electrophysiology of opioids. Receptor binding of opioids triggers complex processes that inhibit depolarization and transmitter release (Jaffe and Martin, 1985; Duggan and North, 1984; Cooper et al., 1986; Kaczmarek and Levitan, 1987). Opioid signals are mediated by many second messengers, and their definition is an intimidating prospect in view of the number and complexity of these systems (Cohen and Houslay, 1985; Cabot and McKeehan, 1987).

Calcium is a key second messenger of opioid actions in vitro (Ross and Cardenas, 1979; Bradford et al., 1986; Werz and Macdonald, 1983) and in vivo (Chapman and Way, 1982). Intracellular calcium mediates essential cellular processes such as neurotransmitter release or action potential generation both directly and after binding to regulatory proteins such as calmodulin. Opioids influence not only calcium flux but also the effects of those fluxes, such as calmodulin activation (Ross and Cardenas, 1987). Opioid–calcium interactions are now being probed in detail through the application of selective calcium channel antagonists. In vivo, calcium channel blockers potentiate opioid analgesia produced by drugs (Hoffmeister and Tettenborn, 1986) or environmental stress (Kavaliers, 1987) and suppress the morphine withdrawal syndrome (Bongianni et al., 1986; Ramkumar and El-Fakahany, 1988). In conjunction with kappa opioid agonists, these salutary actions may reflect the direct binding of opioids to the calcium channels themselves (Macdonald and Werz, 1986; Gandhi and Ross, 1988), or even to a specific subtype of calcium channel (Gross and Macdonald, 1987).

In contrast, mu or delta opioid agonists primarily increase potassium conductance, thereby shortening the duration of the action potential, and secondarily decrease calcium conductance (North and Williams, 1983; North, 1986). The potassium channels coupled to mu and delta receptors appear identical not only to each other but also to potassium channels coupled to other neurotransmitter receptors for acetylcholine, norepinephrine, dopamine, adenosine, and somatostatin (North et al., 1987). As has occurred for adrenergic receptors, "designer" ion channels containing specific amino acid substitutions are now being synthesized to study these effector mechanisms (Lear et al., 1988).

A guanine nucleotide regulatory (G or N) protein appears to be the locus of the coupling between the opioid receptor and potassium channel (North et al., 1987). The G proteins are a widely distributed second messenger system of profound importance to opioid and other neurotransmitter action (Jaffe and Martin, 1985; Cohen and Houslay, 1985; Cabot McKeehan, 1987; Dolphin, 1987). The G proteins are important to opioid actions because of their association with ion channels and their regulation of intracellular cyclic adenosine $5'$-monophosphate (cAMP) levels through effects on the catalytic subunit of adenylate cyclase. Since the active form of adenylate cyclase is coupled to guanosine triphosphate (GTP), and the inactive form to guanosine diphosphate, each of the G proteins is a GTPase.

Changes in intracellular cAMP, cyclic guanine monophosphate, calcium, or calmodulin levels activate diverse protein kinases, which are enzymes that phosphorylate substrates ranging from hormone receptors to ion channels to G proteins (Jaffe and Martin, 1985; Cooper *et al.*, 1986; West and Miller, 1983). Protein kinases are thus cellular effectors, regulated by second messengers and influenced by opioids, among many other drugs and hormones (Kaczmarek and Levitan, 1987; Cohen and Houslay, 1985; West and Miller, 1983; Clouet and O'Callaghan, 1979). The functions of a multitude of key biological molecules, and excitable membrane proteins in particular (Robertson, 1983), are altered and thereby regulated by protein kinase-dependent phosphorylation.

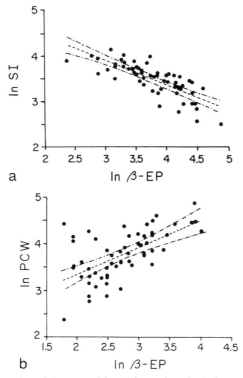

Figure 5 (a) Scatter plot of the natural logarithms of stroke index and immunoactive beta-endorphin in preoperative cardiac surgical patients. Ninety-five percent confidence limits for the regression line are drawn. The linear regression line formula is (In SI) = 5.7 − (0.60)(In iBE). (b) Scatter plot of the natural logarithms of pulmonary capillary wedge pressure and immunoactive beta-endorphin in preoperative cardiac surgical patients. Ninety-five percent confidence limits for the regression line are drawn. Linear regression line formula is (In PCW) = 1.7 + (0.79)(In iBE). Reprinted with permission from the International Anesthesia Research Society from Carr *et al.* (1989).

VI. Peripheral Opioid Interactions

It is reasonable to question whether secretion of opioids into the peripheral circulation during stress may result in an endogenous antiarrhythmic effect. The recent investigation by Carr *et al.* (1989) provides direct experimental evidence for a closely coupled quantitative regulation of beta-endorphin secretion into the periphery in parallel with elevated filling pressure or diminished stroke index (Figure 5). This observation is consistent with the concept that opioid secretion into the periphery increases to accommodate to changes in myocardial distension and in the level of adrenergic tone.

A number of investigators have underscored the potential importance of the peripheral actions of opioids (Fields *et al.*, 1980; Mays *et al.*, 1987; Joris *et al.*, 1987; Ferreira and Nakamura, 1979; Kosterlitz and Wallis, 1964). Intriguing interactions between the pain and cardiovascular regulatory systems have been illustrated in the excellent review by Randich and Maixner (1984). Thus, based on the available information, it seems reasonable to postulate that the antiarrhythmic effects of opioids derive from peripheral as well as central mechanisms.

VII. Summary and Conclusion

Opioids appear to confer protection against the arrhythmias that arise during stress. The mechanisms of these effects are still undergoing clarification and may vary according to the stressor. This disparity is illustrated by morphine's protective effect during aversive stress, which is due to vagal efferent activation, and alternatively by the baroceptor afferent mediation of fentanyl's protective effect during hemorrhage.

The research strategies suggested by our current state of knowledge include the following. First, we need to explore the effects of various opioids upon VF during ischemia and other pathologic states. Recent evidence indicates that opioid agonists may exert stress-specific antifibrillatory effects. In the context of hemorrhage, the baroreceptor arc influences are primary (Saini *et al.*, 1988), whereas during acute myocardial ischemia, enhanced vagal efferent activity is the main factor (Saini *et al.*, 1989). As these mechanisms are better understood, clinicians will be enabled to select particular agents (e.g., mixed agonist–antagonists to avert respiratory compromise or pain) based on the clinical context and the specific nature of hemodynamic compromise. Second, we need to extend consideration to other ligand subtypes, such as the kappa agonists. From such work could result the refinement of structure–activity relationships based on central nervous system effects rather than direct actions on the myocardium. Third, it would ap-

pear promising to search for possible antifibrillatory roles among other neu-
rohormones that participate in the global stress response (e.g., atrial peptides or corticotropin-releasing factor, CRF), that modify that response
(e.g., gamma-aminobutyric acid, GABA), that are present in the nerves sup-
plying the myocardium and coronary vasculature [e.g., substance P (Weihe
et al., 1981), vasoactive intestinal peptide (Weihe *et al.*, 1984), neurotensin
(Reinecke *et al.*, 1982), and neuropeptide Y (Allen *et al.*, 1985)], or that are
analgesic (e.g., somatostatin or calcitonin gene-related peptide, CGRP).
This will be a major task but will likely result in the development of new
antiarrhythmic agents as well as an improved understanding of electrophysiology. Finally, we need to apply the knowledge gained in these initial studies concomitantly with more sophisticated models of behavioral stress. For
the clinician, such basic research would have obvious relevance in view of
the wide use of opiates in anesthesia and intensive care, often in an older
population at risk for infarction or sudden death. Moreover, the supple-
mentation of standard antiarrhythmic regimens with neuropeptide agents
may allow clinicians to avert the toxicities of membrane active drugs and
to permit more specific antagonism in the event of therapeutic overshoot.
The development of modalities for the treatment of cardiac arrhythmias at
central nervous system sites would be the ultimate fruition of neurocardi-
ology.

Acknowledgment

This research was supported by grants HL-33567 and HL-35138 from the National Heart,
Lung and Blood Institute, National Institutes of Health, Bethesda, Maryland.

References

Allen, J. M., Polak, J. M., Rodrigo, J., Darcy, K., and Bloom, S. R. (1985). Localisation of
    neuropeptide Y in nerves of the rat cardiovascular system and the effect of 6-hydroxy-
    dopamine. *Cardiovasc. Res.* **19**, 570–577.
Atweh, S. F., and Kuhar, M. J. (1977a). Autoradiographic localization of opiate receptors in
    rat brain. I. Spinal cord and lower medulla. *Brain Res.* **124**, 53–67.
Atweh, S. F., and Kuhar, M. J. (1977b). Autoradiographic localization of opiate receptors in
    rat brain. II. The brain stem. *Brain Res.* **129**, 1–12.
Atweh, S. F., and Kuhar, M. J. (1977c). Autoradiographic localization of opiate receptors in
    rat brain. III. The telencephalon. *Brain Res.* **134**, 393–405.
Bergey, J. L., and Beil, M. E. (1983). Antiarrhythmic evaluation of naloxone against acute
    corollary occlusion-induced arrhythmias in pigs. *Eur. J. Pharmacol.* **90**, 427–431.
Billman, G. E., Schwartz, P. J., and Stone, H. L. (1982). Baroreceptor reflex control of heart
    rate: A predictor of sudden cardiac death. *Circulation* **66**, 874–880.

Bongianni, F., Carla, V., Moroni, F., and Pellegrini-Giampetro, D. E. (1986). Calcium channel inhibitors suppress the morphine-withdrawal syndrome in rats. Br. J. Pharmacol. 88, 561–567.

Bradford, H. F., Crowder, J. M., and White, E. J. (1986). Inhibitory actions of opioid compounds on calcium fluxes and neurotransmitter release from mammalian cerebral cortical slices. Br. J. Pharmacol. 88, 87–93.

Brodsky, M. A., Sato, D. A., Iseri, L. T., Wolff, L. J., and Allen, B. J. (1987). Ventricular tachyarrhythmia associated with psychological stress: The role of the sympathetic nervous system. JAMA, J. Am. Med. Assoc. 257, 2064–2067.

Cabot, M. C., and McKeehan, W. L., eds. (1987). "Mechanisms of Signal Transduction by Hormones and Growth Factors." Alan R. Liss, New York.

Caffrey, J. L., Gaugl, J. F., and Jones, C. E. (1985a). Local endogenous opiate activity in dog myocardium: Receptor blockade with naloxone. Am. J. Physiol. 248, H382–H388.

Caffrey, J. L., Wooldridge, C. B., and Gaugl, J. F. (1985b). The interaction of endogenous opiates with autonomic circulatory control in the dog. Circ. Shock 17, 233–242.

Caffrey, J. L., Wooldridge, C. B., and Gaugl, J. F. (1986). Naloxone enhances myocardial responses to isoproterenol in dog isolated heart-lung. Am. J. Physiol. 250, H749–H754.

Cagin, N. A., and Natelson, B. H. (1981). Cholinergic activation produces psychosomatic digitalis toxicity. J. Pharmacol. Exp. Ther. 218, 709–711.

Carr, D. B. (1984). Endorphins in psychiatry: The next five years. Drug Ther. 10, 109–126.

Carr, D. B., Bergland, R., Hamilton, A., Blume, H., Kasting, N., Arnold, M., Martin, J. B., and Rosenblatt, M. (1982). Endotoxin-stimulated opioid peptide secretion: Two secretory pools and feedback control in vivo. Science 217, 845–848.

Carr, D. B., Jones, K. J., Bergland, R. M., Hamilton, A., Kasting, N. W., Fisher, J. E., and Martin, J. B. (1985). Causal links between plasma and CSF endorphin levels in stress: Vector-ARMA analysis. Peptides (N.Y.) 6, Suppl. 1, 5–10.

Carr, D. B., Athanasiadis, C. G., Skourtis, C. T., Fishman, S. M., Fahmy, N. R., and Lappas, D. G. (1989). Quantitative relationships between plasma beta-endorphin immunoactivity and hemodynamic performance in preoperative cardiac surgical patients. Anesth. Analg. (Cleveland) 68, 77–82.

Chapman, D. B., and Way, E. L. (1982). Modification of endorphin/enkephalin analgesia and stress-induced analgesia by divalent cations, a cation chelator and an ionophore. Br. J. Pharmacol. 75, 389–396.

Clo, C., Muscari, C., Tantini, B., Pignatti, C., Bernardi, P., and Ventura, C. (1985). Reduced mechanical activity of perfused rat heart following morphine or enkephalin peptides administration. Life Sci. 37, 1327–1333.

Clouet, D. H., and O'Callaghan, J. P. (1979). Role of protein kinases in opiate actions in brain. In "Neurochemical Mechanisms of Opiates and Endorphins" (H. H. Loh and D. H. Ross, eds.), pp. 281–300. Raven Press, New York.

Cohen, P., and Houslay, M. D., eds. (1985). "Molecular Mechanisms of Transmembrane Signalling." Am. Elsevier, New York.

Cooper, J. R., Bloom, F. E., and Roth, R. H. (1986). "The Biochemical Basis of Neuropharmacology," 5th ed. Oxford Univ. Press, New York.

DeSilva, R. A., Verrier, R. L., and Lown, B. (1978a). Protective effect of the vagotonic action of morphine sulphate on ventricular vulnerability. Cardiovasc. Res. 2, 167–172.

DeSilva, R. A., Verrier, R. L., and Lown, B. (1978b). The effects of psychological stress and vagal stimulation with morphine on vulnerability to ventricular fibrillation (VF) in the conscious dog. Am. Heart J. 95, 197–203.

Dolphin, A. C. (1987). Nucleotide binding proteins in signal transduction and disease. Trends Neurosci. 10, 53–57.

Duggan, A. W., and North, R. A. (1984). Electrophysiology of opioids. *Pharmacol. Rev.* 35, 219–281.

Dworkin, B. R., Filewich, R. J., Miller, N. E., Craigmyle, N., and Pickering, T. G. (1979). Baroreceptor activation reduces reactivity to noxious stimulation: Implications for hypertension. *Science* 205, 1299–1301.

Engel, G. L. (1971). Sudden and rapid death during psychological stress: Folklore or folk wisdom? *Ann. Intern. Med.* 74, 771–782.

Eyster, J. A. E., and Meek, W. J. (1912). Cardiac irregularities in morphine poisoning in the dog. *Heart* 4, 59–66.

Faden, A. I., and Holaday, J. W. (1979). Opiate antagonists: A role in the treatment of hypovolemic shock. *Science* 205, 317–318.

Fagbemi, O., Lepran, I., Parratt, J. R., and Szekeres, L. (1982). Naloxone inhibits early arrhythmias resulting from acute coronary ligation. *Br. J. Pharmacol.* 76, 504–506.

Fagbemi, O., Kane, K. A., Lepran, I., Parratt, J. R., and Szekeres, L. (1983). Antiarrhythmic actions of meptazinol, a partial agonist at opiate receptors in acute myocardial ischaemia. *Br. J. Pharmacol.* 78, 455–460.

Farsang, C., and Kunos, G. (1979). Naloxone reverses the antihypertensive effect of clonidine. *Br. J. Pharmacol.* 67, 161–164.

Farsang, C., Ramirez-Gonzales, M. D., Mucci, L., and Kunos, G. (1980). Possible role of an endogenous opiate in the cardiovascular effects of central alpha adrenoceptor stimulation in spontaneously hypertensive rats. *J. Pharmacol. Exp. Ther.* 214, 203–208.

Ferreira, S. H., and Nakamura, M. (1979). Prostaglandin hyperalgesia: The peripheral analgesic activity of morphine, enkephalins and opioid antagonists. *Prostaglandins* 18, 191–200.

Feuerstein, C. (1985). The opioid system and central cardiovascular control: Analysis of controversies. *Peptides (N.Y.)* 6, Suppl. 2, 51–58.

Fields, H. L., Emson, P. C., Gilbert, R. L., and Iversen, L. L. (1980). Multiple opiate receptor sites on primary afferent fibers. *Nature (London)* 284, 351–353.

Frame, L. H., and Argentieri, T. M. (1985). Naloxone has local anesthetic effects on canine cardiac Purkinje fibers. *Circulation* 72, Suppl. III, 234 (abstr.).

Gandhi, V. C., and Ross, D. H. (1988). The effect of kappa agonist U50-488H on [^{3}H] nimodipine receptor binding in rat brain regions. *Eur. J. Pharmacol.* 150, 51–57.

Gautret, B., and Schmitt, H. (1985). Multiple sites for the cardiovascular actions of fentanyl in rats. *J. Cardiovasc. Pharmacol.* 7, 649–652.

Gross, R. A., and Macdonald, R. L. (1987). Dynorphin A selectively reduces a large transient (N-type) calcium current of mouse dorsal root ganglion neurons in cell culture. *Proc. Natl. Acad. Sci. U.S.A.* 84, 5469–5473.

Haddad, G. G., Jeng, H. J., and Lai, T. L. (1986). Effect of endorphins on heart rate and blood pressure in adult dogs. *Am. J. Physiol.* 250, H796–H805.

Harvey, W. P., and Levine, S. A. (1952). Paroxysmal ventricular tachycardia due to emotion: Possible mechanisms of death from fright. *JAMA, J. Am. Med. Assoc.* 150, 479–480.

Hoffmeister, F., and Tettenborn, D. (1986). Calcium agonists and antagonists of the dihydropyridine type: Antinociceptive effects, interference with opiate-mu-receptor agonists and neuropharmacological actions in rodents. *Psychopharmacology* 90, 299–307.

Holaday, J. W. (1983). Cardiovascular effects of endogenous opiate systems. *Annu. Rev. Pharmacol. Toxicol.* 23, 541–594.

Huang, X. D., Lee, A. Y. S., Wong, T. M., Zhan, C. Y., and Zhao, Y. Y. (1986). Naloxone inhibits arrhythmias induced by coronary artery occlusion and reperfusion in anaesthetized dogs. *Br. J. Pharmacol.* 87, 475–477.

Jaffe, J. H., and Martin, W. R. (1985). Opioid analgesics and antagonists. *In* "The Pharmacological Basis of Therapeutics" (A. G. Gilman, L. S. Goodman, T. W. Rall, and F. Murad, eds.), 7th ed., pp. 491–531. Macmillan, New York.

Johnson, M. W., Mitch, W. E., and Wilcox, C. S. (1985). The cardiovascular actions of morphine and the endogenous opioid peptides. *Prog. Cardiovasc. Dis.* **27**, 435–442.

Joris, J., Dubner, R., and Hargreaves, K. M. (1987). Opioid analgesia at peripheral sites. *Anesth. Analg. (Cleveland)* **66**, 1277–1281.

Kaczmarek, L. K., and Levitan, I. B, eds. (1987). "Neuromodulation." Oxford Univ. Press, New York.

Kavaliers, M. (1987). Stimulatory influences of calcium channel antagonists on stress-induced opioid analgesia and locomotor activity. *Brain Res.* **408**, 403–407.

Kent, K. M., Epstein, S. E., Cooper, T., and Jacobowitz, D. M. (1974). Cholinergic innervation of the canine and human ventricular conducting system: Anatomic and electrophysiologic correlations. *Circulation* **50**, 948–955.

Klupp, H., Knappen, F., Otsuka, Y., Streller, I., and Teichmann, H. (1970). Effects of clonidine on central sympathetic tone. *Eur. J. Pharmacol.* **10**, 225–229.

Kosterlitz, H. W., and Wallis, D. I. (1964). The action of morphine-like drugs on impulse transmission in mammalian nerve fibers. *Br. J. Pharmacol.* **22**, 499–510.

Kunos, G., Ramirez-Gonzalez, M. D., and Farsang, C. (1984). Adrenergic-opioid interactions and the central control of blood pressure in hypertension. *In* "Norepinephrine" (M. G. Ziegler and C. R. Lake, eds.), p. 414. Williams & Wilkins, Baltimore, Maryland.

Laubie, M., Schmitt, H., Canellas, J., Roquebert, J., and Demichel, P. (1974). Centrally mediated bradycardia and hypotension induced by narcotic analgesics: Dextromoramide and fentanyl. *Eur. J. Pharmacol.* **28**, 66–75.

Laurent, S., Marsh, J. D., and Smith, T. W. (1985). Enkephalins have a direct positive inotropic effect on cultured cardiac myocytes. *Proc. Natl. Acad. Sci. U.S.A.* **82**, 5930–5934.

Laurent, S., Marsh, J. D., and Smith, T. W. (1986). Enkephalins increase cyclic adenosine monophosphate content, calcium uptake, and contractile state in cultured chick embryo heart cells. *J. Clin. Invest.* **77**, 1436–1440.

Lear, J. D., Wasserman, Z. R., and DeGrado, W. F. (1988). Synthetic amphiphilic peptide models for protein ion channels. *Science* **240**, 1177–1181.

Liang, C.-S., Imai, N., and Stone, C. K. (1987). The role of endogenous opioids in congestive heart failure: Effects of nalmephene on systemic and regional hemodynamics in dogs. *Circulation* **75**, 443–448.

Lowenstein, E., Hallowell, P., Levine, F. H., Daggett, W. M., Austen, W. G., and Laver, M. B. (1969). Cardiovascular responses to large doses of intravenous morphine in man. *N. Engl. J. Med.* **281**, 333–338.

Lowenstein, E., Whiting, R. B., Bittar, D. A., Sanders, C. A., and Powell, W. J., Jr. (1972). Local and neurally mediated effects of morphine on skeletal muscle vascular resistance. *J. Pharmacol. Exp. Ther.* **180**, 359–367.

Lown, B. (1987). Sudden cardiac death: Biobehavioral perspective. *Circulation* **76**, Suppl. I, I-186–I-196.

Lown, B., and Verrier, R. L. (1976). Neural activity and ventricular fibrillation. *N. Engl. J. Med.* **294**, 1165–1170.

Macdonald, R. L., and Werz, M. A. (1986). Dynorphin A decreases voltage-dependent calcium conductance of mouse dorsal root ganglion neurones. *J. Physiol. (London)* **377**, 237–249.

Mays, K. S., Lipman, J. J., and Schnapp, M. (1987). Local analgesia without anesthesia using peripheral perineural morphine injections. *Anesth. Analg. (Cleveland)* **66**, 417–420.

Montastruc, J., Montastruc, P., and Morales-Olivas, F. (1981). Potentiation by naloxone of pressor reflexes. *Br. J. Pharmacol.* **74**, 105–109.

Natelson, B. H., and Cagin, N. A. (1981). The role of shock predictability during aversive conditioning in producing psychosomatic digitalis toxicity. *Psychosom. Med.* **43**, 191–197.

Natelson, B. H., Cagin, N. A., Tufts, M., Ferrara, M., Biehl, D., and Abramson, M. (1982). Bidirectional effect of naloxone on emotionally conditioned digitalis toxicity. *Psychosom. Med.* **44**, 397–400.

Nathan, M. A., and Reis, D. J. (1977). Chronic labile hypertension produced by lesions of the nucleus tractus solitarii in the cat. *Circ. Res.* **40**, 72–81.

Nathan, M. A., Tucker, L. W., Severini, W. H., and Reis, D. J. (1978). Enhancement of conditioned arterial pressure responses in cats after brainstem lesions. *Science* **201**, 71–73.

North, R. A. (1986). Opioid receptor types and membrane ion channels. *Trends Neurosci.* **9**, 114–117.

North, R. A., and Williams, J. T. (1983). Opiate activation of potassium conductance inhibits calcium action potentials in rat locus coeruleus neurones. *Br. J. Pharmacol.* **80**, 225–228.

North, R. A., Williams, J. T., Suprenant, A., and Christie, M. (1987). Mu and delta receptors belong to a family of receptors that are coupled to potassium channels. *Proc. Natl. Acad. Sci. U.S.A.* **84**, 5487–5491.

Petty, M. A., and Reid, J. L. (1981). Opiate analogs, substance P, and baroreceptor reflexes in the rabbit. *Hypertension* **3**, I-142–I-147.

Pinto, J. M. B., Kirby, D. A., and Verrier, R. L. (1989). Abolition of clonidine's effects on ventricular refractoriness by naloxone in the conscious dog. *Life Sci.* **45**, 413–420.

Rabkin, S. W. (1987). The effect of D-Ala-2-Me-Phe-4-Met-(0)-01-enkephalin on blood pressure, heart rate, and digoxin-induced arrhythmias in the guinea pig. *Life Sci.* **41**, 1109–1116.

Rabkin, S. W., Einzig, S., and Benditt, D. G. (1987). Morphine suppression of digitalis-induced arrhythmias. *Arch. I. Phar.* **289**, 267–277.

Rabkin, S. W., and Roob, O. (1986). Effect of the opiate antagonist naloxone on digitalis-induced cardiac arrhythmias. *Eur. J. Pharmacol.* **130**, 47–55.

Ramkumar, V., and El-Fakahany, E. E. (1988). Prolonged morphine treatment increases rat brain dihydropyridine binding sites: Possible involvement in development of morphine dependence. *Eur. J. Pharmacol.* **146**, 73–83.

Randich, A., and Maixner, W. (1984). Interactions between cardiovascular and pain regulatory systems. *Neurosci. Biobehav. Rev.* **8**, 343–367.

Reinecke, M., Weihe, E., Carraway, R. E., Leeman, S. E., and Forssmann, W. G. (1982). Localisation of neurotensin immunoreactive nerve fibers in the guinea-pig heart. *Neuroscience* **7**, 1785–1795.

Robertson, R. N. (1983). "The Lively Membranes." Cambridge Univ. Press, New York.

Rosow, C. E. (1985). Cardiovascular effects of narcotics. *In* "Effects of Anesthesia" (B. G. Covino, H. A. Fozzard, and K. Rehder, eds.), pp. 195–213. Am. Physiol. Soc., Bethesda, Maryland.

Ross, D. H., and Cardenas, H. L. (1979). Nerve cell calcium as a messenger for opiate and endorphin actions. *In* "Neurochemical Mechanisms of Opiates and Endorphins" (H. H. Loh and D. H. Ross, eds.), pp. 301–336. Raven Press, New York.

Ross, D. H., and Cardenas, H. L. (1987). Opiates inhibit calmodulin activation of a high-affinity Ca^{2+}-stimulated Mg^{2+}-dependent ATPase in synaptic membranes. *Neurochem. Res.* **12**, 41–48.

Rotenberg, F. A., Verrier, R. L., Lown, B., and Sole, M. J. (1978). Effects of clonidine on vulnerability to fibrillation in the normal and ischemic canine ventricle. *Eur. J. Pharmacol.* **47**, 71–79.

Ruth, J. A., and Eiden, L. E. (1984). Leucine-enkephalin modulation of catecholamine positive chronotropy in rat atria is receptor-specific and calcium-dependent. *Neuropeptides* **4**, 101–108.

Saini, V., Carr, D. B., Hagestad, E. L., Lown, B., and Verrier, R. L. (1988). Antifibrillatory mechanism of the narcotic agonist fentanyl. *Am. Heart J.* **115**, 598–605.

Saini, V., Carr, D. B., and Verrier, R. L. (1989). Comparative effects of the opioids fentanyl and buprenorphine on ventricular vulnerability during acute coronary artery occlusion. *Cardiovasc. Res.* **23**, 1001–1006.

Sawynok, J., Pinsky, C., and LaBella, F. S. (1979). Minireview on the specificity of naloxone as an opiate antagonist. *Life Sci.* **25**, 1621–1632.

Shepherd, J. T., and Weiss, S. M., eds. (1987). "Conference on Behavioral Medicine and Cardiovascular Disease," *Circulation,* Vol. 76, Suppl. I. Am. Heart Assoc., Dallas, Texas.

Skinner, J. E., Lie, J. T., and Entman, M. L. (1975). Modification of ventricular fibrillation latency following coronary artery occlusion in the conscious pig. The effects of psychological stress and beta-adrenergic blockade. *Circulation* **51**, 656–667.

Vargish, T., Reynolds, D. G., Gurll, N. J., Lechner, R. B., Holaday, J. W., and Faden, A. I. (1980). Naloxone reversal of hypovolemic shock in dogs. *Circ. Shock* **7**, 31–38.

Verrier, R. L. (1987). Mechanisms of behaviorally induced arrhythmias. *Circulation* 76, Suppl. I, I-48–I-56.

Verrier, R. L. (1988). Autonomic substrates for arrhythmias. *Prog. Cardiol.* **1**, 65–85.

Verrier, R. L. (1990). Behavioral stress, myocardial ischemia, and arrhythmias. *In* "Cardiac Electrophysiology and Arrhythmias: From Cell to Bedside" (D. P. Zipes and J. Jalife, eds.). Saunders, Philadelphia, Pennsylvania.

Verrier, R. L., Hagestad, E. L., and Lown, B. (1987). Delayed myocardial ischemia induced by anger. *Circulation* **75**, 249–254.

Walland, A., Kobinger, W., and Csongrady, A. (1974). Action of clonidine on baroreceptor reflexes in conscious dogs. *Eur. J. Pharmacol.* **26**, 184–190.

Weihe, E., Reinecke, M., Opherk, D., and Forssmann, W. G. (1981). Peptidergic innervation (substance P) in the human heart. *J. Mol. Cell. Cardiol.* **13**, 331–333.

Weihe, E., Reinecke, M., and Forssmann, W. G. (1984). Distribution of vasoactive intestinal polypeptide-like immunoreactivity in the mammalian heart. *Cell Tissue Res.* **236**, 527–540.

Weinstock, M., Schorer-Apelbaum, D., and Rosin, A. J. (1984). Endogenous opiates mediate cardiac sympathetic inhibition in response to a pressor stimulus in rabbits. *J. Hypertens.* **2**, 639–646.

Werz, M. A., and Macdonald, R. L. (1983). Opioid peptides with differential affinity for mu and delta receptors decrease sensory neuron calcium-dependent action potentials. *J. Pharmacol. Exp. Ther.* **227**, 394–402.

West, R. E., and Miller, R. J. (1983). Opiates, second messengers and cell response. *Br. Med. Bull.* **39**, 53–58.

Wolf, S. (1969). Psychosocial forces in myocardial infarction and sudden death. *Circulation* **39/40**, Suppl. IV, IV-74–IV-81.

Zhan, Z. Y., Lee, A. Y. S., and Wong, T. M. (1985). Naloxone blocks the cardiac effects of myocardial ischemia and reperfusion in the rat isolated heart. *Clin. Exp. Pharmacol. Physiol.* **12**, 373–378.

20

The Role of Endogenous Opioids in Chronic Congestive Heart Failure

*Robert P. Frantz**
Cardiology Unit
University of Rochester Medical Center
Rochester, New York 14642

Chang-seng Liang
Cardiology Unit
University of Rochester Medical Center
Rochester, New York 14642

I. Introduction
II. The Endogenous Opioid System in a Canine Model of CHF
   A. Evidence That the Opioid System Is Activated in CHF
   B. Effects of Opioid System Inhibition in Experimental CHF
III. Effect of Opioids and Opioid Antagonists on Myocardial Contractility
IV. Studies of Opioid Antagonists in Humans with CHF
V. Implications and Future Directions
   References

I. Introduction

Many investigators have shown that endogenous opioids play a role in modulating the cardiovascular response to circulatory stressors, and that administration of opiate antagonists may have beneficial effects in certain disease states. Opiate antagonists have salutary effects on blood pressure in animal models of hemorrhagic and endotoxic shock (Curtis and Lefer, 1980; D'Amato and Holaday, 1984; Sandor *et al.*, 1987; Schadt and York, 1980). Naloxone administration has also been shown to result in significant increases in blood pressure in patients with septic shock (Peters *et al.*, 1981). There is also evidence that endogenous opioids are involved in baroreflex function in normal humans (Rubin *et al.*, 1983). However, relatively little investigation has been done with regard to the endogenous opioid system in chronic congestive heart failure (CHF).

    Because CHF represents a form of chronic circulatory stress, it is reasonable to postulate that endogenous opioids are involved in the cardiovas-

*Present address: Division of Cardiovascular Diseases, Mayo Clinic, Rochester, Minnesota 55905.

cular changes that accompany CHF. Therefore, we have been investigating the role of endogenous opioids in a canine model of chronic stable right-sided CHF. These animals exhibit many of the neurohormonal and circulatory changes of clinical heart failure. They also have a depressed left ventricular function, but differ from patients with left heart failure in that their left ventricular filling pressure is not elevated. In this chapter, we will review the available experimental and clinical evidence regarding the role of endogenous opioids in CHF, discuss the mechanisms involved in their action, and describe avenues for future exploration.

II. The Endogenous Opioid System in a Canine Model of CHF

A. Evidence That the Opioid System Is Activated in CHF

We have studied the hemodynamic and biochemical effects of chronic right-sided CHF produced in dogs by a modification of the Barger technique (Barger et al., 1952; Higgins et al., 1973). This technique utilizes a two-step surgical procedure. Initially the tricuspid valve is rendered incompetent by rupturing the chordae tendineae of the anterior tricuspid leaflet. Two weeks later, a silicone rubber hydraulic occluder is placed around the pulmonary artery. Following a 2-week recovery period, the occluder is gradually inflated until right atrial pressure stabilizes at 14–17 mm Hg. CHF is manifested by resting tachycardia, reduced cardiac output, ascites formation, and diminished right and left ventricular contractile function (Liang et al., 1987).

Our initial investigation of the endogenous opiate system in this model (Liang et al., 1987) involved measurement of beta-endorphin levels in sham-operated and CHF dogs. Adrenocorticotropic hormone (ACTH) and cortisol levels were also measured, since beta-endorphin and ACTH secretion are known to be linked (Guillemin et al., 1977). Plasma norepinephrine levels were also measured. Following baseline measurement of heart rate, aortic pressure, cardiac output, and left ventricular dP/dt (a measure of left ventricular contractile function), we administered the long-acting opiate receptor antagonist nalmefene to the animals. We also administered nalmefene to a separate group of sham-operated and CHF animals after pretreatment with propranolol or propranolol plus prazosin, in order to determine whether the effects of opiate receptor inhibition are mediated via the adrenergic receptors. We administered two doses of nalmefene (0.2 mg/kg and 1.0 mg/kg) intravenously 20 min apart. Hemodynamic measurements were made before and after each intervention. Regional blood flows were measured utilizing radioactive microspheres before and after each dose of nalmefene. Blood samples for beta-endorphin, ACTH, cortisol, and norepinephrine levels were obtained before and after nalmefene administration in

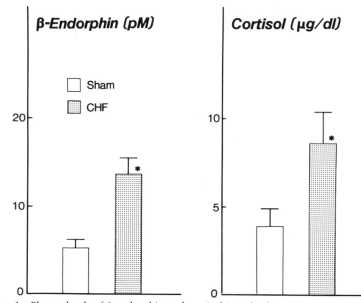

Figure 1 Plasma levels of β-endorphin and cortisol in eight sham-operated dogs and 11 dogs with CHF at rest.

the two groups of animals not pretreated with either propranolol or prazosin.

As shown in Figure 1, plasma beta-endorphin and cortisol levels were significantly elevated in dogs with CHF, while the ACTH levels in CHF were not significantly different from the sham group. Administration of nalmefene resulted in significant increases in beta-endorphin, ACTH, and cortisol levels in the CHF group, but not in the sham group. Plasma norepinephrine levels were elevated in the CHF group, and rose significantly following nalmefene administration, while no such effect was seen in the sham group. These results clearly demonstrate that the opioid system is activated in this model of CHF. Moreover, since plasma beta-endorphin is increased further after opiate receptor antagonist administration, it appears that activation of the endogenous opioid system exerts a negative feedback effect on the production of endogenous opioids.

B. Effects of Opioid System Inhibition in Experimental CHF

1. Hemodynamic Effects

Figure 2 shows that nalmefene caused an increase in aortic pressure, cardiac output, and left ventricular dP/dt in a dog with CHF. These changes were

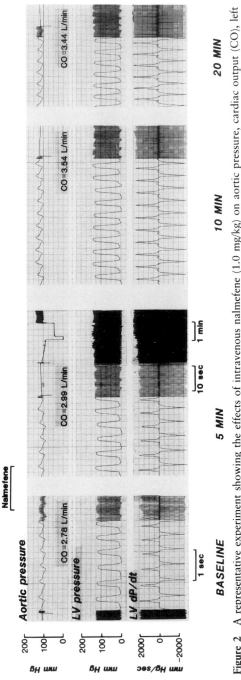
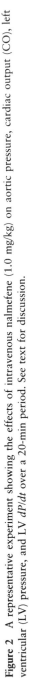

Figure 2 A representative experiment showing the effects of intravenous nalmefene (1.0 mg/kg) on aortic pressure, cardiac output (CO), left ventricular (LV) pressure, and LV dP/dt over a 20-min period. See text for discussion.

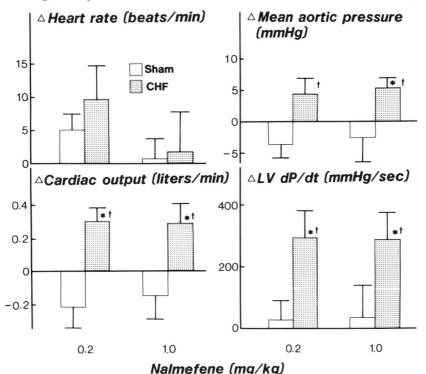

Figure 3 Changes in heart rate, mean aortic pressure, cardiac output, and left ventricular (LV) *dP/dt* produced by two doses of nalmefene in 11 dogs with CHF and eight sham-operated dogs. Bars indicate SE. Asterisks denote values that differ significantly from the baseline at $p < 0.05$. Daggers indicate values that differ from those in the sham-operated group at $p < 0.05$. [Taken with permission from Liang *et al.* (1987).]

evident within 5 min, and reached a plateau 10–20 minutes after nalmefene administration. Heart rate increased transiently after nalmefene administration, but the increase was not statistically significant 10–20 min after administration. Values obtained between 10 and 20 min after drug administration were averaged for statistical analyses. The group results of the CHF dogs are shown in Figure 3. The figure shows that nalmefene caused an increase in mean aortic pressure, cardiac output, and left ventricular *dP/dt*. In contrast, nalmefene resulted in no hemodynamic effects in sham-operated dogs. Propranolol pretreatment in CHF abolished the increases in heart rate, cardiac output, and left ventricular *dP/dt*, but did not attenuate the pressor response to nalmefene. The pressor response was abolished, however, by the addition of prazosin.

434 Robert P. Frantz and Chang-seng Liang

2. Effects on Regional Blood Flow

Nalmefene caused a redistribution of cardiac output in dogs with CHF, but had no such a effect in the sham group. In CHF, nalmefene increased blood flow to the ventricular muscle (Figure 4), quadriceps muscle (Figure 5), and kidneys (Figure 6), and decreased the organ vascular resistances. Figure 4 also shows that beta-receptor blockade attenuated the increase in myocardial blood flow, and addition of prazosin abolished the increase. Propranolol also abolished the increase in skeletal muscle and renal blood flow that occurred after nalmefene in dogs with CHF (Figures 5 and 6).

The effects of opiate receptor antagonism in this model are similar to those previously demonstrated to occur in shock (Curtis and Lefer, 1980; Holaday and Faden, 1978; Vargish et al., 1980). We have also demon-

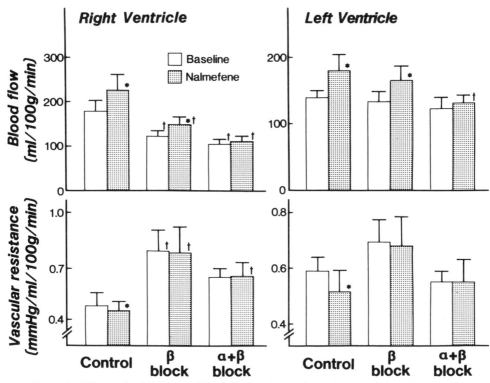

Figure 4 Effects of nalmefene on blood flow and vascular resistance of the left and right ventricles in three groups of dogs with CHF. Bars indicate SE. Asterisks indicate values that differ significantly from the baseline at $p < 0.05$. Daggers indicate values that differ from the corresponding values in the control group at $p < 0.05$. [Taken with permission from Liang et al. (1987).]

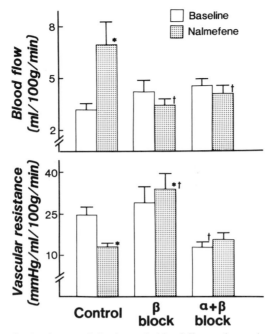

Figure 5 Effects of nalmefene on skeletal muscle blood flow and vascular resistance in three groups of dogs with CHF. Bars indicate SE. Asterisks indicate values that differ significantly from the baseline at $p < 0.05$. Daggers indicate values that differ from the corresponding values in the control group at $p < 0.05$. [Taken with permission from Liang et al. (1987).]

strated that the effect of endogenous opioids are probably mediated through the sympathetic nervous system, since adrenergic receptor blockade abolished the effects of opiate antagonism. The similarity to results of studies in shock is again striking, as adrenergic blockade or surgical disruption of sympathetic outflow have been shown to abolish the effect of naloxone in anaphylactic shock (Amir, 1984). However, our initial study did not address specifically whether the effects of opiate antagonism are primarily mediated via the central nervous system or peripherally; therefore further investigation was performed in order to address this question.

3. Demonstration of the CNS Action of Opioid Antagonism

We compared the effects of an opiate receptor antagonist that crosses the blood–brain barrier (naloxone HCl) with the effects of one that does not (naloxone methylbromide, a quaternary opiate antagonist). Naloxone was administered intravenously at two different doses utilizing a bolus/infusion technique (0.275 μmol/kg bolus over 1 min followed by a continuous infu-

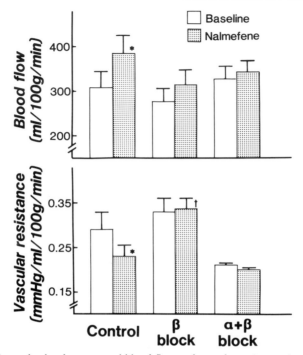

Figure 6 Effects of nalmefene on renal blood flow and vascular resistance in three groups of dogs with CHF. Bars indicate SE. Asterisks indicate values that differ significantly from the baseline at $p < 0.05$. The dagger indicates value from that in the control group at $p < 0.05$. [Taken with permission from Liang *et al.* (1987).]

sion of 13.77 pmol/kg for 20 min). Then a fivefold higher dose was given in the same manner. Naloxone methylbromide was administered in equimolar doses on a separate occasion. We found that naloxone HCl had effects in CHF dogs that were similar to those obtained with nalmefene, causing increases in plasma beta-endorphin, ACTH, and norepinephrine, and increasing aortic pressure, cardiac output, and left ventricular *dP/dt*, while total peripheral resistance fell. Naloxone methylbromide produced no significant changes in these parameters; a transient decrease in mean aortic pressure and left ventricular *dP/dt* occurred after the higher dose (Sakamoto *et al.*, 1989). Other investigators have shown a dose-dependent hypotensive effect of naloxone methylbromide (Giles *et al.*, 1983). At higher doses, naloxone methylbromide increases heart rate (Giles *et al.*, 1983), due to baroreflex-mediated sympathetic stimulation or a direct anticholinergic action (Willette *et al.*, 1983). Since the quaternary opiate receptor antagonist did not show effects similar to naloxone HCl, it appears that the effects of naloxone

HCl in our model are primarily mediated via the central nervous system. It is also reassuring to observe that nalmefene and naloxone HCl had similar effects; this indicates that the observed effects are indeed mediated via the opiate receptor system, and not some direct effect of the drugs that is unrelated to opiate antagonism.

4. Studies in Anesthetized Dogs

To determine whether the effects of opiate receptor antagonists in our model were due in part to abolition of the opioid-induced antinociception, we also studied the effect of anesthesia on the animal's response to naloxone HCl. We administered pentobarbital to dogs with CHF in a dose sufficient to abolish physical and hemodynamic responses to nociceptive stimuli, without depressing spontaneous respiration. These animals still responded to naloxone HCl with an increase in mean aortic pressure, cardiac output, left ventricular dP/dt, and plasma catecholamines. The changes in aortic pressure and plasma norepinephrine were similar to those in conscious animals, suggesting that anesthesia did not affect the sympathetic stimulation produced by naloxone. However, the anesthetized dogs showed smaller increases in cardiac output and left ventricular dP/dt than conscious dogs, and plasma epinephrine rose less as well. The greater cardiac and adrenal responses to naloxone in conscious dogs probably were related to abolition of the antinociceptive effects of endogenous opioids. However, we did observe that anesthetized dogs had a diminished inotropic response to isoproterenol when compared with conscious dogs, raising the possibility that naloxone had a diminished inotropic effect in the anesthetized dogs because of a myocardial depressant effect of the pentobarbital.

5. Opioid Antagonists Improve Baroreflex Function in CHF

Baroreflex function is abnormal in patients with heart failure (Eckberg *et al.*, 1971; Ferguson *et al.*, 1984). It is also abnormal in the Barger dog model of CHF (Higgins *et al.*, 1972). The mechanisms underlying this abnormality are incompletely understood. Because endogenous opioids have been shown to depress baroreflex function, we elected to look for a possible role of the endogenous opiate system in mediating baroreflex abnormalities in the dogs with heart failure. These animals slow their heart rates less in response to phenylephrine-induced hypertension than do normal dogs. We studied this parameter of baroreflex function in CHF dogs pretreated with naloxone HCl or an equivalent volume of saline (Sakamoto and Liang, 1989). Figure 7 shows the relationship between R–R interval and phenylphrine-induced elevation in blood pressure in a dog with CHF after pretreatment with either saline or naloxone HCl. The slope of the linear relationship is taken as a measure of baroreflex sensitivity. Compared to saline

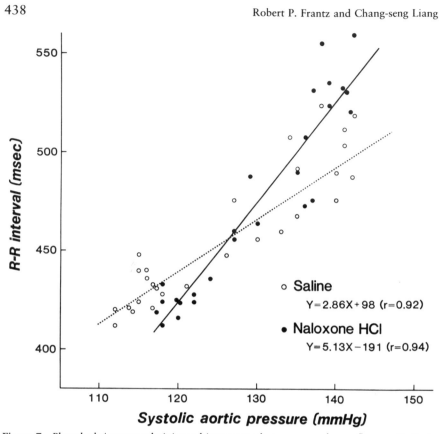

Figure 7 Phenylephrine was administered intravenously to measure baroreflex sensitivity in a dog with CHF 10 min after administration of either normal saline or naloxone (1.0 mg/kg). The cardiac cycle length was plotted on a beat-to-beat basis against the systolic aortic pressure of the preceding beat. Correlation and regression analyses were performed. The figure gives correlation coefficients (*r*) and equations of the regression lines. The slopes of the regression lines are taken as a measure of baroreflex sensitivity.

pretreatment, naloxone HCl increased baroreflex sensitivity in CHF, but it did not restore the baroreflex sensitivity to normal values (10.9 ± 1.2 ms/ mm Hg). In order to determine which opiate receptor subtype mediated the improvement, we compared the effects of naloxone HCl, a relatively nonselective antagonist, with the effects of naloxonazine (a mu-receptor-selective antagonist), ICI 154129 (a delta-receptor-selective antagonist), and the quaternary compound naloxone methylbromide. The results of this study are illustrated in Figure 8. Naloxone HCl and naloxonazine had similar effects, while ICI 154129 and naloxone methylbromide did not improve baroreflex function, indicating that the involved opiate receptors are in the central nervous system and are mu receptors. The degree of improvement

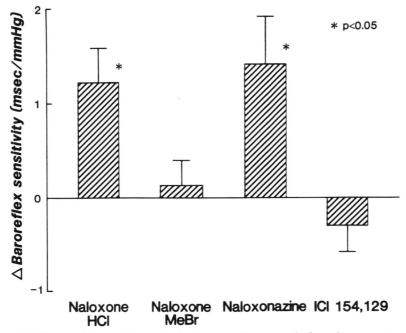

Figure 8 Changes in baroreflex sensitivity (compared to control after saline pretreatment) produced by naloxone, HCl, naloxone methylbromide (MeBr), naloxonazine, and ICI 154, 129. Bars indicate SE. Asterisks indicate values that differ significantly from the control at $p < 0.01$. Analysis of variance showed the results differ among the groups at $p < 0.05$. [Taken with permission from Sakamoto and Liang (1989).]

in baroreflex function with naloxone in CHF correlated with the extent of preexisting elevation in plasma beta-endorphin (Figure 9). Naloxone had no effects in sham-operated dogs with normal beta-endorphin levels. Thus it appears that the increased activity of the endogenous opiate system is in part responsible for the abnornal baroreflex responses observed in chronic CHF.

III. Effects of Opioids and Opioid Antagonists on Myocardial Contractility

Intracoronary administration of naloxone has been shown to increase myocardial contractile force in anesthetized dogs (Caffrey *et al.*, 1985). Caffrey *et al.* (1985) also demonstrated that the opiate peptide dynorphin had a negative inotropic effect that could be reversed by naloxone HCl. They suggest that opioids may suppress myocardial contractility by inhibiting nor-

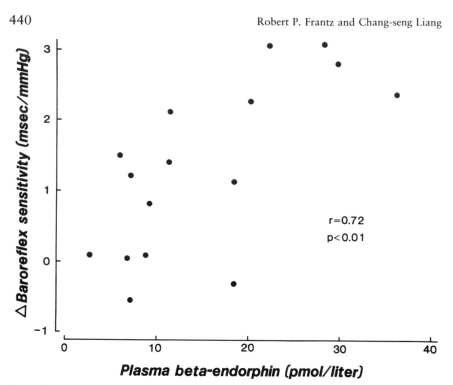

Figure 9 Correlation between naloxone- and naloxonazine-induced changes in baroreflex sensitivity and plasma β-endorphin levels in dogs with CHF; r, correlation coefficient. [Taken with permission from Sakamoto and Liang (1989).]

epinephrine release from sympathetic nerve terminals, and that naloxone exerts its effect by blocking this inhibitory effect of opiates. Sagy and colleagues (1987) have found that naloxone may also enhance myocardial contractility via a nonopiate mechanism in the isolated rat heart. They found that *l*-naloxone, which has opioid antagonist properties, and *d*-naloxone, which is not active as an opioid antagonist, had similar positive inotropic properties that were not attenuated by morphine. These effects also were not prevented by alpha- and beta-receptor blockade, indicating that the action is not mediated via the adrenergic receptors. This study raises the possibility that at least part of naloxone's effects on the heart may not be related to opiate-receptor antagonism, and illustrates the important maxim that demonstration of an effect with naloxone is necessary but not sufficient evidence for opiate system involvement (Hayes *et al.*, 1977; Sawynok *et al.*, 1979). However, Lechner and colleagues (1985a) have demonstrated that the increase in myocardial contractility produced by intracoronary administration of naloxone in dogs is indeed stereospecific. This strongly supports the concept that naloxone works primarily via opiate receptor antagonism.

The nonspecific inotropic effects of naloxone reported by Sagy *et al.* (1987) have not been demonstrated in other animal models.

Morphine and other opiates have been shown to have negative inotropic and chronotropic properties in an isolated rat heart model, although the cellular mechanism by which this occurs is uncertain (Vargish and Beamer, 1989). Lechner *et al.* (1985b,c) have extensively studied the effects of naloxone in a canine model of hemorrhagic shock in an effort to understand the mechanisms by which opiate antagonists improve cardiovascular function. Based upon this work and the findings of other investigators, they have proposed an intriguing interaction between opioids and catecholamines. They suggest that the effects of opioids are not simply due to inhibition of sympathetic activity; rather, opioids may also attenuate the cellular response to a given level of sympathetic activity (Gurll, 1988). They propose that opioids stimulate production of inhibitory G protein, thereby blunting the ability of catecholamines to stimulate adenylate cyclase; naloxone blocks the opioid receptor, preventing opioid stimulation of inhibitory G protein, and allowing full activation of adenylate cyclase by catecholamines. Enkephalins have been shown to inhibit adenylate cyclase activity in mouse neuroblastoma–glioma hybrid cells via a process that is Na^+ and GTP dependent (Blume *et al.*, 1979). This hypothesis is further supported by the demonstration that naloxone potentiates the effect of epinephrine in a monkey model of hemorrhagic shock (Modin *et al.*, 1985).

Interestingly, enkephalins have been shown to have positive inotropic effects when studied in cultured chick embryo myocytes (Laurent *et al.*, 1985). This effect appears to be mediated via stimulation of adenylate cyclase (Laurent *et al.*, 1986). The authors propose that the net observed effect of opiates on myocardium *in vivo* or in isolated whole heart preparations may be a combination of bidirectional effects: (1) direct positive inotropic effects and (2) indirect negative inotropic effects mediated via inhibition of norepinephrine release. Whether enkephalins will be shown to have positive inotropic properties in other myocardial cell preparations (e.g., adult myocyte preparations) remains to be seen. The opposite effects of opioids on adenylate cyclase activity and contractility in different cell types emphasize the importance of further investigation utilizing adult myocyte preparations, in order to substantiate the opioid–catecholamine interaction proposed by Gurll (1988).

IV. Studies of Opioid Antagonists in Humans with CHF

Remarkably few studies have addressed the endogenous opiate system in patients with primary myocardial dysfunction. A case report of naloxone use in cardiogenic shock following cardiac surgery is available (Unzueta

Merino *et al.*, 1987). Salutary effects on blood pressure were observed following administration of two 0.8-mg doses of intravenous naloxone. Another series of patients with refractory shock included two patients with cardiogenic shock; they received approximately 5 mg of intravenous naloxone without apparent effect (Allolio *et al.*, 1987). In addition, a study by Kindman and Fowler (1989) showed no acute hemodynamic effects of naloxone, at doses as high as 1 mg/kg, in six patients with stable New York Heart Association Functional Class II and III CHF. These findings suggest that the endogenous opiate system may not be activated in all patients with left ventricular dysfunction.

V. Implications and Future Directions

The available evidence indicates that the endogenous opiate system is activated in experimental CHF. The principal effect of this activation is to suppress sympathetic outflow from the cardiovascular centers within the central nervous system. Opiate antagonists have salutary acute effects on cardiac function, hemodynamics, and baroreflex function in experimental CHF. Future investigation should seek to answer several questions:

1. Is the endogenous opioid system activated in patients with CHF? A few relatively simple studies could address this question. Simply measuring plasma beta-endorphin levels in patients with CHF and age-matched controls would be a first step. A study of baroreflex function before and after a dose of naloxone in such patients would address whether endogenous opioids play a role in the abnormal baroreflex function that accompanies CHF.
2. Does administration of an opiate antagonist have salutary hemodynamic effects in patients with heart failure?
3. Do opioids or opiate antagonists have positive inotropic effects on isolated adult cardiac myocytes, and if so, what are the mechanisms involved? Do opioids stimulate production of inhibitory G proteins in adult myocytes?

It is likely that future investigation will provide further understanding of the role of endogenous opioids in CHF. Whether this understanding will lead to clinically useful new therapies is uncertain, but understanding the pathophysiology and receptor pharmacology is a necessary step toward the ultimate goal of improving the treatment of patients with CHF.

References

Allolio, B., Fischer, H., Kaulen, D., Deuss, U., and Winkelmann, W. (1987). Naloxone in treatment of circulatory shock resistant to conventional therapy. *Klin. Wochenshr.* **65**, 213–217.

Amir, S. (1984). Beneficial effect of i.c.v. naloxone in anaphylactic shock is mediated through peripheral beta-adrenoceptive mechanisms. *Brain Res.* **290**, 191–194.

Barger, A. C., Roe, B. B., and Richardson, G. S. (1952). Relation of valvular lesions and of exercise to auricular pressure, work tolerance and to development of chronic, congestive failure in dogs. *Am. J. Physiol.* **169**, 384–399.

Blume, A. J., Lichtshtein, D., and Boone, G. (1979). Coupling of opiate receptors to adenylate cyclase: Requirement for Na^+ and GTP. *Proc. Natl. Acad. Sci. U.S.A.* **76**, 5626–5630.

Caffrey, J. L., Gaugl, J. F., and Jones, C. E. (1985). Local endogenous opiate activity in dog myocardium: Receptor blockade with naloxone. *Am. J. Physiol.* **248**, H382–H388.

Curtis, M. T., and Lefer, A. M. (1980). Protective actions of naloxone in hemorrhagic shock. *Am. J. Physiol.* **239**, H416–H421.

D'Amato, R., and Holaday, J. W. (1984). Multiple opioid receptors in endotoxic shock: Evidence for δ involvement and μ-δ interactions *in vivo*. *Proc. Natl. Acad. Sci. U.S.A.* **81**, 2898–2901.

Eckberg, D. L., Drabinsky, M., and Braunwald, E. (1971). Defective cardiac parasympathetic control in patients with heart disease. *N. Engl. J. Med.* **285**, 877–883.

Ferguson, D. W., Abboud, F. M., and Mark, A. L. (1984). Selective impairment of baroreflex-mediated vasoconstrictor responses in patients with ventricular dysfunction. *Circulation* **69**, 451–460.

Giles, T., Sander, G., and Merz, H. (1983). Quaternary opiate antagonists lower blood pressure and inhibit leucine-enkephalin responses. *Eur. J. Pharmacol.* **95**, 247–252.

Guillemin, R., Vargo, T., Rossier, J., Minick, S., Ling, N., Rivier, C., Vale, W., and Bloom, F. (1977). Beta-endorphin and adrenocorticotropin are secreted concomitantly by the pituitary gland. *Science* **197**, 1367–1369.

Gurll, N. J. (1988). Opioid-catecholamine interactions in circulatory shock. *In* "Perspectives in Shock Research" (R. F. Bond, ed.), pp. 255–263. Alan R. Liss, New York.

Hayes, R., Price, D. D., and Dubner, R. (1977). Naloxone antagonism as evidence for narcotic mechanisms. *Science* **196**, 600.

Higgins, C. B., Vatner, S. F., Eckberg, D. L., and Braunwald, E. (1972). Alterations in the baroreceptor reflex in conscious dogs with heart failure. *J. Clin. Invest.* **51**, 715–724.

Higgins, C. B., Pavelec, R., and Vatner, S. F. (1973). Modified technique for production of experimental right-sided congestive heart failure. *Cardiovasc. Res.* **7**, 870–874.

Holaday, J. W., and Faden, A. I. (1978). Naloxone reversal of endotoxin hypotension suggests role of endorphins in shock. *Nature (London)* **275**, 450–451.

Kindman, L. A., and Fowler, M. B. (1989). Hemodynamic effects of high dose naloxone in congestive heart failure. *Am. J. Cardiol.* **64**: 542–544.

Laurent, S., Marsh, J. D., and Smith, T. W. (1985). Enkephalins have a direct positive inotropic effect on cultured cardiac myocytes. *Proc. Natl. Acad. Sci. U.S.A.* **82**, 5930–5934.

Laurent, S., Marsh, J. D., and Smith, T. W. (1986). Enkephalins increase cyclic adenosine monophosphate content, calcium uptake, and contractile state in cultured chick embryo heart cells. *J. Clin. Invest.* **77**, 1436–1440.

Lechner, R. B., Gurll, N. J., and Reynolds, D. G. (1985a). Intracoronary naloxone in hemorrhagic shock: Dose-dependent stereospecific effects. *Am. J. Physiol.* **249**, H272–H277.

Lechner, R. B., Gurll, N. J., and Reynolds, D. G. (1985b). Role of the autonomic nervous system in mediating the response to naloxone in canine hemorrhagic shock. *Circ. Shock* **16**, 279–295.

Lechner, R. B., Gurll, N. J., and Reynolds, D. G. (1985c). Naloxone potentiates the cardiovascular effects of catecholamines in canine hemorrhagic shock. *Circ. Shock* **16**, 347–361.

Liang, C.-S., Imai, N., Stone, C.K., Woolf, P.D., Kawashima, S., and Tuttle, R.R. (1987). The role of endogenous opioids in congestive heart failure: Effects of nalmefene on systemic and regional hemodynamics in dogs. *Circulation* **75**, 443–451.

Modin, B. E., Ganes, E., Reynolds, D. G., and Gurll, N. J. (1985). Naloxone requires circulating catecholamines for efficacy in primate hemorrhagic shock. *Fed. Proc., Fed. Am. Soc. Exp. Biol.* **44**, 1574.

Peters, W. P., Friedman, P. A., Johnson, M. W., and Mitch, W. E. (1981). Pressor effect of naloxone in septic shock. *Lancet* **1**, 529–532.

Rubin, P. C., McLean, K., and Reid, J. L. (1983). Endogenous opioids and baroreflex control in humans. *Hypertension* **5**, 535–538.

Sagy, M., Shavit, G., Oron, Y., Vidne, V. A., Gitter, S., and Sarne, Y. (1987). Nonopiate effect of naloxone on cardiac muscle contractility. *J. Cardiovasc. Pharmacol.* **9**, 682–685.

Sakamoto, S., and Liang, C.-S. (1989). Opiate receptor inhibition improves the blunted baroreflex function in dogs with right sided congestive heart failure. *Circulation,* **80**, 1010–1015.

Sakamoto, S., Stone, C. K., Woolf, P. D., and Liang, C.-S. (1989). Opiate receptor antagonism in right-sided congestive heart failure: Naloxone exerts salutary hemodynamic effects via its action on the central nervous system. *Circ. Res.* **65**, 103–114.

Sandor, P., de Jong, W., Wiegant, V., and de Wied, D. (1987). Central opioid mechanisms and cardiovascular control in hemorrhagic hypotension. *Am. J. Physiol.* **253**, H507–H511.

Sawynok, J., Pinsky, C., and LaBella, F. S. (1979). Minireview on the specificity of naloxone as an opiate antagonist. *Life Sci.* **25**, 1621–1632.

Schadt, J. C., and York, D. H. (1980). The reversal of hemorrhagic hypotension by naloxone in conscious rabbits. *Can. J. Physiol. Pharmacol.* **59**, 1208–1213.

Unzueta Merino, M. C., Bonnin, O., Cabrera Ruiz, J. C., and Villar Landeira, J. M. (1987). Naloxona y shock cardiogenico. *Rev. Esp. Anestesiol. Reanim,* **34**, 446–449.

Vargish, T., and Beamer, K. C. (1989). Delta and mu receptor agonists correlate with greater depression of cardiac function than morphine sulfate in perfused rat hearts. *Circ. Shock* **27**, 245–251.

Vargish, T., Reynolds, D. G., Gurll, N. J., Lechner, R. B., Holaday, J. W., and Faden, A. I. (1980). Naloxone reversal of hypovolemic shock in dogs. *Circ. Shock* **7**, 31–38.

Willette, R. N., Krieger, A. J., and Sapru, H. N. (1983). Evidence for anticholinergic effects of naloxone methylbromide. *Res. Commun. Subst. Abuse* **4**, 325–338.

21

Diminished Opioid Inhibition of Blood Pressure and Pituitary Function in Hypertension Development

James A. McCubbin
Department of Behavioral Science
University of Kentucky College of Medicine
Lexington, Kentucky 40536-0086

I. Introduction

The early stages of essential hypertension are characterized by altered autonomic cardiovascular tone and exaggerated blood pressure reactions during psychological stress (Nestel, 1969; Julius, 1976). The apparent abnormalities of catecholaminergic function and the obvious efficacy of sym-

Stress, Neuropeptides, and Systemic Disease

patholytic pharmacotherapy suggest a neurogenic component in the developmental etiology of some types of hypertensive disease. However, it is inappropriate to conclude that mild hypertension in young people represents a primary derangement of the sympathetic nervous system. In fact, evidence of reciprocal alteration in both sympathetic and parasympathetic tone in borderline hypertension (Julius, 1976) suggests a more proximal neurophysiological irregularity.

The opioid neuropeptides are involved in various reactions to aversive stimulation with impact on the balance of autonomic tone and subsequent effects on the organ systems under autonomic neural control. If opioidergic neurochemical processing can affect autonomic outflow, then it is conceivable that altered opioid function could impair blood pressure homeostasis, especially during stress. In some circles, this blood pressure dysregulation is considered benign. However, a growing body of scientists and clinicians believes that these repeated pressor episodes, when maintained over a prolonged period of time, are instrumental in the developmental process that may ultimately result in fixed essential hypertension.

This chapter will explore the hypothesis that altered opioidergic control of autonomic outflow results in blood pressure dysregulation, altered responses to stress, and enhanced risk for hypertension development. The anatomical proximity of opioid mechanisms to major cardiovascular control nuclei will be briefly reviewed, and evidence will be presented for the importance of opioid mechanisms in regulation of blood pressure and neuroendocrine responses during psychological stress. A series of studies examining the effects of opioid antagonism on responses during stress in young people with mildly elevated blood pressure will be presented, further supporting the contention that opioidergic control of circulatory reactivity is altered in some young adults at enhanced risk for hypertension development.

II. Anatomical Distribution of Opioid Peptides and Receptors

The anatomical distribution of opioid-containing cell bodies and terminals and opioid-sensitive receptors indicates multiple sites for potential interaction with circulatory control mechanisms. The abundance of opioids in central and peripheral baroreflex nuclei suggests the potential importance of these substances in reflex control of blood pressure. Moreover, evidence has been found for opioid pathways in supramedullary nuclei indirectly controlling circulatory responses via more highly integrated neuroendocrine mechanisms.

A. Central Cardiovascular Control

Dense representation of opioid ligands and receptors in central baroreflex nuclei suggests that these peptides may have direct impact on circulatory reflex integrity. For example, opioid peptides and/or receptors have been localized in nucleus tractus solitarius, locus ceruleus, dorsal motor nucleus of the vagus, nucleus intermediolateralis, and other nuclei involved in central baroreflex circuitry (Lang et al., 1983; Romagnano et al., 1984; Akil et al., 1981). Enkephalin-containing perikarya are abundant throughout the brain, including hypothalamus, limbic system, and brainstem (Lang et al., 1983). Cell bodies exhibiting beta-endorphin-like immunoreactivity have been localized in the arcuate nucleus of the mediobasal hypothalamus, nucleus tractus solitarius, and nucleus commissuralis (Akil et al., 1984). In addition to beta-endorphin in brain, significant quantities are found in both anterior and intermediate lobes of pituitary. Beta-endorphin and corticotropin (ACTH) are costored and concomitantly released from pituitary in nearly equimolar concentrations (Voigt et al., 1984). Diencephalic peptides apparently regulate release of both ACTH and beta-endorphin from the pituitary.

B. Peripheral Autonomic Nervous System

Opiate-like immunoreactivity has been detected throughout the autonomic nervous system of humans and other animals. In humans, immunohistochemistry has localized enkephalin-like staining in thoracic, cervical, and paravertebral sympathetic ganglia (Hervonen et al., 1981). Additionally, opiate-like immunoreactivity has been found in catecholamine-containing cells of the carotid body and adrenal medullae as well as in pheochromocytoma (Varndell et al., 1982). Consistent with these anatomical findings are physiological studies of the effects of opioids on autonomic ganglionic function. Opiates inhibit cholinergic neurotransmission in mesenteric ganglia of guinea pigs (Konishi et al., 1979) and produce dose-dependent, naloxone-reversible decreases in release of norepinephrine and dopamine beta-hydroxylase upon stimulation of the isolated, perfused cat spleen (Gaddis and Dixon, 1982).

III. Functional Significance of Opioid Mechanisms

The complexity of opioidergic cardiovascular control results in pressor or depressor actions of opioid agonists and antagonists, depending on the

dose, site of action, behavioral state, and the particular species under investigation (Mosqueda-Garcia and Kunos, 1987; Golanov *et al.*, 1987; Natelson *et al.*, 1982; Kapusta *et al.*, 1989). Therefore, the interpretation of the
action of nonselective antagonists must be made with caution. Despite these
difficulties, several studies have noted the ability of some opioid pathways
to alter the perception of pain, influence aversively motivated behaviors,
inhibit release of important stress hormones, and lower blood pressure during various provocative challenges.

A. Pain Mechanisms

Behavioral studies indicate the importance of endogenous opioid pathways
in the motivational impact of environmental stressors. Decreases in pain
sensitivity occur after exposure to various intense stimuli, including electric
footshock (Akil *et al.*, 1976a; Jackson *et al.*, 1979) and heat stress (Kulkarni, 1976). Opioid blockade with naloxone or naltrexone can partially
reverse these antinociceptive responses. Furthermore, opioid antagonism in-
terferes with analgesia from electric brain stimulation (Akil *et al.*, 1976b),
acupuncture (Pomeranz and Chiu, 1976), and classical aversive conditioning (Olivero and Castellano, 1982). In humans, opioid analgesia follows
nociceptive stimuli (Willer *et al.*, 1981), exercise (Haier *et al.*, 1981), and
clinical pain (Cohen *et al.*, 1982). Reversal of stress-induced analgesia in
humans is associated with subjective changes characterized by increased
negative affect and increased anxiety (File and Silverstone, 1981). Furthermore, naloxone reverses antinociceptive responses and exaggerates heart-
rate responses to painful stimuli in both humans and horses (Willer *et al.*,
1981; Lagerweij *et al.*, 1984).

B. Aversively Motivated Behaviors

Opioid systems influence performance in behavioral tasks and are important in learning and memory (McCubbin *et al.*, 1984; Kelleher and Goldberg, 1977). In rabbits, naloxone decreases the magnitude of bradycardia
during classical aversive conditioning (Hernandez and Powell, 1980). In
rats, naltrexone prevents footshock-induced performance deficits (McCubbin *et al.*, 1984), and these effects are believed to be independent of nociceptive changes. The protective significance of opioidergic neuromodulation
is suggested by naloxone effects on digitalis-induced cardiotoxicity during
classical aversive conditioning in guinea pigs (Natelson *et al.*, 1982). Therefore, endogenous opioids have an important physiological role in the motivational aspects of experience with intense stimuli as well as in more generalized learning phenomena. The ultimate impact of these opioidergic

neurobehavioral mechanisms on responses during stress has been largely unexplored despite the importance to understanding functional disorders of the autonomic nervous system.

C. Endocrine Mechanisms

The functional significance of opioids as hypophyseal hormones remains to be fully characterized, but these substances appear to play an important role in the integration of neural and endocrine responses to stress. For example, acute opioid antagonism alters basal levels and response characteristics of important stress hormones. Peripheral administration of naloxone in the rat enhances release of ACTH and corticosterone during footshock (Siegel *et al.*, 1982) and retards the fall in corticosterone after immobilization (Tapp *et al.*, 1981). In humans, naloxone increases basal levels of ACTH, cortisol, growth hormone, and luteinizing hormone (Volauka *et al.*, 1980). Furthermore, painful stimuli exaggerate the adrenocortical effects of opioid antagonism. Therefore, at least some endogenous opioid pathways inhibit the secretion of important stress hormones with significant effects on target organs.

D. Cardiovascular Responses

The importance of opioids in regulation of autonomic neurotransmission suggests that these neuropeptides may have a significant role in blood pressure control. Moreover, opioids have been implicated in the pathophysiology of circulatory shock. For example, Faden, Holaday, and co-workers have shown that naloxone reverses hypotension induced by endotoxin, hypovolemia, and spinal transection (Faden and Holaday, 1979; Faden *et al.*, 1980; Holaday, 1983). The effect of naloxone is antagonized by atropine (Faden *et al.*, 1980) and enhanced by thyrotropin-releasing hormone (Holaday *et al.*, 1983). Studies of hypovolemic shock in rabbits suggest that the effects of opiate blockade depend on both sympathetic and parasympathetic branches of the autonomic nervous system (Schadt and York, 1982).

Direct evidence for a role of opioids in baroreflex modulation has been shown in different models of experimental hypertension. Administration of opioid agonists and antagonists to nucleus tractus solitarius produces differential cardiovascular responsivity in hypertensive versus normotensive rats (de Jong *et al.*, 1983). Additionally, baroreflexes are altered by systemic and central administration of enkephalin and by naloxone in spontaneously hypertensive rats (Schaz *et al.*, 1980). In normotensive, pentobarbital-anesthetized rats, the hypotensive effects of D-Ala^2-Met^5-enkephalinamide is antagonized by naloxone as well as by lesions of nucleus reticularis gigantocellularis (Wont *et al.*, 1984). A series of studies by Kunos and co-workers (Kunos *et al.*, 1980; Farsang *et al.*, 1980) demonstrates that naloxone antagonizes the hypotensive effects of clonidine in spontaneously hypertensive rats. Taken together, these studies demonstrate important opioidergic inhibitory input to baroreflex and peripheral autonomic pathways, and furthermore, these systems are altered in some forms of experimental hypertension.

IV. Opioids and Hypertension

Essential hypertension is characterized by sustained elevations in systemic arterial pressure of unknown etiology. Its prevalence is widespread, and secondary complications of coronary and cerebral vascular involvement make this chronic degenerative disease a major medicoeconomic problem. Sustained hypertension is a developmental disorder, and the physiological profile of the established disease may be radically different from that seen in early stages. Additionally, prolonged high blood pressure can produce neurophysiological abnormalities that may obscure the primary pathophysiological process. Therefore, studies of the physiological profile of prehypertensive populations are necessary to isolate etiologic mechanisms.

A. Stress Reactivity and Hypertension

Early stages of essential hypertension are characterized by functional derangement of the autonomic nervous system. Studies of hypertension in young patients show propranolol and metoprolol-sensitive elevations in blood pressure, heart rate, left ventricular performance, and cardiac output (Julius, 1976; Frolich *et al.*, 1969; Alicandri *et al.*, 1983; Verdecchia *et al.*, 1983). Additionally, young hypertensives have elevations of norepinephrine in plasma (Falkner *et al.*, 1979) and urine (Nestel, 1969) as well as elevations in plasma renin activity (Esler *et al.*, 1979). This aberration of sympathetic circulatory control results in exaggerated physiological responses to behavioral stressors. Falkner and associates (1979) demonstrated that children of hypertensive parents have exaggerated blood pressure and catecholamine responses to a mental arithmetic challenge. Young adults with a positive family history of hypertension (Hastrup *et al.*, 1982) and type A individuals (Glass *et al.*, 1980) respond during stress with exaggerated heart rate and blood pressure changes. As with the hemodynamics of hypertension, exaggerated reactivity can be attenuated with adrenergic blocking drugs (Obrist, 1976). Additionally, stress-induced changes in heart rate, systolic blood pressure, and systolic time intervals correlate with plasma catecholamine levels (McCubbin *et al.*, 1983). Several studies suggest that pharmacotherapy initiated during the early stages of hypertension development can prevent the major complications of sustained high blood pressure (Berenson *et al.*, 1983). This lends credibility to the notion that the autonomic sympathoadrenomedullary reactivity in the early stages of hypertension directly contributes to later cardiovascular morbidity. However, the precise neuroendocrine mechanism that underlies sympathoadrenomedullary lability has not been previously characterized.

B. Laboratory Methods

A series of studies has been initiated in my laboratory to determine the role of opioid mechanisms in the autonomic lability of hypertension development. The specific hypothesis is that diminished activity of an opioidergic depressor pathway underlies the exaggerated sympathoadrenomedullary and circulatory reactivity characteristic of the early stages of hypertension. This exaggerated reactivity and resultant periodic pressor episodes, when maintained over a prolonged interval, may ultimately result in sustained hypertension. Since opioid abnormalities could result from the hypertensive process, I chose to study young adults with mildly elevated casual arterial pressures. Although these individuals are normotensive by clinical criteria, their pressures are high relative to their age group. Previous longitudinal studies indicate that the level of pressure in college-aged males predicts both the level of pressure and the incidence of hypertension later in life (Rabkin *et al.*, 1982; Paffenbarger *et al.*, 1968). Furthermore, these high-risk individuals show exaggerated blood pressure responses during standardized behavioral stressors compared with low blood pressure controls.

Semiquantitative measurement of opioid function in humans is a difficult methodology, especially when the precise anatomical structures are unknown. Measurement of opioid substances in plasma is not an economical approach for preliminary studies, since beta-endorphin released in blood may not necessarily reflect the hypothesized deficit. If an enkephalinergic system is involved, the levels in plasma may not be quantitatively sensitive, especially with their characteristically short half-life in blood. Therefore, a receptor antagonist strategy has been employed. Naloxone HCl (Narcan, DuPont, Manati, Puerto Rico), the wide-spectrum opioid blocker, is relatively devoid of agonist activity and can be safely administered to opiate-naive humans. High doses can effectively block both mu and delta receptors, and if either of these receptor subtypes is responsible for exaggerated blood pressure reactivity in high-risk subjects, then high doses of naloxone should eliminate or attenuate the reactivity differences between high- and low-risk groups.

1. Subject Selection

Research participants were normal male volunteers from 18 to 26 years old. Subjects reported no major medical problems, and were taking no prescription medication at time of testing. Volunteers were recruited from a casual blood pressure screening conducted in a quiet semidarkened room in the Student Activity Center on the Duke University campus. Participants in the screening completed a brief family and personal medical history and rested 5 min prior to blood pressure measurement. Four blood pressure determinations were made at 1-min intervals via an automated oscillometric device (Dinamap Adult/Pediatric Vital Signs Monitor, Critikon, Inc., Tampa, Florida). When 100 individuals had been screened, the distribution of mean arterial pressures was examined, and subjects were rank-ordered by the mean of their third and fourth pressure determination and divided into quintiles before recruitment for in-laboratory procedures. Participants with pressure values falling in the upper (High BP), middle (Mid BP), and lower (Low BP) quintiles were recruited for counterbalanced, placebo-controlled, in-laboratory naloxone/stress challenges.

2. Procedures

In-laboratory stress testing entailed entry to the Duke Medical Center Clinical Research Unit for a brief medical exam and insertion of an indwelling intravenous cannula for later drug infusion and blood sampling. Subjects were then seated upright in a quiet, semidarkened chamber and told to rest until the experimental task began. A 1-h rest interval allowed recovery from the venipuncture. Oscillometric blood pressure determinations were made throughout the experiment at 1-min intervals. Following a preinfusion rest, 8 mg naloxone HCl (Narcan) or saline placebo was slowly infused over 10 min. A 10-min prestress rest period followed infusion. The behavioral stressor was 10 min of performance on a self-paced arithmetic task with monetary incentive for speed and accuracy. This task is a cognitive stressor that requires active coping by the subjects. The arithmetic stressor was chosen because tasks of this type are known to be effective in revealing individual differences in blood pressure reactivity, especially in groups that are characterized by blood pressure instability (Obrist, 1976). Following task performance, a final rest allowed parameters to return to baseline. Participants returned for a similar stress test approximately 1 week later. All subjects received naloxone on one visit and saline on the other visit with the order counterbalanced within blood pressure subgroups. Subjects were unaware of the order of administration.

Systolic, diastolic, and mean arterial pressures were obtained as well as heart rate. In some subjects, blood was sampled and assayed for catecholamines, ACTH, cortisol, and beta-endorphin. Reactivity data were derived for each subject by subtraction of prestress scores from values obtained during stress.

C. Blood Pressure Responses during a Psychological Stressor

The first experiment examined the effect of naloxone on blood pressure responses to an arithmetic stressor in persons from the high, middle, and low blood pressure quintiles from the on-campus screening (McCubbin *et al.*, 1985). As expected, the arithmetic stressor produced significant differences in magnitude of blood pressure response in the three groups, with the High BP group showing the largest responses. For example, despite their higher initial blood pressure levels, the High BP group response averaged 11 ± 2.7 mm Hg diastolic pressure versus 4.3 ± 2.2 mm Hg ($p < 0.05$) in the Low BP group during saline tests. This differential blood pressure response to the arithmetic stressor supports the concurrent validity of casual blood pressure subgrouping. The exaggerated blood pressure response in subjects with mildly elevated casual pressure is similar to responses observed in offspring of hypertensive patients, young adults with elevated catecholamine levels, and type A coronary-prone persons.

Infusion of 8 mg naloxone produced no significant effect on resting blood pressures in the three groups. In contrast, during stress opioid blockade increased the blood pressure response in the Low BP group, resulting in a significant group multi drug interaction for mean pressure reactivity ($F[2,7] = 9.06, p < 0.05$). Naloxone produced no noticeable effect in Mid and High BP groups, but significantly increased the magnitude of response in the Low BP group. The results are similar for diastolic pressure as well. Two subsequent studies have confirmed the pressor effect of naloxone on responses to stress in Low BP groups and the relative absence of a pressor effect in High BP groups. Figure 1 shows the effect of naloxone on the change in mean arterial pressure.

The positive pressor effect of naloxone indicates inhibitory opioidergic tone during stress in the Low BP group. A differential effect of opioid antagonism suggests different levels of opioid tone during stress in the different BP subgroups. Absence of a pressor response to naloxone in the High BP group suggests that these individuals may be characterized by a preexisting state of functional opioid blockade. This could result from a defect in opioid biosynthesis, a deficiency in number or sensitivity of opioid receptors, or an overproduction of an endogenous opioid antagonist. Regardless of precise mechanism, these findings suggest a possible protective effect of opioidergic modulation of cardiovascular responses to psychological stress in persons with the lowest risk for development of hypertension.

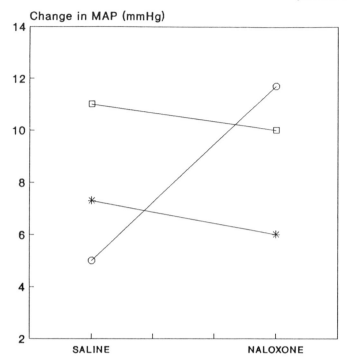

Figure 1   Effects of opioid antagonism with naloxone on mean arterial blood pressure (MAP) response to behavioral stress in young adults with different levels of casual arterial pressure. Data are expressed as response magnitude on drug and placebo days. Naloxone pretreatment significantly increased mean arterial pressure reactivity in the low blood pressure quintile (Low BP) only ($p < 0.05$). ○, Low BP; *, Mid BP; □, High BP. Reprinted with permission from McCubbin *et al.* (1985).

D. Blood Pressure Responses during an Orthostatic Stressor

The effects of naloxone suggest an opioid-mediated depressor mechanism that is variably effective in groups with differing levels of casual arterial pressure. However, the precise level of integration of opioid/autonomic interaction remained to be outlined. The opioid depressor mechanism in the Low BP group could affect blood pressure control at the baroreflex level or at higher levels of central autonomic outflow. Therefore, the next experiment was designed to examine the role of altered baroreflex function in the differential pressor effect of naloxone. If the opioid anomaly is in series with baroreflex circuits, then the effects of naloxone on an orthostatic baroreflex challenge should mimic its pressor effects on the cognitive challenge. If, however, the peptide anomaly resides in the adrenal medullae, or at levels of central autonomic control that are parallel with, or rostral to, baroreflex circuits, then there should be no abnormal pressor effect of naloxone during an orthostatic challenge in persons at risk for hypertension. The original experiment was repeated with the addition of a simple orthostatic baroreflex challenge, that is, postural change from sitting to standing upright (McCubbin *et al.*, 1988). Although baroreflexes could have been studied by examination of heart rate changes following infusion of a pressor agent, the gravitational stress of orthostasis is a sympathoexcitatory challenge and more appropriate for the study of opioidergic sympathoinhibition.

Comparison of arithmetic versus orthostatic responses was facilitated by calculation of an index of drug effect on response magnitude, that is, the difference in response magnitude between the saline test and the naloxone test for each task. These response differences were averaged by risk group and task. For systolic reactivity differences, there was a significant group × task interaction ($F[2,26] = 3.44, p < 0.05$). During minutes 1–3 and minutes 6–8 of the arithmetic stressor (MATH1 and MATH2 respectively), there are positive pressor drug effects in the Low BP group and either no change or depressor drug effects in the High BP group. This pattern is reversed during the standing orthostatic challenge (see Figure 2). These data suggest that abnormal systolic responses to the arithmetic stressor in the High BP group cannot be explained by altered opioidergic control of baroreflexes.

E. Opioidergic Inhibition of Sympathoadrenomedullary and Hypothalamo–Pituitary–Adrenocortical Axes

A third experiment was designed to determine the effects of opioid antagonism on sympathoadrenomedullary and hypothalamo–pituitary–adrenocortical (HPA) function (McCubbin *et al.*, 1989). As in previous studies, this experiment examined the effects of naloxone on responses to the arithmetic stressor in young adults with high and low casual arterial blood pressures. Blood was sampled throughout the experiment for later determination of plasma concentration of adrenocorticotropin (ACTH), cortisol, and beta-endorphin as well as the sympathetic and adrenomedullary catecholamines, epinephrine and norepinephrine.

Blood samples were obtained at the end of each rest period, and twice during the arithmetic stressor. Whole blood was drawn into sample tubes containing ethylenediamine tetraacetic acid (EDTA) for ACTH and beta-endorphin assay and separate tubes containing reduced glutathione for catecholamine assay. All samples were immediately centrifuged and the plasma supernate frozen at −90°C until assay. ACTH was determined by the method of Gutkowska, Julesz, St. Louis, and Genest (1982), cortisol was

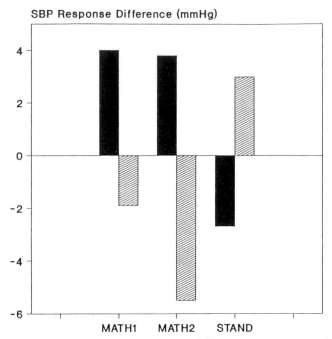

SBP Response Difference (mmHg)

Figure 2 Systolic blood pressure (SBP) response differences (response magnitude during placebo test minus response magnitude during naloxone test) for the average of minutes 1–3 (MATH1) and 6–8 (MATH2) of mental arithmetic stress and minutes 1–3 of orthostatic stress (STAND) in young adults with high (High BP, hatched bars) and low (Low BP, solid bars) casual arterial pressure. Reprinted with permission from McCubbin *et al.* (1988).

assayed by the method of Murphy (1967), and beta-endorphin by the method of Wardlaw and Franz (1979). Catecholamines were determined by high-pressure liquid chromatography (HPLC) methods of Kilts, Gooch, and Knopes (1984) using electrochemical detection.

1. Sympathoadrenomedullary Catecholamines

Figure 3 shows the effect of naloxone on plasma epinephrine responses during the arithmetic stressor in High and Low BP groups. Preinfusion resting epinephrine levels were comparable in High and Low BP groups, but after saline infusion, the High BP group had significantly higher levels than those obtained from Low BP subjects ($F[1,15] = 7.835$, $p < 0.025$). Infusion of naloxone significantly increased plasma epinephrine concentrations during

Figure 3 Effects of opioid antagonism with 0.1 mg/kg naloxone on plasma epinephrine (pg/ml) in young adults with (A) low and (B) high levels of casual arterial pressure; * $p < 0.05$ compared with saline. □, Saline; ○ naloxone. Reprinted with permission from McCubbin *et al.* (1989).

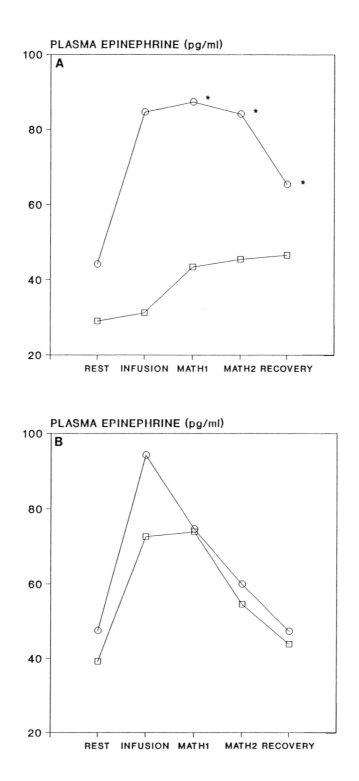

stress in the Low BP group only. The effect of naloxone on plasma epinephrine concentration was significantly correlated with the effect of naloxone
on mean arterial pressure in the Low BP group only. There were no consistent effects of naloxone on plasma norepinephrine responses.

These findings suggest that the pressor effect of naloxone may relate
to opioid inhibition, either direct or indirect, of sympathoadrenomedullary
responses to stress. These data indicate that individuals with low casual
arterial pressures have moderate sympathoadrenomedullary and circulatory
responses during psychological stress. Naloxone-sensitive opioid receptors
apparently inhibit responses in these individuals, since opioid blockade significantly potentiates both blood pressure and epinephrine reactivity. The
High BP group is characterized by exaggerated epinephrine and blood pressure responses, and these responses are relatively unaffected by opioid antagonism. This indicates that one difference between High and Low BP
groups is the relative efficacy of opioidergic inhibition of the sympathoadrenomedullary axis during psychological stress. The contribution of peripheral noradrenergic sympathetic fibers remains to be determined.

2. Anterior Pituitary Hormones

The effect of naloxone on plasma ACTH levels during stress is seen in Figure 4. Although naloxone had no apparent effect on basal plasma ACTH
concentrations in the High BP group ($t < 1$), it marginally increased resting
ACTH concentrations in the Low BP group [$t(9) = 2.167$, $p = 0.058$].
Multivariate analysis of variance utilizing drug-effect scores revealed a significant groups $\times$ periods interaction for the ACTH-stimulating effect of
naloxone (F[4,15] = 3.24, $p < 0.05$). Opioid blockade with naloxone significantly increased plasma ACTH concentrations during both stress periods as well as during recovery in the Low BP group. In contrast, naloxone
was a relatively poor stimulus for ACTH release in the High BP group.
These results are comparable with the findings for plasma cortisol, suggesting that the effects of naloxone on ACTH concentration had observable
activity at the adrenal cortex.

The results with plasma beta-endorphin-like immunoreactivity are
summarized in Figure 5. Infusion of naloxone significantly increased plasma
beta-endorphin-like immunoreactivity in the Low BP group only ($p <
0.005$), with no effect in the High BP group. The group difference in the
endorphin-releasing effect of naloxone was maintained across postinfusion

Figure 4   Effects of opioid antagonism with naloxone on plasma ACTH-like immunoreactivity (fmol/ml) in young adults with (A) low and (B) high levels of casual arterial pressure; * $p
< 0.05$, ** $p < 0.01$ compared with saline. □, saline; ○, naloxone. Reprinted with permission
from McCubbin et al. (1989).

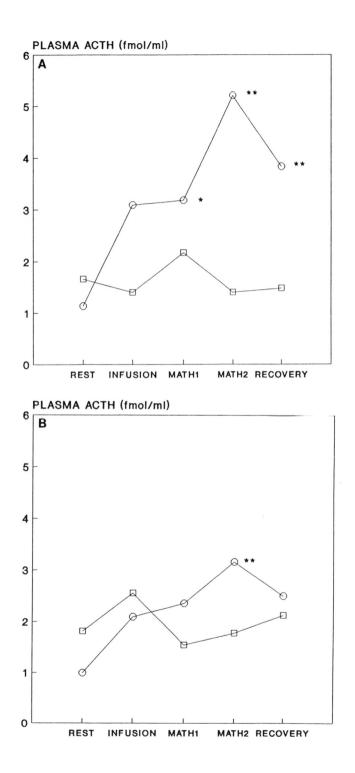

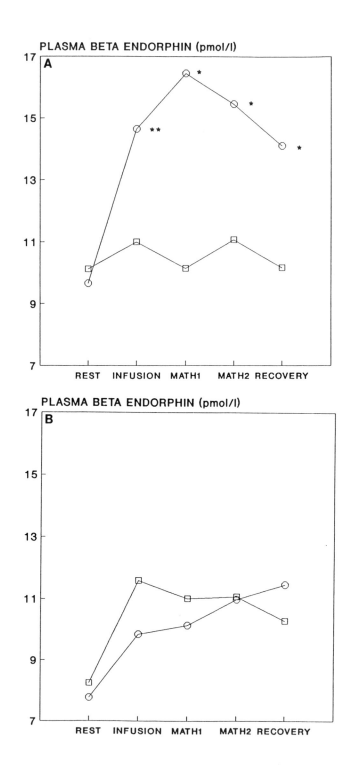

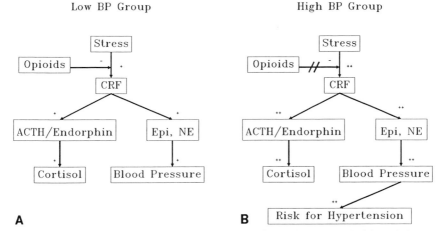

Figure 6 Schematic diagram of the postulated role of opioids in control of hypothalamo–pituitary–adrenocortical and sympathoadrenomedullary responses during stress in young adults with (A) low and (B) high levels of casual arterial pressure. CRF, corticotropin releasing factor; Epi, epinephrine; NE, norepinephrine. See text for explanation.

samples ($F[1,8] = 5.718$, $p < 0.05$). There were no consistent effects of stress or BP grouping on the ratio of ACTH to beta-endorphin in plasma.

F. Discussion

Endogenous opioid peptides appear to have an important inhibitory role during psychological stress in young adults. However, the efficacy of opioidergic inhibition appears to vary with the level of casual arterial pressure and possibly other risk factors for essential hypertension. Young adults with elevated casual pressures are at enhanced risk for development of essential hypertension later in life (Rabkin et al., 1982; Paffenbarger et al., 1968). Their pattern of exaggerated sympathoadrenomedullary and circulatory reactivity is believed to be one possible etiologic mechanism in the sequence of events that may eventually result in fixed essential hypertension (Obrist, 1976; Julius, 1976). The differences in blood pressure reactivity between High and Low BP groups are significantly reduced by opioid receptor antagonism with naloxone, suggesting that these reactivity differences are mediated by naloxone-sensitive opioid receptors. Comparison of results with arithmetic versus orthostatic stressors, combined with the effects of nalox-

Figure 5 Effects of opioid antagonism with naloxone on plasma beta-endorphin-like immunoreactivity (pmol/1) in young adults with (A) low and (B) high levels of casual arterial pressure; * $p < 0.05$, ** $p < 0.01$ compared with saline. □, saline; ○, naloxone. Reprinted with permission from McCubbin et al. (1989).

one on sympathoadrenomedullary and pituitary adrenocortical function, suggests that the group differences in opioid inhibition of stress reactivity may be integrated centrally.

One possible mechanism for integration of HPA and central autonomic outflow is via hypothalamic peptidergic neurons, especially those containing corticotropin-releasing factor (CRF) (Swanson and Sawchenko, 1980; Fisher and Brown, 1983). Paraventricular CRF-containing cell bodies are believed to stimulate the hypothalamospinal upper motoneurons of the sympathetic nervous system (Palkovitz, 1987). The effects of naloxone on pituitary function and blood pressure responses may be mediated via direct or indirect opioidergic input to hypothalamic CRF neurons. Although paraventricular CRF control of central sympathetic outflow and ACTH/endorphin secretion may reflect two distinct populations of neurons (see Chapter 1 by Sawchenko, this volume), these two CRF systems may have a common opioidergic input, possibly via limbic, brainstem, or intrinsic afferents. This is plausible given the correlations between HPA and sympathoadrenomedullary function. Moreover, this is consistent with the effect of naloxone on blood pressure responses during the orthostatic baroreflex challenge, suggesting that impaired opioidergic inhibition of blood pressure responses during psychological stress is not simply a characteristic of reflex-stimulated sympathetic nerve discharge. The results of these studies, taken together, suggest altered opioidergic input to both sympathoadrenomedullary and the HPA axes in young persons at enhanced risk for hypertension development.

V. A Model of Opioid Dysfunction in Hypertension Development

A working model for the role of opioids in stress reactivity and risk for hypertension is illustrated in Figure 6. Although this diagram is oversimplified and highly speculative, it can serve as a heuristic model for analyzing the possible relationships between opioidergic inhibition of the HPA and the sympathoadrenomedullary axes in the regulation of blood pressure. Corticotropin-releasing factor is one possible mediator of the effects of environmental stimulation on the integrated defense reflex pathway. The Low BP group is characterized by effective modulatory inhibition from a naloxone-sensitive and presumably opioidergic input to the HPA axis and central autonomic control nuclei. Functional impairment of the inhibitory opioidergic tone in the High BP group results in disinhibition of both the HPA and the sympathoadrenomedullary axes. The diminished inhibitory input results in a magnified HPA and sympathoadrenomedullary cascade, ultimately producing blood pressure dysregulation and exaggerated pressor responses during psychological stress. Although activity of the HPA axis does not appear to be exaggerated in High BP subjects in the present experiment, this may reflect the efficacy of cortisol-mediated feedback inhibition of ACTH release.

The exaggeration of blood pressure responses during stress may contribute to the expression of risk for essential hypertension. Recent studies have shown normalization of plasma beta-endorphin and enkephalin levels after treatment with clonidine, suggesting that some antihypertensive therapies may work via opioidergic mechanisms (Kraft *et al.*, 1987). This is consistent with the ability of naloxone to antagonize the blood pressure-lowering effects of clonidine. These findings indicate that novel pharmaceutical and behavioral antihypertensive therapies may be strategically designed to stimulate endogenous sympathoinhibitory opioid systems, thereby reducing inappropriate pressor episodes and the subsequent circulatory sequelae.

Acknowledgments

These studies have been supported by NHLBI awards HL35195 and HL32738 as well as NIH grant RR-30 from the Division of Research Resources, General Clinical Research Centers Program. I would like to express grateful appreciation to Paul A. Obrist, John S. Kizer, Richard S. Surwit, Redford B. Williams, and Elizabeth Harlan for their help in various aspects of this work.

References

Akil, H., Madden, J., Patrick, R., and Barchas, J. (1976a). Stress-induced increase in endogenous opiate peptides: Concurrent analgesia and its partial reversal by naloxone. *In* "Opiates and Endogenous Opioid Peptides," pp. 63–70. Elsevier, Amsterdam
Akil, H., Mayer, D., and Liebeskind, J. (1976b). Antagonism of stimulation produced analgesia by naloxone, a narcotic antagonist. *Science* 191, 961–962.
Akil, H., Ueda, Y., Lin, H., Lewis, J., Walker, J., Shiomi, H., Liebeskind, J., and Watson, S. (1981). Multiple forms of beta-endorphin in pituitary and brain. *In* "Advances in Endogenous and Exogenous Opioids" (H. Tagaki and E. Simon, eds), pp. 116–118. Kodansha, Tokyo.
Akil, H., Watson, S. J., Young, E., Lewis, M. E., Khachaturian, H., and Walker, M. J. (1984). Endogenous opioids: Biology and function. *Annu. Rev. Neurosci.* 7, 223–255.
Alicandri, C., Fetnat, M., Tarazi, R., Bravo, E., and Greenstreet, R. (1983). Sympathetic contribution to the cardiac response to stress in hypertension. *Hypertension* 5, 147–154.
Berenson, G. S., Voors, A. W., Webber, L. S., Frank, G. C., Farris, R. P., Hyg, M. S., Tobian, L., and Aristimuno, G. G. (1983). A model of intervention for prevention of early essential hypertension in the 1980s. *Hypertension* 5, 41–53.
Cohen, M., Pikar, D., Dubois, M., and Bunney, W. (1982). Stress-induced plasma beta-endorphin immunoreactivity may predict postoperative morphine usage. *Psychiatr. Res.* 6, 7–12.

de Jong, W., Petty, M., and Sitzen, J. (1983). Role of opioid peptides in brain mechanisms regulating blood pressure. *Chest* 2, 306–308.

Esler, M., Zweifler, A., Randall, O., Julius, S., and DeQuattro, V. (1979). The determinants of plasma-renin activity in essential hypertension. *Ann. Intern. Med.* 88, 746–752.

Faden, A., and Holaday, J. W. (1979). Opiate antagonists: A role in treatment of hypovolemic shock. *Science* 205, 317–318.

Faden, A., Jacobs, T., and Holaday, J. W. (1980). Endorphin-parasympathetic interaction in spinal shock. *J. Auton. Nerv. Syst.* 2, 295–304.

Falkner, B., Onesti, G., Angelakos, E., Fernandez, M., and Langman, C. (1979). Cardiovascular response to mental stress in normal adolescents with hypertensive parents. *Hypertension* 1, 23–30.

Farsang, C., Ramirez-Gonzales, M. D., and Kunos, G. (1980). Possible role of an endogenous opiate in the cardiovascular effects of central alpha adrenoreceptor stimulation in spontaneously hypertensive rats. *J. Pharmacol. Exp. Ther.* 214, 203–208.

File, S., and Silverstone, T. (1981). Naloxone changes self-ratings but not performance in normal subjects. *Psychopharmacology (Berlin)* 74, 353–354.

Fisher, L. A., and Brown, M. R. (1983). Corticotropin-releasing factor: Central nervous system effects on the sympathetic nervous system and cardiovascular regulation. *In* "Central Cardiovascular Control" (D. Ganten and D. Pfaff, eds.), pp. 87–101. Springer-Verlag, Berlin and New York.

Frolich, E., Tarazi, R., and Dustan, H. (1969). Hyperdynamic beta adrenergic state. *Arch. Intern. Med.* 123, 1–7.

Gaddis, R. R., and Dixon, W. R. (1982). Modulation of peripheral adrenergic neurotransmission by methionine-enkephalin. *J. Pharmacol. Exp. Ther.* 221, 282–288.

Glass, D., Krakoff, L., Contrada, R., Hilton, W., Kehoe, K., Manucci, E., Collins, C., Snow, B., and Elting, E. (1980). Effects of harassment and competition on cardiovascular and catecholaminergic responses in Type A and Type B individuals. *Psychophysiology* 17, 453–463.

Golanov, E. V., Fufacheva, A. A., Cherkovich, G. M., and Parin, S. B. (1987). The effect of opioid receptor ligands on the alteration of emotiogenic cardiovascular reactions in monkeys. *Byull. Eksp. Biol. Med.* 4, 424–427.

Gutkowska, J., Julesz, J., St. Louis, J., and Genest, J. (1982). Radioimmunoassay of corticotropin from plasma. *Clin. Chem. (Winston-Salem, N.C.)* 28, 2229–2234.

Haier, R., Quaid, K., and Mills, J. (1981). Naloxone alters pain perception after jogging. *Psychiatr. Res.* 5, 231–232.

Hastrup, J., Light, K. C., and Obrist, P. A. (1982). Parental hypertension and cardiovascular response to stress in healthy young adults. *Psychophysiology* 19, 615–622.

Hernandez, L., and Powell, D. (1980). Effects of naloxone on Pavlovian conditioning of eyeblink and heart-rate reponses in rabbits. *Life Sci.* 27, 863–869.

Hervonen, A., Linnoila, I., Pickel, V. M., Helen, P., Pelto-Huikko, M., Alho, H., and Miller, R. J. (1981). Localization of met- and leu-enkephalin-like immunoreactivity in nerve terminals in human paravertebral sympathetic ganglia. *Neuroscience* 6, 323–330.

Holaday, J. W. (1983). Cardiovascular effects of endogenous opiate systems. *Annu. Rev. Pharmacol. Toxicol.* 23, 541–594.

Holaday, J. W., D'Amato, R., Ruvio, B., and Faden, A. (1983). Action of naloxone and TRH on the autonomic regulation of circulation. *In* "Regulatory Peptides from Molecular Biology to Function" (E. Costa and M. Trabucchi, eds.), pp. 353–361. Raven Press, New York.

Jackson, R., Maier, S., and Coon, D. (1979). Long term analgesic effects of inescapable shock and learned helplessness. *Science* 206, 91–93.

Julius, S. (1976). Neurogenic component in borderline hypertension. *In* "The Nervous System and Arterial Hypertension" (S. Julius and M. Esler, eds.), pp. 301–330. Thomas, Springfield, Illinois.

Kapusta, D. R., Jones, S. Y., and DiBona, G. F. (1989). Opioids in the systemic hemodynamic and renal responses to stress in conscious spontaneously hypertensive rat. *Hypertension* 13, 808–816.

Kelleher, R., and Goldberg, W. (1977). Effects of naloxone on schedule-controlled behavior in monkeys. *In* "Endorphins and Mental Health Research" (E. Usdin, W. Bunney, and N. Kline, eds.), p. 461–472. Oxford Univ. Press, New York.

Kilts, C. D., Gooch, M. D., and Knopes, K. D. (1984). Quantitation of plasma catecholamines by online trace enrichment high performance liquid chromatography with electrochemical detection. *J. Neurosci. Methods* 11, 257–273.

Konishi, S., Tsuno, A., and Otsuka, M. (1979). Enkephalins presynaptically inhibit cholinergic transmission in sympathetic ganglia. *Nature (London)* 282, 515–516.

Kraft, K., Theobald, R., Kolloch, R., and Stumpe, K. O. (1987). Normalization of blood pressure and plasma concentrations of beta-endorphin and leucine-enkephalin in patients with primary hypertension after treatment with clonidine. *J. Cardiovasc. Pharmacol.* 10, Suppl. 12, S147–S151.

Kulkarni, S. (1976). Heat and other physiological stress-induced analgesia: Catecholamine mediated and naloxone reversable response. *Life Sci.* 19.

Kunos, G., Farsang, C., and Ramirez-Gonzales, M. D. (1980). Beta-endorphin: Possible involvement in the anti-hypertensive effect of central alpha-receptor activation. *Science* 211, 82–84.

Lagerweij, E., Nelis, P., Wiegant, V., and Van Ree, J. (1984). The twitch in horses: A variant of acupuncture. *Science* 225, 1172–1174.

Lang, R. E., Gaida, W., Ganten, D., Hermann, K., Kraft, K., and Unger, T. (1983). Neuropeptides and central blood pressure regulation. *In* "Central Cardiovascular Control" (D. Ganten and D. Pfaff, eds.), pp. 103–123. Springer-Verlag, Berlin and New York.

McCubbin, J. A., Richardson, J., Langer, A. W., Kizer, J. S., and Obrist, P. A. (1983). Sympathetic neuronal function and left ventricular performance during behavioral stress in humans: The relationship between plasma catecholamines and systolic time intervals. *Psychophysiology* 20, 102–110.

McCubbin, J. A., Kizer, J. S., and Lipton, M. A. (1984). Naltrexone prevents footshock-induced performance deficit in rats. *Life Sci.* 34, 2057–2066.

McCubbin, J. A., Surwit, R. S., and Williams, R. B. (1985). Endogenous opiates, stress reactivity, and risk for hypertension. *Hypertension* 7, 808–811.

McCubbin, J. A., Surwit, R. S., and Williams, R. B. (1988). Opioid dysfunction and risk for hypertension: Naloxone and blood pressure responses during different types of stress. *Psychosom. Med.* 50, 8–14.

McCubbin, J. A., Surwit, R. S., Williams, R. B., Nemeroff, C. B., and McNeilly, M. (1989). Altered pituitary hormone response to naloxone in hypertension development. *Hypertension* 14, 636–644.

Mosqueda-Garcia, R., and Kunos, G. (1987). Opiate receptors and the endorphin-mediated cardiovascular effects of clonidine in rats: Evidence for hypertension-induced mu-receptor to delta-subtype changes. *Proc. Natl. Acad. Sci. U.S.A.* 84, 8637–8641.

Murphy, B. E. P. (1967). Some studies of the protein binding of steroids and their application to the routine micro and vitramicro measurement of various steroids in body fluids by competitive protein binding radioimmunoassay. *J. Clin. Endocrinol. Metab.* 27, 973–990.

Natelson, B. H., Cagin, N., Tufts, M., Ferrara, M., Biehl, D., and Abramson, M. (1982). Bidirectional effect of naloxone on emotionally conditioned digitalis toxicity. *Psychosom. Med.* 44, 397–400.

Nestel, P. (1969). Blood pressure and catecholamine excretion after mental stress in labile hypertension. *Lancet* **5**, 692–694.

Obrist, P. A. (1976). The cardiovascular-behavioral interaction—As it appears today. *Psychophysiology* **13**, 95–107.

Olivero, A., and Castellano, C. (1982). Classical conditioning of stress-induced analgesia. *Physiol. Behav.* **25**, 171–172.

Paffenbarger, R. S., Thorne, M. C., and Wing, A. L. (1968). Chronic disease in former college students. VIII. Characteristics in youth predisposing to hypertension in later years. *Am. J. Epidemiol.* **88**, 25–32.

Palkovits, M. (1987). Organization of the stress response at the anatomical level. *In* "Progress in Brain Research Vol. 72, Neuropeptides and Brain Function" (E. De Kloet, V. Weigant, and D. De Weid, eds.), pp. 47–55. Elsevier, Amsterdam.

Pomeranz, B., and Chiu, D. (1976). Naloxone blockade of acupuncture analgesia: Endorphin implicated. *Life Sci.* **19**, 1757–1762.

Rabkin, S. W., Mathewson, F. A., and Tate, R. B. (1982). Relationship of blood pressure in 20-39-year old men to subsequent blood pressure and incidence of hypertension over a 30 year observation period. *Circulation* **65**, 291–300.

Romagnano, M., and Hamill, R. (1984). Spinal sympathetic pathway. *Science* **225**, 737–738.

Schadt, J., and York, D. (1982). Involvement of both adrenergic and cholinergic receptors in the cardiovascular effects of naloxone during hemorrhagic hypotension in the conscious rabbit. *J. Auton. Nerv. Syst.* **6**, 237–251.

Schaz, K., Stock, G., Simon, W., Schlor, K., Unger, T., Rockhold, R., and Ganten, D. (1980). Enkephalin effects on blood pressure, heart rate, and baroreflex. *Hypertension* **2**, 395–407.

Siegel, R., Chowers, I., Confortti, N., Feldman, S., and Weidenfield, J. (1982). Effects of naloxone on basal and stress induced ACTH and corticosterone secretion in the male rat—Site and mechanism of action. *Brain Res.* **249**, 103–109.

Swanson, L. W., and Sawchenko, P. E. (1980). Paraventricular nucleus: A site for integration of neuroendocrine and autonomic mechanisms. *Neuroendocrinology* **31**, 410–417.

Tapp, W., Mittler, J., and Natelson, B. (1981). Effects of naloxone on corticosterone response to stress. *Pharmacol., Biochem. Behav.* **14**, 749–751.

Varndell, I. M., Tapia, F. J., De Mey, J., Rush, R. A., Bloom, S. R., and Polak, J. M. (1982). Electron immunocytochemical localization of enkephalin-like material in catecholamine-containing cells of the carotid body, the adrenal medulla, and in pheochromocytomas of man and other mammals. *J. Histochem. Cytochem.* **30**, 682–690.

Verdecchia, P., Brignole, M., Delfine, G., Queirolo, C., Marchi, G., and Vertulla, A. (1983). Systolic time intervals and possible predictors of pressure response to sustained beta adrenergic blockade in arterial hypertension. *Hypertension* **5**, 140–146.

Voigt, K., Weber, E., Fehm, H., and Martin, R. (1984). The concomitant storage and simultaneous release of ACTH and beta-endorphin. *In* "Brain and Pituitary Peptides" (W. Wuttke, A. Weindl, Voigt, K., and R. Dries, eds.), pp. 54–58. Karger, Basil.

Volauka, J., Bauman, J., Bevnick, J., Reker, D., James, B., and Cho, D. (1980). Short-term hormonal effects of naloxone in man. *Psychoneuroendocrinology* **5**, 225–234.

Wardlaw, S. L., and Franz, A. G. (1979). Measurement of beta-endorphin in human plasma. *J. Clin. Endocrinol. Metab.* **48**, 176–180.

Willer, J., Dehen, H., and Cambier, J. (1981). Stress-induced analgesia in humans: Endogenous opioids and naloxone-reversible depression of pain reflexes. *Science* **212**, 689–691.

Wont, T. M., Chan, S. H., and Tse, S. Y. (1984). Central cardiovascular actions of D-Ala2-Met5-enkephalinamide in the rat: Effects of naloxone and nucleus reticularis gigantocellularis lesion. *Neurosci. Lett.* **46**, 246–254.

Index

467